# ALCOHOL *and* *the* GASTROINTESTINAL TRACT

*Edited by*

VICTOR R. PREEDY
RONALD R. WATSON

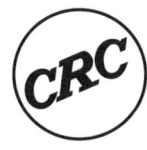

**CRC Press**
**Boca Raton   New York   London   Tokyo**

**Library of Congress Cataloging-in-Publication Data**

Alcohol and the gastrointestinal tract / edited by Victor R. Preedy
  and Ronald R. Watson.
       p.   cm.
    Includes bibliographical references and index.
    ISBN 0-8493-2480-7 (alk. paper)
    1. Gastrointestinal system—Pathophysiology.   2. Alcohol-
-Toxicology.   I. Preedy, Victor R.   II. Watson, Ronald R. (Ronald
Ross)
    [DNLM:   1. Gastrointestinal System—drug effects.
2. Gastrointestinal Diseases—chemically induced.   3. Alcohol,
Ethyl—adverse effects.   4. Alcohol Drinking—epidemiology.   WI 100
A353 1995]
RC802.A35   1995
616.3′3071—dc20
DNLM/DLC
for Library of Congress                                                    95-24883
                                                                              CIP

No claim to original U.S. Government works
International Standard Book Number 0-8493-2480-7
Library of Congress Card Number 95-24883
Printed in the United States of America   1  2  3  4  5  6  7  8  9  0
Printed on acid-free paper

# PREFACE

Virtually every organ in the body is targeted by the deleterious effects of ethanol or its catabolites. Paradoxically, most attention has focused on a few tissues or organs, especially the liver and nervous system. However, there are a number of other tissues that are especially affected by ethanol, and the gastrointestinal tract is included in this category. Derangements occur in virtually all regions of the digestive system, including the salivary glands, esophagus, and stomach as well as the small and large bowel. The pancreas is also subject to the injurious effects of ethanol. Furthermore, different layers of the individual tissues are heterogeneous, which is reflected in the fact that they display an assortment of responses. Thus, in the small bowel both the seromuscular layer and the mucosa are adversely affected. The transformations induced by ethanol range from gross defects in functional abilities, such as malabsorption, electrolyte imbalance and exchange, to gross necrosis, hemorrhagic erosions and other morphological abnormalities. Many of these changes contribute to the malnutrition frequently observed in alcoholics. Up to one-third to one-half of alcohol misusers have gastrointestinal disturbances. The incidence of cancer is also particularly high in patients suffering from ethanol misuse.

The mechanisms responsible for the above abnormalities are complex. They range from defects in intermediary metabolism to protein synthesis; from the genesis of free radicals to changes in antioxidant capacity; from microvascular changes to alterations in whole organ blood flow. The activities of enzymes such as the peptidases of the brush-border membrane are also impaired. Cancers may involve the activation of procarcinogens and immune function is also adversely affected in alcoholics. Ethanol studies are also useful for elucidating the mechanism of biochemical control. For example, many of the model systems of the last three or four decades utilized either starvation or hormonal dysfunction, such as diabetes, i.e., the absence of controlling factors. In alcohol studies the investigation of regulatory process occurs under strictly defined criteria, where the perturbant is given in precisely defined amounts. It is necessary to bring these complex facets of alcohol-toxicity together to help one understand the disease process per se. Furthermore, the chapters of this book offer an insight into pathological mechanisms that may be applicable to other gastrointestinal diseases.

The ensuing chapters have been divided into the following categories: (1) Epidemiology of alcohol misuse and general pathological mechanisms. These chapters essentially define the magnitude and extent of the problems, and describe specific processes and mechanisms of disease that may apply to other ethanol-induced disorders; and (2) Biochemistry and physiology of the intestinal tissues and organ-specific reactions. Some chapters describe normal metabolism in the gastrointestinal tract and how it is altered in other disease conditions. Overall, the text should provide informative reading for both the clinician and experimental scientist alike.

*Dr. Victor R. Preedy*
*Professor Ronald R. Watson*

# THE EDITORS

**Victor R. Preedy** is currently a lecturer in the Department of Clinical Biochemistry, King's College School of Medicine and Dentistry, London. He also holds Honorary Appointments in The Roehampton Institute, the School of Pharmacy and the Persistent Viral Disease Research Foundation. He directs studies regarding protein turnover, cardiology, nutrition, and the biochemical aspects of alcoholism, in particular.

Dr. Preedy graduated in 1974 from the University of Aston with a Combined Honors Degree in Biology and Physiology with Pharmacology. He gained his Ph.D. in 1981, in the field of Nutrition and Metabolism, specializing in protein turnover. In 1992 he received his Membership of the Royal College of Pathologists, based on his published works and in 1993 he gained a D.Sc. degree for his outstanding contribution to protein and metabolism. At the time, he was one of the university's youngest recipients of this distinguished award.

Dr. Preedy is a member of the Bone and Tooth Society, the Biochemical Society, the Laboratory Animal Science Association, the Medical Research Society, the European Society for Biomedical Research into Alcoholism, International Society for Biomedical Research into Alcoholism, the Research Defense Society, and the European Biomedical Research Association (Founder Member).

Dr. Preedy has published over 250 articles which includes over 80 peer reviewed manuscripts based on original research and 25 reviews. He lectures nationally and internationally and the venues of his recent guest lectures and presentations have included Hong Kong, Australia, Germany, and the U.S.

His current major research interests include protein turnover with reference to enteral nutrition, messenger, transfer, and ribosomal RNA degradation products, and the molecular mechanisms responsible for alcoholic muscle damage and the interaction of alcohol-induced intestinal pathologies with infection.

**Ronald R. Watson, Ph.D.,** initiated and directed the National Institute of Alcohol Abuse and Alcoholism (NIAAA) Alcohol Research Center at the University of Arizona College of Medicine. The main goal of the Center was to understand the role of ethanol-induced immunosuppression on immune function and disease resistance in animals. Dr. Watson has edited 35 books, including 10 on alcohol abuse and 4 on other drugs of abuse. He has worked for several years on research for the U.S. Navy Alcohol and Substance Abuse Program.

Dr. Watson attended the University of Idaho but graduated from Brigham Young University in Provo, Utah, with a degree in Chemistry in 1966. He completed his Ph.D. degree in 1971 in Biochemistry from Michigan State University. His postdoctoral schooling was completed at the Harvard School of Public Health in Nutrition and Microbiology, including a two-year postdoctoral research experience in immunology. He was an Assistant Professor of Immunology and did research at the University of Mississippi Medical Center in Jackson from 1973 to 1974. He was an Assistant Professor of Microbiology and Immunology at the Indiana University Medical School from 1974 to 1978 and an Associate Professor at Purdue University in the Department of Food and Nutrition from 1978 to 1982. In 1982, he joined the faculty at the University of Arizona in the Department of Family and Community Medicine, Nutrition Section, and is a research Professor. He has published 275 research papers and review chapters.

Dr. Watson is a member of several national and international nutrition, immunology, and cancer societies and research societies on alcoholism.

# CONTRIBUTORS

**Emanuele Albano, M.D., Ph.D.**
Department of Medical Sciences
University of Turin
Novara, Italy

**Ivan T. Beck, M.D., Ph.D.**
Gastrointestinal Diseases Research Unit
Hotel Dieu Hospital
Kingston, Ontario, Canada

**Ingvar Bjarnason, M.D.**
Department of Clinical Biochemistry
King's College School of Medicine and
  Dentistry
London, England

**Paolo Clot, M.D.**
Department of Experimental Medicine and
  Oncology
University of Turin
Torino, Italy

**Jaume Farrés, M.D.**
Department of Biochemistry and Molecular
  Biology
Faculty of Sciences
University Autonoma de Barcelona
Bellaterra, Spain

**Jeremy Z. Fields, M.D.**
Department of Medicine
Loyola University School of Medicine
Maywood, Illinois

**George K. Grimble, M.D.**
Addictive Behavior Center
Roehampton Institute
London, England

**Richard F. Harty, M.D.**
Department of Medicine
Oklahoma Health Sciences Center
Oklahoma City, Oklahoma

**Hiroshi Hayashi, M.D.**
Department of Internal Medicine
Yokohama Red Cross Hospital
Yokohama, Japan

**Laura C. Heap, Ph.D.**
Wyeth Research (U.K.), Ltd.
Maidenhead, England

**Ikuko Kato, M.D.**
Department of Environmental Medicine
New York University Medical Center
New York, New York

**Ali Keshavarzian, M.D.**
Department of Medicine
Loyola University School of Medicine
Maywood, Illinois

**Jan W. Konturek, M.D.**
Institute of Physiology
Faculty of Medicine
Jagiellonian University School of Medicine
Krakow, Poland

**Stanisław J. Konturek, M.D.**
Institute of Physiology
Faculty of Medicine
Jagiellonian University School of Medicine
Krakow, Poland

**Charles S. Lieber, M.D.**
Mount Sinai School of Medicine
Veteran Affairs Medical Center
Bronx, New York

**Andrew Macpherson, M.D.**
Department of Medicine
King's College School of Medicine
London, England

**Jaspaul S. Marway, Ph.D.**
Tissue Pathology Unit
Roehampton Institute
London, England

**Siraj I. Mufti, M.D.**
College of Pharmacy
University of Arizona
Tucson, Arizona

**Ian D. Norton, F.R.A.C.P.**
Department of Gastroenterology
Prince of Wales Hospital
Sydney, Australia

**Harry S. Ojeas, M.D.**
Department of Medicine
Oklahoma Health Sciences Center
Oklahoma City, Oklahoma

**Xavier Parés, Ph.D.**
Department of Biochemistry and Molecular
  Biology
Faculty of Sciences
University Autonoma de Barcelona
Bellaterra, Spain

**Jeremy Powell-Tuck, M.D.**
Rank Department of Human Nutrition
London Hospital Medical College
London, England

**Victor R. Preedy, Ph.D.**
Department of Clinical Biochemistry
King's College of Medicine and Dentistry
London, England

**Gordon B. Proctor, Ph.D.**
Department of Oral Pathology
King's College School of Medicine and
  Dentistry
London, England

**Helmut K. Seitz, M.D.**
Department of Medicine
Salem Medical Center
Heidelberg, Germany

**Deepak K. Shori, M.D.**
Department of Oral Pathology
King's College School of Medicine and
  Dentistry
London, England

**Ulrich A. Simanowski, M.D.**
Department of Medicine
Salem Medical Center
Heidelberg, Germany

**Jerzy Stachura, M.D.**
Institute of Physiology
Faculty of Medicine
Jagiellonian University School of Medicine
Krakow, Poland

**A. D. Thomson, Ph.D.**
Department of Gastroenterology
Greenwich District Hospital
London, England

**Roberta J. Ward, Ph.D.**
Department of Clinical Biochemistry
King's College School of Medicine and
  Dentistry
London, England

**David Van Thiel, M.D.**
Department of Transplantation Medicine
Oklahoma Transplantation Institute
Oklahoma City, Oklahoma

**Ronald R. Watson, Ph.D.**
Department of Family and Community
  Medicine
University of Arizona
Tucson, Arizona

**Jeremy S. Wilson, M.D.**
Department of Gastroenterology
Prince of Wales Hospital
Sydney, Australia

# TABLE OF CONTENTS

# 1

# The Extent of the Problems and the Epidemiological Aspects of Alcohol Drinking

Ikuko Kato

## CONTENTS

## 1.1   COMPOSITION OF ALCOHOLIC BEVERAGES

Ethanol, formed by the fermentation of carbohydrates with yeast, is usually the second largest component of alcoholic beverages following water, although in some very sweet liqueurs the sugar content can be higher than the ethanol content.[1] A wide variety of organic materials, including grain (beer, shochu), fruit (wine, cider), sap (palm wine, pulque), and honey (mead), are used as sources of the carbohydrates. Table 1.1 summarizes the average ethanol concentration and content per glass in three major types of alcoholic beverages: wine, beer, and distilled spirits.[1] It is worth noting that the amount of ethanol consumed in a standard measure of drinks is approximately the same for each type of beverage. The ethanol content can be expressed either by weight or by volume, the conversion factor being 1 ml = 789 mg.

0-8493-2480-7/96/$0.00+$.50

**TABLE 1.1  Approximate Ethanol Content of the Three Major Groups of Alcoholic Beverages**

| Type of beverage | Ethanol content (%) | | Average standard glass | | Ethanol per drink | |
|---|---|---|---|---|---|---|
| | Volume | Weight | U.S. [oz (ml)] | Europe (ml) | ml | g |
| Beer | 5 | 4 | 12 (350) | 250 | 12–17.5 | 10–14 |
| Wine | 12 | 10 | 4 (120) | 100 | 12–14.5 | 10–12 |
| Spirits | 40 | 32 | 1.5 (45) | 35 | 14–18 | 11–14.2 |

Adapted from Hoofdproduktschap voor Akkerbouwprodukten (1984); IARC (1988).

Besides ethanol, water, and sugar, alcoholic beverages contain a wide range of volatile and nonvolatile flavor compounds, at concentrations that vary with the type of beverage.[1] The volatiles include aliphatic carbonyl compounds, other alcohols, monocarboxylic acids and their esters, nitrogen- and sulfur-containing compounds, hydrocarbons, terpenic compounds, and heterocyclic and aromatic compounds. Nonvolatile compounds comprise di- and tribasic carboxylic acids, coloring substances, tannic and polyphenolic substances, and inorganic salts. These substances can also have physiological and pathological effects, so that epidemiological findings on effects of consuming alcoholic beverages do not necessarily indicate the effect of ethanol itself.

## 1.2    TRENDS IN PRODUCTION AND CONSUMPTION OF ALCOHOLIC BEVERAGES BY COUNTRY

Total alcohol consumption per person is usually calculated by dividing the difference between the quantities produced and imported and the quantities exported and in stock (or sales statistics collected for taxation purpose), by the total population. Therefore, statistics on alcohol consumption have been limited to commercial products, although homemade alcohol may be more common than commercial alcohol in some developing countries. Since World War II, the production and estimated consumption of alcoholic beverages have increased in almost all countries. Table 1.2 shows annual per capita consumption of alcohol (liters) by country in 1960, 1970, 1977, and 1990.[1-4] The rate of increase slowed during the 1970s and, in some developed countries, leveled off and slightly declined. In general, higher rates of growth were recorded in countries that started from a relatively low level of average consumption. As a result, the difference in average consumption between countries has narrowed. There are still wide variations, however, in the rates of consumption between countries and regions. The highest levels have been recorded in European countries and the lowest in Asian and African countries. According to the latest statistics, the estimated consumption is highest in France, followed by Luxemburg, East Germany, and Switzerland.[4] As far as the preferred choice of beverage, countries have also had a tendency to be more alike in their patterns of drinking,[1] with the proportion of beer, wine, and spirits in the total consumption being very similar in most countries. In other words, local predominances of particular types of beverage (e.g., wine in Europe, beer in America, and spirits in the former Soviet Union) relative to the others are becoming less pronounced. Despite this convergence, strong preferences still remain in the choice of beverage, and the traditional beverages have not been replaced by other drinks. The change has been one of addition rather than substitution.

## 1.3    PREVALENCE AND EXTENT OF ALCOHOL DRINKING

The prevalence of alcohol drinking is also important when estimating the impact of alcohol drinking in a population. Population-based epidemiological surveys have provided such data.

**TABLE 1.2  International Statistics: Consumption of Commercial Alcohol (as ethanol) for 1960, 1970, 1977, and 1990**

| Country[a] | Ethanol (liters per person) | | | |
|---|---|---|---|---|
| | 1960 | 1970 | 1977 | 1990 |
| Argentina | 9.7 | 13.1 | 14.0 | 7.5 |
| Australia | 6.5 | 8.2 | 9.8 | 8.0 |
| Austria | 8.7 | 11.9 | 11.5 | 10.4 |
| Belgium | 6.4 | 8.9 | 10.1 | 9.9 |
| Brazil | 0.7 | 2.2 | 2.4 | — |
| Bulgaria | 3.8 | 7.2 | — | 8.9 |
| Canada | 4.8 | 6.5 | 8.5 | 7.5 |
| Chile | 7.0 | 6.5 | 7.1 | — |
| Cyprus | 3.3[b] | 3.3 | 3.8 | 7.7 |
| Czechoslovakia | 5.5 | 9.1 | 9.9 | 8.8 |
| Denmark | 4.2 | 6.3 | 8.8 | 9.7 |
| East Germany | 4.6 | 6.3 | 9.1 | 11.8 |
| Finland | 1.8 | 4.5 | 6.9 | 7.7 |
| France | 17.3 | 19.6 | 17.3 | 12.7 |
| Gambia | 0.2 | 2.0 | 1.3 | — |
| Greece | — | 5.9 | 6.3 | 5.4[d] |
| Hungary | 6.2 | 10.1 | 13.6 | 10.8 |
| Iceland | 1.7 | 2.7 | 3.2 | 3.9[c] |
| Ireland | 3.4 | 4.2 | 5.8 | 7.2[c] |
| Israel | 2.3[b] | 2.8 | 2.9 | — |
| Italy | 12.2 | 14.5 | 12.4 | 8.7 |
| Japan | 3.6 | 4.9 | — | 6.5 |
| Luxemburg | 8.3 | 10.2 | 14.4 | 12.2 |
| Mexico | 1.5 | 2.1 | 2.4 | — |
| Netherlands | 2.5 | 5.7 | 8.9 | 8.2 |
| New Zealand | 6.5 | 6.7 | 8.4 | 7.8 |
| Norway | 2.6 | 3.6 | 4.5 | 4.0[c] |
| Poland | 3.8 | 5.1 | 8.2 | 6.2 |
| Portugal | 10.4 | 9.9 | 14.0 | 9.8 |
| Romania | 4.1 | 6.3 | — | 7.6[d] |
| South Africa | 1.8 | 4.3 | 5.2 | 4.8 |
| South Korea | 0.8 | 3.6 | 7.0 | — |
| Spain | 10.3[b] | 11.3 | 12.8 | 10.8 |
| Sweden | 3.7 | 5.6 | 6.0 | 5.3 |
| Switzerland | 9.8 | 10.5 | 10.6 | 10.8 |
| Turkey | 0.3[b] | 0.5 | — | 1.0[c] |
| U.K. | 5.1 | 5.2 | 6.8 | 7.6 |
| Uruguay | — | 5.6 | — | 5.5[d] |
| U.S. | 5.2 | 6.8 | 8.1 | 7.5 |
| Former Soviet Union | 3.7 | 5.1 | 5.2 | 8.4[c] |
| West Germany | 6.9 | 11.2 | 12.2 | 10.6 |
| Yugoslavia | 4.7 | 7.6 | 6.9 | 6.1 |

[a] Names of some countries have subsequently changed.

[b] 1963.

[c] 1985.

[d] 1987.

From IARC (1988), Walsh and Grant (1985), Pyörärlä (1990), and Systembolaget (1993).

**TABLE 1.3  The Prevalence of Drinkers and Mean Intake of Alcohol (g/day) in Various Populations**

| Country (area) | No. of study subjects | Prevalence of drinkers (%) | Mean alcohol intake (g/day) |
|---|---|---|---|
| Intersalt Cooperative Research Group (1988) | | | |
| Argentina | 200 | 79 | 22.7 |
| Belgium (Charleroi, Ghent) | 357 | 79 | 12.3 |
| Canada (Labrador, St John's) | 361 | 57 | 16.2 |
| China (Beijing, Nanning, Tianjin) | 600 | 32 | 3.8 |
| Colombia | 191 | 51 | 12.8 |
| Denmark | 199 | 90 | 16.6 |
| Finland (Joensuu, Turku) | 400 | 60 | 10.7 |
| Germany (East Germany, Bernried, Heidelberg) | 591 | 86 | 16.7 |
| Hungary | 200 | 58 | 10.5 |
| Iceland | 200 | 53 | 7.2 |
| India (Ladakh, New Delhi) | 399 | 36 | 18.1 |
| Italy (Bassiano, Gubbio, Mirano, Naples) | 798 | 88 | 23.0 |
| Japan (Osaka, Tochigi, Toyama) | 591 | 60 | 14.3 |
| Kenya | 176 | 31 | 8.2 |
| Malta | 200 | 73 | 17.0 |
| Mexico | 172 | 87 | 61.2 |
| Netherlands | 199 | 68 | 12.2 |
| Papua New Guinea | 162 | 9 | 0.9 |
| Poland (Krakow, Warsaw) | 400 | 55 | 6.4 |
| Portugal | 198 | 55 | 25.1 |
| South Korea | 198 | 24 | 3.0 |
| Soviet Union | 194 | 33 | 2.4 |
| Spain (Manresa, Torrejon) | 400 | 73 | 18.3 |
| Taiwan | 181 | 20 | 3.3 |
| Trinidad and Tobago | 176 | 36 | 8.3 |
| U.K. (Belfast, Birmingham, South Wales) | 598 | 70 | 17.7 |
| U.S. (Chicago, Goodman, Hawaii, Jackson) | 1150 | 44 | 11.9 |
| Zimbabwe | 195 | 44 | 19.4 |
| Péquignot et al. (1988) | | | |
| Italy (Torino, Varese) | 1596 | 89 | 33.5 |
| Spain (Navarra, Zaragoza) | 1363 | 67 | 26.4 |
| Switzerland | 575 | 92 | 28.1 |
| France | 1800 | 89 | 28.4 |
| Pinn and Bovet (1991) | | | |
| Australia | 1071 | 52 | 35.3 |

Table 1.3 lists the results from three studies.[5-7] In the INTERSALT Study, an international study on blood pressure and electrolyte excretion, various behavioral factors, including alcohol intake, were recorded from 200 men and women aged 20 to 50 years at each of 52 centers in 32 countries. The prevalence of alcohol drinking ranged from 8.7% (Papua New Guinea) to 90% (Denmark). Another survey conducted in four European countries found the highest rate in Switzerland (92%). Mean daily intake of alcohol ranged from 1 g (Papua New Guinea) to 61 g (Mexico). This corresponds to 0 to 5 drinks per day assuming that one drink equals 12 g alcohol. These epidemiological measurements include intakes from homemade products and exclude amounts used for purposes other than drinking such as cooking, but are prone to sampling variations. For example, study subjects of a relatively small sample in each area may not be representative of

the general population of the entire country. In addition, results may not be comparable across studies where different methods were used to collect data on alcohol intake. However, when self-reported alcohol consumption data were compared with per capita sales of alcoholic beverages in 21 states of the U.S., there was a good correlation ($r = 0.81$).[8] Therefore, both types of data are useful in estimating the level of alcohol consumption in a population.

The definition of heavy drinking seems to depend on the average alcohol consumption in a population. In the Behavior Risk Factor Surveillance in the U.S., heavier drinking was defined as consumption of 60 or more drinks in the past month, which is equal to two or more drinks per day. In this survey, 6% met this criterion.[9] In European countries where the average consumption is much higher, five or more drinks per day is used as the definition of heavy drinking, but still more than 20% of men fall into this category.[6]

## 1.4   FACTORS INFLUENCING ALCOHOL USE AND ABUSE

Many factors, including both social and personal characteristics, have been identified as determinants of alcohol drinking and alcohol abuse.[10] The increased availability of alcohol due to a drop in real cost, a weakening of restrictions, the substitution of industrial techniques of production for traditional methods of brewing and distilling, and improvements in transport and distribution have contributed to an increase in consumption since World War II. The relation of urbanization to patterns of drinking depends on geographical areas. It is associated with not only the availability of alcohol but also lifestyles in urban and rural areas. In the U.S., abstention and absence from heavy drinking tend to be strongly associated with rural areas, but this is not seen in European countries. Among personal characteristics, sex is the strongest determinant. In nearly all populations, women are less frequent drinkers and less likely to drink heavily than men. The tendency seems to be more marked at heavier levels. Except for childhood and adolescent years, the prevalence of alcohol drinking generally declines with age, while the proportion of ex-drinkers increases. Compared with married individuals, the never married, separated, divorced, or widowed are more likely to develop alcohol abuse. Social class and educational level are generally inversely associated with prevalence of alcohol abuse.[11] Most of these factors were found to be significantly associated with the 1-month prevalence of alcohol abuse or dependence in five areas of the U.S.[12] (Table 1.4). An important determinant of abstention from drinking is religion. Certain sects of Christians (such as Seventh Day Adventists and Mormons) and Muslims abstain from alcohol because of a religious proscription,[1] and therefore have often been used to study the effect of abstinence.

## 1.5   EXTENT OF ALCOHOL-RELATED PROBLEMS

The range and severity of alcohol-related problems vary considerably from country to country as well as within countries. According to Grant and Riston, the problems associated with excessive alcohol drinking, alcohol abuse, and intoxication are classified as follows[2]:

a. Medical problems: Cancers of the mouth, pharynx, and esophagus, gastritis, peptic ulcers, stomach hemorrhage, pancreatitis, diabetes, feminization, sexual impotence, testicular atrophy, anemia, chronic myopathy, cardiomyopathy, peripheral neuritis, Wernicke's encephalopathy, Korsakoff's psychosis, minor brain damage, dementia, fatty liver, alcoholic hepatitis, liver cirrhosis, liver cancer, fat metabolism diseases, gout, fetal alcohol syndrome, epilepsy, depression, anxiety, phobic illness, hallucinations, paranoid states, delirium tremens, withdrawal epilepsy, alcoholic psychosis, acute alcohol poisoning, drug overdose, suicidal behavior, trauma, head injury, accidents, hangover, etc.
b. Social problems: Debt, homelessness, family problems, marital problems, sexual problems, absenteeism, employment problems, etc.
c. Legal problems: Driving offenses, drunkenness offenses, theft, assault, homicide, criminal damage to property, etc.

**TABLE 1.4  Standardized 1-Month Prevalence Rates and Adjusted Odds Ratios of Alcohol Abuse or Dependence by Demographic Variables in the U.S.**

| Characteristics | Rate (%) (SE) | Odds ratio |
|---|---|---|
| Age | | |
| 18–24 | 4.1 (0.6) | 1.00 |
| 25–44 | 3.6 (0.3) | 1.04 |
| 45–64 | 2.1 (0.3) | 0.57 |
| 65+ | 0.9 (0.2) | 0.20[a] |
| Sex | | |
| Male | 5.0 (0.4) | 1.00 |
| Female | 0.9 (0.1) | 0.16[a] |
| Race | | |
| Nonblack/nonhispanic | 2.7 (0.2) | 1.00 |
| Black | 3.4 (0.4) | 0.87 |
| Hispanic | 3.6 (0.6) | 0.96 |
| Marital status | | |
| Married | 2.0 (0.2) | 1.00 |
| Single | 4.2 (0.5) | 1.51 |
| Separated/divorced | 5.9 (0.7) | 3.23[a] |
| Widowed | 1.3 (0.3) | 2.07 |
| Socioeconomic status | | |
| 1 (high) | 2.3 (0.3) | 1.00 |
| 2 | 3.0 (0.3) | 1.38 |
| 3 | 3.0 (0.3) | 1.68 |
| 4 (low) | 3.0 (0.4) | 2.53[a] |
| Total | 2.8 (0.2) | 1.00 |

[a] $p < 0.01$.

From Regier et al. (1993).[12]

The remainder of the chapter focuses mainly on medical problems. The alcohol-attributable fraction, a best estimate of the proportion of diseases or injuries that would be eliminated if alcohol did not exist, relies on not only the prevalence of alcohol drinking but also those of other risk factors, and so varies with country and time. By using these fractions, it has been estimated that in 1987 there were 105,095 (60,168 males and 34,927 females) alcohol-related deaths in the U.S. (Table 1.5).[13] This corresponded to 4.9% of total national mortality and the average number of years of potential life lost was 25.9 years. Injuries (both unintentional and intentional combined) ranked first, causing 46% of alcohol-related deaths and 65% of the years of potential life lost. Digestive disease including cancers of digestive organs ranked second, accounting for 33,815 deaths (32%) of the total alcohol-related mortality. Among these, alcoholic liver cirrhosis was the most common followed by cancer of the esophagus. Using the same method, the alcohol-related mortality in Spain was estimated to be 6.1% of the total number of deaths in 1986.[14] These estimates could be conservative, since some conditions that have been associated with alcohol consumption relatively recently were not included. In addition, the impact on less fatal diseases and injuries cannot be assessed properly. Gorsky et al. estimated that alcohol-attributable direct health costs in New Hampshire, U.S. amounted to 10% of total health care costs, 40% of which were for digestive diseases excluding cancer.[15]

## 1.6  ALCOHOL AND TOTAL MORTALITY

Most evidence on the relationship between alcohol consumption and total mortality has been derived from prospective studies conducted in various geographical areas, mostly in developed countries.[16-32] The types of study population include the general population of a defined area, or

**TABLE 1.5   Alcohol-Attributable Fractions and Estimated Alcohol-Related Mortality by Diagnosis, U.S. (1987)**

| Diagnosis | AAFs | ARM | Diagnosis | AAFs | ARM |
|---|---|---|---|---|---|
| Malignant neoplasms | | (15.2%) | Digestive diseases | | (18.7%) |
| Mouth, pharynx | 0.50[a] | 3,679 | Other diseases of esophagus, stomach, and duodenum | 0.10 | 907 |
| Esophagus | 0.75 | 6,803 | Alcoholic gastritis | 1.00 | 73 |
| Stomach | 0.20 | 2,722 | Alcoholic fatty liver | 1.00 | 914 |
| Liver | 0.15 | 1,057 | Acute alcoholic hepatitis | 1.00 | 794 |
| Larynx | 0.50[a] | 1,760 | Alcoholic liver cirrhosis | 1.00 | 7,508 |
| | | | Unspecified alcoholic liver damage | 1.00 | 2,049 |
| Mental disorders | | (5.1%) | Other liver cirrhosis | 0.50 | 6,303 |
| Alcohol psychoses | 1.00 | 382 | Acute pancreatitis | 0.42 | 891 |
| Alcohol dependence syndrome | 1.00 | 4,261 | Chronic pancreatitis | 0.60 | 117 |
| Alcohol abuse | 1.00 | 673 | Unintentional injuries | | (28.7%) |
| Cardiovascular diseases | | (10.2%) | Motor vehicle accidents | 0.42 | 20,282 |
| Essential hypertension | 0.08 | 306 | Other road vehicle accidents | 0.20 | 46 |
| Alcoholic cardiomyopathy | 1.00 | 797 | Water transport accidents | 0.20 | 190 |
| Cerebrovascular disease | 0.07 | 9,644 | Air/space transport accidents | 0.16 | 202 |
| | | | Alcohol poisonings | 1.00 | 188 |
| Respiratory diseases | | (3.5%) | Accidental falls | 0.35 | 4,052 |
| Respiratory tuberculosis | 0.25 | 327 | Accidents caused by fires | 0.45 | 2,119 |
| Pneumonia, influenza | 0.05 | 3,362 | Accidental drowning | 0.38 | 1,657 |
| Other alcohol-related diagnoses | | (1.8%) | Other injuries | 0.25 | 1,470 |
| Diabetes mellitus | 0.05 | 1,888 | Intentional injuries | | (16.8%) |
| Alcoholic polyneuropathy | 1.00 | 4 | Suicide | 0.28 | 8,552 |
| Excess blood alcohol level | 1.00 | 11 | Homicide | 0.46 | 9,107 |
| | | | Total | 0.05 | 105,095 |

*Note:*  AAFs, alcohol-attributable fractions; ARM, alcohol-related mortality.

[a] 0.40 for females.

From CDC (1990).[13]

random samples of it: volunteers, conscripts, participants in a health check-up program, physicians, civil servants, and a specific ethnic group and are mostly middle-aged men. The length of follow-up ranges from 5 to more than 20 years. In almost all studies, a U- or J-shaped mortality curve was observed with alcohol consumption. In other words, the mortality is lowest in light to moderate drinkers and increased in both nondrinkers and heavy drinkers (Table 1.6). One exception is the study of Swedish conscripts, in which the subjects were apparently younger than those in the other studies, and more than 70% of the deaths were caused by violence.[29] Usually, heavy drinkers have a higher mortality rate than do nondrinkers and the increased mortality of alcoholics compared with the general population supports this finding.[33-35] It has been suggested that one of the reasons for the increased mortality in nondrinkers is that ex-drinkers are not usually separated out from never-drinkers.[23] Drinkers often must abstain from alcohol because of their health problems. When ex-drinkers were examined separately, their mortality was as high as that among heavy drinkers in the Japanese Physicians Study.[32] Other studies have shown that ex-drinkers have higher rates of certain symptoms of chronic diseases and physician-diagnosed medical conditions than never-drinkers.[30,36] Therefore, the lower mortality among light to moderate drinkers as compared to nondrinkers is likely to be exaggerated. Another factor determining the mortality curve is the distribution of causes of death, particularly the proportion of coronary heart disease, which is significantly reduced by alcohol drinking.

## 1.7  IMPACT OF ALCOHOL DRINKING ON MAJOR CAUSES OF DEATH

### 1.7.1  Coronary Heart Disease

Most prospective studies have found that alcohol drinkers have a lower risk of coronary heart disease than nondrinkers.[17-22,26,30,32,37-40] In some studies the risk decreased progressively with increased levels of alcohol consumption[30,37-40] and in the others a reverse J- or U-shaped incidence or mortality curve was observed.[17-22,26,32] The reductions in risk have been 20 to 70% compared with nondrinkers. The most plausible explanation for the protective effects of moderate alcohol drinking is that it elevates levels of high-density lipoprotein cholesterol which is inversely associated with the risk of coronary heart disease. In addition, alcohol is associated with an increased prostacyclin/thromboxane ratio and a decreased platelet aggregability. It also interacts with aspirin to prolong bleeding time. Alcohol also increases the release of plasminogen activator and lowers the level of fibrinogens, a potent risk factor for coronary heart disease.[39] The biological plausibility and the consistent results in past epidemiological studies suggest a causal relationship.

### 1.7.2  Stroke

Several prospective studies have found that heavy drinkers are at an increased risk of stroke. When all types of stroke were combined, relative risks of 1.5 to 1.9 were observed in American volunteers,[20] Japanese Americans in Hawaii,[41] Japanese male physicians,[32] and Swedish middle-aged men,[42] while another cohort study in Canada found three times the risk among persons who consumed three or more drinks per day.[43] The risk tends to be particularly elevated for hemorrhagic stroke and subarachnoid hemorrhage (relative risks of 3 to 4).[18,39,41] In contrast, alcohol consumption was associated with a decreased risk of ischemic stroke in studies of American nurses[39] and participants in a health check-up program.[18] The effect of alcohol on platelets and clotting discussed in the above section may increase the risk of hemorrhagic stroke. In addition, alcohol raises the risk of hypertension and in experimental animals, it can induce spasm in the cerebral vasculature.

### 1.7.3  Cancer

Excessive alcohol drinking has been associated with increased mortality and incidence for all cancers combined in various types of prospective study, including studies of alcoholics,[34,44-46]

**TABLE 1.6  The Relation Between Alcohol Consumption and Total Mortality in the Selected Prospective Studies**

| Country/area | No. and characteristics of study population | Age at entry | Follow-up length (years) | Drinking category with the lowest mortality | RR[a] for other drinking levels Non/minimum | Highest | Reference no. |
|---|---|---|---|---|---|---|---|
| U.S. | 5,209 men and women in Framingham | 29–62 | 22 | 30–59 oz/month | 1.2 | 1.0 | 16 |
| | 4,590 residents of Alameda County | 35+ | 15 | 1–30 drinks/month  (M) | 1.2 | 2.3 | 17 |
| | | | | (F) | 1.1 | 1.5 | |
| | 123,840 participants in multiphasic health check-ups | 40.5 | 5.3 | >1 drink/month and <1 drink/day | 1.1 | 1.6 | 18 |
| | 1,823 male volunteers in Boston | 42.0 | 12 | 25–1094 drinks/year | 1.6 | 1.4 | 19 |
| | 276,802 male volunteers | 40–59 | 12 | 1 drink/day | 1.2 | 1.6 | 20 |
| | 1,910 male civil service employees | 38–55 | 18 | 1–9 oz/month | 2.0 | 3.6 | 21 |
| | 1,832 white male employees at Chicago Western Electric Company | 40–55 | 17 | 1 drink/day | 1.1 | 3.0 | 22 |
| U.K. | 7,735 men in 24 towns | 40–59 | 7.5 | 16–42 drinks/week | 1.5[b] | 1.3[b] | 23 |
| | 1,422 male civil servants | 40–64 | 10 | 0.1–9 g/day | 1.6 | 1.5 | 24 |
| Denmark | 7,234 women and 6,051 men in a defined area of Copenhagen | 30–79 | 10–12 | 1–6 drinks/week | 1.4 | 2.3 | 25 |
| Yugoslavia | 11,121 men in three areas | 35–62 | 7 | 1–6 drinks/week | 1.4 | 1.5 | 26 |
| Italy | 1,536 men in two villages | 45–64 | 15 | 56.4 g/day | 1.2 | 1.7 | 27 |
| Switzerland | 419 men of a community sample | 30–69 | 13 | 20–80 ml/day | 1.2 | 1.6 | 28 |
| Sweden | 49,464 male conscripts | 18–19 | 20 | Nondrinker | 1.0 | 1.6 | 29 |
| Trinidad | 1,341 men in a defined area | 35–69 | 7.5 | Not alcoholic | 1.5 | 2.1 | 30 |
| Hawaii | 8,006 Japanese men | 45–68 | 8 | 1–10 ml/day | 1.4[b] | 1.5[b] | 31 |
| Japan | 5,135 male physicians | 25+ | 19 | <54 ml/day | 1.1 | 1.4 | 32 |

[a] Relative risk compared with the lowest mortality.

[b] Calculated based on the crude death rates (%), no age- or other covariate-adjusted mortality was available in the original papers.

brewery workers,[47] volunteers,[20] physicians,[32] participants in a health check-up program,[48] and the general population.[42,49] Other prospective studies and a number of case-control studies have also found an increased risk for cancer of specific sites in relation to alcohol use.[1] Among a variety of cancer sites studied, an association has been established for cancers of the upper aerodigestive tract and liver, while for cancers of the stomach and pancreas, results have been inconsistent and have often failed to show a dose–response trend.[1] Accumulated evidence suggests that alcohol may increase the risk of colorectal cancer, especially rectal cancer.[47] Likewise, a consistent positive association has recently been observed between moderate alcohol consumption and breast cancer.[1] If these associations are causal, the impact of alcohol use on cancer morbidity and mortality would become much larger than estimated in Section 5. Although some investigators have also found a positive association between alcohol consumption and lung cancer, this is probably due to insufficient adjustment for cigarette smoking.

### 1.7.4    Infection

Follow-up studies of alcoholics have found an increased risk of death from all infectious diseases combined, and tuberculosis, pneumonia, bronchitis, other pulmonary diseases or all respiratory diseases,[33,34,46] and an increased rate of hospitalization for pneumonia.[50] A follow-up study of participants in a health check-up program has also confirmed a higher death rate from respiratory diseases in heavy drinkers compared with nondrinkers and light drinkers.[48] Frequent hangover was associated with an increased mortality from respiratory diseases in Finland.[51] Alcohol ingestion broadly suppresses the various host defenses, including polymorphonuclear neutrophil function, cell-mediated immune function, reticuloendothelial system function, and humoral immunity,[52] thus increasing susceptibility to infection.

### 1.7.5    Accidents

Several cohort studies have shown that alcoholics have from 3 to 9 times the risk of death or hospitalization from accidents compared with reference populations,[33,34,46,50] and that brewery workers[53,54] are more likely to die from motor vehicle accidents than the general population. Other prospective studies of nonalcoholic populations have confirmed that heavy drinkers have an increased risk of deaths from accidents.[20,48] In a case-control study of fatal two-car crashes, there was a significant increasing trend in risk for crash initiation as the level of blood alcohol concentrations increased. Compared with drivers with no detectable alcohol, those with blood alcohol of 100 to 149, 150 to 299, 200 to 249, and 250 mg/dl or more had odds ratios of being involved in an accident of 10.0, 13.9, 32.4, and 36.2, respectively.[55] The risk of injurious falls leading to hospitalization or deaths was also associated with alcohol consumption in a prospective study conducted in Finland. For consumptions of 100 to 499, 500 to 999, and 1000 g or more per month, the relative risk was elevated to 1.4, 2.5, and 3.6 respectively, compared with nondrinkers.[56]

## 1.8    IMPACT OF ALCOHOL USE ON OFFSPRING

Children of alcoholics are a high-risk group in terms of various outcomes including child abuse and incest, emotional disturbance, delinquency, and poor school performance. In particular, children of alcoholic mothers are at risk for fetal alcohol syndrome, characterized by prenatal and postnatal growth deficiency, a pattern of abnormalities including short palpebral fissures, epicanthic folds, ear anomalies, maxillary hypoplasia, minor joint and limb anomalies, cardiac defects, and mental retardation.[57] A prospective study at the Boston City Hospital showed that 32% of infants born to heavy drinkers had congenital anomalies, as compared with 9% in the abstinent and 14% in the moderate drinking group.[58] Even moderate alcohol drinking during pregnancy has been associated with decreased infant birth weight.[59-61] There is evidence that ethanol and/or its metabolic products exert a direct toxic effect on the fetus in animal studies.[62] Another experimental study has shown that exposure to alcohol via the mother's milk leads to long-term deficits in cellular immunity.[63]

Much of the evidence has suggested that alcohol not only adversely affects female reproductive function when ingested during pregnancy, but is also detrimental to male reproductive function, manifested by sexual impotence, feminization, hypogonadism, and sterility.[62] Although these phenomena are mainly attributable to alcohol-induced hepatic damage, direct inhibitory effects of ethanol on testicular steroidogenesis and on the hypothalamic pituitary axis have also been identified.[62] In animal studies, substantial evidence has been accumulated which associates paternal alcohol consumption with anomalies in subsequent offspring.[62]

## 1.9 ALCOHOL AND GASTROINTESTINAL DISEASE

### 1.9.1 Esophagus

Although there are various mechanisms by which alcohol consumption could increase the risk of esophagitis, epidemiological evidence has been limited.[64] In a survey at nine clinics in Argentina, the prevalence of chronic esophagitis increased progressively with the level of alcohol consumption. Adjusted for cigarette smoking, men who consumed 80 g or more alcohol per day had 2.5 times the risk of chronic esophagitis compared with those who consumed less than 40 g per day.[65] Gray et al. reported that patients with severe esophagitis drank statistically significantly more than those with Barrett's columnar lined esophagus and even more than patients with adenocarcinoma of the esophagus.[66] In a study in the former Soviet Union, the relative risk of chronic esophagitis was about two in current smokers who drank, but the effect of alcohol drinking alone was not reported.[67] No association was found between the prevalence of chronic esophagitis and alcohol consumption in a survey in France.[68] Mallory-Weiss syndrome has been recognized to occur frequently in alcoholics. According to Shay and Johnson, the incidence of recent alcoholism in the affected patients is 53 to 73%.[64] No data are available from epidemiological studies with adequate control groups. In a follow-up study of alcoholics in U.S. veterans, the relative risk for deaths from any benign esophageal disease was 3.3.[33] Because of the small number of cases ($n = 3$), statistical evaluation was impossible.

### 1.9.2 Stomach/Duodenum

Although excessive alcohol intake is described as an important cause of acute gastritis, little evidence is available from epidemiological studies. In a clinical survey on hemorrhagic gastritis in Sweden, bleeding episodes were frequently associated with alcohol intake (35%).[69] For all types of gastritis and duodenitis combined, a significantly increased hospitalization rate was observed in alcoholics compared with controls.[49] More epidemiological data are available for chronic gastritis. In an earlier study by Edwards and Coghill, the prevalence of chronic gastritis, analyzed by drinking habit, was highest in regular and irregular heavy drinkers.[70] Fontham et al. found that patients with chronic atrophic gastritis consumed more alcohol than controls diagnosed with normal gastric mucosa or superficial gastritis by gastric biopsy.[71] An endoscopic survey in seven areas of France also found that the proportion of heavy drinkers was twice as high in patients with chronic gastritis as in those without.[72] In support of these findings, decreased gastric secretory capacity has been demonstrated in alcoholics compared with controls.[73]

An increased risk of death or hospitalization from gastric and duodenal ulcer was found in three follow-up studies of alcoholics in the U.S.[33,50] and Canada[34] and in another cohort study of Danish brewery workers.[53] The relative risk compared with the comparison population ranged from 1.6 to 4.4. However, other cohort studies of general populations in Japan[49,74] and Denmark,[75] college students in the U.S.[76] and Japanese Americans in Hawaii,[77] and cross-sectional studies in the U.S.[78] and Japan[79] did not find any significant association between alcohol consumption and gastric and duodenal ulcer risk. These findings may suggest that excessive alcohol consumption increases the risk of dying from these diseases but that moderate consumption does not.

### 1.9.3    Large Intestine

In agreement with the positive association between colorectal cancer and alcohol consumption,[47] it has been suggested that alcohol consumption may also increase the risk of colorectal adenoma. In a prospective autopsy study among Japanese Americans in Hawaii, the mean number of adenomatous polyps increased with increasing level of alcohol consumption. Men at the highest quartile of alcohol consumption had more than twice the number of adenomatous polyps compared with those at the lowest consumption level.[80] Sandler et al. reported that the risk of colonic adenoma progressively increased with the level of alcohol consumption in males, but not in females. The relative risk for the highest quartile compared with nondrinkers was around four in males.[81] A similar trend was observed in Japan. Male military officials who consumed 60 ml or more alcohol per day had 2.4 times the risk of sigmoid colon adenoma compared with those who never drank.[82] Another study showed that daily drinkers had about twice the risk of proximal colon adenoma compared with never-drinkers.[83] Beer consumption was also associated with an increased risk of colonic adenoma in a case-control study in the U.S.[84] Recently, a large prospective study in the U.S. confirmed the association between alcohol consumption and distal colon adenoma. The risk was almost doubled at the highest level of consumption (>30 g/day) compared with nondrinkers.[85]

### 1.9.4    Biliary Tract

Evidence suggests that alcohol intake may protect against gallbladder diseases. Earlier studies including both prospective and case-control studies found that patients with gallbladder disease or cholesterol stones consumed less alcohol than those without.[86,87] A recent case-control study in Australia showed that the risk of gallstone disease was inversely associated with alcohol consumption in both men and women.[88] In a follow-up study of American nurses, the risk of symptomatic gallstones decreased with increasing levels of alcohol consumption. The relative risk for the highest level of consumption was 0.7 compared with nondrinkers.[89] When cases were limited to gallstone disease requiring surgery in a case-control study in Italy, the reduction in risk was more clear: consumption of three drinks or more a day yielded an odds ratio of 0.5 compared with nondrinkers.[90] A similar decreasing trend in risk was observed for gallstone disease ascertained by ultrasonography in a Danish population[91] and in a case-control study of roentgenographically confirmed gallbladder disease among Greek women.[92] Among Japanese male military officials, the inverse association with alcohol was observed only for men who had undergone cholecystectomy, but not for those with prevalent gallstones.[93] In a cross-sectional study in Mexican Americans, the protective effect of alcohol was seen only in women,[94] whereas it was found only for men in another cross-sectional analysis in the San Antonio Heart Study.[95] Although there is still inconsistency in the results from epidemiological studies, a possible effect of alcohol on cholesterol metabolism could be involved in the association.

### 1.9.5    Pancreas

Pancreatitis has long been associated with excessive alcohol drinking, evidenced mainly on the basis of clinical observations. Because of the relatively low frequency of the disease, epidemiological evidence has been rather limited. In a follow-up study of alcoholics who were U.S. veterans, there were six deaths from benign pancreatic diseases, compared with one in the comparison group, giving a relative risk of 6.6.[33] Alcoholics also had a significantly higher rate of hospitalization for pancreatic diseases than controls in another study.[50] In two other follow-up studies of Swedish conscripts and a random sample from the male general population in Finland, pancreatitis was analyzed combined with liver cirrhosis. In the Swedish study, the relative risk for liver cirrhosis and pancreatitis combined was 11.0 for men who consumed 250 g or more alcohol per week as compared with men who consumed 100 g or less alcohol per week.[29] In the Finnish study, the consumption of at least five bottles of beer per week yielded a relative risk of 3.7 for deaths due to liver cirrhosis and acute pancreatitis combined.[96] Neither of these studies reported how many pancreatitis cases were included. Yen et al. conducted a case-control study at 11 hospitals in eastern Massachusetts. They confirmed that alcohol was an independent risk factor for pancreatitis in men, providing a relative risk of 2.2 for regular drinkers.[97] Another case-control study in France also found that the alcohol intake per day was directly associated with the risk of chronic pancreatitis.[98]

## 1.10   CONFOUNDING FACTORS WITH ALCOHOL DRINKING

Alcohol drinking is not independent of other personal habits in humans. Alcohol use is known to be associated with other drug use,[11] among which cigarette smoking is the most common. Consumption of alcohol and tobacco is strongly correlated in most societies. Kato et al. reported that the prevalence of moderate to heavy drinkers increased with the number of cigarettes per day and that the prevalence of current smokers increased with increasing alcohol consumption.[99] A similar trend was observed in middle-aged British men.[100] Among 36,656 white men and women who participated in a multiphasic health check-up program, the proportion of heavy drinkers was three to four times higher in smokers than in nonsmokers.[78] Since cigarette smoking is a risk factor for most of the conditions discussed above, inadequate adjustment leads to an over- or underestimation of the effects of alcohol consumption.

Nutritional deficiencies of both macro- and micronutrients are frequently found in alcoholics[101] and are likely to play an important role in the pathogenesis of alcohol-related diseases. The principal cause of the nutritional deficiencies has been considered to be low dietary intake.[101] With increasing alcohol consumption, the proportion of calories from major nutrients automatically decreases. Consequently, the intake of micronutrients per calorie decreases. As long as total calorie intake is not increased by alcohol intake, most micronutrients, including calcium, vitamins A and C, thiamin and fiber, are found to be significantly lower in heavy drinkers than in nondrinkers to light drinkers.[102] Even when total energy intake is increased, intakes of fresh fruits, dairy products, vitamins A and C, β-carotene, and total fiber per calorie tend to be lower in heavy drinkers than in nondrinkers and light drinkers.[103-105] In addition, malabsorption and increased requirements reinforce the nutritional deficiencies.[101] The effect of these nonalcoholic factors is usually much greater for heavy drinkers than it is for moderate drinkers. As a result, some discrepancies in health effects of alcohol consumption between them could be due to the extent of confounding. One should remember that the health consequences of excessive alcohol drinking in humans are multifactorial.

## REFERENCES

1. **IARC,** *IARC Monograph on the Evaluation of Carcinogenic Risks to Humans, Vol 44. Alcohol Drinking,* IARC, Lyon, 1988.
2. **Walsh, B. and Grant, M.,** *Public Health Implications of Alcohol Production and Trade,* World Health Organization, Geneva, 1985.
3. **Pyörälä, E.,** Trends in alcohol consumption in Spain, Portugal, France and Italy from the 1950s until the 1980s, *Br. J. Addict.,* 85, 469, 1990.
4. **Systembolaget,** *Annual Report 1992,* Stockholm, 1993.
5. **Intersalt Cooperative Research Group,** Intersalt: an international study of electrolyte excretion and blood pressure: results for 24 hour urinary sodium and potassium excretion, *Br. Med. J.,* 297, 319, 1988.
6. **Péquignot, G., Crosingnani, P., Terracini, B., Ascunce, N., Zubiri, A., Raymond, L., Estève, J., and Tuyns, A. J.,** A comparative study of smoking, drinking and dietary habits in population samples in France, Italy, Spain and Switzerland. III. Consumption of alcohol, *Rev. Epidemiol. Sante Publ.,* 36, 177, 1988.
7. **Pinn, G. and Bovet, P.,** Alcohol-related cardiomyopathy in the Seychelles, *Med. J. Australia,* 155, 529, 1991.

8. **Smith, P. F., Remington, P. L., Williamson, D. F., and Anda, R. F.,** A comparison of alcohol sales data with survey data on self-reported alcohol use in 21 states, *Am. J. Public Health*, 80, 309, 1990.

9. **CDC,** Behavioral risk factor surveillance, 1988, *CDC MMWR*, 39, 1, 1990.

10. **Edwards, G., Gross, M. M., Keller, M., Moser, J., and Room, R.,** *Alcohol-Related Disabilities*, World Health Organization, Geneva, 1977.

11. **Crum, R. M., Helzer, J. E., and Anthony, J. C.,** Level of education and alcohol abuse and dependence in adulthood: a further inquiry, *Am. J. Public Health*, 83, 830, 1993.

12. **Regier, D. A., Farmer, M. E., Rae, D. S., Myers, J. K., Kramer, M., Robins, L. N., George, L. K., Karno, M., and Locke, B. Z.,** One-month prevalence of mental disorders in the United States and sociodemographic characteristics: the Epidemiologic Catchment Area study, *Acta Psychiatr. Scand.*, 88, 35, 1993.

13. **CDC,** Alcohol-related mortality and years of potential life lost — United States, 1987, *CDC MMWR*, 39, 173, 1990.

14. **Yañez, J. L., Del Rio, M. C., and Alvarez, F. J.,** Alcohol-related mortality in Spain, *Alcohol Clin. Exp. Res.*, 17, 253, 1993.

15. **Gorsky, R. D., Schwartz, E., and Dennis, D.,** The mortality, morbidity, and economic costs of alcohol abuse in New Hampshire, *Prev. Med.*, 17, 736, 1988.

16. **Gordon, T. and Kannel, W. B.,** Drinking and mortality. The Framingham study, *Am. J. Epidemiol.*, 120, 97, 1984.

17. **Camacho, T. C., Kaplan, G. A., and Cohen, R. D.,** Alcohol consumption and mortality in Alameda County, *J. Chron. Dis.*, 40, 229, 1987.

18. **Klatsky, A. L., Armstrong, M. A., and Friedman, G. D.,** Risk of cardiovascular mortality in alcohol drinkers, ex-drinkers and nondrinkers, *Am. J. Cardiol.*, 66, 1237, 1990.

19. **De Labry, L. O., Glynn, R. J., Levenson, M. R., Hermos, J. A., LoCastro, J. S., and Vokonas, P. S.,** Alcohol consumption and mortality in an American male population: recovering the U-shaped curve — findings from the Normative Aging study, *J. Stud. Alcohol*, 53, 25, 1992.

20. **Bofetta, P. and Garfinkel, L.,** Alcohol drinking and mortality among men enrolled in an American Cancer Society prospective study, *Epidemiology*, 1, 342, 1990.

21. **Gordon, T. and Doyle, J. T.,** Drinking and mortality. The Albany study, *Am. J. Epidemiol.*, 125, 263, 1987.

22. **Dyer, A. R., Stamler, J., Paul, O., Lepper, M., Shekelle, R. B., McKean, H., and Garside, D.,** Alcohol consumption and 17-year mortality in the Chicago Western Electric Company study, *Prev. Med.*, 9, 78, 1980.

23. **Shaper, A. G., Wannamethee, G., and Walker, M.,** Alcohol and mortality in British men: explaining the U-shaped curve, *Lancet*, 2, 1267, 1988.

24. **Marmot, M. G., Rose, G., Shipley, M. J., and Thomas, B. J.,** Alcohol and mortality: a U-shaped curve, *Lancet*, 1, 580, 1981.

25. **Gronbek, M., Deis, A., Sorensen, T. I. A., Becker, U., Borch-Johnsen, K., Müller, C., Schnohr, P., and Jensen, G.,** Influence of sex, age, body mass index, and smoking on alcohol intake and mortality, *Br. Med. J.*, 308, 302, 1994.

26. **Kozarevic, D., Vojvodic, N., Gordon, T., Kaelber, C. T., McGee, D., and Zukel, W. J.,** Drinking habits and death, *Int. J. Epidemiol.*, 12, 145, 1983.

27. **Frachi, G., Fidanza, F., Mariotti, S., and Menotti, A.,** Alcohol and mortality in the Italian rural cohorts of the Seven Countries study, *Int. J. Epidemiol.*, 21, 74, 1992.

28. **Rehm, J., Fichter, M. M., and Elton, M.,** Effects on mortality of alcohol consumption, smoking, physical activity, and close personal relationships, *Addiction*, 88, 101, 1993.

29. **Andréasson, S., Romelsjö, A., and Allebeck, P.,** Alcohol, social factors and mortality among young men, *Br. J. Addict.*, 86, 877, 1991.

30. **Miller, G. J., Beckles, G. L. A., Maude, G. H., and Carson, D. C.,** Alcohol consumption: protection against coronary heart disease and risks to health, *Int. J. Epidemiol.*, 19, 923, 1990.

31. **Blackwelder, W. C., Yano, K., Rhoads, G. G., Kagan, A., Gordon, T., and Palesch, Y.,** Alcohol and mortality: the Honolulu Heart Study, *Am. J. Med.*, 68, 164, 1980.

32. **Kono, S., Ikeda, M., Tokudome, S., Nishizumi, M., and Kuratsune, M.,** Alcohol and mortality: a cohort study of male Japanese physicians, *Int. J. Epidemiol.*, 15, 527, 1986.

33. **Robinette, C. D., Hrubec, Z., and Fraumeni, J. F., Jr.,** Chronic alcoholism and subsequent mortality in World War II veterans, *Am. J. Epidemiol.*, 109, 687, 1979.

34. **Schmidt, W. and Popham, R. E.,** The role of drinking and smoking in mortality from cancer and other causes in male alcoholics, *Cancer*, 47, 1031, 1981.

35. **Finney, J. W. and Moos, R. H.,** The long-term course of treated alcoholism: I. Mortality, relapse and remission rates and comparison with community controls, *J. Stud. Alcohol*, 52, 44, 1991.

36. **Wannamethee, G. and Shaper, A. G.,** Men who do not drink: a report from the British Regional Heart study, *Int. J. Epidemiol.*, 17, 307, 1988.

37. **Yano, K., Rhoads, G. G., and Kagan, A.,** Coffee, alcohol and risk of coronary heart disease among Japanese men living in Hawaii, *N. Engl. J. Med.*, 297, 405, 1977.

38. **Rimm, E. B., Giovannucci, E. L., Willett, W. C., Colditz, G. A., Ascherio, A., Rosner, B., and Stampfer, M. J.,** Prospective study of alcohol consumption and risk of coronary disease in men, *Lancet*, 338, 464, 1991.

39. **Stampfer, M. J., Colditz, G. A., Willett, W. C., Speizer, F. E., and Hennekens, C. H.,** A prospective study of moderate alcohol consumption and the risk of coronary disease and stroke in women, *N. Engl. J. Med.*, 319, 267, 1988.

40. **Konishi, M., Iso, H., Iida, M., Naito, Y., Sato, S., Komachi, Y., Shimamoto, T., Doi, M., and Ito, M.,** Trends for coronary heart disease and its risk factors in Japan: epidemiologic and pathologic studies, *Jpn. Circ. J.*, 54, 428, 1990.

41. **Donahue, R. P., Abbott, R. D., Reed, D. M., and Yano, K.,** Alcohol and hemorrhagic stroke, *JAMA*, 255, 2311, 1986.

42. **Rosengren, A., Wilhelmsen, L., and Wedel, H.,** Separate and combined effects of smoking and alcohol abuse in middle-aged men, *Acta Med. Scand.*, 223, 111, 1988.

43. **Semenciw, R. M., Morrison, H. I., Mao, Y., Johansen, H., Davies, J. W., and Wigle, D. T.,** Major risk factors for cardiovascular disease mortality in adults: results from the Nutritional Canada Survey cohort, *Int. J. Epidemiol.*, 17, 317, 1988.

44. **Adami, H.-O., McLaughlin, J. K., Hsing, A. W., Wolk, A., Ekbom, A., Holmberg, L., and Persson, I.,** Alcoholism and cancer risk: a population-based cohort study, *Cancer Causes Control*, 3, 419, 1992.

45. **Tonnesen, H., Moller, H., Andersen, J. R., Jensen, E., and Juel, K.,** Cancer morbidity in alcohol abusers, *Br. J. Cancer*, 69, 327, 1994.

46. **Berglund, M.,** Mortality in alcoholics related to clinical state at first admission, *Acta Psychiatr. Scand.*, 70, 407, 1984.

47. **Carstensen, J. M., Bygren, L. O., and Hatschek, T.,** Cancer incidence among Swedish brewery workers, *Int. J. Cancer*, 45, 393, 1990.

48. **Klatsky, A. L., Friedman, G. D., and Siegelaub, A. B.,** Alcohol and mortality. A ten-year Kaiser-Permanente experience, *Ann. Intern. Med.*, 95, 139, 1981.

49. **Hirayama, T.,** Direct tobacco diseases and indirect tobacco diseases, *Shindan To Chiryo*, 69, 881, 1981.

50. **Kolb, D. and Gunderson, E. K. E.,** Alcohol-related morbidity among older career Navy men, *Drug Alcohol Depend.*, 9, 181, 1982.

51. **Poikolainen, K.,** Inebriation and mortality, *Int. J. Epidemiol.*, 12, 151, 1983.

52. **MacGregor, R. R.,** Alcohol and immune defense, *JAMA*, 256, 1474, 1986.

53. **Jensen, O. M.,** Cancer morbidity and causes of death among Danish brewery workers, *Int. J. Cancer*, 23, 454, 1979.

54. **Dean, G., MacLennan, R., McLoughlin, H., and Shelley, E.,** Causes of death of blue-collar workers at a Dublin brewery, 1954–1973, *Br. J. Cancer*, 40, 581, 1979.

55. **Perneger, T. and Smith, G. S.,** The driver's role in fatal two-car crashes: a paired "case-control" study, *Am. J. Epidemiol.*, 134, 1138, 1991.

56. **Malmivaara, A., Heliövaara, M., Knekt, P., Reunanen, A., and Aromaa, A.,** Risk factors for injurious falls leading hospitalization or death in a cohort of 19,500 adults, *Am. J. Epidemiol.*, 138, 384, 1993.

57. **Streissguth, A. P.,** Fetal alcohol syndrome: an epidemiologic perspective, *Am. J. Epidemiol.*, 107, 467, 1978.

58. **Ouellette, E. M., Rosett, H. L., Rosman, N. P., and Weiner, L.,** Adverse effects on offspring of maternal alcohol abuse during pregnancy, *N. Engl. J. Med.*, 297, 528, 1977.

59. **Little, R. E.,** Moderate alcohol use during pregnancy and decreased infant weight, *Am. J. Public Health*, 67, 1154, 1977.

60. **Wright, J. T., Waterson, E. J., Barrison, I. G., Toplis, P. J., Lewis, I. G., Gordon, M. G., MacRae, K. D., Morris, N. F., and Murray-Lyon, I. M.,** Alcohol consumption, pregnancy, and low birthweight, *Lancet*, 1, 663, 1983.

61. **Kariniemi, V. and Rosti, J.,** Maternal smoking and alcohol consumption as determinants of birth weight in an unselected study population, *J. Perinat. Med.*, 16, 249, 1988.

62. **Anderson, R. A., Jr.,** The possible role of paternal alcohol consumption in the etiology of the fetal alcohol syndrome, in *Fetal Alcohol Syndrome, Vol III. Animal Studies*, Abel, E. L., Ed., CRC Press, Boca Raton, FL, 1982, 83.

63. **Gottesfeld, Z. and LeGrue, S. J.,** Lactational alcohol exposure elicits long-term immune deficits and increased noradrenergic synaptic transmission in lymphoid organs, *Life Sci.*, 47, 457, 1990.

64. **Weinbeck, M. and Berges, W.,** Esophageal and gastric lesions in the alcoholic, in *Alcohol Related Diseases in Gastroenterology*, Seitz, H. K. and Kommerell, B., Eds., Springer-Verlag, Berlin, 1985, 361.

65. **Castelletto, R., Muñoz, N., Landoni, N., Jmelnitzky, A., Crespi, M., Belloni, P., Chopita, N., and Teuchmann, S.,** Pre-cancerous lesions of the oesophagus in Argentina: prevalence and association with tobacco and alcohol, *Int. J. Cancer*, 51, 34, 1992.

66. **Gray, M. R., Donnelly, R. J., and Kingsnorth, A. N.,** The role of smoking and alcohol in metaplasia and cancer in Barrett's columnar lined oesophagus, *Gut*, 34, 727, 1993.

67. **Zaridze, D. G., Blettner, M., Trapeznikov, N. N., Kuvshinov, J. P., Matiakin, E. G., Poljakov, B. P., Poddubni, B. K., Parshikova, S. M., Rottenberg, V. I., Chamrakulov, F. S., Chodjaeva, M. C., Stich, H. F., Rosin, M. P., Thurnham, D. I., Hoffmann, D., and Brunnemann, K. D.,** Survey of a population with a high incidence of oral and oesophageal cancer, *Int. J. Cancer*, 36, 153, 1985.

68. **Jacob, J. H., Riviere, A., Mandard, A. M., Muñoz, N., Crespi, M., Etienne, Y., Castellsagué, X., Marnay, J., Lebigot, G., and Qiu, S. L.,** Prevalence survey of precancerous lesions of the oesophagus in a high-risk population for oesophageal cancer in France, *Eur. J. Cancer Prev.*, 2, 53, 1993.

69. **Borch, K., Jansson, L., Sjödahl, R., and Anderberg, B.,** Haemorrhagic gastritis, *Acta Chir. Scand.*, 154, 211, 1987.

70. **Edwards, F. C. and Coghill, N. F.,** Aetiological factors in chronic gastritis, *Br. Med. J.*, 2, 1409, 1966.

71. **Fontham, E., Zavala, D., Correa, P., Rodriguez, E., Hunter, F., Haenszel, W., and Tannenbaum, S. R.,** Diet and chronic atrophic gastritis: a case-control study, *J. Natl. Cancer Instit.*, 76, 621, 1986.

72. **Potet, F., Florent, C., Benhamou, E., Cabrières, F., Bommelaer, G., Hostein, J., Bigard, M.-A., Bruley de Varannes, S., Colombel, J.-F., and Rampal, P.,** Chronic gastritis: prevalence in the French population, *Gastroenterol. Clin. Biol.*, 17, 103, 1993.

73. **Segawa, K., Nakazawa, S., Tsukamoto, Y., Goto, H., Yamao, K., Hase, S., Osada, T., and Arisawa, T.,** Chronic alcohol abuse leads to gastric atrophy and decreased gastric secretory capacity: a histological and physiological study, *Am. J. Gastroenterol.*, 83, 373, 1988.

74. **Kato, I., Tominaga, S., and Matsuoka, I.,** A prospective study on the relationship between lifestyle and major adult diseases, *Jpn. J. Public Health*, 36, 662, 1989.

75. **Ostensen, H., Gudmundsen, T. E., Ostensen, P., Burhol, P. G., and Bonnevie, O.,** Smoking, alcohol, coffee, and familial factors: any association with peptic ulcer disease? A clinically and radiologically prospective study, *Scand. J. Gastroenterol.*, 20, 1227, 1985.

76. **Paffenbarger, R. S., Wing, A. L., and Hyde, R. T.,** Chronic disease in former college students. XIII. Early precursors of peptic ulcer, *Am. J. Epidemiol.*, 100, 307, 1974.

77. **Kato, I., Nomura, A. M. Y., Stemmermann, G. N., and Chyou, P.-H.,** A prospective study of gastric and duodenal ulcer and its relation to smoking, alcohol and diet, *Am. J. Epidemiol.*, 135, 521, 1992.

78. **Friedman, G. D., Siegelaub, A. B., and Seltzer, C. C.,** Cigarettes, alcohol and peptic ulcer, *N. Engl. J. Med.*, 290, 469, 1974.

79. **Kato, I., Tominaga, S., Ito, Y., Kobayashi, S., Yoshii, Y., Matsuura, A., Kano, T., and Kameya, A.,** Comparative case-control analysis of gastric and duodenal ulcers, *Jpn. J. Public Health*, 37, 919, 1990.

80. **Stemmermann, G. N., Heilbrun, L. K., and Nomura, A. M. Y.,** Association of diet and other factors with adenomatous polyps of the large bowel: a prospective autopsy study, *Am. J. Clin. Nutr.*, 47, 312, 1988.

81. **Sandler, R. S., Lyles, C. M., McAuliffe, C., Woosley, J. T., and Kupper, L. L.,** Cigarette smoking, alcohol, and the risk of colorectal adenoma, *Gastroenterology*, 104, 1445, 1993.

82. **Kono, S., Ikeda, N., Yanai, F., Shinchi, K., and Imanishi, K.,** Alcoholic beverages and adenomatous polyps of the sigmoid colon: a study of male self-defence officials in Japan, *Int. J. Epidemiol.*, 19, 848, 1990.

83. **Kato, I., Tominaga, S., Matsuura, A., Yoshii, Y., Shirai, M., and Kobayashi, S.,** A comparative case-control study of colorectal cancer and adenoma, *Jpn. J. Cancer Res.*, 81, 1101, 1990.

84. **Kikendall, J. W., Bowen, P. E., Burgess, M. B., Magnetti, C., Woodward, J., and Langenberg, P.,** Cigarettes and alcohol as independent risk factors for colonic adenomas, *Gastroenterology*, 97, 660, 1989.

85. **Giovannucci, E., Stampfer, M. J., Colditz, G. A., Rimm, E. B., Trichopoulos, D., Rosner, B. A., Speizer, F. E., and Willett, W. C.,** Folate, methionine, and alcohol intake and risk of colorectal adenoma, *J. Natl. Cancer Instit.*, 85, 875, 1993.

86. **Friedman, G. D., Kannel, W. B., and Dawber, T. B.,** The epidemiology of gallbladder disease: observation in the Framingham study, *J. Chron. Dis.*, 19, 273, 1966.

87. **Wheeler, M., Hills, L. L., and Laby, B.,** Cholelithiasis: a clinical and dietary survey, *Gut*, 11, 430, 1970.

88. **Scragg, R. K. R., McMichael, A. J., and Baghurst, P. A.,** Diet, alcohol, and relative weight in gall stone disease: a case-control study, *Br. Med. J.*, 288, 1113, 1984.

89. **MacLure, K. M., Hayes, K. C., Colditz, G. A., Stampfer, M. J., Speizer, F. E., and Willett, W. C.,** Weight, diet, and the risk of symptomatic gallstones in middle-aged women, *N. Engl. J. Med.*, 321, 563, 1989.

90. **La Vecchia, C., Negri, E., D'Avanzo, B., Franceschi, S., and Boyle, P.,** Risk factors for gallstone disease requiring surgery, *Int. J. Epidemiol.*, 20, 209, 1991.

91. **Jorgensen, T. and Jorgensen, L. M.,** Gallstones and diet in a Danish Population, *Scand. J. Gastroenterol.*, 24, 821, 1989.

92. **Pastides, H., Tzonou, A., Trichopoulos, D., Katsouyanni, K., Trichopoulou, A., Kefalogiannis, N., and Manousos, O.,** A case-control study of the relationship between smoking, diet and gallbladder disease, *Arch. Intern. Med.*, 150, 1409, 1990.

93. **Kono, S., Shinchi, K., Ikeda, N., Yanai, F., and Imanishi, K.,** Prevalence of gallstone disease in relation to smoking, alcohol use, obesity, and glucose tolerance: a study of self-defense officials in Japan, *Am. J. Epidemiol.*, 136, 787, 1992.

94. **Maurer, K. R., Everhart, J. E., Knowler, W. C., Shawker, T. H., and Roth, H. P.,** Risk factors for gallstone disease in the Hispanic population of the United States, *Am. J. Epidemiol.*, 131, 836, 1990.

95. **Diehl, A. K., Haffner, S. M., Hazuda, H. P., and Stern, M. P.,** Coronary risk factors and clinical gallbladder disease: an approach to the prevention of gallstones?, *Am. J. Public Health*, 77, 841, 1987.

96. **Salonen, J. T., Puska, P., and Nissinen, A.,** Intake of spirits and beer and risk of myocardial infarction and death — a longitudinal study in Eastern Finland, *J. Chron. Dis.*, 36, 533, 1983.

97. **Yen, S., Hsieh, C.-C., and MacMahon, B.,** Consumption of alcohol and tobacco and other risk factors for pancreatitis, *Am. J. Epidemiol.*, 116, 407, 1982.

98. **Bourliere, M., Barthet, M., Berthezene, P., Durbec, J. P., and Sarles, H.,** Is tobacco a risk factor for chronic pancreatitis and alcoholic cirrhosis?, *Gut*, 32, 1392, 1991.

99. **Kato, I., Tominaga, S., and Matsuoka, I.,** Characteristics of life style of smokers and drinkers, *Jpn. J. Public Health*, 34, 692, 1987.

100. **Cummins, R. O., Shaper, A. G., Walker, M., and Wale, C. J.,** Smoking and drinking by middle-aged British men: effects of social class and town of residence, *Br. Med. J.*, 283, 1497, 1981.

101. **Morgan, M. Y.,** Alcohol and nutrition, *Br. Med. Bull.*, 38, 21, 1982.

102. **Hillers, V. N. and Massey, L. K.,** Interrelationships of moderate and high alcohol consumption with diet and health status, *Am. J. Clin. Nutr.*, 41, 356, 1985.

103. **Toniolo, P., Riboli, E., and Cappa, A. P. M.,** A community study of alcohol consumption and dietary habits in middle-aged Italian women, *Int. J. Epidemiol.*, 20, 663, 1991.

104. **Hebert, J. R. and Kabat, G. C.,** Implications for cancer epidemiology of differences in dietary intake associated with alcohol consumption, *Nutr. Cancer*, 15, 107, 1991.

105. **Herbeth, B., Didelot-Barthelemy, L., Lemoine, A., and Le Devehat, C.,** Dietary behavior of French men according to alcohol drinking pattern, *J. Stud. Alcohol*, 49, 268, 1988.

# 2

# The Metabolism of Alcohol and Its Implications for the Pathogenesis of Disease

Charles S. Lieber

## CONTENTS

## 2.1   INTRODUCTION

The demonstration that alcohol exerts some intrinsic hepatotoxicity independent of nutritional deficiencies (reviewed recently elsewhere[1]) led to a broad-based search for the mechanism involved. One of the most promising leads was that many of the metabolic and toxic effects of alcohol in the liver can be linked to its metabolism in that organ. Indeed, ethanol is readily absorbed from the gastrointestinal tract. Only 2 to 10% of that absorbed is eliminated through the

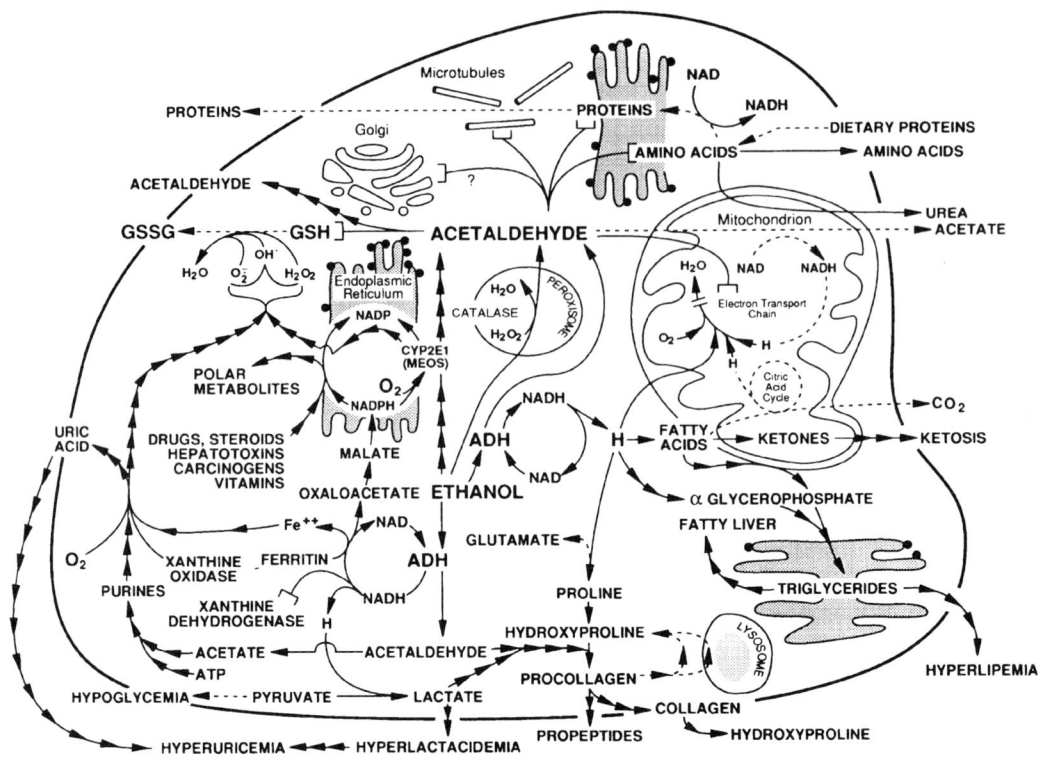

**FIGURE 2.1** Oxidation of ethanol in the hepatocyte. Many disturbances in intermediary metabolism and toxic effects can be linked to (1) ADH-mediated generation of NADH, (2) the induction of the activity of microsomal enzymes, especially the MEOS containing P-4502E1 (CYP2E1), and (3) acetaldehyde, the product of ethanol oxidation. GSH, reduced glutathione; GSSG, oxidized glutathione; - - - -, pathways that are depressed by ethanol; →→→→, stimulation or activation; -[, interference or binding. (From Lieber, C. S., *Gastroenterology*, 106, 1085, 1994.)

kidneys and lungs; the rest is oxidized in the body, principally in the liver. Except for the stomach, extrahepatic metabolism of ethanol is small. This relative organ specificity coupled with the high energy content of ethanol (each gram provides 7.1 kcal) and the lack of effective feedback control of its rate of hepatic metabolism may result in a displacement of up to 90% of the liver's normal metabolic substrates and probably explains why ethanol disposal produces striking metabolic imbalances in the liver.

The hepatocyte contains three main pathways for ethanol metabolism, each located in a different subcellular compartment: (1) the alcohol dehydrogenase (ADH) pathway of the cytosol or the soluble fraction of the cell, (2) the microsomal ethanol oxidizing system located in the endoplasmic reticulum, and (3) catalase located in the peroxisomes[2] (Figure 2.1). Each pathway produces a specific metabolic and toxic disturbance and all three result in the production of acetaldehyde, a highly toxic metabolite.

Bacterial fermentation in the gut is one way in which alcohol is produced in the body; consequently, the enzyme alcohol dehydrogenase may function to rid the body of this alcohol.

## 2.2   THE ALCOHOL DEHYDROGENASE (ADH) PATHWAY

A major pathway for alcohol metabolism involves ADH, an enzyme that catalyzes the conversion of alcohol to acetaldehyde.

## 2.2.1 Multiple Forms of ADH

Human ADH is a dimeric zinc metalloenzyme for which five classes have been distinguished. Subunits hybridize within classes but not between classes. Human liver ADH exists in multiple molecular forms which arise from the association of different types of subunits into active dimeric molecules. A genetic model accounts for this multiplicity as products of seven gene loci, ADH1 through ADH7.[3] Polymorphism occurs at two loci, ADH2 and ADH3, which encode the β and γ subunits. There are three types of subunits, α, β, and γ in class I. The primary structures of all three forms have been established as well as the overall properties and the effects of the amino acid substitutions between the various forms. Each subunit has 374 residues, of which 35 exhibit differences among the α, β, and γ chains. Corresponding cDNA structures are also known, as is the genetic organization and details of the gene structures. Allelic variants occur at the β and γ loci. Corresponding amino acid substitutions have been characterized, and enzymatic differences between the allelic forms are explained by defined residue exchanges. The subunits of class I are derived from at least three genetic loci[4-6] and constitute the α subunit (the major form expressed in fetal liver), different β subunits, distributed nonidentically in various populations (β1 common in Caucasian populations, β2 common in Oriental populations, and β3 found at least in some African populations),[7-9] and the two allelic types of γ subunits (γ1 and γ2, both of high frequency). Von Wartburg et al.[7] first differentiated the normal ADH of human liver (pH optimum 10.5) from the so-called atypical type (pH optimum 8.8), which shows a several-fold higher activity. The main normal human ADH has only the β1 subunit, whereas the atypical type also has the β2 subunit. Both subunits are controlled by the ADH2 locus. The atypical form of ADH occurs in frequencies between 5 and 20% in European populations: English (10%),[4] Swiss (20%),[10] and Germans (9%).[11] In Oriental populations, the frequency is up to 90%.[12] Class II isozymes generally have low $K_m$ values for alcohol, class II (or π) ADH has a relatively high $K_m$ (34 m$M$) and an insensitivity to 4-methylpyrazole inhibition. Class III (χADH) does not participate in the oxidation of alcohol in the liver because of its very low affinity for the substrate. Recently, a new class (IV) of ADH has been identified in human stomach,[13] so-called σ or μ-ADH[14,15] for which a full-length cDNA has been obtained.[16] A cDNA encoding yet another new class of ADH (V) in liver and stomach was also reported.[17]

## 2.2.2 Acinar Distribution of ADH

Immunohistochemical techniques have shown that ADH is located mainly in the zone 3 hepatocytes.[18] In microdissected tissue samples from the whole length of the sinusoid,[19] the ADH activity in men <50 years of age showed an increase in the gradient from zone 1 to zone 3; furthermore, ADH activity was significantly higher in women. The sex difference in the distribution profiles was no longer apparent after age 53 in men and age 50 in women.

## 2.2.3 Redox Change

In ADH-mediated oxidation of alcohol, hydrogen is transferred from the substrate to the cofactor nicotinamide adenine dinucleotide (NAD), converting it to its reduced form (NADH), and acetaldehyde is produced. Thus, the first step in the oxidation of alcohol generates an excess of reducing equivalents in the cytosol, primarily as NADH with a marked shift in the redox potential of the cytosol as measured by changes in the lactate and pyruvate ratio.[20] The altered redox state, in turn, is responsible for a variety of metabolic abnormalities (*vide infra*). Some of these, such as hyperlactacidemia, are linked to the utilization of the excess NADH in the cytosol (Figure 2.2). The reducing equivalents can also be transferred to NADPH, and the increased NADPH can be utilized for synthetic pathways in the cytosol and microsomal functions.

Some hydrogen equivalents formed in this reaction are transferred from the cytosol into the mitochondria. The mitochondrial membrane is impermeable to NADH and the reducing equivalents

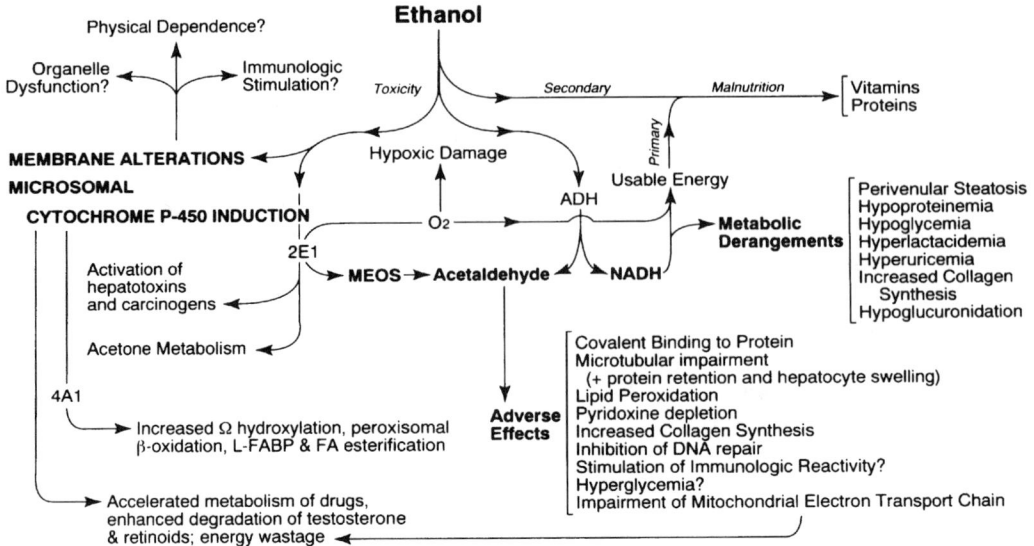

**FIGURE 2.2**  Hepatic, nutritional, and metabolic abnormalities after ethanol abuse. Malnutrition, whether primary or secondary, has been differentiated from direct toxicity. The latter has been attributed to redox changes, or effects secondary to microsomal induction, acetaldehyde, direct membrane alterations, or hypoxia. (From Lieber, C. S., in *The Biology of Alcohol Problems,* Saunders, J. B. and Whitfield, J. B., Eds., Elsevier, Oxford, UK, 1995.

are thought to enter the mitochondria via shuttle mechanisms such as the malate cycle (quantitatively, probably the most important), the fatty acid elongation cycle, and the α-glycerophosphate cycle. Normally, fatty acids are oxidized via β-oxidation and the citric acid cycle of the mitochondria, which serves as a "hydrogen donor" for the mitochondrial electron transport chain. When alcohol is oxidized, the generated hydrogen equivalents, which are shuttled into the mitochondria, supplant the citric acid cycle as the source of hydrogen. Following the administration of alcohol, the mitochondria shift to a more reduced redox state as measured by changes in the ratio of β-hydroxybutyrate to acetoacetate.[20]

### 2.2.4   Gastric ADH

At least three different forms of ADH exist in the human stomach (with the γγ, σσ, and χχ isoenzymes) with either high or low $K_m$s for ethanol.[13] Because of the extraordinary high gastric alcohol concentration after alcohol ingestion, even the gastric ADH with the high $K_m$ for alcohol can become active and significant gastric alcohol metabolism may ensue,[21,22] resulting in first-pass metabolism of ethanol. Ethnic variability is possibly involved, since 80% of Japanese were found to be deficient in one of the gastric isozyme activities.[23] The concentration of alcohol in the beverage affects the amount metabolized in the stomach. Consequently, in the rat, which has only the high $K_m$ enzyme, relatively high concentrations of alcohol are required for significant first-pass metabolism to be observed.[24] When only 2.5% alcohol was used, no first-pass metabolism was measurable.[25] Also, when low concentrations are used, relatively large volumes are involved, which may accelerate gastric emptying, thereby also resulting in less gastric metabolism.

The first-pass metabolism decreases the bioavailability of alcohol and represents a "protective barrier" against systemic effects, at least when alcohol is consumed in small amounts as in "social drinking." This "gastric barrier" disappears after gastrectomy[26] and may be decreased in the alcoholic,[27,28] in part, because of a decrease in gastric ADH activity. Some commonly used drugs inhibit gastric ADH activity *in vitro*, e.g., aspirin[29] and $H_2$-blockers, such as cimetidine,[30,31] and result in increased blood alcohol levels[30,32]; this interaction is particularly apparent at low doses of alcohol.[13,30] Whether the effect of $H_2$-blockers on blood alcohol can be demonstrated with higher doses of alcohol has been the subject of controversy,[33] but a positive interaction has been reported by several groups.[32,34]

Women have a lower gastric ADH activity than men,[28] at least below the age of 50.[35] As a consequence, for a given intake, their blood alcohol levels are higher, an increase that is compounded by differences in body composition (women have more fat and less water) and, on the average, a lower body weight. The higher blood alcohol level, in turn, may contribute to the greater susceptibility of women to alcohol.

## 2.2.5 Rate-Limiting Factors in ADH-Mediated Alcohol Metabolism

In the process of alcohol oxidation, ADH itself may not be the major rate-limiting factor, provided at least that a normal amount of ADH is present. Under these conditions, velocities may depend on availability of the cofactor NAD and the capacity of the cell to dissociate the ADH-NADH complex and reoxidize NADH.

Although ADH activity above normal may not increase the rate of alcohol oxidation, diminution of ADH activity can reduce it, e.g., a low-protein diet has been shown to diminish hepatic ADH levels in rats[36-38] and to considerably slow the metabolism of alcohol — both in rats[37-39] and humans.[40] Bode and Thiele[41] showed that prolonged fasting markedly slows the metabolism of alcohol. In liver cells isolated from fed rats, the rate of alcohol oxidation increased to about twice that in the fasting state. Because the concentrations of malate, aspartate, and $\alpha$-glycerophosphate in liver cells from fed rats were higher than in the cells from starved rats, it seems likely that the higher rate of alcohol oxidation in the liver cells from fed rats were caused by increased activities of the hydrogen-transport cycles.

ADH activity is also affected by sex hormones, with inhibition by testosterone and stimulation by estradiol.[42] Estradiol increased the hepatic activities of ADH and catalase in both ovariectomized and sham-operated female rats on a control diet, whereas the enhancing property was virtually lost in animals on an alcohol diet. According to Lumeng and Crabb,[43] changes in alcohol elimination rates produced by fasting and castration mainly reflected changes in the $V_{max}$ of liver ADH. A decrease in the rate of degradation has been shown to be the principal cause for the increase in liver ADH following castration.[44] Similarly, stimulation of protein degradation (or possibly effects on translation) may explain why corticosterone induces rat liver ADH mRNA but not enzyme protein or activity.[45] In mice, changes in the mRNA levels after alcohol feeding could not be directly related to the changes seen in enzyme activity.[46] In general, in most species tested, alcohol feeding apparently reduces hepatic ADH enzyme activity regardless of corresponding mRNA changes.

Another key factor in the rate of alcohol metabolism is the accumulation of acetaldehyde. In hepatocytes from fed rats, the "flux control coefficient" for ADH decreased with increasing acetaldehyde concentration, suggesting that, as acetaldehyde concentrations rise, control of the pathway shifts from ADH to other enzymes, particularly aldehyde dehydrogenase.[47] Thus, there does not appear to be a single rate-determining step for the alcohol metabolism pathway via ADH.

## 2.2.6 Metabolic Changes Associated With ADH-Mediated Alcohol Oxidation

In ADH-mediated oxidation of alcohol, acetaldehyde is produced and hydrogen is transferred from alcohol to the cofactor nicotinamide adenine dinucleotide (NAD), which is converted to its reduced form (NADH) (Figure 2.1). The acetaldehyde produced again loses hydrogen and is converted to acetate, most of which is released into the bloodstream. As a net result, alcohol oxidation generates an excess of reducing equivalents in the liver, primarily as NADH. The large amounts of reducing equivalents overwhelm the ability of the hepatocyte to maintain redox homeostasis and thus a number of metabolic disorders ensue.

### 2.2.6.1    Hyperlactacidemia, Hyperuricemia, Ketonemia, and Acidosis

The enhanced NADH/NAD ratio is shown in an increased lactate/pyruvate ratio that results in hyperlactacidemia because of both decreased utilization,[48] and enhanced production of lactate by the liver. The hyperlactacidemia contributes to the acidosis and also reduces the capacity of the kidney to excrete uric acid, leading to secondary hyperuricemia.[49] Alcohol-induced ketosis[50] and enhanced purine breakdown[51] may also promote the hyperuricemia. Another possible consequence of enhanced purine degradation is increased production of activated oxygen species by xanthine oxidase, as suggested by the protective effect of allopurinol against the alcohol-induced lipid peroxidation.[52] Hyperuricemia may be related to the clinical observation that excessive consumption of alcoholic beverages commonly aggravates or precipitates gouty attacks.

### 2.2.6.2    Enhanced Lipogenesis, Depressed Lipid Oxidation, and Hypoglycemia

The increased NADH/NAD ratio raises the concentration of $\alpha$-glycerophosphate, which favors hepatic triglyceride accumulation by trapping fatty acids. In addition, excess NADH may promote fatty acid synthesis. Theoretically, enhanced lipogenesis can be considered a means for disposing of the excess hydrogen. The activity of the citric acid cycle is depressed, partly because of a slowing of the reactions of the cycle that require NAD; the mitochondria use the hydrogen equivalents originating from ethanol, rather than those derived from the oxidation of fatty acids that normally serve as the main energy source of the liver. Fatty acids of different sources can accumulate as triglycerides in the liver because of different metabolic disturbances: enhanced hepatic lipogenesis, decreased hepatic release of lipoproteins, increased mobilization of peripheral fat, enhanced hepatic uptake of circulating lipids, and, most importantly, decreased fatty acid oxidation, whether as a result of the reduced citric acid cycle activity secondary to the altered redox potential (*vide supra*) or as a consequence of permanent changes in mitochondrial structure and functions,[53] as documented by breath analysis in alcoholics.[54] In cultured hepatocytes, the increased intracellular accumulation of triacylglycerol in the presence of ethanol was quantitatively accounted for by increased fatty acid uptake, decreased fatty acid oxidation in the tricarboxylic acid cycle, and decreased lipoprotein secretion.[55]

A characteristic feature of liver injury in the alcoholic is the predominance of steatosis and other lesions in the perivenular zone, also known as centrilobular or zone 3 of the hepatic acinus. The mechanism for this zonal selectivity of the toxic effects involves several distinct but not mutually exclusive mechanisms. The hypoxia hypothesis originated from the observation that liver slices from rats fed alcohol chronically consume more oxygen than those of controls. It was then postulated that the enhanced consumption of oxygen would increase the gradient of oxygen tension along the sinusoids to the extent of producing anoxic injury of perivenular hepatocytes.[56] Indeed in human alcoholics[57] and in animals fed alcohol chronically,[58,59] decreases in either hepatic venous oxygen saturation[57] or $PO_2$[58] and in tissue oxygen tension[59] have been found during the withdrawal state. However, the changes in hepatic oxygenation found during the withdrawal state disappeared[58,60] or decreased[59] when alcohol was present in the blood. Acute ethanol administration increased splanchnic oxygen consumption in alcohol-naive baboons, but the consequences of this effect on oxygenation in the perivenular zone were offset by increased blood flow resulting in unchanged hepatic venous oxygen tension.[58] In fact, ethanol increases portal hepatic blood flow.[58,60-63] In cats[48] and in baboons[63] fed alcohol chronically, defective oxygen utilization rather than lack of blood oxygen supply characterized liver injury produced by high concentrations of ethanol. The low oxygen tension normally prevailing in perivenular zones exaggerates the redox shift produced by ethanol.[58] Hypoxia (by increasing NADH), may in turn inhibit the activity of $NAD^+$-dependent xanthine dehydrogenase (XD), thereby favoring that of oxygen-dependent xanthine oxidase (XO).[52] Purine metabolism via XO may lead to the production of oxygen radicals which can mediate toxic effects toward liver cells, including peroxidation. Physiological substrates for XO, hypoxanthine, and xanthine, as well as AMP, significantly increased in the liver after ethanol, together with an enhanced urinary output of allantoin (a final product of xanthine metabolism). Allopurinol pretreatment resulted in 90% inhibition of XO activity, and also significantly decreased ethanol-induced lipid peroxidation.[52]

Short-term alcohol intoxication occasionally causes severe hypoglycemia, which can result in sudden death. As reviewed elsewhere,[53] hypoglycemia is due to the block of hepatic gluconeo-genesis by ethanol, again as a consequence of the increased NADH/NAD ratio in subjects whose glycogen stores are already depleted by starvation or who have preexisting abnormalities in carbohydrate metabolism. Depending on the conditions, ethanol may accelerate rather than inhibit gluconeogenesis. Hyperglycemia may also occur in association with alcoholism. Although its mechanism is still obscure, glucose intolerance may be due, at least in part, to decreased peripheral glucose utilization.

### 2.2.6.3   Alcohol and Protein Metabolism

Inhibition of protein synthesis has been observed after the addition of alcohol to various preparations *in vitro*.[64,65] *In vivo*, the acute effects of alcohol on protein synthesis have been less consistent. The perivenular region of the hepatic acinus, which is already somewhat hypoxic in the normal state, may represent an area of exaggerated toxicity.[58] Indeed, this zone has a striking exaggeration of the alcohol-induced redox changes; the latter may be sufficient to impair protein synthesis.

## 2.3   MICROSOMAL ETHANOL OXIDIZING SYSTEM (MEOS)

### 2.3.1   Characterization of the MEOS and Its Role in Ethanol Metabolism

The first indication of an interaction of alcohol with the microsomal fraction of the hepatocyte was provided by the morphologic observation that in rats, alcohol feeding results in a prolifera-tion of the smooth endoplasmic reticulum (SER).[66-68] This increase in SER resembles that seen after the administration of a wide variety of hepatotoxins,[69] therapeutic agents,[70] and food additives.[71] Since most of the substances that induce a proliferation of the SER are metabolized, at least in part, by the cytochrome P-450 enzyme system that is located on the SER, the possibility that alcohol may also be metabolized by enzymes was suggested. Such a system was indeed demonstrated in liver microsomes *in vitro* and was found to be inducible by chronic alcohol feeding *in vivo*[72] and was named the microsomal ethanol oxidizing system (MEOS).[72,73] Its distinct nature was shown by (1) isolation of a P-450-containing fraction from liver microsomes which, although devoid of any ADH or catalase activity, could still oxidize ethanol as well as higher aliphatic alcohols (e.g., butanol, which is not a substrate for catalase),[74,75] and (2) reconstitution of ethanol-oxidizing activity using NADPH-cytochrome P-450 reductase, phos-pholipid, and either partially purified or highly purified microsomal P-450 from untreated[76] or phenobarbital-treated[77] rats. Ohnishi and Lieber,[76] using a liver microsomal P-450 fraction isolated from ethanol-treated rats, showed that chronic ethanol consumption results in the induction of a unique P-450. An ethanol-inducible form of P-450, purified from rabbit liver microsomes,[78] catalyzed ethanol oxidation at rates much higher than other P-450 isozymes, and also had an enhanced capacity to oxidize 1-butanol, 1-pentanol and aniline,[79] acetaminophen,[80] $CCl_4$,[79] acetone,[81,82] and N-nitrosodimethylamine (NDMA).[83] The purified human protein (now called CYP2E1 or 2E1) was obtained in a catalytically active form, with a high turnover rate for ethanol and other specific substrates.[84] MEOS has a relatively high $K_m$ for ethanol (8 to 10 m$M$ compared with 0.2 to 2 m$M$ for hepatic ADH) and thus ADH normally accounts for the bulk of ethanol oxidation at low blood ethanol concentrations (Figure 2.3A), but not necessarily at high ethanol levels (Figure 2.3B), especially during long-term use of alcohol (Figure 2.3D), in view

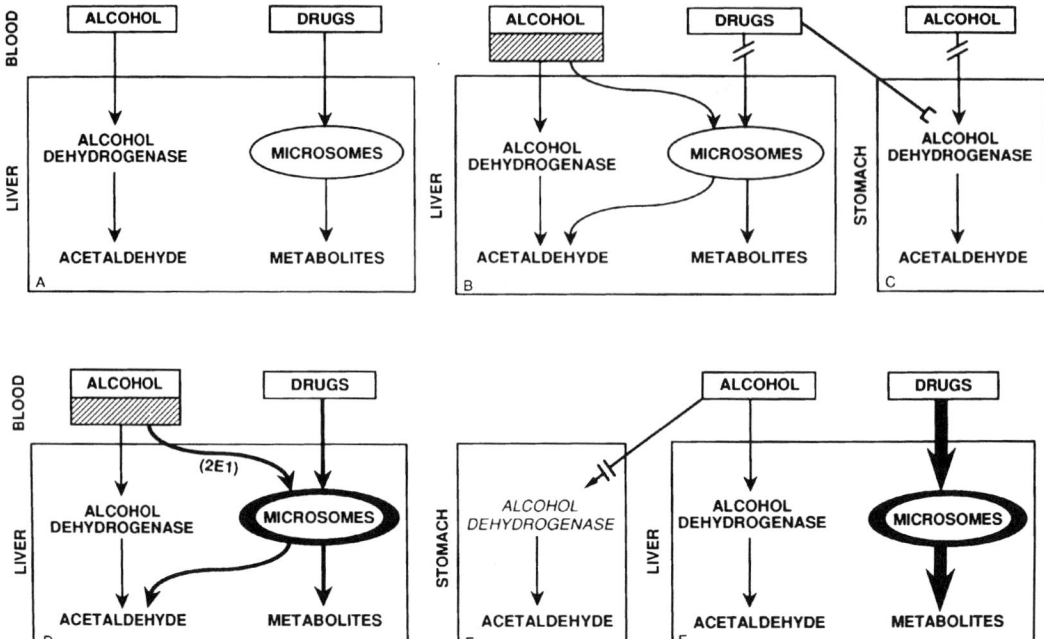

**FIGURE 2.3**   Schematic representation of ethanol-drug interactions involving the ADH pathway and microsomes. (A) Hepatic metabolism of alcohol by ADH and drugs by microsomes; (B) inhibition of hepatic microsomal drug metabolism in the presence of high concentrations of ethanol, in part through competition for a common microsomal detoxification process; (C) inhibition of gastric ethanol metabolism by drugs; (D) microsomal induction after chronic alcohol consumption and its contribution to accelerated hepatic metabolism of ethanol at high blood levels; (E) decreased gastric ADH activity and gastric ethanol metabolism after chronic alcohol abuse; (F) increased hepatic drug metabolism and xenobiotic activation because of the persisting microsomal induction after withdrawal from long-term alcohol consumption. (From Lieber, C. S., *Gastroenterology*, 106, 1085, 1994.)

of the inducibility of the MEOS.[72,73] Indeed, contrasting with hepatic ADH, which is not inducible in primates as well as most other animal species, a 5- to 10-fold induction of 2E1 was found in biopsies from recently drinking subjects using specific antibodies against this 2E1 and the western blot technique.[85] Compounds other than ethanol (e.g., acetone) can also be 2E1 inducers, but their change is not essential for the ethanol effect since 2E1 can be induced after short-term and relatively light consumption of ethanol, even in the absence of increased acetonemia or hepatic steatosis.[86]

The molecular mechanism underlying 2E1 induction remains disputed.[87] Investigations using rabbits (and some involving rats) appeared to have ruled out transcriptional activation of the 2E1 gene or stabilization of 2E1 mRNA as possible mechanisms since ethanol and similar agents (acetone, imidazole, 4-methylpyrazole, pyrazole, and pyridine) had little effect on 2E1 transcript content in liver.[88-92] A posttranslational mechanism, namely protein stabilization, was thus proposed since: (a) ethanol and imidazole were found to prevent the rapid decrease in 2E1 enzyme levels that occurs in rat hepatocytes on primary culture[93]; and (b) acetone treatment was shown to prolong the *in vivo* half-life of 2E1 in rat liver by eliminating the fast-phase component associated with the enzyme's normal degradation.[94] Yet other studies support the role of enhanced *de novo* enzyme synthesis and/or increased mRNA in the 2E1 induction process. Kim and Novak[95] observed increased rates of [14C]leucine incorporation into 2E1 protein after treating rats with pyridine, a phenomenon attributed to the enhancement, by pyridine, of 2E1 mRNA translational efficiency.[96] Kubota et al.[97] found that induction of 2E1 protein in hamsters by ethanol and pyrazole was associated with an increase in translatable 2E1 mRNA, while Diehl et al.[98]

described elevated levels of hepatic 2E1 mRNA in alcohol-treated rats. Enhanced levels of both hepatic 2E1 protein and mRNA were also found in actively drinking patients,[99] indicating that mRNA stabilization and/or transcriptional activation are involved in ethanol-mediated 2E1 induction in humans. Furthermore, by measuring both the synthesis and the degradation of radiolabeled 2E1 protein at induced high steady-state levels in the rat, ethanol stimulated rates of *de novo* 2E1 synthesis but did not affect rates of enzyme degradation.[100] It is therefore reasonable to assume that the enhancement of *de novo* 2E1 synthesis noted in ethanol-treated rats results from increased steady-state levels of 2E1 message and/or the increased efficiency with which this mRNA is translated.

The conflicting results with regard to the 2E1 induction process may stem from differences among species, the duration and/or manner of inducer treatment and/or distinct mechanisms of induction by the various compounds, since the commonly used 2E1 inducing agents other than ethanol, such as acetone, pyrazole, or pyridine, may differ in their mode of action. Obviously the most clinically relevant results are those obtained with alcohol in humans. The dose of the inducer is also important, because 2E1 induction appears to occur via two steps: (1) a posttranslational mechanism at low ethanol concentrations, and (2) an additional transcriptional mechanism at high ethanol levels.[101,102]

## 2.3.2   Interactions of Ethanol With Other Microsomal Substrates, Including Drugs

The microsomal induction resulting from chronic alcohol consumption not only accelerates the oxidation of ethanol, but also increases the metabolism of many other microsomal substrates, including the synthesis of triacylglycerols.[103] Its main interaction, however, is with other drugs such as warfarin, phenytoin, tolbutamide, propranolol, and rifampin.[53] Ethanol administration to volunteers under metabolic-ward conditions increased the rate of blood clearance of meprobamate and pentobarbital.[104] The metabolic drug tolerance persists several days to weeks after the cessation of alcohol abuse, and the duration of recovery varies with each drug.[105] During that period, the dosage of these drugs has to be raised to offset the increased breakdown.

Contrasting with the inductive effect of long-term ethanol consumption, after short-term administration, inhibition of hepatic drug metabolism is seen, primarily because of its direct competition for a common metabolic process involving cytochrome P-450[53] (Figure 2.3B). Methadone provides a cogent example of this dual interaction; whereas long-term ethanol consumption increases hepatic microsomal metabolism of methadone and decreases levels in the brain and liver. Short-term administration has the opposite effect: it inhibits microsomal demethylation of methadone and enhances brain and liver concentrations of the drug.[106] These effects may be clinically relevant, since approximately 50% of the patients taking methadone are alcohol abusers. The combination of ethanol with tranquilizers and barbiturates increases drug concentrations in the blood, sometimes to dangerously high levels, which is commonly seen in successful suicides.

## 2.3.3   Increased Xenobiotic Toxicity and Carcinogenicity in Alcoholics

Frequently, the metabolites produced in the microsomes are more toxic than the precursor compounds. Much of the medical significance of MEOS (and its ethanol-inducible 2E1) results not only from the oxidation of ethanol but also from the unusual and unique capacity of 2E1 to generate reactive oxygen intermediates, such as superoxide radicals (Figure 2.1)[107] and to activate many xenobiotic compounds to toxic metabolites. This pertains, for instance, to carbon tetrachloride and other industrial solvents such as bromobenzene[108] and vinylidene chloride,[109] as well as anesthetics such as enflurane[110] and halothane.[111] Ethanol also markedly increased the activity of microsomal low $K_m$ benzene metabolizing enzymes[112] and aggravated the hemopoietic toxicity of benzene. Enhanced metabolism (and toxicity) pertains also to a variety of prescribed drugs, including isoniazid and phenylbutazone[113] and some over-the-counter medications. Among alcoholic patients, hepatic injury associated with acetaminophen (paracetamol, N-acetyl-p-aminophenol) has been described following repetitive intake for headaches (including those associated with withdrawal symptoms), dental pain, or the pain of pancreatitis, which leads some patients to take high daily doses.[114]

An association exists between alcohol misuse and an increased incidence of upper alimentary and respiratory tract cancers.[115] Many factors have been implicated, one of which is the effect of ethanol on enzyme systems involved in the cytochrome P-450-dependent activation of carcinogens. This effect has been demonstrated with the use of microsomes derived from a variety of tissues, including the liver (the principal site of xenobiotic metabolism),[116,117] lung,[116,117] and intestines[118,119] (the chief portals of entry for tobacco smoke and dietary carcinogens, respectively), and the esophagus[120] (where ethanol consumption is a major risk factor for development of cancer). Alcoholics are commonly heavy smokers, and a synergistic effect of alcohol consumption and smoking on cancer development has been described, as reviewed elsewhere.[115] Indeed, long-term ethanol consumption was found to enhance the mutagenicity of tobacco-derived products.[115] Alcohol may also influence carcinogenesis in many other ways,[121] one of which involves vitamin A (*vide infra*).

### 2.3.4    Interactions With Retinoids and Carotenoids

Depressed hepatic levels of vitamin A were observed even when alcohol was given to subjects with diets containing large amounts of vitamin A.[122] New hepatic enzyme pathways of retinol metabolism, induced by either alcohol or drug administration, have been discovered.[123,124] Hepatic vitamin A depletion is associated with lysosomal lesions[125] and decreased detoxification of NDMA.[126] Although vitamin A deficiency might adversely affect the liver,[125] an excess of vitamin A is also known to be hepatotoxic.[127] Long-term ethanol consumption enhances this effect, resulting in striking morphologic and functional alterations of the mitochondria,[128] along with hepatic necrosis and fibrosis.[129] Hypervitaminosis A can induce fibrosis and even cirrhosis, as reviewed elsewhere.[128] Unlike retinoids, for which the case for interactive hepatotoxicity with ethanol is well established, the case for the possible interaction between β-carotene and liver disease, alcohol and/or drugs are virtually uncharted but cannot be excluded since enhanced hepatic toxicity of β-carotene in the presence of ethanol has been observed recently with the possible existence of a defect in utilization and/or excretion associated with liver injury and/or alcohol abuse.[130-132] Similarly, in men, heavy drinking was associated with a relative increase in serum β-carotene.[133] Recent epidemiologic studies have revealed that β-carotene supplementation may increase the incidence of pulmonary cancer and cardiovascular complications in smokers who were also drinkers.[134] Thus, in heavy drinkers there is a narrowed therapeutic window for vitamin A and β-carotene.

### 2.4    ROLE OF CATALASE

Catalase is capable of oxidizing alcohol *in vitro* in the presence of an $H_2O_2$-generating system[135] (Figure 2.1). However, under physiological conditions, catalase does not appear to play a major role and cannot account quantitatively for the ADH-independent pathway of alcohol metabolism. Most patients with acetalasemia are also asymptomatic.[136]

The catalase contribution might be enhanced if significant amounts of $H_2O_2$ become available through β-oxidation of fatty acids such as octanoate, palmitate, and oleate in peroxisomes.[137] However, the peroxisomal enzymes do not oxidize short chain fatty acids such as octanoate and this phenomenon was observed only in the absence of ADH activity. Otherwise the rate of alcohol metabolism is reduced by adding fatty acids,[138] and β-oxidation of fatty acids is inhibited by NADH produced from alcohol metabolism via ADH.[138] Similarly, generation of reducing equivalents from alcohol by ADH in the cytosol inhibits $H_2O_2$ generation leading to significantly diminished rates of peroxidation of alcohols via catalase.[139] Various other results have indicated that peroxisomal fatty acid oxidation does not play a major role in alcohol metabolism.[140] Furthermore, when Handler and Thurman[137] used fatty acids to stimulate alcohol oxidation, this effect was very sensitive to inhibition by aminotriazole — a catalase inhibitor. Therefore, if this mechanism plays an important role *in vivo*, one would expect a significant inhibition of alcohol metabolism after aminothiazole administration *in vivo*, when physiologic amounts of fatty acids and other substrates for $H_2O_2$ generation are present. A number of studies, however, have shown that aminotriazole treatment has little, if any, effect on alcohol oxidation *in vivo*, as reviewed by Takagi et al.[141] and Kato et al.,[142,143] who have confirmed this effect, while also verifying its inhibitory effect on catalase mediated alcohol peroxidation *in vitro*. Despite the considerable controversy that originally surrounded this issue, it is now agreed by the principal contenders involved that catalase cannot account for microsomal ethanol oxidation.[144,145] However, catalase could contribute to fatty acid oxidation. Indeed, long-term ethanol consumption is associated with increases in the content of a specific cytochrome (P-450 4A1) which promotes microsomal ω-hydroxylation of fatty acids. Products of ω-oxidation increase liver cytosolic fatty acid-binding protein (L-FABPc) content and peroxisomal β-oxidation,[146] an alternate pathway for fatty acid disposition. ω-Oxidation may compensate at least in part for the deficit in fatty acid oxidation due to the ethanol-induced injury of the mitochondria.[53]

## 2.5 NONOXIDATIVE METABOLISM

The possible pathogenic role of a nonoxidative pathway of alcohol metabolism to form fatty acid ethyl esters was suggested by Laposata and Lange.[147] The capacity of alcohol to form ethyl esters *in vivo* had been demonstrated by Goodman and Deykin[148] and also by Lange[149] who purified the enzyme.[150] Laposata and Lange[147] found that in acutely intoxicated subjects, concentrations of fatty acid ethyl esters in pancreas, liver, heart, and adipose tissue were significantly higher than in controls. Since this nonoxidative alcohol metabolism occurs in humans in the organs most commonly injured by alcohol abuse, and since some of these organs lack oxidative alcohol metabolism, Laposata and Lange[147] postulated that fatty acid ethyl esters may have a role in the production of alcohol-induced injury. Further experiments are needed to verify this interesting hypothesis.

## 2.6 EFFECTS OF LIVER DISEASE, CIRCADIAN RHYTHM, AND OTHER FACTORS ON HEPATIC ALCOHOL METABOLISM

Chronic ethanol consumption is associated with an increased rate of alcohol disappearance from the blood (Figure 2.4), primarily at high ethanol consumption. Because of the activity of the microsomal system, which has a higher $K_m$ (8 to 10 m$M$ or 37 to 46 mg/100 ml) than the bulk of hepatic ADH ($K_m$ of 0.5 to 1.0 m$M$), the rate of alcohol disappearance from the bloodstream is significantly greater at higher than at lower alcohol concentrations. This is particularly evident after chronic alcohol consumption (Figure 2.4). The observation of an acceleration of alcohol disappearance from the blood at high alcohol concentrations is particularly significant for the medicolegal application of blood alcohol measurements. Heretofore, a common procedure to determine retrospectively the blood alcohol concentrations was to linearly extrapolate from a subsequent determination with assumption of a standard rate of metabolism. In view of the nonlinear disappearance of ethanol and the adaptive increase after chronic consumption, conventional calculations should be applied with caution. In the presence of severe alcoholic liver disease this acceleration disappears, and on occasion there may be an actual reduction in blood alcohol clearance. This occurs, however, only with very severe liver disease, which is shown to be associated with reduced liver ADH.[151] In patients with cirrhosis, the rate of alcohol metabolism may be normal.[152] In addition to the activity of the alcohol-metabolizing enzymes the total hepatic mass is an important parameter which is not often measurable. Other key factors in alcohol

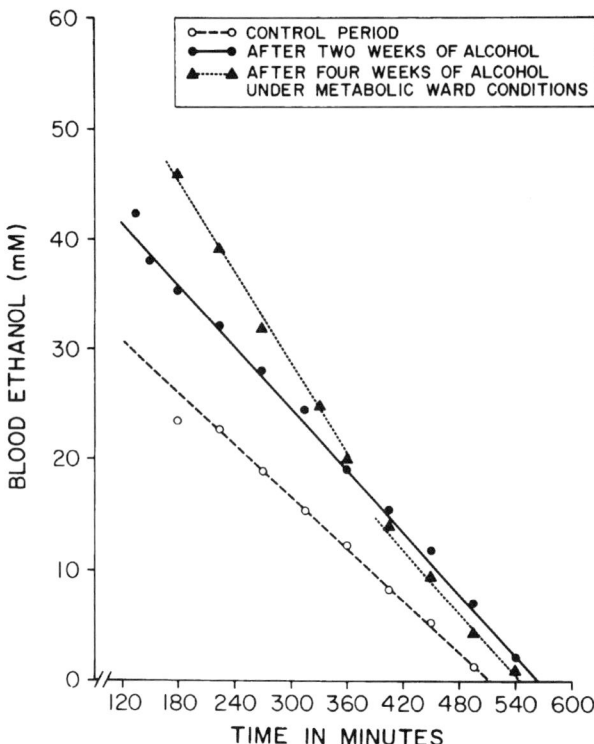

**FIGURE 2.4**   The effect of chronic alcohol consumption on the blood ethanol elimination curve in a human volunteer. The dose of alcohol administration was 1.0 g/kg in the first experiment, 1.3 g/kg after 2 weeks of alcohol, and 1.5 g/kg after 4 weeks of alcohol. (From Salaspuro, M. P. and Lieber, C. S., *Ann. Clin. Res.*, 10, 294, 1978.)

metabolism *in vivo* include availability of cofactors, and the capacity of the liver to dispose of the metabolic products (NADH and acetaldehyde). In addition to activation of MEOS, high alcohol concentrations inhibit ADH activity (substrate inhibition).[153,154]

Another factor that is difficult to assess is blood flow. Chronic alcohol consumption tends to increase hepatic blood flow in the baboon.[86] Acutely, the results depend on the dose used, some investigations showing no effect or even a decrease, whereas most studies reported an increase, as discussed elsewhere.[53] The increase in portal blood flow after alcohol administration was attributed to a preportal vasodilatory effect of adenosine formed from acetate metabolism in extrahepatic tissues.[155] In general, when unchanged or decreased flow was observed, this was associated with low blood alcohol levels. Conflicting reports on the effects of alcohol on hepatic hemodynamics may be related to the dose of alcohol administered.[156] Such experiments are difficult to control, especially since very large doses of alcohol may also produce hypothermia.[157] Hypothermia, in turn, has been found to decrease liver blood flow[158] and to slow alcohol metabolism.[159,160]

Most studies do not mention the time of day that the experiments were carried out. Such information is important, in view of the circadian variation of alcohol metabolism,[161-163] which is particularly manifested and perhaps even altered in the alcoholic.[164] Stress associated with the experimental conditions is rarely described, but it may significantly affect alcohol metabolism.[165]

## 2.7   ACETALDEHYDE: ITS METABOLISM AND TOXICITY

Acetaldehyde is produced from ethanol in both the ADH and MEOS pathways. It is highly toxic and is rapidly metabolized to acetate, mainly by a mitochondrial low $K_m$ aldehyde dehydrogenase

(ALDH), the activity of which is significantly reduced by chronic ethanol consumption.[166] The decreased capacity of mitochondria of alcohol-fed subjects to oxidize acetaldehyde, associated with unaltered or even enhanced rates of ethanol oxidation (and therefore acetaldehyde generation because of MEOS induction: *vide supra*), results in an imbalance between production and disposition of acetaldehyde. The latter causes the elevated acetaldehyde levels observed after chronic ethanol consumption in humans[27] and in baboons, which revealed a tremendous increase of acetaldehyde in hepatic venous blood,[63] reflecting high tissue levels.

Acetaldehyde's toxicity (Figure 2.2) is due, in part, to its capacity to form protein adducts, resulting in antibody production, enzyme inactivation, and decreased DNA repair.[63,167] It is also associated with a striking impairment of the capacity of the liver to utilize oxygen. Moreover, acetaldehyde promotes GSH depletion, free radical-mediated toxicity, and lipid peroxidation. The decrease in glutathione is associated with *S*-adenosylmethione depletion and can be partly corrected by *S*-adenosyl-*L*-methione replenishment.[168] In addition, acetaldehyde affects hepatic collagen synthesis: cultured lipocytes respond with increase in collagen accumulation,[169] with increased mRNA for collagen.[170] Other aldehydes (such as malonaldehyde) are produced from lipid peroxidation and they may also stimulate collagen production. Acetaldehyde stimulates collagen synthesis in cultured myofibroblasts as well[103] and a similar effect was observed with lactate. These cells were shown to proliferate in the perivenular zones of the liver after chronic alcohol consumption; they are similar to "activated" lipocytes, although they can be differentiated by ultrastructural and cytochemical characteristics.

Collagen accumulation reflects not only enhanced synthesis, but results from an imbalance between collagen degradation and collagen production. Thus, cirrhosis might, in part, represent a relative failure of collagen degradation to keep pace with synthesis. Interestingly, polyunsaturated lecithin may affect this balance. Indeed, addition of polyunsaturated lecithin to transformed lipocytes prevented the acetaldehyde-mediated increase in collagen accumulation, possibly by stimulation of collagenase activity.[171] The active ingredient was identified as dilinoleoyl-phosphatidylcholine.[172] The role of collagenase was also shown indirectly in humans by the correlation of the development of alcoholic fibrosis with increased activity of the circulating tissue inhibitor of metalloproteinase (TIMP).[173] Another beneficial effect is the partial correction of the activity of phosphatidyl-ethanolamine methyltransferase, which is depressed by alcohol.[174]

The stimulation of collagenase activity may explain, at least in part, why polyunsaturated lecithin attenuates the development of fibrosis (including cirrhosis) after chronic alcohol administration,[175] an effect confirmed using more purified lecithin extracts, which again pointed to dilinoleoyl-phosphatidylcholine as the active ingredient of the polyunsaturated lecithin.[172] In the latter studies, the control livers remained normal whereas 10 of 12 baboons fed alcohol without phosphatidylcholine developed septal fibrosis or cirrhosis, with transformation of $81 \pm 3\%$ of the hepatic lipocytes to collagen producing transitional cells. By contrast, none of the eight animals fed alcohol with phosphatidylcholine developed septal fibrosis or cirrhosis, and only $48 \pm 9\%$ of their lipocytes were transformed. Recently, the polyunsaturated lecithin, also called polyenylphosphatidylcholine, was shown to not only prevent cirrhosis but also to reduce preexisting fibrosis as demonstrated in rats treated with either carbon tetrachloride or human albumin.[176]

Acetaldehyde is converted to acetate, which is not an inert product; its various metabolic effects have been described elsewhere.[53,177]

## 2.8 INTERACTIONS OF ETHANOL CONSUMPTION WITH ENERGY BALANCE

Although ethanol is rich in energy (7.1 kcal/g), chronic consumption of substantial amounts of alcohol is not associated with the expected effect on body weight.[178] Furthermore, isocaloric substitution of carbohydrates by ethanol under metabolic ward conditions results in weight loss, and addition of ethanol to an otherwise normal diet does not produce the expected weight gain.[179] This energy deficit cannot be explained merely on the basis of maldigestion or malabsorption but has been attributed primarily to induction of MEOS (a metabolic pathway which oxidizes ethanol without associated chemical energy production; Figure 2.1). Alternate or additional mechanisms invoked include increased sympathetic tone and associated thermogenesis, and/or enhanced ATP breakdown (with increased purine catabolism) secondary to the acetate produced from ethanol (*vide supra*). Although attractive, these hypotheses do not fully explain the lack of weight loss when alcohol is consumed with a very low fat diet (5% of energy),[86] which suggests that an alteration in the energy utilization derived from fat plays a major role in the ethanol-induced energy deficit. One possible mechanism is uncoupling of oxidation with phosphorylation in mitochondria damaged by chronic ethanol consumption, in part because of the acetaldehyde generated, as reviewed elsewhere.[2] Thus, the energy wastage may be due to a cooperative effect between poor energy conservation in the induced microsomes coupled with inefficient mitochondrial oxidative phosphorylation (Figure 2.2).

## 2.9 SUMMARY

Alcohol oxidation, once thought to be a simple, one enzyme-mediated reaction, has now been shown to be a complex process affected by a variety of enzyme systems, the nutritional status, the presence of liver disease, genetic factors, and prior history of alcohol and drug use. Advances in our knowledge of hepatic metabolism of alcohol enable us to understand a number of metabolic alterations associated with the oxidation of alcohol that develop in the alcoholic. We have also gained better insight into various consequences of chronic alcoholic consumption, including the metabolic tolerance to alcohol that develops in the alcoholic. The acceleration of blood alcohol clearance after chronic alcohol consumption is highest at high alcohol blood levels, which may have some forensic importance. The acute and chronic interactions between alcohol and drug metabolism are now better understood on the basis of the existence of an inducible non-ADH pathway of alcohol metabolism, namely the microsomal ethanol oxidizing system involving a unique cytochrome P-450, namely 2E1, the induction of which not only increases acetaldehyde production, but also generates oxygen radicals and activates many xenobiotics to toxic metabolites, thereby explaining the increased vulnerability of heavy drinkers to industrial solvents, anesthetics, commonly used drugs, over-the-counter medications, and carcinogens as well as toxic interactions with vitamin A and β-carotene. Conversely, nutritional deficits may affect the toxicity of ethanol and acetaldehyde, as illustrated by the depletion in glutathione, ameliorated by *S*-adenosyl-*L*-methionine, as well as by polyunsaturated lecithin, shown to correct the alcohol-induced hepatic phosphatidylcholine depletion and to prevent alcoholic cirrhosis in nonhuman primates. Thus, elucidation of the metabolism of ethanol has provided a better understanding of the associated pathology and is now generating improved prospects for therapy.

## 2.10 ACKNOWLEDGMENTS

Original studies cited were supported, in part, by the Department of Veterans Affairs and DHHS Grants AA03508, AA07802, AA09479, AA05934, and AA07275. The author thanks Ms. R. Cabell for her skillful typing of the manuscript.

## REFERENCES

1. **Lieber, C. S. and DeCarli, L. M.,** Hepatotoxicity of ethanol, *J. Hepatol.*, 12, 392, 1991.
2. **Lieber, C. S.,** Hepatic, metabolic and toxic effects of ethanol: 1991 update, *Alcoholism: Clin. Exp. Res.*, 15, 573, 1991.
3. **Bosron, W. F., Ehrig, T., and Li, T.-K.,** Genetic factors in alcohol metabolism and alcoholism, *Semin. Liver Dis.*, 13, 126, 1993.
4. **Smith, M., Hopkins, D. A., and Harris, H.,** Developmental changes and polymorphism in human alcohol dehydrogenase, *Annu. Human Genet. (London)*, 34, 251, 1971.

5. **von Bahr-Lindstrom, H., von Hoog, J. O., Heden, L. O., Kaiser, R., Fleetwood, L., Larsson, K., Lake, M., Holmquist, B., Holmgren, A., and Hempel, J.,** cDNA and protein structure for the subunit of human liver alcohol dehydrogenase, *Biochemistry*, 25, 2465, 1986.

6. **Duester, G., Smith, M., Bilanchone, V., and Hatfield, G. W.,** Molecular analysis of the human class I alcohol dehydrogenase gene family and nucleotide sequence of the gene encoding the subunit, *J. Biol. Chem.*, 261, 2027, 1986.

7. **von Wartburg, J. P., Papenberg, J., and Aebi, H.,** An atypical human alcohol dehydrogenase, *Can. J. Biochem.*, 43, 889, 1965.

8. **Jornvall, H., Hempel, J., Vallee, B. L., Bosron, W. F., and Li, T.-K.,** Human liver alcohol dehydrogenase: amino acid substitution in the $\beta_2\beta_2$ Oriental isozymes explains functional properties, establishes an active site structure, and parallels mutational exchanges in the yeast enzyme, *Proc. Natl. Acad. Sci. U.S.A.*, 81, 3034, 1984.

9. **Bosron, W. F., Magnes, L. J., and Li, T. K.,** Human liver alcohol dehydrogenase: ADH Indianapolis results from genetic polymorphism at the ADH2 gene locus, *Biochem. Genet.*, 21, 735, 1983.

10. **von Wartburg, J. P. and Schurch, P. M.,** Atypical human liver alcohol dehydrogenase, *Ann. N.Y. Acad. Sci.*, 151, 936, 1968.

11. **Harada, S., Agarwal, D. P., and Goedde, H. W.,** Human liver alcohol dehydrogenase isoenzyme variations: improved separation methods using prolonged high voltage starch gel electrophoresis and isoelectric focusing, *Human Genet.*, 40, 215, 1978.

12. **Stamatoyannopolos, G., Chen, S., and Fukui, M.,** Liver alcohol-dehydrogenase in Japanese: high population frequency of atypical form and its possible role in alcohol sensitivity, *Am. J. Human Genet.*, 27, 789, 1975.

13. **Hernandez-Munoz, R., Caballeria, J., Baraona, E., Uppal, R., Greenstein, R., and Lieber, C. S.,** Human gastric alcohol dehydrogenase: its inhibition by $H_2$-receptor antagonists, and its effect on the bioavailability of ethanol, *Alcohol. Clin. Exp. Res.*, 14, 946, 1990.

14. **Yin, S.-J., Wang, M.-F., Liao, C.-S., Chen, C.-M., and Wu, C.-W.,** Identification of a human stomach alcohol dehydrogenase with distinctive kinetic properties, *Biochem. Int.*, 22, 829, 1990.

15. **Moreno, A. and Parés, X.,** Purification and characterization of a new alcohol dehydrogenase from human stomach, *J. Biochem.*, 266, 1128, 1991.

16. **Yokoyama, H., Baraona, E., and Lieber, C. S.,** Molecular cloning of human class IV alcohol dehydrogenase, *Biochem. Biophys. Res. Commun.*, 103, 219, 1994.

17. **Yasunami, M., Chen, C.-S., and Yoshida, A.,** A human alcohol dehydrogenase gene (ADH6) encoding an additional class of isozyme, *Proc. Natl. Acad. Sci. U.S.A.*, 88, 7610, 1991.

18. **Buehler, R., Hess, M., and von Wartburg, J. P.,** Immunohistochemical localization of human liver alcohol dehydrogenase in liver tissue, cultured fibroblasts and hela cells, *Am. J. Pathol.*, 108, 89, 1982.

19. **Maly, I. P. and Sasse, D.,** Interacinar profiles of alcohol dehydrogenase and aldehyde dehydrogenase activities in human liver, *Gastroenterology*, 101, 1716, 1991.

20. **Domschke, S., Domschke, W., and Lieber, C. S.,** Hepatic redox state: attenuation of the acute effects of ethanol induced by chronic ethanol consumption, *Life Sci.*, 15, 1327, 1974.

21. **Julkunen, R. J. K., DiPadova, C., and Lieber, C. S.,** First pass metabolism of ethanol: a gastrointestinal barrier against the systemic toxicity of ethanol, *Life Sci.*, 37, 567, 1985.

22. **Julkunen, R. J. K., Tannenbaum, L., Baraona, E., and Lieber, C. S.,** First pass metabolism of ethanol: an important determinant of blood levels after alcohol consumption, *Alcohol*, 2, 437, 1985.

23. **Baraona, E., Yokoyama, A., Ishii, H., Hernandez-Munoz, R., Takagi, T., Tsuchiya, M., and Lieber, C. S.,** Lack of alcohol dehydrogenase isoenzyme activities in the stomach of Japanese subjects, *Life Sci.*, 49, 1929, 1991.

24. **Roine, R. P., Gentry, R. T., Lim, R. T., Jr., Baraona, E., and Lieber, C. S.,** Effect of concentration of ingested ethanol on blood alcohol levels, *Alcoholism: Clin. Exp. Res.*, 15, 734, 1991.

25. **Smith, T., DeMaster, E. G., Furne, J. K., Springfield, J., and Levitt, M. D.,** First-pass gastric mucosal metabolism of ethanol is negligible in the rat, *J. Clin. Invest.*, 89, 1801, 1992.

26. **Caballeria, J., Frezza, M., Hernandez-Munoz, R., DiPadova, C., Korsten, M. A., Baraona, E., and Lieber, C.S.,** The gastric origin of the first pass metabolism of ethanol in man: effect of gastrectomy, *Gastroenterology* 97, 1205, 1989.

27. **Di Padova, C., Worner, T. M., Julkunen, R. J. K., and Lieber, C. S.,** Effects of fasting and chronic alcohol consumption on the first pass metabolism of ethanol, *Gastroenterology*, 92, 1169, 1987.

28. **Frezza, M., Di Padova, C., Pozzato, G., Terpin, M., Baraona, M., and Lieber, C. S.,** High blood alcohol levels in women: role of decreased gastric alcohol dehydrogenase activity and first pass metabolism, *N. Engl. J. Med.*, 322, 95, 1990.

29. **Roine, R., Gentry, R. T., Hernández-Muñoz, R., Baraona, E., and Lieber, C. S.,** Aspirin increases blood alcohol concentrations in human after ingestion of ethanol, *JAMA*, 264, 2406, 1990.

30. **Caballeria, J., Baraona, E., Rodamilans, M., and Lieber, C. S.,** Effects of cimetidine on gastric alcohol dehydrogenase activity and blood ethanol levels, *Gastroenterology*, 96, 388, 1989.

31. **Caballeria, J., Baraona, E., Deulofeu, R., Hernandez-Munoz, R., Rodes, J., and Lieber, C. S.,** Effects of $H_2$ receptor antagonists on gastric alcohol dehydrogenase activity, *Dig. Dis. Sci.*, 36, 1673, 1991.

32. **Di Padova, C., Roine, R., Frezza, M., Gentry, R. T., Baraona, E., and Lieber, C. S.,** Effects of ranitidine on blood alcohol levels after ethanol ingestion: comparison with other $H_2$-receptor antagonists, *JAMA*, 267, 83, 1992.

33. **Roine, R. P., Hernandez-Munoz, R., Gentry, R. T., Baraona, E., and Lieber, C. S.,** $H_2$ antagonists and blood alcohol levels, *Dig. Dis. Sci.,* 37, 891, 1992.

34. **Seitz, H. K., Veith, S., Czygan, P., Bosche, J., Simon, B., Gugler, R., and Kommerell, B.,** *In vivo* interactions between $H_2$-receptor antagonists and ethanol metabolism in man and in rats, *Hepatology*, 4, 1231, 1984.

35. **Seitz, H. K., Egerer, G., Simanowski, U.A., Waldherr, R., Eckey, R., Agarwal, D. P., Goedde, H. W., and von Wartburg, J. P.,** Human gastric alcohol dehydrogenase activity: effect of age, gender and alcoholism, *Gut*, 34, 1433, 1993.

36. **Horn, R. S. and Manthei, R. W.,** Ethanol metabolism in chronic protein deficiency, *J. Pharmacol. Exp. Ther.*, 147, 385, 1965.

37. **Bode, Ch., Goebell H., and Stähler, M.,** Änderungen der Alkoholdehydrogenase-Aktivität in der Rattenleber durch Eiweissmangel und Äthenol, *Z. Gesamte Inn. Med.*, 151, 111, 1970.

38. **Wilson, J. S., Korsten, M. A., and Lieber, C. S.,** The combined effects of protein deficiency and chronic ethanol administration on rat ethanol metabolism, *Hepatology*, 6, 823, 1986.

39. **Pekkanen, L., Eriksson, K., and Silivonen, M. L.,** Dietarily-induced changes in voluntary ethanol consumption and ethanol metabolism in the rat, *Br. J. Nutr.*, 40, 103, 1978.

40. **Bode, Ch., Buchwald, B., and Goebell, H.,** Inhibition of ethanol breakdown due to protein deficiency in man, *Ger. Med Mon.*, 1, 149, 1971.

41. **Bode, J. C. and Thiele, D.,** Hemmung des Äthanolabbaus beim Menschen durch Fasten: Reversibilitat durch Fructose-Infusion, *Dtsch. Med. Wochenschr.*, 100, 1849, 1975.

42. **Rachmamin, G., MacDonald, J. A., Wahid, S., Clapp, J. J., Khanna, J. M., and Israel, Y.,** Modulation of alcohol dehydrogenase and ethanol metabolism by sex hormones in the spontaneously hypertensive rat. Effect of chronic ethanol administration, *Biochem. J.*, 186, 483, 1980.

43. **Lumeng, L. and Crabb, D. W.,** Rate determining factors for ethanol metabolism in fasted and castrated male rats, *Biochem. Pharmacol.*, 33, 2623, 1984.

44. **Mezey, E. and Potter, J. J.,** Effect of castration on the turnover of rat liver alcohol dehydrogenase, *Biochem. Pharmacol.*, 34, 369, 1985.

45. **Qulali, M. and Crabb, D. W.,** Corticosterone induces rat liver alcohol dehydrogenase mRNA but not enzyme protein or activity, *Alcoholism: Clin. Exp. Res.*, 16, 427, 1992.

46. **Bond, S. L. and Singh, S. M.,** Studies with cDNA probes on the *in vivo* effect of ethanol on expression of the genes of alcohol metabolism, *Alcohol Alcohol.*, 25, 385, 1990.

47. **Page, R. A., Kitson, K. E., and Hardman, M. J.,** The importance of alcohol dehydrogenase in regulation of ethanol metabolism in rat liver cells, *Biochem. J.*, 278, 659, 1991.

48. **Greenway, C. V. and Lautt, W. W.,** Acute and chronic ethanol on hepatic oxygen ethanol and lactate metabolism in cats, *Am. J. Physiol.*, 258, G411, 1990.

49. **Lieber, C. S., Jones, D. P., Losowsky, M. S., and Davidson, C. S.,** Interrelation of uric acid and ethanol metabolism in man, *J. Clin. Invest.*, 41, 1863, 1962.

50. **Lefevre, A., Adler, H., and Lieber, C. S.,** Effect of ethanol on ketone metabolism, *J. Clin. Invest.*, 49, 1775, 1970.

51. **Faller, J. and Fox, I. H.,** Evidence for increased urate production by activation of adenine nucleotide turnover, *N. Engl. J. Med.*, 307, 1598, 1982.

52. **Kato, S., Kawase, T., Alderman, J., Inatomi, N., and Lieber, C. S.,** Role of xanthine oxidase in ethanol-induced lipid peroxidation in rats, *Gastroenterology*, 98, 203, 1990.

53. **Lieber, C. S.,** *Medical and Nutritional Complications of Alcoholism: Mechanisms and Management*, New York, Plenum Press, 1992, 579.

54. **Lauterburg, B. H., Liang, D., Schwarzenbach, F. A., and Breen, K. J.,** Mitochondrial dysfunction in alcoholic patients as assessed by breath analysis, *Hepatology*, 17, 418, 1993.

55. **Grunnet, N., Kondrup, J., and Dich, J.,** Effect of ethanol on lipid metabolism in cultured hepatocytes, *Biochem. J.*, 228, 673, 1985.

56. **Israel, Y., Kalant, H., Orrego, H., Khanna, J. M., Videla, I., and Phillips, J. M.,** Experimental alcohol-induced hepatic necrosis: suppression by propylthiouracil, *Proc. Natl. Acad. Sci. U.S.A.*, 72, 1137, 1975.

57. **Kessler, B. J., Lieber, J. B., Bronfin, G. J., and Sass, M.,** The hepatic blood flow and splanchnic oxygen consumption in alcohol fatty liver, *J. Clin. Invest.*, 33, 1338, 1954.

58. **Jauhonen, P., Baraona, E., Miyakawa, H., and Lieber, C. S.,** Mechanism for selective perivenular hepatotoxicity of ethanol, *Alcoholism: Clin. Exp. Res.*, 6, 350, 1982.

59. **Sato, N., Kamada, T., Kawano, S., Hayashin, N., Kishida, Y., Meren, H., Yoshihara, H., and Abe, H.,** Effect of acute and chronic ethanol consumption on hepatic tissue oxygen tension in rats, *Pharmacol. Biochem. Behav.*, 18, 443, 1983.

60. **Shaw, S., Heller, E. A., Friedman, H. S., Baraona, E., and Lieber, C. S.,** Increased hepatic oxygenation following ethanol administration in baboon, *Proc. Soc. Exp. Biol. Med.*, 156, 509, 1977.

61. **Stein, S. W., Lieber, C. S., Cherrick, G. R., Leevy, C. M., and Ablemann, W. H.,** The effect of ethanol upon systemic hepatic blood flow in man, *Am. J. Clin. Nutr.*, 13, 68, 1973.

62. **Carmichael, F. J., Saldivia, V., Israel, Y., McKaigney, J. P., and Orrego, H.,** Ethanol-induced increase in portal hepatic blood flow: interference by anesthetic agents, *Hepatology*, 97, 89, 1987.

63. **Lieber, C. S., Baraona, E., Hernandez-Munoz, R., Kubota, S., Sato, N., Kawano, S., Matsumura, T., and Inatomi, N.,** Impaired oxygen utilization: a new mechanism for the hepatotoxicity of ethanol in sub-human primates, *J. Clin. Invest.*, 83, 1682, 1989.

64. **Rothschild, M. A., Oratz, M., Mongelli, J., and Schreiber, S. S.,** Alcohol induced depression of albumin synthesis: reversal by tryptophan, *J. Clin. Invest.*, 50, 1812, 1971.

65. **Jeejeeboy, K. N., Bruce-Robertson, A., Ho, J., and Sodtke, U.,** The effect of ethanol on albumin and fibrinogen synthesis *in vivo* and in hepatocyte suspension, in *Alcohol and Abnormal Protein Synthesis*, Rothschild M. A., Oratz, M., and Schreiber, S. S., Eds., Pergamon Press, New York, 1975, 373.

66. **Iseri, O. A., Gottlieb, L. S., and Lieber, C. S.,** The ultrastructure of ethanol-induced fatty liver, *Fed. Proc.*, 23, 579, 1964.

67. **Iseri, O. A., Lieber, C. S., and Gottlieb, L. S.,** The ultrastructure of fatty liver induced by prolonged ethanol ingestion, *Am. J. Pathol.*, 48, 535, 1966.

68. **Lane, B. P. and Lieber, C. S.,** Ultrastructural alterations in human hepatocytes following ingestion of ethanol with adequate diets, *Am. J. Pathol.*, 49, 593, 1966.

69. **Meldolesi, J.,** On the significance of the hypertrophy of the smooth endoplasmic reticulum in liver cells after administration of drugs, *Biochem. Pharmcol.*, 16, 125, 1967.

70. **Conney, A. H.,** Pharmacological implications of microsomal enzyme induction, *Pharmacol. Rev.*, 19, 317, 1967.

71. **Lane, B. P. and Lieber, C. S.,** Effects of butylated hydroxytoluene on the ultrastructure of rat hepatocytes, *Lab. Invest.*, 16, 341, 1967.

72. **Lieber, C. S. and DeCarli, L. M.,** Ethanol oxidation by hepatic microsomes: adaptive increase after ethanol feeding, *Science*, 162, 917, 1968.

73. **Lieber, C. S. and DeCarli, L. M.,** Hepatic microsomal ethanol oxidizing system: *in vitro* characteristics and adaptive properties *in vivo*, *J. Biol. Chem.*, 245, 2505, 1970.

74. **Teschke, R., Hasumura, Y., Joly, J. G., Ishii, H., and Lieber, C. S.,** Microsomal ethanol-oxidizing system (MEOS): purification and properties of a rat liver system free of catalase and alcohol dehydrogenase, *Biochem. Biophys. Res. Commun.*, 49, 1187, 1972.

75. **Teschke, R., Hasumura, Y., and Lieber, C. S.,** Hepatic microsomal alcohol oxidizing system solubilization, isolation and characterization, *Arch. Biochem. Biophys.*, 163, 404, 1974.

76. **Ohnishi, K. and Lieber, C. S.,** Reconstitution of the microsomal ethanol-oxidizing system: qualitative and quantitative changes of cytochrome P-450 after chronic ethanol consumption, *J. Biol. Chem.*, 252, 7124, 1977.

77. **Miwa, G. T., Levin, W., Thomas, P. E., and Lu, A. Y. H.,** The direct oxidation of ethanol by catalase- and alcohol dehydrogenase-free reconstituted system containing cytochrome P-450, *Arch. Biochem. Biophys.*, 187, 464, 1978.

78. **Koop, D. R., Morgan, E. T., Tarr, G. E., and Coon, M. J.,** Purification and characterization of a unique isozyme of cytochrome P-450 from liver microsomes of ethanol-treated rabbits, *J. Biol. Chem.*, 257, 8472, 1982.

79. **Morgan, E. T., Koop, D. R., and Coon, M. J.,** Catalytic activity of cytochrome P-450 isozyme 3a isolated from liver microsomes of ethanol-treated rabbits, *J. Biol. Chem.*, 257, 13951, 1982.

80. **Morgan, E. T., Koop, D. R., and Coon, M. J.,** Comparison of six rabbit liver cytochrome P-450 isozymes in formation of a reactive metabolite of acetaminophen, *Biochem. Biophys. Res. Commun.*, 112, 8, 1983.

81. **Ingelman-Sundberg, M. and Johansson, I.,** Mechanisms of hydroxyl radical formation and ethanol oxidation by ethanol-inducible and other forms of rabbit liver microsomal cytochromes P-450, *J. Biol. Chem.*, 259, 6447, 1984.

82. **Koop, D. R. and Casazza, J. P.,** Identification of ethanol-inducible P-450 isozyme 3a as the acetone and acetol monooxygenase of rabbit microsomes, *J. Biol. Chem.*, 260, 13607, 1985.

83. **Yang, C. S., Tu, Y. Y., Koop, D. R., and Coon, M. J.,** Metabolism of nitrosamines by purified rabbit liver cytochrome P-450 isozymes, *Cancer Res.*, 45, 1140, 1985.

84. **Lasker, J. M., Raucy, J., Kubota, S., Bloswick, B. P., Black, M., and Lieber, C. S.,** Purification and characterization of human liver cytochrome P-450-ALC, *Biochem. Biophys. Res. Commun.*, 148, 232, 1987.

85. **Tsutsumi, M., Lasker, J. M., Shimizu, M., Rosman, A. S., and Lieber, C. S.,** The intralobular distribution of ethanol-inducible P450IIE1 in rat and human liver, *Hepatology*, 10, 437, 1989.

86. **Lieber, C. S., Lasker, J. M., DeCarli, L. M., Saeli, J., and Wojtowicz, T.,** Role of acetone, dietary fat, and total energy intake in the induction of the hepatic microsomal ethanol oxidizing system, *J. Pharmacol. Exp. Ther.*, 247, 791, 1988.

87. **Koop, D, R. and Tierney, D. J.,** Multiple mechanism in the regulation of ethanol-inducible cytochrome P450IIE1, *Bioessays*, 12, 429, 1990.

88. **Song, B. J., Gelboin, H. V., Park, S.-S., Yang, C. S., and Gonzalez, F. J.,** Complementary DNA and protein sequences of ethanol-inducible rat and human cytochrome P-450s: transcriptional and post-transcriptional regulation of the rat enzyme, *J. Biol. Chem.*, 261, 16689, 1986.

89. **Song, B. J., Matsunaga, T., Hardwick, J., Park, S. S., Veech, R. I., Yang, C. S., Gelboin, H. V., and Gonzalez, F. J.,** Stabilization of cytochrome P450j messenger ribonucleic acid in the diabetic rat, *Mol. Endocrinol.*, 1, 542, 1987.

90. **Khani, S. C., Zaphiropoulos, P. G., Fujita, V. S., Porter, T. D., Koop, D. R., and Coon, M. J.,** cDNA and derived amino acid sequence of ethanol-inducible rabbit liver cytochrome P-450 isozyme 3a (P450ALC), *Proc. Natl. Acad. Sci. U.S.A.*, 84, 638, 1987.

91. **Johansson, I. J., Ekstrom, G., Scholte, B., Puzycki, D., Jornvall, H., and Ingleman-Sundberg, M.,** Ethanol-, fasting, and acetone-inducible cytochromes P-450 in rat liver: regulation and characteristics of enzymes belonging to the IIB and IIE gene subfamilies, *Biochemistry*, 27, 1925, 1988.

92. **Porter, T. D., Khani, S. C., and Coon, M. J.,** Induction and tissue-specific expression of rabbit cytochrome P450IIE1 and IIE2 genes, *Mol. Pharmacol.*, 36, 61, 1989.

93. **Eliasson, E., Johansson, I., and Ingelman-Sundberg, M.,** Ligand-dependent maintenance of ethanol-inducible cytochrome P-450 in primary rat hepatocyte cell cultures, *Biochem. Biophys. Res. Commun.*, 150, 436, 1988.

94. **Song, B. J., Veech, R. I., Park, S. S., Gelboin, H. V., and Gonzalez, F. J.,** Induction of rat hepatic N-nitrosodimethylamine demethylase by acetone is due to protein stabilization, *J. Biol. Chem.*, 264, 3568, 1989.

95. **Kim, S. G. and Novak, R. F.,** Induction of rat hepatic P450IIE1 (CYP 2E1) by pyridine: evidence for a role of protein synthesis in the absence of transcriptional activation, *Biochem. Biophys. Res. Commun.*, 166, 1072, 1990.

96. **Kim, S. G., Shehin, S. E., States, J. C., and Novak, R. F.,** Evidence for increased translational efficiency in the induction of P450IIE1 by solvents: analysis of P450IIE1 mRNA polyribosomal distribution, *Biochem. Biophys. Res. Commun.*, 172, 767, 1990.

97. **Kubota, S., Lasker, J. M., and Lieber, C. S.,** Molecular regulation of ethanol inducible cytochrome P450-IIE1 in hamsters, *Biochem. Biophys. Res. Commun.*, 150, 304, 1988.

98. **Diehl, A. M., Bisgaard, H. C., Kren, B. T., and Steer, C. J.,** Ethanol interferes with regeneration-associated changes in biotransforming enzymes: a potential mechanism underlying ethanol's carcinogenicity?, *Hepatology*, 13, 722, 1991.

99. **Takahashi, T., Lasker, J. M., Rosman, A. S., and Lieber, C. S.,** Induction of P4502E1 in human liver by ethanol is due to a corresponding increase in encoding mRNA, *Hepatology*, 17, 236, 1993.

100. **Tsutsumi, M., Lasker, J. M., Takahashi, T., and Lieber, C. S.,** *In vivo* induction of hepatic P4502E1 by ethanol: role of increased enzyme synthesis, *Arch. Biochem. Biophys.*, 304, 209, 1993.

101. **Ronis, M. J., Huang, J., Crouch, J., Mercado, C., Irby, D., Valentine, C. R., Lumpkin, C. K., Ingelman-Sundberg, M., and Badger, T. M.,** Cytochrome P450 CYP 2E1 induction during chronic alcohol exposure occurs by a two-step mechanism associated with blood alcohol concentration in rats, *J. Pharmacol. Exp. Ther.*, 264, 944, 1993.

102. **Badger, T. M., Huang, J., Ronis, M., and Lumpkin, C. K.,** Induction of cytochrome P450 2E1 during chronic ethanol exposure occurs via transcription of the CYP 2E1 gene when blood alcohol concentrations are high, *Biochem. Res. Commun.*, 190, 780, 1993.

103. **Savolainen, E.-R., Leo, M. A., Timple, R., and Lieber, C. S.,** Acetaldehyde and lactate stimulate collagen synthesis of cultured baboon liver myofibroblasts, *Gastroenterology*, 87, 777, 1984.

104. **Misra, P. S., Lefèvre, A., Ishii, H., Rubin, E., and Lieber, C. S.,** Increase of ethanol meprobamate and pentobarbital metabolism after chronic ethanol administration in man and in rats, *Am. J. Med.*, 51, 346, 1971.

105. **Hetu, C. and Joly, J.-G.,** Differences in the duration of the enhancement of liver mixed-function oxidase activities in ethanol-fed rats after withdrawal, *Biochem. Pharmacol.*, 34, 1211, 1985.

106. **Borowsky, S. A. and Lieber, C. S.,** Interaction of methadone and ethanol metabolism, *J. Pharmacol. Exp. Ther.*, 207, 123, 1978.

107. **Dai, Y., Rashba-Step, J., and Cederbaum, A. I.,** Stable expression of human cytochrome P4502E1 in HepG2 cells: characterization of catalytic activities and production of reactive oxygen intermediates, *Biochemistry*, 32, 6928, 1993.

108. **Hetu, C., Dumont, A., and Joly, J.-G.,** Effect of chronic ethanol administration on bromobenzene liver toxicity in the rat, *Toxic Appl. Pharmacol.*, 67, 166, 1983.

109. **Siegers, C. P., Heidbuchel, K., and Younes, M.,** Influence of alcohol, dithiocard and (+)-catechin on the hepatotoxicity and metabolism of vinylidene chloride in rats, *J. Appl. Toxicol.*, 3, 90, 1983.

110. **Tsutsumi, R., Leo, M. A., Kim, C., Tsutsumi, M., Lasker, J. M., Lowe, N., and Lieber, C. S.,** Interaction of ethanol with enflurane metabolism and toxicity: role of P450IIE1, *Alcohol. Clin. Exp. Res.*, 14, 174, 1990.

111. **Takagi, T., Ishii, H., Takahashi, H., Kato, S., Okuno, F., Ebihara, Y., Yamauchi, H., Nagata, Y., Tashiro, M., and Tsuchiya, M.,** Potentiation of halothane hepatotoxicity by chronic ethanol administration in rat: an animal model of halothane hepatitis, *Pharmacol. Biochem. Behav.*, 18(Suppl 1), 461, 1983.

112. **Nakajima, T., Okino, T., and Sato, A.,** Kinetic studies on benzene metabolism in rat liver — possible presence of three forms of benzene metabolizing enzymes in the liver, *Biochem. Pharmacol.*, 36, 2799, 1987.

113. **Beskid, M., Bialck, J., Dzieniszewski, J., Sadowski, J., and Tlalka, J.,** Effect of combined phenylbutazone and ethanol administration on rat liver, *Exp. Pathol.*, 18, 487, 1980.

114. **Seef, L. B., Cuccherini, B. A., Zimmerman, H. J., Alder, E., and Benjamin, S. B.,** Acetaminophen hepatotoxicity in alcoholics (clinical review), *Ann. Intern. Med.*, 104, 399, 1986.

115. **Lieber, C. S., Garro, A., Leo, M. A., Mak, K. M., and Worner, T. M.,** Alcohol and cancer, *Hepatology*, 6, 1005, 1986.

116. **Garro, A. J., Seitz, H. K., and Lieber, C. S.,** Enhancement of dimethylnitrosamine metabolism and activation to a mutagen following chronic ethanol consumption, *Cancer Res.*, 41, 120, 1981.

117. **Seitz, H. K., Garro, A. J., and Lieber, C. S.,** Enhanced pulmonary and intestinal activation of procarcinogens and mutagens after chronic ethanol consumption in the rat, *Eur. J. Clin. Invest.*, 11, 33, 1981.

118. **Seitz, H. K., Czygan, P., Waldherr, K., Veith, S., and Kommerell, B.,** Ethanol and intestinal carcinogenesis in the rat, *Alcohol*, 2, 491, 1985.

119. **Shimizu, M., Lasker, J. M., Tsutsumi, M., and Lieber, C. S.,** Immunohistochemical localization of ethanol-inducible P450IIE1 in the rat alimentary tract, *Gastroenterology*, 99, 1044, 1990.

120. **Farinati, F., Zhou, Z., Bellah, J., Lieber, C. S., and Garro, A. J.,** Effect of chronic ethanol consumption on activation of nitrosopyrrolidine to a mutagen by rat upper alimentary tract, lung and hepatic tissue, *Drug Metab. Dispos.*, 13, 210, 1985.

121. **Garro, A. J. and Lieber, C. S.,** Alcohol and cancer, *Annu. Rev. Pharmacol. Toxicol.*, 30, 219, 1990.

122. **Sato, M. and Lieber, C. S.,** Hepatic vitamin A depletion after chronic ethanol consumption in baboons and rats, *J. Nutr.*, 111, 2015, 1981.

123. **Leo, M. A. and Lieber, C. S.,** New pathway for retinol metabolism in liver microsomes, *J. Biochem.*, 260, 5228, 1985.

124. **Leo, M. A., Kim, C. I., and Lieber, C. S.,** NAD$^+$-dependent retinol dehydrogenase in liver microsomes, *Arch. Biochem. Biophys.*, 259, 241, 1987.

125. **Leo, M. A., Sato, M., and Lieber, C. S.,** Effect of hepatic vitamin A depletion on the liver in men and rats, *Gastroenterology*, 84, 562, 1983.

126. **Leo, M. A., Lowe, N., and Lieber, C. S.,** Interaction of drugs and retinol, *Biochem. Pharmacol.*, 35, 3949, 1986.

127. **Leo, M. A. and Lieber, C. S.,** Hypervitaminosis A: a liver lover's lament, *Hepatology*, 8, 412, 1988.

128. **Leo, M. A., Arai, M., Sato, M., and Lieber, C. S.,** Hepatotoxicity of vitamin A and ethanol in the rat, *Gastroenterology*, 82, 194, 1982.

129. **Leo, M. A. and Lieber, C. S.,** Hepatic fibrosis after long term administration of ethanol and moderate vitamin A supplementation in the rat, *Hepatology*, 2, 1, 1983.

130. **Leo, M. A., Kim, C. I., Lowe, N., and Lieber, C. S.,** Interaction of ethanol with β-carotene: Delayed blood clearance and enhanced hepatotoxicity, *Hepatology*, 15, 883, 1992.

131. **Leo, M. A., Rosman, A., and Lieber, C. S.,** Differential depletion of carotenoids and tocopherol in liver diseases, *Hepatology*, 17, 977, 1993.

132. **Leo, M. A., Aleynik, S., Aleynik, M., and Lieber, C. S.,** Hepatotoxicity of alcohol is potentiated by β-carotene beadlets, *Gastroenterology*, 108, A1109, 1995.

133. **Ahmed, S., Leo, M. A., and Lieber, C. S.,** Interactions between alcohol and β-carotene in patients with alcoholic liver disease, *Am. J. Clin. Nutr.*, 60, 430, 1994.

134. Alpha-Tocopherol, β-carotene and Cancer Prevention Study Group, *N. Engl. J. Med.*, 330, 1029, 1994.

135. **Keilin, D. and Hartree, E. F.,** Properties of catalase: catalysis of coupled oxidation of alcohols, *Biochem. J.*, 39, 293, 1945.

136. **Moser, H. W. and Moser, A. B.,** Long chain fatty acids and peroxisomal disorders, in *Polyunsaturated Fatty Acids in Human Nutrition*, Bracco, U. and Deckelbaum, R. J., Eds., Nestec Ltd., Vevey/Raven Press, New York, 1992, 65–79.

137. **Handler, J. A. and Thurman, R. G.,** Fatty acid-dependent ethanol metabolism, *Biochem. Biophys. Res. Commun.*, 133, 44, 1985.

138. **Williamson, J. R., Scholz, R., Browning, E. T., Thurman, R. G., and Fukami, M. H.,** Metabolic effects of ethanol in perfused rat liver, *J. Biol. Chem.*, 25, 5044, 1969.

139. **Handler, J. A. and Thuamn, R. G.,** Redox interactions between catalase and alcohol dehydrogenase pathways of ethanol metabolism in the perfused rat liver, *J. Biol. Chem.*, 265, 1510, 1990.

140. **Inatomi, N., Kato, S., Ito, D., and Lieber, C. S.,** Role of peroxisomal fatty acid beta-oxidation in ethanol metabolism, *Biochem. Biophys. Res. Commun.*, 163, 418, 1989.

141. **Takagi, T., Alderman, J., Geller, J., and Lieber, C. S.,** Assessment of the role of non-ADH ethanol oxidation *in vivo* and in hepatocytes from deermice, *Biochem. Pharmacol.*, 35, 3601, 1986.

142. **Kato, S., Alderman, J., and Lieber, C. S.,** Ethanol metabolism in alcohol dehydrogenase deficient deermice is mediated by the microsomal ethanol oxidizing system, not by catalase, *Alcohol Alcohol.*, (Suppl)1, 231, 1987.

143. **Kato, S., Alderman, J., and Lieber, C. S.,** Respective roles of the microsomal ethanol oxidizing system (MEOS) and catalase in ethanol metabolism by deer mice lacking alcohol dehydrogenase, *Arch. Biochem. Biophys.*, 254, 586, 1987.

144. **Thurman, R. G. and Brentzel, H. J.,** The role of alcohol dehydrogenase in microsomal ethanol oxidation and the adaptive increase in ethanol metabolism due to chronic treatment with ethanol, *Alcoholism: Clin. Exp. Res.*, 1, 33, 1977.

145. **Teschke, R., Matsuzaki, S., Ohnishi, K., DeCarli, L. M., and Lieber, C. S.,** Microsomal ethanol oxidizing system (MEOS): current status of its characterization and its role, *Alcoholism: Clin. Exp. Res.*, 1, 7, 1977.

146. **Kaikaus, R. M., Chan, W. K., Lysenko, N., Ortiz, P., Montellano, D., and Bass, N. M.,** Induction of liver fatty acid binding protein (l-FABP) and peroxisomal fatty acid β-oxidation by peroxisome proliferators (PP) is dependent on cytochrome p-450 activity, *Hepatology*, 12, A248, 1990.

147. **Laposata, E. A. and Lange, L. G.,** Presence of nonoxidative ethanol metabolism in human organs commonly damaged by ethanol abuse, *Science*, 231, 497, 1986.

148. **Goodman, D. W. and Deykin, D.,** Fatty acid ethyl ester formation during ethanol metabolism *in vivo*, *Proc. Soc. Exp. Biol.*, 113, 65, 1963.

149. **Lange, L. G.,** Nonoxidative ethanol metabolism: formation of fatty acid ethyl esters by cholesterol esterase, *Proc. Natl. Acad. Sci. U.S.A.*, 79, 3954, 1982.

150. **Mogelson, S. and Lange, L. G.,** Nonoxidative ethanol metabolism in rabbit myocardium: purification to homogeneity of fatty acyl ethyl ester synthase, *Biochemistry*, 23, 4075, 1984.

151. **Dow, J., Krasner, N., and Goldberg, A.,** Relation between hepatic alcohol dehydrogenase activity and the ascorbic acid in leucocytes of patients with liver disease, *Clin. Sci. Mol. Med.*, 49, 603, 1975.

152. **Dacruz, A. G., Correia, J. P., and Menezes, L.,** Ethanol metabolism in liver cirrhosis and chronic alcoholism, *Acta Hepato-Gastroenterol.*, 22, 369, 1975.

153. **Theorell, H., Nygaard, A. P., and Bonnichsen, R.,** Studies on liver alcohol dehydrogenase. III. The influence of pH and some anions on the reaction velocity constants, *Acta Chem. Scand.*, 9, 1148, 1955.

154. **von Wartburg, J. P., Bethune, J. L., and Vallee, B. L.,** Human liver-alcohol dehydrogenase. Kinetic and physiochemical properties, *Biochemistry*, 3, 1175, 1964.

155. **Carmichael, F. J., Saldivida, V., Varghese, G. A., Israel, Y., and Orrego, H.,** Ethanol-induced increase in portal blood flow: role of acetate and $A_1$- and $A_2$-adenosine receptors, *Am. J. Physiol.*, 255, G417, 1988.

156. **Jenkins, S. A., Baxter, J. N., Devitt, P., Taylor, I., and Shields, R.,** Effects of alcohol on hepatic haemodynamics in the rat, *Digestion*, 34, 236, 1986.

157. **Nikki, P., Vapaatalo, H., and Karppanen, H.,** Effect of ethanol on body temperature, postanaesthetic shivering and tissue monoamines in halothane-anesthetized rats, *Ann. Med. Exp. Biol. Fenn.*, 49, 157, 1971.

158. **Brauer, R. W., Holloway, R. J., Krebs, J. S., Leong, G. F., and Carrol, H. W.,** The liver in hypothermia, *Ann. N.Y. Acad. Sci.*, 80, 395, 1958.

159. **Larsen, J. A.,** The effect of cooling on liver function in cats, *Acta Physiol. Scand.*, 81, 197, 1971.

160. **Krarup, N. and Larsen, J. A.,** The effect of slight hypothermia on liver function as measured by the elimination rate of ethanol, the hepatic uptake and excretion of indocyanine green and bile formation, *Acta Physiol. Scand.*, 84, 396, 1972.

161. **Wilson, R. H. L., Newman, E. J., and Newman, H. W.,** Diurnal variation in rate of alcohol metabolism, *J. Appl. Physiol.*, 8, 556, 1956.

162. **Sturtevant, F. M., Sturtevant, R. P., Scheving, L. E., and Pauly, J. E.,** Chronopharmacokinetics of ethanol. II. Circadian rhythm in rate of blood level decline in a single subject, *Naunyn Schmiedebergs Arch. Pharmacol.*, 293, 203, 1976.

163. **Pinkston, J. N. and Soniman, K. F. A.,** Effect of light and fasting on the circadian variation of ethanol metabolism in the rat, *J. Interdiscip. Cycle Res.*, 10, 185, 1979.

164. **Jones, B. M. and Paredes, A.,** Circadian variation of ethanol metabolism in alcoholics, *Br. J. Addict.*, 69, 3, 1974.

165. **Mezey, E., Potter, J. J., and Kvetransky, R.,** Effect of stress by repeated immobilization on hepatic alcohol dehydrogenase and ethanol metabolism, *Biochem. Pharmacol.*, 28, 657, 1979.

166. **Hasumura, Y., Teschke, R., and Lieber, C. S.,** Hepatic microsomal ethanol oxidizing system (MEOS): dissociation from reduced nicotinamide adenine dinucleotide phosphate-oxidase and possible role of form 1 of cytochrome P-450, *J. Pharmacol. Exp. Ther.*, 194, 469, 1975.

167. **Espina, N., Lima, V., Lieber, C. S., and Garro, A. J.,** *In vitro* and *in vivo* inhibitory effect of ethanol and acetaldehyde on $O^6$-methylguanine transferase, *Carcinogenesis*, 9, 761, 1988.

168. **Lieber, C. S., Casini, A., DeCarli, L. M., Kim, C., Lowe, N., Sasaki, R., and Leo, M. A.,** S-adenosyl-L-methionine attenuates alcohol-induced liver injury in the baboon, *Hepatology*, 11, 165, 1990.

169. **Moshage, H., Casini, A., and Lieber, C. S.,** Acetaldehyde stimulates collagen production in cultured rat liver fat-storing cells but not in hepatocytes, *Hepatology*, 12, 511, 1990.

170. **Casini, A., Cunningham, M., Rojkind, M., and Lieber, C. S.,** Acetaldehyde increases procollagen type I and fibronectin gene transcription in cultured rat fat-storing cells through a protein synthesis-dependent mechanism, *Hepatology*, 13, 758, 1991.

171. **Li, J.-J., Kim, C.-I., Leo, M. A., Mak, K. M., Rojkind, M., and Lieber, C. S.,** Polyunsaturated lecithin prevents acetaldehyde-mediated hepatic collagen accumulation by stimulating collagenase activity in cultured lipocytes, *Hepatology*, 15, 373, 1992.

172. **Lieber, C. S., Robins, S., Li, J., DeCarli, L. M., Mak, K. M., Fasulo, J. M., and Leo, M. A.,** Phosphatidyl-choline protects against fibrosis and cirrhosis in the baboon, *Gastroenterology*, 106, 161, 1994.

173. **Li, J.-J., Rosman, A. S., Leo, M. A., Nagai, Y., and Lieber, C. S.,** Tissue inhibitor of metalloproteinase (TIMP) is increased in the serum of precirrhotic and cirrhotic alcoholic patients, and can serve as a marker of fibrosis, *Hepatology*, 19, 1418, 1994.

174. **Lieber, C. S., Robins, S. J., and Leo, M. A.,** Hepatic phosphatidylethanolamine methyltransferase activity is decreased by ethanol and increased by phosphatidylcholine, *Alcoholism: Clin. Exp. Res.*, 1106, 161, 1994.

175. **Lieber, C. S., DeCarli, L. M., Mak, K. M., Kim, C.-I., and Leo, M. A.,** Attenuation of alcohol-induced hepatic fibrosis by polyunsaturated lecithin, *Hepatology*, 12, 1390, 1990.

176. **Ma, X., DeCarli, L. M., and Lieber, C. S.,** Polyenylphosphatidylcholine attenuates nonalcoholic hepatic fibrosis, *Gastroenterology*, 106, 936, 1994.

177. **Israel, Y., Orrego, H., and Carmichael, F. J.,** Acetate-mediated effects of ethanol, *Alcohol. Clin. Exp. Res.*, 18, 144, 1994.

178. **Pirola, R. C. and Lieber, C. S.,** The energy cost of the metabolism of drugs, including ethanol, *Pharmacology*, 7, 185–196, 1972.

179. **Lieber, C. S.,** Perspectives: do alcohol calories count?, *Am. J. Clin. Nutr.*, 54, 976, 1991.

180. **Lieber, C. S.,** Alcohol and the liver: 1994 update, *Gastroenterology*, 106, 1085, 1994.

181. **Lieber, C. S.,** Susceptibility to alcohol-related liver injury, in *The Biology of Alcohol Problems,* Saunders, J. B. and Whitfield, J. B., Eds., Elsevier, Oxford, UK, 1995.

182. **Salaspuro, M. P. and Lieber, C. S.,** Non-uniformity of blood ethanol elimination: its exaggeration after chronic consumption, *Ann. Clin. Res.*, 10, 294, 1978.

# 3

# Alcohol and Aldehyde Dehydrogenases in the Gastrointestinal Tract

Xavier Parés and Jaume Farrés

## CONTENTS

## 3.1  INTRODUCTION

The existence of ethanol metabolism in the gastrointestinal tract depends on the presence of suitable enzymatic systems to oxidize the alcohol to aldehyde. These systems are the microsomal cytochrome P-450 dependent system, catalase, and alcohol dehydrogenase. These three systems exist in the gastrointestinal tract, although their relative contribution is still controversial. Recently, different levels of alcohol dehydrogenase activity and different enzyme forms in the various digestive organs have been described, suggesting that they can be sites of active ethanol oxidation. The second step in ethanol metabolism, the oxidation of acetaldehyde to acetic acid, can be also locally performed due to the presence of aldehyde dehydrogenase in the gastrointestinal tract. This chapter describes the functional and structural characteristics of the gastrointestinal forms of both dehydrogenases and their distribution in human gut. Data from the rat species are also included where the corresponding information from the human enzyme is not available.

## 3.2   THE ALCOHOL DEHYDROGENASE SYSTEM

More than 30 years of continuous and intensive research on human alcohol dehydrogenase (EC 1.1.1.1) (ADH)[1] have resulted in the present complex picture of the enzyme. Human ADH exhibits different molecular forms that have been grouped in classes.[2,3] These classes differ from each other in more than 30% of their amino acid sequence and exhibit distinct kinetic properties and specific tissue distribution.[4,5] Class I is composed of isozymes with $\alpha$, $\beta$, and $\gamma$ subunits, encoded by the *ADH1*, *ADH2*, and *ADH3* gene loci, respectively. Most of the class I isozymes show low $K_m$ for ethanol (0.05 to 5 m$M$, at pH 7.5), a high sensitivity to inhibition by 4-methylpyrazole (Ki <3 $\mu$M), and are mostly localized in liver but are also present in the gastrointestinal tract and kidney. Class II consists of only one form with $\pi$ subunits, encoded by the *ADH4* gene; it has been also described in liver, exhibits high $K_m$ for ethanol (34 m$M$) and has a low sensitivity to 4-methylpyrazole (Ki = 2 m$M$).[6,7] Class III has a ubiquitous distribution in tissues, is formed by $\chi$ subunits encoded by *ADH5*, is not inhibited by 4-methylpyrazole, exhibits a very low activity with ethanol because it cannot be saturated by this substrate, effectively oxidizes long-chain alcohols, such as $\omega$-hydroxy fatty acids, and shows the best kinetic constants as a glutathione-dependent formaldehyde dehydrogenase, suggesting that the elimination of formaldehyde is the main physiological function of class III.[8-10] Class IV was initially described in stomach mucosa,[11,12] consisting of a homodimer with $\sigma$ subunits encoded by *ADH7*. Although $K_m$ for ethanol of $\sigma\sigma$-ADH is high (37 m$M$), $k_{cat}$ is also very high (1510 min$^{-1}$), suggesting an effective contribution to ethanol metabolism. Evidence suggests that a new class may be present in liver and gastric tissues, which would be encoded by *ADH6*, although only data on its cDNA and the *in vitro* expressed protein are available.[13,14] ADH forms homologous to human classes have been described in many mammals, although class II appears to have a low level of expression in some species, since it has been only possible to study it at the cDNA level in the rat.[15] Recently, one more class (class VI) has been characterized, thus far only from deermouse cDNA[16] and rat cDNA.[17] The separate class nomenclatures have been reviewed.[18]

## 3.3   ALCOHOL DEHYDROGENASE IN THE GASTROINTESTINAL TRACT

Alcohol dehydrogenase of human stomach was investigated several years ago, and the presence of distinct isozymes was clearly recognized.[19,20] The initial effort in fully describing ADH in the digestive tract was performed, however, in the rat[21-23] and mouse[24] species. The most characteristic ADH in rat digestive tract organs, not detected in liver, was named ADH-1 because it showed the most anodic mobility in starch gel electrophoresis. ADH-1 is present in the upper part of the digestive tract, from mouth to stomach, and in rectum, while other parts of the intestine contain the cathodic migrating form ADH-3, also present in liver. In addition, all rat tissues contain ADH-2, with intermediate electrophoretic mobility. The three rat ADHs were characterized both enzymatically[22] and structurally.[25-28] It was demonstrated that ADH-3, ADH-2, and ADH-1 corresponded to class I, III, and IV enzymes, respectively. Because each rat ADH class contains a single isozyme, they will be referred to by their class to avoid nomenclature confusion and to make a clear correlation with the homologous human classes.

A more complete study of ADH in the human gastrointestinal tract has started recently.[11,12,29] The composition and distribution of ADH classes parallels that of the rat with some additional

**TABLE 3.1 Kinetic Constants for Ethanol Oxidation for Human Gastrointestinal ADH, at pH 7.5**

| Class | Allele | Enzyme | $K_m$ (m$M$) | $k_{cat}$ (min$^{-1}$) | $k_{cat}/K_m$ (m$M^{-1} \times$ min$^{-1}$) | $K_m$ (NAD) ($\mu M$) |
|-------|--------|--------|--------------|------------------------|---------------------------------------------|------------------------|
| I | *ADH2*1* | $\beta_1\beta_1$ | 0.049 | 18.4 | 375 | 7.4 |
| | *ADH2*2* | $\beta_2\beta_2$ | 0.94 | 800 | 850 | 180 |
| | *ADH2*3* | $\beta_3\beta_3$ | 36 | 600 | 17 | 712 |
| | *ADH3*1* | $\gamma_1\gamma_1$ | 1 | 174 | 174 | 7.9 |
| | *ADH3*2* | $\gamma_2\gamma_2$ | 0.63 | 70 | 110 | 8.7 |
| III | *ADH5* | $\chi\chi$ | N.S. | — | 0.006 | 64 |
| IV | *ADH7* | $\sigma\sigma$ | 37 | 1510 | 40 | 180 |

*Note:* Kinetic constants were determined in 0.1 $M$ sodium phosphate/NaOH, pH 7.5, at 25°C. $k_{cat}$ values are expressed per dimer. N.S., no saturation.

Values for class I are from Burnell and Bosron,[31] and values for class III and class IV from Farrés et al.[5]

complexity as a result of the isoenzymatic multiplicity of the human class I. Class IV ADH is characteristic of the upper gastrointestinal tract; classes IV and I coexist in the stomach, while intestinal ADH is essentially composed of class I. Class III is present in all organs. Levels of enzymatic activity and the isozyme composition, however, are difficult to determine in humans because of the low amount of enzyme in the digestive tract and the limitations for obtaining fresh samples of healthy tissue. The mucosa lining the gastrointestinal tract seems the site of highest ADH activity, although the inner tissue layers appear to contain some additional enzyme activity.

### 3.3.1 Properties of the Alcohol Dehydrogenase Forms Present in the Human Gastrointestinal Tract

We will now describe the properties of the enzyme forms that have been usually detected in human digestive tract. Table 3.1 presents a summary of the kinetic constants of the purified enzymes, while Figure 3.1 shows a separation, by starch gel electrophoresis, of the ADH forms using homogenates from mucosal biopsies of various digestive organs.

#### 3.3.1.1 Class I γγ-ADH

The characteristic class I isozymes in gastric and intestinal mucosa are those composed of γ-subunits, encoded by *ADH3*. This locus shows polymorphism in the population (Figure 3.1), with allelic frequencies for *ADH3*1*/*ADH3*2* ranging from about 0.5/0.5 in Caucasians, American Indians, and Asian Indians, to about 0.9/0.1 in Orientals, Brazilians, and Black Americans.[29] The respective homodimers $\gamma_1\gamma_1$ and $\gamma_2\gamma_2$ exhibit different kinetic properties (Table 3.1), suggesting that each phenotype may provide a distinct ethanol oxidizing capability to the digestive tract. Like all other class I isozymes, γγ-ADH shows a wide substrate specificity[30] and, therefore, it can be involved in the metabolism of ingested and endogenous alcohols and aldehydes of different structures. Interestingly, isozymes with γ-subunits are the only human ADHs that can oxidize 3β-hydroxy-5β-steroids,[33] suggesting that these isozymes play a role in steroid metabolism and are inhibited by testosterone,[34] although with a Ki value (3.5 to 16 $\mu M$), probably too high to have any physiological significance.

Retinol can also be a physiological substrate for γγ-ADH[35] in the digestive tract mucosa. Retinol is an important regulator of normal epithelial cell growth, function, and differentiation, and has to be locally converted to retinoic acid, the active compound. This process includes the conversion of retinol to retinal and the further oxidation to retinoic acid. Alcohol dehydrogenase may be involved in the first step, the oxidation of retinol, being both class I and class IV active with retinol.[35,36] In this regard, *ADH3* is the only class I ADH gene that contains a retinoic acid

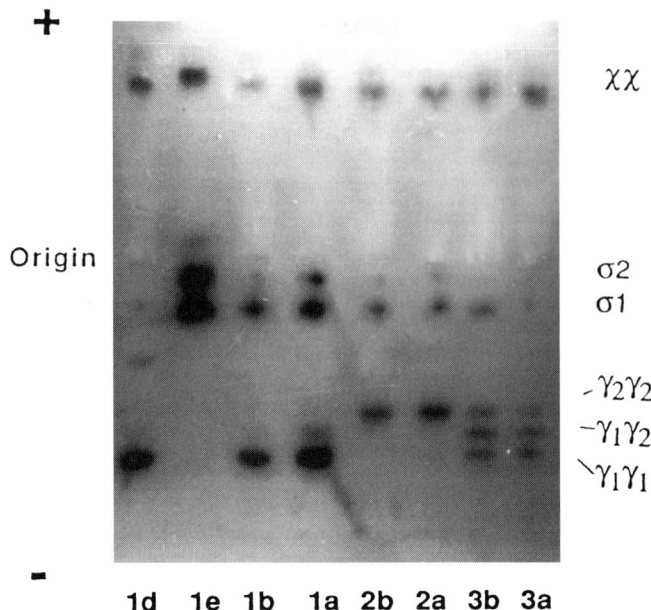

**FIGURE 3.1**  Starch gel electrophoresis of homogenates from gastrointestinal biopsies stained for crotyl alcohol (0.1 *M*) oxidizing activity. Each patient is indicated with a different number while letters indicate the gastrointestinal region analyzed: d, duodenum; e, esophagus; b, gastric body; a, gastric antrum. Polymorphism is observed at the *ADH3* locus: sample 1, *ADH3\*1/\*1*; sample 2, *ADH3\*2/\*2*; and sample 3, *ADH3\*1/\*2*. (From Moreno et al., *Alcohol Alcohol.*, 29, 663, 1994. With permission.)

response element in the promoter region, and it has been suggested that retinoic acid activation of *ADH3* constitutes a positive feedback loop regulating retinoic acid synthesis.[37]

### 3.3.1.2    Class I ββ-ADH

Isozymes with β-subunits are detected in low amount in the digestive tract muscular layers, but not in the mucosa. The undetection of heterodimers with β and γ isozymes evidences that each class I isozyme is expressed in different cell types. The *ADH2* locus shows three alleles in the human population that encode for $\beta_1$, $\beta_2$, and $\beta_3$ subunits. Individuals with $\beta_2$ subunits (atypical ADH) represent less than 20% of Caucasians, but more than 80% of Japanese and Chinese.[7] Isozymes with $\beta_3$ are found in 25% of Black Americans but were not detected in other populations.[7] The distinct β subunits differ in single amino acid residues, but the corresponding homodimers exhibit important differences in enzymatic properties with ethanol (Table 3.1), since the forms with $\beta_2$ or $\beta_3$ are much more active than those with $\beta_1$ at neutral pH. Consequently, although the *ADH2* expression is low in the gastrointestinal tract, individuals with $\beta_2$ or $\beta_3$ can potentially exhibit higher ADH activity than individuals with $\beta_1$ enzymes. The maximal activity, however, will never be reached because of the high $K_m$ for NAD, especially for $\beta_3\beta_3$ (Table 3.1), which would prevent saturation by coenzyme.

### 3.3.1.3    Class III ADH

The χχ-ADH form is detected in all digestive tract organs (Figure 3.1). It is active with ethanol but cannot be saturated by this substrate and its $k_{cat}/K_m$ value is extremely low (Table 3.1). The main function of class III is the elimination of formaldehyde endogenously formed by normal metabolism, acting as a glutathione-dependent formaldehyde dehydrogenase,[10] although a contribution to the oxidation of long-chain alcohols, especially ω-hydroxy fatty acids, cannot be excluded.[36] Some distilled alcoholic beverages contain a proportion of methanol that can be as

**TABLE 3.2  Alcohol Dehydrogenase in Gastrointestinal Tract**

| Organ | *n* | ADH activity (nmol/min/mg protein) | Major ADH forms | References |
|---|---|---|---|---|
| Mouth | 3 | 14 ± 10 | σσ | 32 |
| Esophagus | 4 | 69 ± 14 | σσ | 32 |
| Stomach | 19 | 6.7 ± 1.7 | γγ, σσ | 32 |
|  | 11 | 46 ± 5 |  | 51 |
|  | 11 | 9.5 ± 1.3 |  | 52 |
| Duodenum | 3 | 5.5 ± 3.6 | γγ | 32 |
| Rectum |  | 8.2 ± 1.8 |  | 53 |

*Note:* Activities were measured at 100 to 580 m$M$ ethanol, pH 9.6 to 10.0, using homogenates of endoscopic biopsies, except for oral mucosa samples which were obtained at autopsy. Stomach samples were from men. Isozyme composition was determined by starch gel electrophoresis. χχ-ADH is present in all organs.

high as 0.15 g/l.[38] Methanol can be oxidized by class I ADH[30] and, therefore, a certain amount of formaldehyde will be generated during the absorption of methanol through the gastrointestinal tract. The class III localized in this region may then help eliminate this highly toxic aldehyde.

### 3.3.1.4  Class IV ADH

The σσ-ADH form has been the most recently characterized human ADH.[3,5,12,39,40] Also called μ-ADH,[11] it was isolated and purified from gastric mucosa. The kinetic properties of σσ-ADH showed some similarities with class II,[12] but analysis of its primary structure has proved that σσ-ADH represents a novel ADH class (class IV), with 30 to 41% sequence differences with any of the other human ADH classes.[5,40] The closest related structure is class I, with 30 to 31% differences, which already is a percentage for class distinction. Moreover, the lack of hybridization with the class I γ-subunits in the gastric mucosa supports the separation of σσ-ADH as a distinct class. The homologous rat stomach ADH was previously characterized at the structural level[28,41] and defined as a class IV enzyme. Human σσ-ADH possesses 88% positional identities with the rat enzyme, consistent with the evolutionary relationship between both enzymes and with the proposed classification.

Human class IV exhibits a wide substrate specificity. It uses ethanol (Table 3.1) and short-chain alcohols but is much more specific for medium- and long-chain alcohols, being the $k_{cat}/K_m$ value 1000-fold higher for octanol than for ethanol.[12] The most characteristic property of human class IV is its extraordinarily high activity, exhibiting the highest specific activity (70 μmol/min/ mg)[39] and kcat (1510 min$^{-1}$)[5,39] among the human ADHs. This is a common property with the rat class IV,[5,28] suggesting that it may be typical for this class in mammals. In the rat species, class IV has been localized in the most external epithelia, such as skin and cornea, and in the mucosa of the digestive, respiratory, and sexual tracts. Class IV possibly represents a metabolic barrier to external, potentially toxic, alcohols and aldehydes.[22,36] Distribution of class IV in human tissues is not yet well known, although its presence in the upper gastrointestinal tract (Table 3.2; Figure 3.1) and cornea[42] coincides with that of the rat enzyme, suggesting a similar function in both species. In several human tissues, class IV appears as two bands (σ1 and σ2) in starch gel electrophoresis (Figure 3.1), although the structural relationship between both forms is presently not understood.[43] Rat and human class IV are active with retinoids,[35,36] and with cytotoxic aldehydes generated by lipid peroxidation such as 4-hydroxynonenal,[36] suggesting that class IV helps maintain and protect epithelial tissues.

### 3.3.1.5  Other Gastrointestinal ADHs

A functional new ADH gene, designated *ADH6*, has been characterized and the deduced amino acid sequence showed about 60% positional identity with known human ADHs.[13] Analysis by slot-blot hybridization and polymerase chain reaction (PCR) indicated that both liver and stomach (a surgically removed normal part from a Japanese adult female with adenocarcinoma) contained the *ADH6* mRNA. *In vitro* translation of *ADH6* mRNA produced a 40-kDa subunit, with an isoelectric point of 8.6, a pH optimum of 10 and a $K_m$ for ethanol of 28 m$M$.[14] Although these properties are similar to those of human class IV, the sequence identity is only 60%; therefore, *ADH6* represents a new class, designated class V.[3] The class V ADH protein has not been detected in either liver or in stomach and, therefore, its metabolic significance is not known.

Class II alcohol dehydrogenase is not detected in human or in rat gastrointestinal tissues by electrophoresis, but the corresponding mRNA has reportedly occurred in several of those tissues. Human stomach, ileum, and colon showed a low level of class II mRNA,[44] while rat duodenum exhibited a high mRNA level and it was practically absent in other rat gastrointestinal regions.[15,45] The lack of detection at the protein level makes it difficult to assess the physiological role of class II in the gastrointestinal tract.

### 3.3.1.6    Microbial ADH

Many bacteria possess ADH, which enables them to produce energy anaerobically by fermenting sugars via acetaldehyde to ethanol. Bacterial ethanol production is known to occur in the intestine and this is believed to be the major source of endogenously formed ethanol.[46] Several studies have recently been performed on *Helicobacter pylori* alcohol dehydrogenase.[47-49] This gram negative bacterium colonizes the gastrointestinal tract, and is a major factor behind active chronic gastritis and contributing strongly to peptic ulcer disease. Interestingly, *H. pylori* exhibits much more ADH activity than other common gastrointestinal bacteria and can produce significant amounts of acetaldehyde in presence of excess ethanol. The ADH purified from *H. pylori* shows a subunit molecular weight of 38 kDa and has a strong preference for NADP ($K_m$ = 80 μ$M$) over NAD ($K_m$ = 4.4 m$M$) as a cofactor in alcohol oxidation. At pH 7.4 and 37°C, the enzyme exhibits a $K_m$ for ethanol of 65 m$M$ and a kcat of 530 min$^{-1}$ per active site. As the ethanol concentration is several hundred millimolar that could be found in stomach after ethanol ingestion, the enzyme is probably fully active and produces acetaldehyde effectively. Neither *H. pylori* strain studied showed any NAD-linked aldehyde dehydrogenase, which may favor the accumulation of acetaldehyde in the close vicinity of the bacterial colonies in gastric mucin layer. Although the contribution of *H. pylori* ADH to ingested ethanol oxidation must be minimal because of the small bacterial mass present, this local production of acetaldehyde may constitute a pathogenic mechanism behind mucosal injury associated with this organism.[49]

### 3.3.2    Distribution and Activity of Alcohol Dehydrogenase in the Various Parts of the Gastrointestinal Tract

Activity analysis and immunohistochemical techniques show that the mucosa is the layer with higher ADH content throughout the gastrointestinal tract.[50] Esophagus is the organ of highest ADH activity[32,43] (Table 3.2), with a rate per mg of protein similar to that of the liver. The σσ-ADH form is mainly responsible for this activity.

ADH-specific activity of human stomach is much lower than that of esophagus (Table 3.2). However the larger mass of stomach mucosa and the longer time of exposure of ingested ethanol to the gastric ADH makes this enzyme suitable for playing a role in ethanol metabolism. Mean values ranging from 6.6 nmol/min/mg protein to 46 nmol/min/mg protein have been reported at pH 9.6 to 10.0 for gastric biopsy homogenates[32,51,52,54] (Table 3.2). The largest sample (290 patients) has been studied by Seitz et al.,[52] who reported values from 3.7 to 9.5 nmol/min/mg protein, with 580 m$M$ ethanol, similar to those found with 100 m$M$ ethanol by Moreno et al.[32] The σσ-ADH and γγ-ADH are the characteristic enzymatic forms in gastric mucosa,[32] while a small amount of ββ-ADH has been detected in the muscular layer.[29]

Mucosa biopsies from duodenum contain similar ADH-specific activity to that of stomach, about 5 nmol/min/mg (Table 3.2). Most of this activity corresponds to γγ-ADH. An activity of 8 nmol/min/mg has been detected in rectal biopsies.[53]

### 3.3.2.1 Variability of Gastric ADH Activity

Different parameters have been found to influence gastric ADH activity. Conflicting results have been reported regarding the effect of gender. Thus, an initial report indicated that ADH activity in women was 59% of that of men.[51] In another study, activity was decreased in women as compared to men but only in certain groups (less than 50 years of age) and under specific experimental conditions (with 580 m$M$ ethanol but not with 16 m$M$).[52] In a recent report differences in gastric ADH between men and women were not significant.[32]

Most of the studies on the effect of age on gastric ADH indicate a decrease of activity in older individuals,[31,52,55] concluding that age is a strong determinant of gastric ADH levels. A higher activity in gastric body with respect to antrum has been reported by two groups,[31,55] although no differences were found in another study.[52] Polymorphism at the *ADH3* locus seems an obvious source of gastric ADH variability since kinetic constants differ between the corresponding allelozymes γ$_1$γ$_1$ and γ$_2$γ$_2$ (Table 3.1), and a study on gastric biopsies supports this possibility.[32] Differences in *ADH7* expression have been suggested in stomach of Orientals[43,56] but it has not been confirmed by another report.[55]

ADH activity is generally considered to be low in chronic alcoholics.[51,52] Gastritis and *H. pylori* infection also appear to be factors that negatively influence gastric ADH activity.[57] Effect of treatment by H$_2$-receptor antagonists on gastric ADH is probably small because they exhibit high inhibition constants (from 0.1 to >5 m$M$) with the isolated ADH forms.[58-60] Assessment of the physiological significance of inhibition by H$_2$-receptor antagonists on gastric ADH would require precise information about the pharmacological levels of these drugs in mucosa. In conclusion, several factors appear to influence gastric ADH activity, with age[31,52,55] and stomach pathology[51,52,57] the most consistently reported.

### 3.3.2.2 Gastric ADH Activity at Physiological Conditions

The extensive work by Lieber, Baraona and co-workers[51,61-63] has shown that a certain amount of orally administered ethanol is metabolized before it reaches the peripheral circulation. This first-pass metabolism occurs predominantly in the stomach,[62,63] essentially because of gastric ADH. It has been argued, however, that the liver rather than the stomach is the site of the first-pass effect.[64]

At physiological pH, gastric ADH activity is lower than that at pH 9.6 or 10.0 used in the activity assays. Thus, at pH 7.5, χχ-ADH exhibits about one-twentieth the activity seen at pH 10.0, indicating that physiological contribution of class III to gastric ethanol metabolism, even at high ethanol concentrations, is minimal.[9] At saturating ethanol concentrations and, therefore, taking into account only the k$_{cat}$ value[12,65] (Table 3.1), activity at pH 7.5 of the γγ-ADH isozymes is 2.5 to 3.5 times lower than the activity at pH 10.0, while activity at pH 7.5 of σσ-ADH is about one-half the activity at pH 10.0. An additional factor that should decrease σσ-ADH activity at physiological conditions is the high K$_m$ for NAD (0.18 m$M$; Table 3.1), suggesting that σσ-ADH will not be saturated by the cofactor in the mucosal cell. It can be estimated that the activity under these conditions is not higher than 4 nmols/min/mg of protein for the most active gastric mucosa specimens, which corresponds approximately to 0.3 μmol/min/g of mucosa. Assuming 50 g of mucosa in a 150 g stomach, total activity is 15 μmol/min, with 100 m$M$ ethanol, at pH 7.5. The contribution of the ββ-ADH from the muscular layer, estimated from very active surgical samples, corresponds to about 5 μmol/min for the whole stomach. Total gastric ADH activity is, therefore, about 20 μmol/min, which corresponds to approximately 1% of the activity of liver with 33 m$M$ ethanol, at pH 7.5. This value agrees with previous calculations[12,39] and does not support an important contribution of stomach to ethanol metabolism.

## 3.4    THE FAMILY OF ALDEHYDE DEHYDROGENASES

Aldehyde dehydrogenases (ALDH, EC 1.2.1.3) catalyze the irreversible oxidation of various aliphatic and aromatic aldehydes, as well as the hydrolysis of activated esters, to their corresponding carboxylic acids.[66] ALDHs are involved in the detoxification of ethanol-derived acetaldehyde, and they could play a role in the conversion of aldehyde intermediates formed during the metabolism of corticosteroids,[67] amino acids,[68,69] biogenic amines,[70] anticancer drugs,[71] retinoids,[71] and products of lipid peroxidation.[72,73]

The family of aldehyde dehydrogenases includes substrate-specific enzymes, such as betaine aldehyde dehydrogenase and various semialdehyde dehydrogenases, as well as enzymes with broad-substrate specificity. Similarly to ADH, mammalian ALDHs have been grouped in different classes,[74,75] based on their structural properties, subcellular localization, and tissue distribution. Class 1 ALDH is represented by the tetrameric enzymes located in the cytosol and is found mainly in the liver but also in many other tissues. In rat liver, the class 1 enzyme is inducible by phenobarbital.[76] Class 2 ALDH includes the tetrameric forms located in the mitochondria.[77] They are most abundant in liver but are expressed in many other organs. Human ALDHx, identified only at gene level, is expressed in liver and testes, and is most similar to class 2 ALDH.[78] Class 3 ALDH refers to the dimeric, cytosolic forms, constitutively expressed in stomach, esophagus, lung, cornea, and, to a much lesser extent, in liver.[73,79,80] The enzyme appears to be induced by various xenobiotics in a number of rodent tissues, and during hepatocarcinogenesis in humans and rats.[74,80,81] A rat liver microsomal ALDH, whose sequence has been recently reported,[82] is essentially a class 3 enzyme.

Recently, many ALDH sequences have become available.[75] Human class 1 and class 2 ALDHs show 68% sequence identity, which is also the level for class distinction in human ADHs. In contrast, human class 3 ALDH shares only 30% sequence identity with class 1 or class 2 ALDH. Homologous ALDHs have been detected and characterized in other mammalian species.[74,83-85]

### 3.4.1    Properties of the Aldehyde Dehydrogenase Forms Present in the Human Gastrointestinal Tract

The human gastrointestinal tract contains ALDHs of the three classes (Figure 3.2), which differ widely in their properties and kinetic constants for acetaldehyde oxidation (Table 3.3).

#### 3.4.1.1    Class 1 ALDH

Class 1 ALDH is found in both the mucosa and the muscular layer of most gastrointestinal tissues.[43,88,89] It has a low $K_m$ for acetaldehyde (Table 3.3) and theoretically could contribute to acetaldehyde elimination when class 2 ALDH is not present, although less efficiently than the class 2 enzyme. For aliphatic aldehydes, the $K_m$ values of class 1 ALDH decrease as the number of carbons increase.[70] This is the only form that oxidizes retinal ($K_m = 0.3$ µM),[71] and has been implicated in the biotransformation of anticancer drugs.[71] Moreover, it has been proposed that class 1 ALDH has a role in the metabolism of monoamines because of high activity toward 3,4-dihydroxyphenylacetaldehyde and 5-hydroxyindoleacetaldehyde.[70]

#### 3.4.1.2    Class 2 ALDH

Class 2 ALDH has a very low $K_m$ for acetaldehyde (Table 3.3), which allows for efficient removal of this compound produced during ethanol consumption. A deficient class 2 variant, with the amino acid substitution E487K,[90,91] has been detected in 50% of Orientals.[92] This ALDH variant is virtually inactive under physiological conditions,[93] thus causing acetaldehyde accumulation and flushing.[94] The lack of human class 2 activity is readily diagnosed by the absence of the most

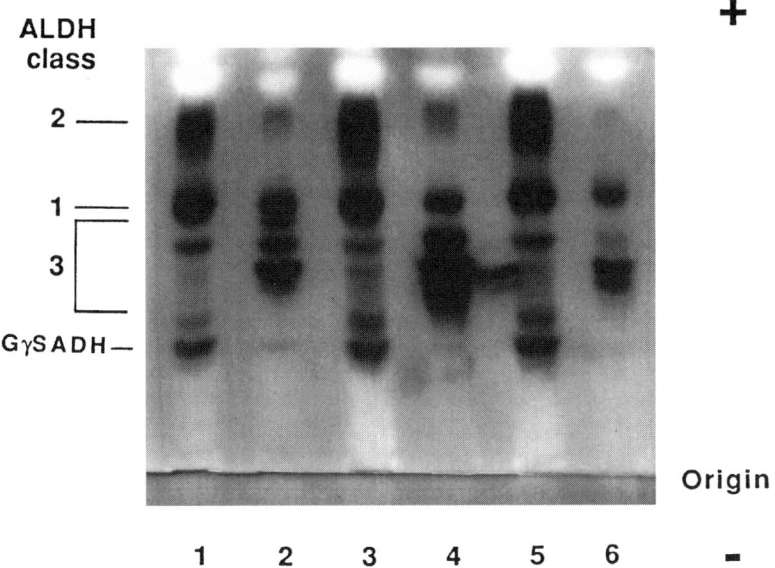

**FIGURE 3.2**  Starch gel electrophoresis of homogenates from liver (lanes 1, 3, and 5) and stomach (lanes 2, 4, and 6) necropsies. The activity staining was performed with 0.11 $M$ propionaldehyde. Gγ SADH, glutamic γ-semialdehyde dehydrogenase.

anodic band in the electrophoretic patterns (Figure 3.2). One study,[29] using human gastroendoscopic biopsies from Chinese subjects, showed that the frequency of the deficient allele was 0.45, similar to what had been found with liver samples. Conceivably, impaired acetaldehyde metabolism could exacerbate the toxic effects of locally generated acetaldehyde leading to tissue damage.[95] In a separate study, the presence of a class 2–deficient genotype was not associated with higher prevalence of diseases of the gastrointestinal tract, including cancer.[96] Similar to class 1 ALDH, the class 2 enzyme oxidizes medium-chain aliphatic aldehydes and monoamine derivatives with high specificity.[70] It is not active with retinal. Class 2 ALDH is present in stomach and intestine, but barely detectable in esophagus (Table 3.4).[88,89,97-99]

### 3.4.1.3   Class 3 ALDH

Class 3 has been found in stomach, esophagus, gingiva, and, recently, in saliva.[100] It is absent or expressed at very low levels in duodenum, jejunum, ileum,[98] and colon (Table 3.4).

Human class 3 ALDH has been purified to homogeneity from human gastric mucosa[87] and cornea,[73] and detailed kinetic studies have been performed. Both stomach and cornea enzymes

**TABLE 3.3   Kinetic Constants for Acetaldehyde Oxidation for Human Gastrointestinal ALDH**

| ALDH class | $K_m$ (μ$M$) | $k_{cat}$ (min$^{-1}$) | $k_{cat}/K_m$ (μm$^{-1}$ × min$^{-1}$) | $K_m$ (NAD) (μ$M$) |
|---|---|---|---|---|
| 1 | 50 | 55 | 1.1 | 40 |
| 2 | 1 | 68 | 68 | 70 |
| 3 | 88000 | 4730 | 0.05 | 15 |

*Note:*   Kinetic constants were determined at pH 7.0 for class 1 and class 2 ALDH, and at pH 8.5 for class 3 ALDH. kcat values are expressed per molecule of enzyme.

From References 70, 86, and 87.

**TABLE 3.4  Distribution of ADH and ALDH Forms
in the Gastrointestinal Tract**

| Organ | ADH class I | ALDH class 2 | ADH class IV | ALDH class 3 |
|---|---|---|---|---|
| Mouth | – | n.d. | + | + |
| Esophagus | – | – | + | + |
| Stomach | + | + | + | + |
| Duodenum | + | + | – | – |
| Jejunum | + | + | – | – |
| Colon | + | + | – | – |

*Note:* Enzymes were detected by gel electrophoresis or
isoelectrofocusing. + indicates a clear detection; –, not
detected or extremely faint band; n.d., not determined.

From References 32, 43, 88, 89, and 97–99.

appear to be identical. $K_m$ values are in the millimolar range for short-chain aliphatic aldehydes but decrease as the number of carbons increase. The products of lipid peroxidation, hexanol, trans-2-hexenal, and 4-hidroxynonenal, are oxidized very efficiently.[73] Aromatic aldehydes, such as benzaldehyde and 4-nitrobenzaldehyde, are also good substrates.[73,87] Class 3 ALDH exhibits very high $k_{cat}$ values as compared to the other ALDH classes (Table 3.3). The enzyme is active with both NAD and NADP as coenzymes, although $K_m$ for NAD is much lower and physiologically significant. Overall kinetic properties are similar to those of rat and mouse stomach class 3 ALDH.[84,101]

Human stomach class 3 ALDH exhibits multiple bands (pI 5.9 to 6.4) by starch-gel electrophoresis (Figure 3.2) and isoelectrofocusing, with various banding patterns in different individuals.[79,97-99] The enzymatic properties of each form have not been studied, and thus it is not known if different phenotypes reflect distinct metabolic capabilities. Recently, based on the dimeric nature of the class 3 ALDH enzyme and the observed patterns in human stomach and liver samples, a two-gene model was proposed.[29] According to this model, human class 3 ALDH would be encoded by two separate gene loci, *ALDH3a* and *ALDH3b* coding for A and B subunits, respectively. In addition, two common alleles, *ALDH3b\*1* and *ALDH3b\*2*, would exist at the *ALDH3b* locus. Stomach contains A and B subunits. The AA form is the only one expressed in liver, while the BB form is predominantly expressed in esophagus.[43] Multiple forms of class 3 ALDH can also be found in lung[102] and cornea.[73]

Other groups have considered the possibility of multiple forms arising from posttranslational modification[103] or from a single gene with two allelic variants.[97,99] In this regard, analysis of human genomic DNA reveals that a single *ALDH3* gene is present.[80] Further genetic analysis will be needed to clarify this point.

### 3.4.2  Acetaldehyde-Metabolizing Capacity of the Human Gastrointestinal Tract

Class 3 ALDH has been estimated to account for more than 80% of the ALDH activity, measured with a high concentration of aldehyde, in human gastric mucosa.[29] Because of its high $K_m$ value for acetaldehyde, however, class 3 ALDH contributes little to the elimination of acetaldehyde.

In order to assess the overall ethanol-metabolizing capacity of the gastrointestinal tissues, it is informative to compare the ethanol-oxidation rate against the acetaldehyde-oxidation rate for a given tissue. Thus, using 200 $\mu M$ acetaldehyde, a concentration that saturates class 2 ALDH and that is the upper intracellular level during ethanol metabolism, the rate of oxidation by human stomach homogenates is $3.06 \pm 0.29$ nmol/min/mg protein (pH 7.5, 30°C).[43] This value is similar to the value reported for ethanol oxidation (Table 3.2), suggesting that acetaldehyde generated by gastric ADH could be oxidized in the same tissue. A different picture is seen in the esophagus, where the ALDH activity measured with 200 $\mu M$ acetaldehyde is only $0.922 \pm 0.058$ nmol/min/mg protein (pH 7.5, 30°C),[43] while the rate of acetaldehyde production is approximately 70 times higher (Table 3.2). Thus, accumulation of acetaldehyde could occur in esophageal tissue, contributing to the alcohol-related damage to it observed among heavy drinkers.[95]

## 3.5 ADH-ALDH METABOLIC RELATIONSHIP IN THE GASTROINTESTINAL TRACT

ADH and ALDH catalyze consecutive reactions in alcohol metabolism. It seems reasonable to assume that enzymatic forms of both dehydrogenases with related specificity will be located in the same tissue and will be involved in common metabolic pathways. The distribution and substrate specificity of ADH and ALDH in the gastrointestinal tract clearly support this assumption and give evidence of the physiological role of these enzymes (Table 3.4). Class I ADH, with low $K_m$ values for ethanol and short-chain alcohols, is detected in stomach and intestine but not in upper digestive organs. Class 1 ALDH and class 2 ALDH, the forms with low $K_m$ for acetaldehyde, are present in all digestive tract organs, but class 2 ALDH, the main form responsible for acetaldehyde oxidation, is barely detected in esophagus.[43] In contrast, the enzymes with high $K_m$ for ethanol (class IV ADH) and acetaldehyde (class 3 ALDH) are expressed in upper digestive tract but not in intestine. Another property shared by class IV ADH and class 3 ALDH is their extremely high $k_{cat}$. It appears, therefore, that stomach and intestine contain an enzymatic system (class I ADH–class 2 ALDH) with broad-substrate specificity, while upper digestive organs including stomach exhibit a metabolizing system more specific for medium, long chain, and aromatic alcohols and aldehydes (class IV ADH–class 3 ALDH). A significant amount of class 1 ALDH is detected in all organs. The class IV ADH–class 3 ALDH system, located only in the mucosa of the most external part of the digestive tract, and also in great amount in the cornea, would play a role as a first metabolic barrier against the exposition to xenobiotic alcohols and aldehydes. Both components are relatively efficient in removing aldehydes derived from lipid peroxidation, and this could also be an important function of the enzymatic system in external mucosa. The class I ADH–class 2 ALDH enzymes, with the addition of class 1 ALDH, are located in both mucosa and muscular layer of more internal gastrointestinal organs, and constitute a system for elimination of ingested alcohols and of those produced by intestinal microorganisms.[46] The system would also play a role in the metabolic conversions of endogenous alcohols or aldehydes such as retinoids, neurotransmitter metabolites, lipid peroxidation products, etc.

## 3.6 CONCLUSIONS

A certain amount of ADH and ALDH is detected in all organs of the gastrointestinal tract. The localization of the enzymes in sites of ethanol absorption, such as stomach and intestine, makes possible their role in first-pass metabolism. However, the low level of ADH would result in a small contribution of the gastrointestinal tract to overall ethanol elimination. This contribution would be higher with factors (i.e., delay of gastric emptying) that reduce the rate of absorption and, therefore, that would increase the time of contact between ethanol and the enzymes. The local ethanol oxidation, with the corresponding acetaldehyde accumulation and redox change, may explain some aspects of tissue injury caused by ethanol. The presence of low-$K_m$ ALDH in the whole gastrointestinal tract suggests that the accumulation of acetaldehyde would not be, in general, large. The organ with the highest ADH activity is esophagus, which, in contrast, exhibits a low acetaldehyde-oxidizing activity. After ingesting beverages of high ethanol concentration, some ethanol absorption occurs during passage through the esophagus, and accumulation of acetaldehyde is then expected, with possible deleterious effects on this organ.

Class IV ADH and class 3 ALDH exhibit similar specificity toward medium- and long-chain substrates and aromatic compounds, and both are expressed in mouth, esophagus, and stomach mucosa. This suggests that they constitute an ADH-ALDH system involved in specific metabolic pathways in these organs, probably related to elimination of xenobiotics and lipid-peroxidation derived compounds. In contrast, class I ADH and class 2 ALDH — both enzymes with broad-substrate specificity and mainly responsible for short-chain alcohol and aldehyde metabolism — are located in mucosa and muscular layer of stomach and intestine. They constitute a distinct enzymatic system involved in the elimination of a variety alcohols and aldehydes, either ingested or produced by intestinal microorganisms, and in the interconversion of endogenous physiological compounds.

## 3.7   ACKNOWLEDGMENTS

The portion of this work performed in the authors' laboratory has been supported by grants from Dirección General de Investigación Científica y Técnica (PB92-0624), Fondo de Investigaciones Sanitarias de la Seguridad Social (94/0796), and the Commission of the European Communities (BMH1-CT93-1601).

## REFERENCES

1. **von Wartburg, J.-P., Bethune, J. L., and Vallee, B. L.,** Human liver-alcohol dehydrogenase. Kinetic and physicochemical properties, *Biochemistry*, 3, 1775, 1964.
2. **Vallee, B. L. and Bazzone, T. J.,** Isozymes of human liver alcohol dehydrogenase, *Isozymes: Curr. Top. Biol. Med. Res.*, 8, 219, 1983.
3. **Parés, X., Cederlund, E., Moreno, A., Saubi, N., Höög, J.-O., and Jörnvall, H.,** Structural analysis of human σσ-ADH reveals class IV to be variable and confirms the presence of a fifth mammalian alcohol dehydrogenase class, *FEBS Lett.*, 303, 69, 1992.
4. **Jörnvall, H.,** The alcohol dehydrogenase system, in *Toward a Molecular Basis of Alcohol Use and Abuse*, Jansson, B., Jörnvall, H., Rydberg, U., Terenius, L., and Vallee, B. L., Eds., Birkhäuser Verlag, Basel, 1994, 221.
5. **Farrés, J., Moreno, A., Crosas, B., Peralba, J. M., Allali-Hassani, A., Hjelmqvist, L., Jörnvall, H., and Parés, X.,** Alcohol dehydrogenase of class IV (σσ-ADH) from human stomach. cDNA sequence and structure/function relationships, *Eur. J. Biochem.*, 224, 549, 1994.
6. **Bosron, W. F., Li, T.-K., Dafeldecker, W. P., and Vallee, B. L.,** Human liver π-alcohol dehydrogenase: kinetic and molecular properties, *Biochemistry*, 18, 1101, 1979.
7. **Bosron, W. F. and Li, T.-K.,** Genetic polymorphism of human liver alcohol and aldehyde dehydrogenases and their relationship to alcohol metabolism and alcoholism, *Hepatology*, 6, 502, 1986.
8. **Parés, X. and Vallee, B. L.,** New human liver alcohol dehydrogenase forms with unique kinetic characteristics, *Biochem. Biophys. Res. Commun.*, 98, 122, 1981.
9. **Wagner, F. W., Parés, X., Holmquist, B., and Vallee, B. L.,** Physical and enzymatic properties of a class III isozyme of human liver alcohol dehydrogenase: χ-ADH, *Biochemistry*, 23, 2193, 1984.
10. **Koivusalo, M., Baumann, M., and Uotila, L.,** Evidence for the identity of glutathione-dependent formaldehyde dehydrogenase and class III alcohol dehydrogenase, *FEBS Lett.*, 257, 105, 1989.
11. **Yin, S.-J., Wang, M.-F., Liao, C.-S., Chen, C.-M., and Wu, C.-W.,** Identification of human stomach alcohol dehydrogenase with distinctive kinetic properties, *Biochem. Int.*, 22, 829, 1990.
12. **Moreno, A. and Parés, X.,** Purification and characterization of a new alcohol dehydrogenase from human stomach, *J. Biol. Chem.*, 266, 1128, 1991.
13. **Yasunami, M., Chen, C.-S., and Yoshida, A.,** A human alcohol dehydrogenase gene *(ADH6)* encoding an additional class of isozyme, *Proc. Natl. Acad. Sci. U.S.A.*, 88, 7610, 1991.
14. **Chen, C.-S. and Yoshida, A.,** Enzymatic properties of the protein encoded by newly cloned human alcohol dehydrogenase *ADH6* gene, *Biochem. Biophys. Res. Commun.*, 181, 743, 1991.
15. **Estonius, M., Danielsson, O., Karlsson, C., Persson, H., Jörnvall, H., and Höög, J.-O.,** Distribution of alcohol and sorbitol dehydrogenases. Assessment of mRNA species in mammalian tissues, *Eur. J. Biochem.*, 215, 497, 1993.
16. **Zeng, Y.-W., Bey, M., Liu, H., and Felder, M. R.,** Molecular basis of the alcohol dehydrogenase-negative deer mouse. Evidence for deletion of the gene for class I enzyme and identification of a possible new enzyme class, *J. Biol. Chem.*, 268, 24933, 1993.
17. **Höög, J.-O. and Brandt, M.,** Mammalian class VI alcohol dehydrogenase, Proc. Seventh International Workshop on Enzymology and Molecular Biology of Carbonyl Metabolism. Palmerston North, New Zealand, 34, 1994.
18. **Jörnvall, H. and Höög, J.-O.,** Nomenclature of alcohol dehydrogenases, *Alcohol Alcohol.*, 30, 153, 1995.

19. **Smith, M., Hopkinson, D. A., and Harris, H.,** Alcohol dehydrogenase isozymes in adult human stomach and liver: evidence for activity of the *ADH3* locus, *Ann. Human Genet.,* 35, 243, 1972.

20. **Hempel, J. D. and Pietruszko, R.,** Human stomach alcohol dehydrogenase: isoenzyme composition and catalytic properties, *Alcoholism: Clin. Exp. Res.,* 3, 95, 1979.

21. **Cederbaum, A. I., Pietruszko, R., Hempel, J., Becker, F. F., and Rubin, E.,** Characterization of a nonhepatic alcohol dehydrogenase from rat hepatocellular carcinoma and stomach, *Arch. Biochem. Biophys.,* 171, 348, 1975.

22. **Julià, P., Farrés, J., and Parés, X.,** Characterization of three isoenzymes of rat alcohol dehydrogenase. Tissue distribution and physical and enzymatic properties, *Eur. J. Biochem.,* 162, 179, 1987.

23. **Boleda, M. D., Julià, P., Moreno, A., and Parés, X.,** Role of extrahepatic alcohol dehydrogenase in rat ethanol metabolism, *Arch. Biochem. Biophys.,* 274, 74, 1989.

24. **Algar, E. S., Seeley, T.-L., and Holmes, R. S.,** Purification and molecular properties of mouse alcohol dehydrogenase isozymes, *Eur. J. Biochem.,* 137, 139, 1983.

25. **Jörnvall, H.,** Functional aspects of structural studies on alcohol dehydrogenases, in *Alcohol and Aldehyde Metabolizing Systems,* Thurman, R. G., Yonetani, T., Williamson, J. R., and Chance, B., Eds., Academic Press, New York, 1974, 23.

26. **Crabb, D. W., Stein, P. M., Dipple, K. M., Hittle, J. B., Sidhu, R., Qulali, M., Zhang, K., and Edenberg, H. J.,** Structure and expression of the rat class I alcohol dehydrogenase gene, *Genomics,* 5, 906, 1989.

27. **Julià, P., Parés, X., and Jörnvall, H.,** Rat liver alcohol dehydrogenase of class III. Primary structure, functional consequences and relationships to other alcohol dehydrogenases, *Eur. J. Biochem.,* 172, 73, 1988.

28. **Parés, X., Cederlund, E., Moreno, A., Hjelmqvist, L., Farrés, J., and Jörnvall, H.,** Mammalian class IV alcohol dehydrogenase (stomach alcohol dehydrogenase): structure, origin, and correlation with enzymology, *Proc. Natl. Acad. Sci. U.S.A.,* 91, 1893, 1994.

29. **Yin, S.-J., Cheng, T.-C., Chang, C.-P., Chen, Y.-J., Chao, Y.-C., Tang, H.-S., Chang, T.-M., and Wu, C.-W.,** Human stomach alcohol and aldehyde dehydrogenases (ALDH): a genetic model proposed for ALDH III isozymes, *Biochem. Genet.,* 26, 343, 1988.

30. **Wagner, F. W., Burger, A. R., and Vallee, B. L.,** Kinetic properties of human liver alcohol dehydrogenase: oxidation of alcohols by class I isozymes, *Biochemistry,* 22 1857, 1983.

31. **Burnell, J. C. and Bosron, W. F.,** Genetic polymorphism of human liver alcohol dehydrogenase and kinetic properties of the isoenzymes, in *Human Metabolism of Alcohol,* Vol. II, Crow, K. E. and Batt, R. D., Eds., CRC Press, Boca Raton, FL, 1989, chap. 5.

32. **Moreno, A., Parés, A., Ortiz, J., Enríquez, J., and Parés, X.,** Alcohol dehydrogenase from human stomach: variability in normal mucosa and effect of age, gender, ADH3 phenotype and gastric region, *Alcohol Alcohol.,* 29, 663, 1994.

33. **McEvily, A. J., Holmquist, B., Auld, D. S., and Vallee, B. L.,** 3$\beta$-Hydroxy-5$\beta$-steroid dehydrogenase activity of human liver alcohol dehydrogenase is specific to $\gamma$-subunits, *Biochemistry,* 27, 4284, 1988.

34. **Mårdh, G., Falchuck, K. H., Auld, D. S., and Vallee, B. L.,** Testosterone allosterically regulates ethanol oxidation by homo and heterodimeric $\gamma$-subunit-containing isozymes of human alcohol dehydrogenase, *Biochemistry,* 83, 2836, 1986.

35. **Yang, Z. N., Davis, G. J., Hurley, T. D., Stone, C. L., Li, T.-K., and Bosron, W. F.,** Catalytic efficiency of human alcohol dehydrogenases for retinol oxidation and retinal reduction, *Alcoholism: Clin. Exp. Res.,* 17, 496, 1994.

36. **Boleda, M. D., Saubi, N., Farrés, J., and Parés, X.,** Physiological substrates for rat alcohol dehydrogenase classes: aldehydes of lipid peroxidation, $\omega$-hydroxy fatty acids, and retinoids, *Arch. Biochem. Biophys.,* 307, 85, 1993.

37. **Duester, G., Shean, M. L., McBride, M. S., and Stewart, M. J.,** Retinoic acid response element in the human alcohol dehydrogenase gene *ADH3*: implications for regulation of retinoic acid synthesis, *Mol. Cell. Biol.,* 11, 1638, 1991.

38. **Kricka, L. J. and Clark, P. M. S.,** *Biochemistry of Alcohol and Alcoholism,* Ellis Horwood, Chichester, 1979, chap. 4.

39. **Stone, C. L., Thomasson, H. R., Bosron, W. F., and Li, T.-K.,** Purification and partial amino acid sequence of a high-activity human stomach alcohol dehydrogenase, *Alcoholism: Clin. Exp. Res.,* 17, 911, 1993.

40. **Satre, M. A., Zgombicknight, M., and Duester, G.,** The complete structure of human class IV alcohol dehydrogenase (retinol dehydrogenase) determined from the *ADH7* gene, *J. Biol. Chem.,* 269, 15606, 1994

41. **Parés, X., Moreno, A., Cederlund, E., Höög, J.-O., and Jörnvall, H.,** Class IV mammalian alcohol dehydrogenase. Structural data of the rat stomach enzyme reveal a new class well separated from those already characterized, *FEBS Lett.* 277, 115, 1990.

42. **Holmes, R. S.,** Alcohol dehydrogenases and aldehyde dehydrogenases of anterior eye tissues from humans and other mammals, in *Biomedical and Social Aspects of Alcohol and Alcoholism,* Kuriyama, K., Takada, A., and Ishii, H., Eds., Elsevier, New York, 1988, 51.

43. **Yin, S.-J., Chou, F. J., Chao, S.-F., Tsai, S.-F., Liao, C.-S., Wang, S. L., Wu, C.-W., and Lee, S.-C.,** Alcohol and aldehyde dehydrogenases in human esophagus: comparison with the stomach enzyme activities, *Alcoholism: Clin. Exp. Res.,* 17, 376, 1993.

44. **Engeland, K. and Maret, W.,** Extrahepatic, differential expression of four classes of human alcohol dehydrogenase, *Biochem. Biophys. Res. Commun.,* 193, 47, 1993.

45. **Höög, J.-O., Estonius, M., and Danielsson, O.,** Site-directed mutagenesis and enzyme properties of mammalian alcohol dehydrogenases correlated with their tissue distribution, in *Toward a Molecular Basis of Alcohol Use and Abuse,* Jansson, B., Jörnvall, H., Rydberg, U., Terenius, L., and Vallee, B. L., Eds., Birkhäuser Verlag, Basel, 1994, 301.

46. **Krebs, H. A. and Perkins, J. R.,** The physiological role of liver alcohol dehydrogenase, *Biochem. J.,* 118, 635, 1970.

47. **Roine, R. P., Salmela, K. S., Höök-Nikanne, J., Kosunen, T. U., and Salaspuro, M.,** Alcohol dehydrogenase mediated acetaldehyde production by *Helicobacter Pylori* — a possible mechanism behind gastric injury, *Life Sci.,* 51, 1333, 1992.

48. **Salmela, K. S., Roine, R. P., Koivisto, T., Höök-Nikanne, J., Kosunen, T. U., and Salapuro, M.,** Characteristics of *Helicobacter pylori* alcohol dehydrogenase, *Gastroenterology,* 105, 325, 1993.

49. **Salaspuro, M.,** *Helicobacter pylori* alcohol dehydrogenase, in *Toward a Molecular Basis of Alcohol Use and Abuse,* Jansson, B., Jörnvall, H., Rydberg, U., Terenius, L., and Vallee, B. L., Eds., Birkhäuser Verlag, Basel, 1994, 185.

50. **Pestalozzi, D. M., Bühler, R., von Wartburg, J. P., and Hess, M.,** Immunohistochemical localization of alcohol dehydrogenase in the human gastrointestinal tract, *Gastroenterology,* 85, 1011, 1983.

51. **Frezza, M., di Padova, C., Pozzato, G., Terpin, M., Baraona, E., and Lieber, C. S.,** High blood alcohol levels in women. The role of decreased gastric alcohol dehydrogenase activity and first-pass metabolism, *N. Engl. J. Med.,* 332, 95, 1990.

52. **Seitz, H. K., Egerer, G., Simanowski, U. A., Waldherr, R., Eckey, R., Agarwal, D. P., Goedde, H. W., and von Wartburg, J.-P.,** Human gastric alcohol dehydrogenase activity: effect of age, sex, and alcoholism, *Gut,* 34, 1433, 1993.

53. **Seitz, H. K., Krämer, S., Egerer, G., Klee, F., Wysocki, S., and Simanowski, U. A.,** Metabolism of ethanol by alcohol dehydrogenase in the human rectum, *Gastroenterology,* 102, A882, 1992.

54. **Hernández-Muñoz, R., Caballería, J., Baraona, E., Uppal, R., Greenstein, R., and Lieber, C. S.,** Human gastric alcohol dehydrogenase: its inhibition by $H_2$-receptor antagonists, and its effect on the bioavailability of ethanol, *Alcoholism: Clin. Exp. Res.,* 14, 946, 1990.

55. **Harada, S. and Okubo, T.,** Investigation of alcohol dehydrogenase isozymes of biopsy gastric mucosa in Japanese, *Alcohol Alcohol.,* 28, 59, 1993.

56. **Baraona, E., Yokoyama, A., Ishii, H., Hernández-Muñoz, R., Takagi, T., Tsuchiya, M., and Lieber, C. S.,** Lack of alcohol dehydrogenase isoenzyme activities in the stomach of Japanese subjects, *Life Sci.,* 49, 1929, 1991.

57. **Thuluvath, P. J., Wojno, K. J., Milligan, F. D., Yardley, J. H., and Mezey, E.,** Effects of *Helicobacter pylori* (HP) infection and gastritis on gastric alcohol dehydrogenase (ADH) activity, *Hepatology,* 18, 151A, 1993.

58. **Allali-Hassani, A., Peralba, J. M., Vidal, J., Richart, C., and Parés, X.,** Inhibition of purified human stomach alcohol dehydrogenase isozymes by $H_2$-receptor antagonists, *Alcohol Alcohol.,* 28, 230, 1993.

59. **Stone, C. L., Davis, G. J., Peggs, C. F., Thomasson, H. R., Yang, Z.-N., Bosron, W. F., and Li, T.-K.,** Inhibition of gastric and liver alcohol dehydrogenase (ADH) isoenzymes by $H_2$-receptor antagonists, *Hepatology,* 18, 151A, 1993.

60. **Stone, C. L., Davis, G. J., Peggs, C. F., Thomasson, H. R., Li, T.-K. and Bosron, W. F.,** Inhibition of gastric and liver alcohol dehydrogenase (ADH) isoenzymes by $H_2$-receptor antagonists, *Alcoholism: Clin. Exp. Res.,* 18, 420, 1994.

61. **Julkunen, R. J. K., di Padova, C., and Lieber, C. S.,** First pass metabolism of ethanol — a gastrointestinal barrier against the systemic toxicity of ethanol, *Life Sci.,* 37, 567, 1985.

62. **Caballería, J., Frezza, M., Hernández-Muñoz, R., Dipadova, C., Korsten, M. A., Baraona, E., and Lieber, C. S.,** Gastric origin of the first-pass metabolism of ethanol in humans: effect of gastrectomy, *Gastroenterology,* 97, 1205, 1989.

63. **Lim, R. T., Gentry, R. T., Jr., Ito, D., Yokoyama, H., Baraona, E., and Lieber, C. S.,** First-pass metabolism of ethanol is predominantly gastric, *Alcoholism: Clin. Exp. Res.,* 17, 1337, 1993.

64. **Levitt, M. D. and Levitt, D. G.,** The critical role of the rate of ethanol absorption in the interpretation of studies purporting to demonstrate gastric metabolism of ethanol, *J. Pharmacol. Exp. Ther.* 269, 297, 1994.

65. **Bosron, W. F., Magnes, L. J., and Li, T.-K.,** Kinetic and electrophoretic properties of native and recombined isoenzymes of human liver alcohol dehydrogenase, *Biochemistry,* 22, 1852, 1983.

66. **Weiner, H.,** Aldehyde dehydrogenase. Mechanism of action and possible physiological roles, in *Biochemistry and Pharmacology of Ethanol,* Majchrowicz, E. and Noble, E. P., Eds., Plenum Press, New York, 1979, chap. 6.

67. **Monder, C., Purkaystha, A. R., and Pietruszko, R.,** Oxidation of the 17-aldol ($20\beta$-hydroxy-21-aldehyde) intermediate of corticosteroid metabolism to hydroxy acids by homogeneous human liver aldehyde dehydrogenases, *J. Steroid Biochem.,* 17, 41, 1982.

68. **Forte-McRobbie, C. M. and Pietruszko, R.,** Purification and characterization of human liver "high $K_m$" aldehyde dehydrogenase and its identification as glutamic $\gamma$-semialdehyde dehydrogenase, *J. Biol. Chem.,* 261, 2154, 1986.

69. **Farrés, J., Julià, P., and Parés, X.,** Aldehyde oxidation in human placenta: purification and properties of 1-pyrroline-5-carboxylate dehydrogenase *Biochem. J.*, 256, 461, 1988.

70. **Ambroziak, W. and Pietruszko, R.,** Human aldehyde dehydrogenase: activity with aldehyde metabolites of monoamines, diamines, and polyamines, *J. Biol. Chem.* 266, 13011, 1991.

71. **Dockham, P. A., Lee, M.-O., and Sladek, N. E.,** Identification of human liver aldehyde dehydrogenases that catalyze the oxidation of aldophosphamide and retinaldehyde, *Biochem. Pharmacol.*, 43, 2453, 1992.

72. **Lindahl, R. and Petersen, D. R.,** Lipid aldehyde oxidation as a physiological role for class 3 aldehyde dehydrogenases, *Biochem. Pharmacol.*, 41, 1583, 1991.

73. **King, G. and Holmes, R. S.,** Human corneal aldehyde dehydrogenase: purification, kinetic characterisation and phenotypic variation, *Biochem. Mol. Biol. Int.*, 31, 49, 1993.

74. **Lindahl, R.,** Aldehyde dehydrogenases and their role in carcinogenesis, *Crit. Rev. Biochem. Mol. Biol.*, 27, 283, 1992.

75. **Hempel, J., Nicholas, H., and Lindahl, R.,** Aldehyde dehydogenases: widespread structural and functional diversity within a shared framework, *Protein Sci.*, 2, 1890, 1993.

76. **Dunn, T. J., Koleske, A. J., Lindahl, R., and Pitot, H. C.,** Phenobarbital-inducible aldehyde dehydrogenase in the rat, *J. Biol. Chem.*, 264, 13057, 1989.

77. **Farrés, J., Guan, K.-L., and Weiner, H.,** Primary structures of rat and bovine liver mitochondrial aldehyde dehydrogenases deduced from cDNA sequences, *Eur. J. Biochem.*, 180, 67, 1989.

78. **Hsu, L. C. and Chang, W.-C.,** Cloning and characterization of a new functional human aldehyde dehydrogenase gene, *J. Biol. Chem.*, 266, 12257, 1991.

79. **Yin, S.-J., Liao, C.-S., Wang, S.-L., Chen, Y.-J., and Wu, C.-W.,** Kinetic evidence for human liver and stomach aldehyde dehydrogenase-3 representing an unique class of isozymes, *Biochem. Genet.*, 27, 321, 1989.

80. **Hsu, L. C., Chang, W.-C., Shibuya, A., and Yoshida, A.,** Human stomach aldehyde dehydrogenase cDNA and genomic cloning, primary structure, and expression in *Escherichia coli, J. Biol. Chem.*, 267, 3030, 1992.

81. **Meier-Tackmann, D., Eckey, R., Wolff, C., Eitzen, R. V., Agarwal, D. P., and Goedde, H. W.,** Tumor-associated aldehyde dehydrogenase (ALDH3): expression in different human tumor cell lines with and without treatment with 3-methylcholanthrene, in *Enzymology and Molecular Biology of Carbonyl Metabolism*, Vol. 4, Weiner, H., Crabb, D. W., and Flynn, T. G., Eds., Plenum Press, New York, 1993, 115.

82. **Miyauchi, K., Masaki, R., Taketani, S., Yamamoto, A., Akayama, M., and Tashiro, Y.,** Molecular cloning, sequencing, and expression of cDNA for rat liver microsomal aldehyde dehydrogenase, *J. Biol. Chem.*, 266, 19536, 1991.

83. **Holmes, R. S. and VandeBerg, J. L.,** Aldehyde dehydrogenases, aldehyde oxidase and xanthine oxidase from baboon tissues: phenotypic variability and subcellular distribution in liver and brain, *Alcohol*, 3, 205, 1986.

84. **Algar, E. M. and Holmes, R. S.,** Purification and properties of mouse stomach aldehyde dehydrogenase. Evidence for a role in the oxidation of peroxidic and aromatic aldehydes, *Biochim. Biophys. Acta*, 995, 168, 1989.

85. **Holmes, R. S., van Oorschot, R. A. H., and VandeBerg, J. L.,** Aldehyde dehydrogenase (ALDH) isozymes in the gray short-tailed opossum (*Monodelphis domestica*): tissue and subcellular distribution and biochemical genetics of ALDH3, *Biochem. Genet.*, 29, 163, 1991.

86. **Greenfield, N. J. and Pietruszko, R.,** Two aldehyde dehydrogenases from human liver, *Biochim. Biophys. Acta*, 483, 35, 1977.

87. **Wang, S.-L., Wu, C.-W., Cheng, T.-C., and Yin, S.-J.,** Isolation of high-$K_m$ aldehyde dehydrogenase isoenzymes from human gastric mucosa, *Biochem. Int.* 22, 199, 1990.

88. **Goedde, H. W. and Agarwal, D. P.,** Polymorphism of aldehyde dehydrogenase and alcohol sensitivity, *Enzyme* 37, 29, 1987.

89. **Yin, S.-J., Wang, S.-L., and Jörnvall, H.,** Human high-Km Aldehyde dehydrogenase (ALDH3): Molecular, kinetic and structural features, in *Enzymology and Molecular Biology of Carbonyl Metabolism*, Vol. 4, Weiner, H., Crabb, D. W., and Flynn, T. G., Eds., Plenum Press, New York, 1993, 87.

90. **Yoshida, A., Huang, I.-Y., and Ikawa, M.,** Molecular abnormality of an inactive aldehyde dehydrogenase variant commonly found in Orientals, *Proc. Natl. Acad. Sci. U.S.A.*, 81, 258, 1984.

91. **Hempel, J., Kaiser, R., and Jörnvall, H.,** Human liver mitochondrial aldehyde dehydrogenase: a C-terminal segment positions and defines the structure corresponding to the one reported to differ in the Oriental enzyme variant, *FEBS Lett.*, 173, 367, 1984.

92. **Agarwal, D. P., Harada, S. H., and Goedde, W. H.,** Racial differences in biological sensitivity to ethanol: the role of alcohol dehydrogenase and aldehyde dehydrogenase isozymes, *Alcoholism: Clin. Exp. Res.* 5, 12, 1981.

93. **Farrés, J., Wang, X., Takahashi, K., Cunningham, S. J., Wang, T. T., and Weiner, H.,** Effects of changing glutamate 487 to lysine in rat and human liver mitochondrial aldehyde dehydrogenase: a model to study human (Oriental type) class 2 aldehyde dehydrogenase, *J. Biol. Chem.*, 269, 13854, 1994.

94. **Mizoi, Y., Ijiri, I., Tatsuno, Y., Kijima, T., Fujiwara, S., and Adachi, J.,** Relationship between facial flushing and blood acetaldehyde levels after alcohol intake, *Pharmacol. Biochem. Behav.*, 10, 303, 1979.

95. **Simanowski, U. A., Suter, P., Stickel, F., Maier, H., Waldherr, R., Smith, D., Russell, R. M., and Seitz, H. K.,** Esophageal epithelial hyperproliferation following long-term alcohol consumption in rats: effects of age and salivary gland function, *J. Natl. Cancer Inst.*, 85, 2030, 1993.

96. **Tsutsumi, M., Takase, S., and Takada, A.,** Genetic factors related to the development of carcinoma in digestive organs in alcoholics, *Alcohol Alcohol.,* 28, S1B, 21, 1993.

97. **Teng, Y.-S.,** Stomach aldehyde dehydrogenase: report of a new locus, *Hum. Hered.,* 31, 74, 1981.

98. **Santisteban, I., Povey, S., West, L. F., Parrington, J. M., and Hopkinson, D. A.,** Chromosome assignment, biochemical and immunological studies on a human aldehyde dehydrogenase, ALDH3, *Ann. Hum. Genet.,* 49, 87, 1985.

99. **Duley, J. A., Harris, O., and Holmes, R. S.,** Analysis of human alcohol- and aldehyde- metabolizing isozymes by electrophoresis and isoelectric focusing, *Alcohol. Clin. Exp. Res.,* 9, 263, 1985.

100. **Dyck, L. E.,** Presence and polymorphism of a class 3 ALDH in human saliva, *Alcoholism: Clin. Exp. Res.,* 18, 14A, 1994.

101. **Koivusalo, M., Aarnio, M., Baumann, M., and Rautoma, P.,** NAD(P)-linked aromatic aldehydes preferring cytoplasmic aldehyde dehydrogenases in the rat. Constitutive and inducible forms in liver, lung, stomach and intestinal mucosa, in *Enzymology and Molecular Biology of Carbonyl Metabolism,* Vol. 2, Weiner, H. and Flynn, T. G., Eds., Alan R. Liss, New York, 1993, 19.

102. **Yin, S.-J., Liao, C.-S., Chen, C.-M., Fan, F.-T., and Lee, S.-C.,** Genetic polymorphism and activities of human lung alcohol and aldehyde dehydrogenases: implications for ethanol metabolism and cytotoxicity, *Biochem. Genet.,* 30, 203, 1992.

103. **Meier-Tackmann, D., Agarwal, D. P., Saha, N., and Goedde, H. W.,** Aldehyde dehydrogenase isozymes in stomach autopsy specimens from Germans and Chinese, *Enzyme,* 32, 170, 1984.

# 4

# Free Radicals and Ethanol Toxicity

Emanuele Albano and Paolo Clot

## CONTENTS

## 4.1   INTRODUCTION

Recently, the possible involvement of free radicals in the pathogenesis of tissue damage associated with a number of human diseases has received increasing attention.[1,2] It is now well established that free radical intermediates and particularly radical species derived from oxygen can be produced in the cells by a variety of enzymatic and nonenzymatic reactions and, by interacting with biological constituents, impair cellular functions.[1]

This chapter will discuss the mechanisms that can lead to the formation of free radical species during ethanol intoxication and the possible involvement of oxidative events in causing ethanol-mediated injury to the gastrointestinal tract.

### 4.1.1   Evidence for the Involvement of Free Radicals in Causing Alcohol-Related Diseases

Several studies have shown that both acute and chronic alcohol administration to rats increases the formation of lipid peroxidation products and decreases tissue levels of antioxidants such as reduced glutathione (GSH) and $\alpha$-tocopherol.[3-5] Furthermore, in an experimental model of intragastric alcohol feeding of rat, the stimulation of lipid peroxidation by ethanol is associated with the development of liver damage and fibrosis.[6,7] Similar studies performed in humans demonstrate that markers of lipid peroxidation such as lipoperoxides and conjugated dienes show higher levels in liver biopsies obtained from heavy drinkers than in specimens from nondrinkers.[8-10] Furthermore, an increased breath exhalation of pentane, another indicator of peroxidative damage, is observed in patients with alcoholic liver disease.[11] Recently, we reported that in heavy drinkers blood levels of malonildialdehyde (MDA) and lipid hydroperoxides are about threefold higher than in moderate drinkers and that the amount of peroxidation products correlates with the daily intake of ethanol, irrespective of the extent of liver injury.[12]

## 4.2    MECHANISMS OF FREE RADICAL FORMATION BY ETHANOL

Most of the current information concerning the generation of free radical species in tissues exposed to ethanol has been obtained in studies performed in the liver; however, many of the enzymatic systems involved are present also in the epithelial cells of the esophagus, stomach, and intestine. Thus, the reactions observed in the liver can occur in other organs of the digestive apparatus.

### 4.2.1    Formation of Reactive Oxygen Species

The formation of reactive oxygen species such as superoxide anion ($O_2^-$) and hydrogen peroxide ($H_2O_2$) represents an important cause of oxidative injury in many diseases associated with free radical formation. In the presence of trace amounts of transition metal, most frequently iron, $O_2^-$ and $H_2O_2$ generated from either enzymatic or nonenzymatic sources might undergo the so-called metal-catalyzed Haber-Weiss reaction, producing highly reactive hydroxyl radicals (OH·), which oxidize biological constituents.[13] Several enzymatic reactions have been proposed as a source of reactive oxygen species during ethanol intoxication and these will be discussed in detail. It is important, however, to stress that the presence of "free" iron represents a critical factor in the generation of hydroxyl radicals as well as in the catalysis of lipid peroxidation reactions. The form of iron associated with free radical reactions seems to be related to a small pool of low molecular weight nonprotein iron complexes with ATP, ADP, or citrate.[14] Alcohol abuse in humans is often associated with an impaired iron utilization and an increased deposition of the element in several tissues.[15,16] At cellular levels ethanol load increases the cytosolic level of low molecular weight iron in liver and cerebellar cells.[17] In the liver, the release of iron from ferritin might be responsible for this effect, since the rise in the cytosolic levels of NADH or the generation of superoxide anion[18] during acetaldehyde oxidation by xanthine oxidase or aldehyde oxidase[19] (see below) has been shown to release catalytically active iron from ferritin.

#### 4.2.1.1    Role of Cytochrome P-450 System

Alcohol exposure has been shown to enhance the activity of a NADPH-dependent ethanol oxidizing system in the endoplasmic reticulum of hepatocytes as well as in other extrahepatic tissues.[20] This system has been characterized in both rodents and humans, showing that it relies on the activity of cytochrome P-4502E1 isozyme (CYP2E1).[20,21] CYP2E1 has an especially high rate of NADPH oxidase activity, even in the absence of substrates, which leads to an extensive production of $O_2^-$ and $H_2O_2$.[22-24] Microsomes obtained from rats chronically exposed to alcohol are more active in producing $O_2^-$, $H_2O_2$, and OH· than microsomes from untreated animals.[25,26] These microsomes also show an enhanced susceptibility to lipid peroxidation which can be selectively inhibited by antibodies directed against CYP2E1.[24] Furthermore, liposome vesicles containing P-450 reductase and CYP2E1 are peroxidized at rates 5- to 10-fold higher than membranes containing other forms of cytochrome P-450.[24] NADH can replace NADPH as cofactor for the microsomal production of reactive oxygen species.[27] Such a peculiarity can be particularly important during ethanol intoxication because alcohol metabolism leads to an excess formation of NADH. A correlation between the CYP2E1 content and increased NADPH-oxidase activity has also been observed in human liver microsomes.[28] Thus, the high efficiency of CYP2E1 in reducing oxygen to superoxide anion and hydrogen peroxide could be regarded as one of the factors contributing to the stimulation of lipid peroxidation during chronic exposure to alcohol.[21]

### 4.2.1.2    Role of Mitochrondria

The respiratory chain of mitochondria represents one of the main sources of superoxide anion in cells.[29] Acute alcohol exposure has been shown to increase superoxide production by submitochrondrial particles.[30] Such an effect coupled with the increased availability of NADH can be responsible for causing oxidative injury to mitochondria.[31] Recently, Kukielka et al.[31] reported that chronic alcohol intake increases the production of reactive oxygen species by intact liver mitochondria incubated with NADH or NADPH. Superoxide formation appears to be independent from the activity of the respiratory chain and depends on the stimulation by ethanol of the activity of rotenone-insensitive NADH-cytochrome c reductase, an enzyme of the outer mitochondrial membrane.[32] The importance of this enzyme in causing ethanol-induced oxidative injury to the mitochondria could be even greater than the respiratory chain because it does not require the transfer of NADH through the mitochondrial membranes.

### 4.2.1.3    Role of Cytosolic Enzymes

Xanthine oxidase is involved in the formation of reactive oxygen species in tissues undergoing reperfusion injury.[33] Several studies have demonstrated that both acute and chronic ethanol intoxication favor the conversion of xanthine dehydrogenase to the oxidase form.[34,35] Moreover, an increase in purine degradation leading to an excess formation of xanthine and hypoxanthine has been documented following alcohol administration.[36] The contribution of this metabolic pathway in causing oxidative damage by alcohol is suggested by the observation that the inhibition of xanthine oxidase by allopurinol prevents the stimulation of ethanol-induced lipid peroxidation in both liver and brain.[36,37]

The oxidation of the excess of acetaldehyde present in the tissues during ethanol metabolism by the enzymes aldehyde oxidase or xanthine oxidase has been suggested as an alternative pathway for the generation of $O_2^-$ and hydroxyl radicals during ethanol metabolism.[38] However, the possibility that acetaldehyde might be an effective substrate for xanthine oxidase is still being debated, since the $K_m$ of the enzyme for acetaldehyde (30 m$M$)[39] exceeds the concentrations of aldehyde present in the liver during alcohol metabolism.[40] Nonetheless, Puntarulo and Cederbaum have reported that concentrations of acetaldehyde close to those present in the liver following alcohol intake (about 0.1 m$M$) can induce the formation of reactive oxygen species by xanthine oxidase.[41] Besides xanthine oxidase, molybdenum-containing aldehyde oxidase, which has a much lower $K_m$ for acetaldehyde (1 m$M$), has also been shown to produce superoxide anion.[42] Consistently, menadione, an inhibitor of aldehyde oxidase, significantly decreased lipid peroxidation when added to isolated hepatocytes incubated with ethanol or acetaldehyde.[43] At present, however, it is not yet clear to what extent the metabolism of acetaldehyde by xanthine oxidase and aldehyde oxidase might contribute to the development of oxidative injury during alcohol abuse. On this respect, a recent study by Nordback et al.[44] has shown that reactive oxygen species produced by xanthine oxidase are responsible for acute pancreatic damage in isolated perfused canine pancreas exposed to acetaldehyde.

### 4.2.1.4    Other Sources of Reactive Oxygen Species

The formation of superoxide anion by activated phagocytes represents an important source of oxidizing species in inflammated tissues.[45] Bautista and Spitzer[46] have observed that acute ethanol administration stimulates superoxide anion production by *in situ* perfused rat liver and have suggested that Kupffer cells are likely responsible for this effect. Consistently, *in vivo* ethanol treatment of mice increases the phagocytic activity of Kupffer cells.[47] Although short-term *in vitro* exposure of macrophages to low doses of ethanol is capable of stimulating the superoxide anion production,[48] the release of arachidonic acid metabolites appears to be involved in the activation of Kupffer cells by ethanol, since ibuprofen, an inhibitor of cyclooxygenase pathway, completely abolishes the production of superoxide anion in perfused liver.[46] The possibility that ethanol might induce the production of chemotactic factors for phagocytes has been extensively studied by Roll and co-workers, who found that a lipid-derived chemotactic factor for neutrophils is formed by rat hepatocytes exposed to alcohol.[49] Further experiments indicate that the formation of such a factor requires free iron and depends on the oxidation of unsaturated lipids by reactive oxygen species generated during acetaldehyde metabolism by cytosolic enzymes, possibly aldehyde oxidase or xanthine oxidase.[50,51] 4-Hydroxynonenal (4-HNE), a reactive aldehyde produced during the peroxidative degradation of unsaturated fatty acids, acts as a powerful chemotactic stimulus for rat neutrophils,[52] and could be responsible for some of the effects observed by Roll's group. Other studies have shown that protein-derived[53] and leucotriene-derived chemotactic factors[54] are also produced by liver cells in the presence of ethanol and that alcohol intereferes with the expression of leukocyte adhesion molecules by the endothelial cells.[55] These findings indicate that ethanol can directly stimulate granulocyte infiltration of the tissues where is metabolized. Thus, the formation of oxygen-free radicals by activated phagocytes might be regarded as an important cause of tissue injury in the gastroenteric tract where ethanol often induces leukocyte infiltration.[56,57]

## 4.2.2    Free Radicals Species Derived From Ethanol or Acetaldehyde

Oxygen-derived free radicals are not the only reactive species produced in relation to alcohol metabolism, and experiments using electron spin resonance (ESR) spectroscopy in combination with spin trapping agents have demonstrated that carbon-centered free radical intermediates are produced during ethanol metabolism.[58-60]

### 4.2.2.1    Hydroxyethyl Free Radicals

We and others have demonstrated that rat liver microsomes incubated in the presence of ethanol and NADPH are able to produce 1-hydroxyethyl free radical intermediates.[58-60] The formation of these radical species has been recently confirmed *in vivo* by detecting hydroxyethyl radicals in either rats and ADH-negative deermice receiving acute doses of ethanol.[61,62] Ethanol can be oxidized by liver microsomes to acetaldehyde through a nonenzymatic pathway involving the presence of hydroxyl radicals (OH·), originating from iron-catalyzed degradation of $H_2O_2$.[25] Although this nonenzymatic pathway can be partially responsible for the formation of hydroxyethyl radicals,[63] other evidence indicates that the production of alcohol-free radicals might be due to an oxidizing species possibly bound to cytochrome P-450 and sufficiently reactive to abstract a proton from the alcohol α-carbon.[64] Indeed, results from our lab indicate that CYP2E1 plays an important role in the formation of hydroxyethyl radicals during ethanol metabolism, since the generation of alcohol-derived free radicals is specifically enhanced following induction of CYP2E1 by chronic ethanol feeding of the rats, while antibodies against CYP2E1 inhibit the spin trapping of alcohol-derived radicals.[64] Furthermore, reconstituted membrane vesicles containing CYP2E1 and cytochrome P-450 reductase, when incubated with NADPH and ethanol, form alcohol-free radicals more efficiently than vesicles containing CYP2B1.[64] The formation of hydroxyethyl free radical has also been observed in microsomes obtained from the liver of kidney donors incubated with ethanol.[65] In human liver microsomes, a direct relationship exists between the levels of CYP2E1 measured in the different microsomal preparations and the capacity of microsomes to generate hydroxyethyl radicals, indicating that CYP2E1 is also responsible for the formation of alcohol radicals in human tissues.

So far the mechanisms by which hydroxyethyl free radicals might contribute to the damaging effects of ethanol have not been elucidated. We have reported that the spin trapping agent 4-pyridyl-N-oxide-t-butyl nitrone (4-POBN) inhibits the covalent binding of ethanol residues to proteins in liver microsomes incubated with NADPH and $^{14}$C-ethanol, without affecting acetaldehyde production.[66] The possibility that hydroxyethyl radicals might be involved in the alkylation of hepatic proteins is supported by the observation that *in vitro* chemically produced hydroxyethyl radicals forms stable adducts with albumin or fibrinogen.[67] Alkylation of proteins by acetaldehyde is one of the mechanisms by which alcohol induces immunologic responses toward liver cells.[68,69] Recently, we have observed that patients with alcoholic cirrhosis, but not cirrhotics without alcohol abuse or healthy subjects, have increased serum levels of both IgG and IgA reacting with proteins of liver microsomes incubated with ethanol and NADPH as well as with human serum albumin modified by the reaction with hydroxyethyl radicals.[67] Although the sera of alcoholic cirrhotics also contains antibodies directed against acetaldehyde-modified proteins,[70,71] they do not cross-react with the epitopes derived from hydroxyethyl radicals.[67] The detection of these specific antibodies confirms that hydroxyethyl radicals are actually produced in humans as a result of alcohol abuse and suggests their involvement in the development of autoimmune reactions observed in alcoholic patients.[72]

### 4.2.2.2   Acetaldehyde-Derived Free Radicals

As mentioned above, xanthine oxidase and aldehyde oxidase metabolize acetaldehyde with the formation of reactive oxygen species. Using ESR spectroscopy coupled with spin trapping technique, we have recently observed the production of a carbon centered free radical during the oxidation of acetaldehyde by xanthine oxidase. This new radical intermediate has been identified as methyl carbonyl species ($CH_3CO$) and originates from the abstraction of an hydrogen atom from the acetaldehyde molecule.[73] The use of superoxide dismutase, catalase, and hydroxyl radical scavengers demonstrates that OH· radicals are responsible for the free radical activation of acetaldehyde, suggesting the possibility that acetaldehyde might act at the same time as source of reactive oxygen species, being a substrate for xanthine oxidase, as well as as target for OH· radicals.[73] The formation of methyl carbonyl radicals by xanthine oxidase is evident using a concentration of the aldehyde as low as 0.1 m$M$, and when acetaldehyde is produced from ethanol in the presence of alcohol dehydrogenase and NAD$^+$.[73] Thus, the formation of radical species from acetaldehyde might contribute to cause the oxidative injury observed during acetaldehyde metabolism by xanthine oxidase or by aldehyde oxidase. Furthermore, by covalent binding to proteins,[73] methyl carbonyl free radicals might also help stimulate the immunological reactions triggered by acetaldehyde alkylation of proteins.[70,71]

## 4.3   POSSIBLE ROLE OF FREE RADICAL FORMATION IN GASTROINTESTINAL TRACT INJURY BY ETHANOL

### 4.3.1   Role of Free Radicals in Gastric Mucosal Injury by Alcohol

The possibility that oxidative injury might be involved in causing gastric mucosal damage associated with alcohol abuse was first suggested because of the fact that oral administration of absolute ethanol to rats resulted in a decrease of nonprotein sulfydrils levels, consisting mainly of reduced glutathione (GSH), and an increase of lipid peroxidation in the stomach mucosa.[74,75] In agreement with these findings, further studies have demonstrated that pretreatment of rats with antioxidant agents, superoxide dismutase, catalase, hydroxyl radical scavengers, and thiol compounds prevents the formation of gastric lesions caused by orally administered ethanol.[74,76-79] Szelenyi and Brune have also shown that the inhibition of superoxide dismutase by diethyldithiocarbamate leads to an extension of hemorrhagic lesions in the stomach of rats receiving ethanol.[79]

Experiments performed with cultured gastric mucosal cells have confirmed that superoxide anion is actually produced following the addition of ethanol and that $O_2^-$ generation increases with the amount of ethanol used.[80] Cellular damage also increases concomitantly with the formation of superoxide anion. The addition of the iron chelator desferrioxamine, or of superoxide dismutase, catalase, and hydroxyl radical scavengers to cultured gastric mucosal cells prevents cell death,[80] suggesting that the intracellular production of reactive oxygen species might be responsible for the ethanol-induced damage of gastric mucosal cells. Ethanol is actively metabolized by gastric mucosa,[81] thus the stimulation in $O_2^-$ production observed in the presence of ethanol could be caused by an increased acetaldehyde oxidation within the mucosal cells by xanthine oxidase or aldehyde oxidase. In support of this possibility, the pretreatment of rats with allopurinol or oxypurinol to block xanthine oxidase protects against the appearance of hemorrhagic lesions due to alcohol administration.[76,77,82] Shaw and co-workers have observed that acute ethanol dosage of rats affects the gastric uptake of vitamin $B_{12}$ by the intrinsic factor and in parallel lowers GSH content of the mucosa.[83] Oxidative damage might be implicated in these effects of alcohol, since the same authors have also reported that in gastric homogenates the formation of oxygen radicals by xanthine oxidase and acetaldehyde also impairs the binding efficiency of the intrinsic factor.[83] Moreover, feeding sodium tungstate to rats (which decreases xanthine oxidase activity) markedly attenuates the effects of ethanol on both intrinsic factor activity and GSH levels.[83]

In contrast to the above results, Kvietys et al.[84] have reported that xanthine oxidase inactivation by rat tungsten feeding or the treatment with superoxide dismutase, catalase, benzoate, or desferrioxamine cannot protect against gastric mucosal injury when the stomach is perfused with 10 to 30% ethanol solutions. In this experimental model, the depletion of circulating neutrophils affords protection, and these findings lead the authors to suggest a preeminent role of leukocyte infiltration in causing ethanol damage to the gastric mucosa.[84] A possible explanation for these conflicting results possibly resides in the fact that Kvietys and co-workers have evaluated the mucosal damage caused by stomach perfusion with 30% ethanol solutions by measuring the leakage into the gastric perfusate of $^{51}$Cr-EDTA injected intravenously.[84] This approach probably allows us to appreciate mucosal damage which is milder than the hemorrhagic lesions observed by others using absolute ethanol.[74-79] Indeed, an increased leakage of $^{51}$Cr-EDTA from the gastric surface occurs in the absence of frank bleeding.[84] Thus, neutrophil infiltration and endogenous production of oxygen radicals might both contribute to the pathogenesis of gastric injury by ethanol. On the other hand, ethanol is able to stimulate the production of neutrophil chemotactic factors through a free radical mechanism[50,51]; and during gastric and intestinal ischemia oxygen radicals generated by xanthine oxidase are involved in the attraction and activation of granulocytes within the mucosa.[85,86]

The lowering of the intracellular levels of GSH is generally believed to be an indicator of oxidative tissue injury, since, as a cofactor of glutathione peroxidase enzymes, GSH is involved in the detoxification of hydrogen peroxide and lipid hydroperoxides.[87] An association between a marked decrease in GSH levels and the appearance of mucosa injury has been documented *in vivo* using canine chambered stomach preparations exposed to 40% ethanol, but not when a lower alcohol concentration (8%) is used.[88] We know little about the mechanisms by which ethanol lowers the GSH content of gastric cells; however, one cannot exclude that other mechanisms beside oxidative reactions might also be involved, since in the liver ethanol affects GSH synthesis[89] and stimulates the efflux of the tripeptide.[90] The importance of GSH in the onset of alcohol-induced gastric mucosal injury in humans has been addressed by recent studies in healthy volunteers undergoing gastric endoscopy. In these subjects a 65% decrease of GSH can be measured in gastric biopsies from the stomach body and antrum after spraying the mucosa with 80% ethanol through the endoscope.[91,92] This effect is associated with a significant increase in the number of hemorrhagic lesions.[91] The parenteral administration of 2.4 g of GSH before ethanol application appreciably reduced both the extent of mucosal lesions and GSH depletion,[92] giving further evidence to the possible occurrence of free radical–mediated processes in human gastric injury by alcohol.

### 4.3.2 Alcohol Damage of the Esophagus and Intestine: Is There a Possible Role for Free Radicals?

The function and structure of intestinal mucosa are often impaired as a result of alcohol abuse.[57] The possibility that free radical mechanisms might be involved in causing ethanol-mediated lesion to intestinal cells can be postulated due to the involvement of oxidative injury in the pathogenesis of intestine damage caused by ischemia-reperfusion or chronic inflammatory diseases.[86] Furthermore, ethanol and oxygen-free radicals similarly increase intestinal mucosa permeability.[93,94] Several studies have demonstrated the presence in the intestinal tract of some enzymes implicated in free radical formation during ethanol exposure. Immunohistochemical studies have shown that CYP2E1 is detectable in duodenal and jejunal villous cells of control rats.[95] Chronic ethanol feeding appreciably increases CYP2E1 expression in these areas and also leads to the appearance of the cytochrome in the surface epithelium of proximal colon.[95] On the other hand, ethanol feeding appears to differently modify the expression of other cytochrome P-450 forms in different parts of the small intestine, since it causes a small elevation of CYP3A2 in microsomes from duodenum and a decrease in the expression of CYP1A2 and CYP3A2 in the jejunal mucosa.[96] These findings along with the observation that microsomes from small intestine of chronic ethanol-fed rats show an increased oxidation of ethanol[97] suggest that free radical species produced by CYP2E1 may play a role in causing ethanol-induced lesions of small intestine. Moreover, oxygen radicals may be also produced within the intestinal mucosa by the action of xanthine oxidase which appears to be located in intestinal epithelial cells.[98]

Recently, Mufti et al.[99] have reported some indirect evidence that free radical mechanisms might play a role in the promoting action exerted by alcohol on esophagus carcinogenesis. They have observed that chronic ethanol feeding of mice increases the number of esophageal cancers induced by different carcinogens, and that the animal supplementation with vitamin E prevents this effect.[99] Furthermore, a relationship exists between the number of tumors in the esophagus and the levels of lipid peroxidation products measured in the liver and in the esophagus.[99] Similar findings have also been obtained in a model of oral carcinogenesis in hamsters where ethanol exerts a promoting effect on tumor growth.[100] The presence of xanthine oxidase has been located in the epithelial cells of the mouth and of the esophagus[98] and chronic ethanol treatment induces the expression of CYP2E1 in squamous epithelial cells of the oral and esophageal mucosa.[95] These enzymes might represent possible sources of reactive oxygen species which have been proposed to exert a promoting effect during epithelial cell carcinogenesis.[101,102] Considering that about 75% of esophageal cancers are associated with alcohol abuse and that ethanol consumption represents a rich factor in the development of cancer in other areas of gastrointestinal tract,[103] the implications of these findings might be of great interest.

## 4.4 CONCLUSIONS

In conclusion, a body of evidence exists that demonstrates that ethanol metabolism is associated with the formation by various mechanisms of free radical intermediates. The data so far available offer some indications that processes involving free radicals might be implicated in causing gastric lesions and also suggest their possible implication in the pathogenesis of toxic as well as carcinogenic actions exerted by alcohol in the esophagus and intestinal tract. However, further studies are needed to clarify the role of oxidative events in the pathogenesis of ethanol-mediated injury to the gatrointestinal apparatus.

## REFERENCES

1. **Kehrer, J. P.,** Free radicals as mediators of tissue injury and disease, *Crit. Rev. Toxicol.,* 23, 21, 1993.
2. **Gutteridge, J. M. C.,** Free radicals in disease processes: a compilation of causes and consequences, *Free Rad. Res. Commun.,* 19, 141, 1993.
3. **Dianzani, M. U.,** Lipid peroxidation in ethanol poisoning: a critical reconsideration, *Alcohol Alcohol.,* 20, 161, 1985.
4. **Albano, E., Ingelman-Sundberg, M., Tomasi, A., and Poli, G.,** Free radical mediated reactions and ethanol toxicity: some considerations on the methodological approaches, in *Alcoholism: A Molecular Perspective,* Palmer, T. N., Ed., Plenum Press, New York, 1991, 45.
5. **Nordmann, R., Ribière, C., and Rouach, H.,** Implication of free radical mechanisms in ethanol induced cellular injury, *Free Rad. Biol. Med.,* 12, 219, 1992.
6. **Kamimura, S., Gall, K., Britton, S. R., Bacon, B. R., Triadafilopulos, G., and Tsukamoto, H.,** Increased 4-hydroxynonenal levels in experimental alcoholic liver disease: association of lipid peroxidation with liver fibrogenesis, *Hepatology,* 16, 448, 1992.
7. **French, S. W., Wong, K., Jui, L., Albano, E., Hagbjörk, A.-L., and Ingelman-Sundberg, M.,** Effect of ethanol on cytochrome P-450 (CYP2E1), lipid peroxidation and serum protein adduct formation in relation to liver pathology pathogenesis, *Exp. Mol. Pathol.,* 58, 61, 1993.
8. **Suematzu, T., Matsumura,T., Sato, N., Miyamoto, T., Ooka, T., Kamada, T., and Abe, H.,** Lipid peroxidation in alcoholic disease in humans, *Alcoholism: Clin. Exp. Res.,* 5, 427, 1981.
9. **Shaw, S., Rubin, K. P., and Lieber, C. S.,** Depressed hepatic glutathione and increased diene conjugates in alcoholic liver disease. Evidence of lipid peroxidation, *Dig. Dis. Sci.,* 28, 585, 1983.
10. **Situnayake, R. D., Crump, B. J., Thurnham, D. I., Davies, J. A., Gearty, J., and Davis, M.,** Lipid peroxidation and hepatic antioxidants in alcoholic liver disease, *Gut,* 31, 1311, 1990.
11. **Letteron, P., Duchettelle, V., Berson, A., Fromenty, B., Fish, C., Degott, C., Benhamou, P. J., and Pessayre, D.,** Increased ethane exhalation, an *in vivo* index of lipid peroxidation, in alcohol abusers, *Gut,* 34, 409, 1993.
12. **Clot, P., Tabone, M., Aricò, S., and Albano, E.,** Monitoring oxidative damage in patients with liver cirrhosis and different daily alcohol intake, *Gut,* 35, 1637, 1994.
13. **Aust, S. D., Morehouse, L. A., and Thomas, C. E.,** Role of metals in oxygen radical reactions, *J. Free Rad. Biol. Med.,* 1, 3, 1985.
14. **Minotti, G., Di Gennaro, M., D'Ugo, D., and Granone, P.,** Possible source of iron for lipid peroxidation, *Free Rad. Res. Commun.,* 12–13, 99, 1991.
15. **Chapman, R. W., Morgan, M. J., Bell, R., and Sherlock, S.,** Hepatic iron uptake in alcoholic liver disease, *Gastroenterology,* 84, 143, 1983.
16. **Irving, M. G., Halliday, J. W., and Powell L. W.,** Association between alcoholism and increased hepatic iron store, *Alcoholism: Clin. Exp. Res.,* 12, 7, 1988.
17. **Rouach, H., Houzè, P., Orfanelli, M. T., Gentil, M., Bourdon, R., and Nordmann, R.,** Effect of acute ethanol administration of the subcellular distribution of iron in rat liver and cerebellum, *Biochem. Pharmacol.,* 39, 1095, 1990.
18. **Tophan, R., Coger, M., Pearce, K., and Schultz, P.,** The mobilization of ferritin by liver cytosol: a comparison of xanthine and NADH as reducing substrates, *Biochem. J.,* 261, 137, 1989.
19. **Shaw, S. and Jayatilleke, E.,** Ethanol-induced iron mobilization: role of acetaldehyde-aldehyde oxidase generated superoxide, *Free Rad. Biol. Med.,* 9, 11, 1990.
20. **Ingelman-Sundberg, M., Johansson, I., Terelius, Y., Eliasson, E., Ekström, G., Bühler, R., and Lindros, K. O.,** Ethanol-inducible CYP2E1: toxicological importance and regulation by nutrients, in *Food, Nutrition and Chemical Toxicity,* Parke, D. V., Ioannides, C., and Walker, R., Eds., Smith-Gordon, London, 1993, 147.
21. **Ingelman-Sundberg, M., Johansson, I., Yin, H., Terelius, Y., Eliasson, E., Clot, P., and Albano, E.,** Ethanol-inducible cytochrome P4502E1: genetic polymorphism, regulation and possible role in the etiology of alcohol-induced liver disease, *Alcohol,* 10, 447, 1993.
22. **Ingelman-Sundberg, M. and Johansson, I.,** Mechanisms of hydroxyl radical formation and ethanol oxidation by ethanol-inducible and other forms of rabbit liver microsomal cytochrome P-450, *J. Biol. Chem.,* 259. 6447, 1984.
23. **Gorsky, L. D., Koop, D. R., and Coon, M. J.,** On the stoichimetry of the oxidase and monoxygenase reactions catalyzed by liver microsomal cytochrome P-450, *J. Biol. Chem.,* 259, 6812, 1984.
24. **Ekström, G. and Ingelman-Sundberg, M.,** Rat liver microsomal NADPH-supported oxidase activity and lipid peroxidation dependent on ethanol-inducible cytochrome P-450, *Biochem. Pharmacol.,* 38, 1313, 1989.
25. **Cederbaum, A. I.,** Oxygen radical generation by microsomes: role of iron and implications for alcohol metabolism and toxicity, *Free Rad. Biol. Med.,* 7, 559, 1989.
26. **Persson, J. O., Terelius, Y., and Ingelman-Sundberg, M.,** Cytochrome P-450-dependent formation of reactive oxygen radicals: isozyme-specific inhibition of P-450-mediates reduction of oxygen and carbon tetrachloride, *Xenobiotica,* 20, 887, 1990.

27. **Dicker, E. and Cederbaum, A. I.,** Increases NADH-dependent production of reactive oxygen interemediates by microsomes after chronic ethanol consumption: comparisons with NADPH, *Arch. Biochem. Biophys.* 293, 274, 1992.

28. **Ekström, G., Von Bahr, C., and Ingelman-Sundberg, M.,** Human liver microsomal cytochrome P450IIE1. Immunological evaluation of its contribution to microsomal ethanol oxidation, carbon tetrachloride reduction and NADPH oxidase activity, *Biochem. Pharmacol.,* 38, 689, 1989.

29. **Forman, H. J. and Boveris, A.,** Superoxide radical and hydrogen peroxide in mitochondria, in *Free Radicals in Biology,* Pryor, W. A., Ed., Academic Press, New York, 1988, 65.

30. **Sinaceur, J., Ribière, C., Sarburault, D., and Nordmann, R.,** Superoxide formation in liver mitochondria during ethanol intoxication: possible role in alcohol hepatotoxicity, in *Free Radicals in Liver Injury,* Poli, G., Cheeseman, K. H., Dianzani, M. U., and Slater, T. F., Eds., IRL Press, Oxford, 1985, 175.

31. **Kukielka, E., Dicker, E., and Cederbaum, A. I.,** Increased production of reactive oxygen species by rat liver mitochondria after chronic ethanol treatment, *Arch. Biochem. Biophys.,* 309, 377, 1994.

32. **Rouach, H., Clément, M., Orfanelli, M. T., Janvier, B., Nordmann, J., and Nordmann, R.,** Hepatic lipid peroxidation and mitochondrial susceptibility to peroxidative attacks during ethanol inhalation and withdrawal, *Biochim. Biophys. Acta,* 753, 439, 1983.

33. **McCord, J.,** Oxygen derived free radicals in postischemic tissue damage, *N. Engl. J. Med.,* 321, 159, 1985.

34. **Sultatos, L. G.,** Effect of acute ethanol administration on the hepatic xanthine dehydrogenase/oxidase system in the rat, *J. Pharmacol. Exp. Ther.,* 246, 946, 1988.

35. **Abbondanza, A., Battelli, M. G., Soffritti, M., and Cessi, C.,** Xanthine oxidase status in ethanol-intoxicated rat liver, *Alcoholism: Clin. Exp. Res.,* 13, 841, 1989.

36. **Kato, S., Kavase, T., Alderman, J., Inatomi, N., and Lieber, C. S.,** Role of xanthine oxidase in ethanol-induced lipid peroxidation, *Gastroenterology,* 98, 203, 1990.

37. **Park, K. M., Rouach, H., Orfanelli, M. T., Janvier, B., and Nordmann, R.,** Influence of allopurinol and desferrioxamine on the ethanol-induced oxidative stress in rat liver and cerebellum, in *Alcohol Toxicity and Free Radical Mechanisms,* Nordmann, R., Ribière, C., and Rouach, H., Eds., Pergamon Press, Oxford, 1988, 135.

38. **Shaw, S.,** Lipid peroxidation, iron mobilization and radical generation induced by alcohol, *Free Rad. Biol. Med.,* 7, 541, 1989.

39. **Fridovich, I.,** Oxygen radicals from acetaldehyde, *Free Rad. Biol. Med.,* 7, 557, 1989.

40. **Stowel, A., Hillbom, M., Salaspuro, M., and Lindros, K.,** Low acetaldehyde levels in blood, breath and cerebrospinal fluid of intoxicated humans assayed by improved methods, *Adv. Exp. Med. Biol.,* 132, 635, 1980.

41. **Puntarulo, S. and Cederbaum, A. I.,** Chemiluminescence from acetaldehyde oxidation by xanthine oxidase involves generation of and interactions with hydroxyl radicals, *Alcoholism: Clin. Exp. Res.,* 13, 84, 1989.

42. **Rajagopalan, K. V. and Handler, P.,** Hepatic aldehyde oxidase. III. The substrate binding site, *J. Biol. Chem.,* 239, 2027, 1964.

43. **Shaw, S. and Jayatilleke, E.,** The role of aldehyde oxidase in ethanol-induced hepatic lipid peroxidation in the rat, *Biochem. J.,* 268, 579, 1990.

44. **Nordback, I. H., MacGowan, S., Potter, J. J., and Cameron, J. L.,** The role of acetaldehyde in the pathogenesis of acute pancreatitis, *Ann. Surg.,* 214, 671, 1991.

45. **Badwey, J. A. and Karnovsky, M. L.,** Active oxygen species and the functions of phagocytic leukocytes, *Annu. Rev. Biochem.,* 49, 696, 1980.

46. **Bautista, A. P. and Spitzer, J. J.,** Acute ethanol intoxication stimulates superoxide anion production by *in situ* perfused rat liver, *Hepatology,* 15, 892, 1992.

47. **Enuchi, H., McCuskey, P. A., and McCuskey, R. S.,** Kupffer cell activity and hepatic microvascular events after acute ethanol ingestion in mice, *Hepatology,* 13, 751, 1991.

48. **Dorio, R. J., Hoek, J. B., Rubin, E., and Forman, H. J.,** Ethanol modulation of rat alveolar macrophage superoxide production. *Biochem. Pharmacol.* 37, 3528, 1988.

49. **Roll, F. J., Alexander, M., and Perez, H. D.,** Generation of chemotactic activity for neutrophils by liver cell metabolizing ethanol, *Free Rad. Biol. Med.,* 7, 549, 1989.

50. **Hultcrantz, R., Bissell, D. M., and Roll, F. J.,** Iron mediates production of a neutrophil chemoattractant by rat hepatocytes metabolizing ethanol, *J. Clin. Invest.* 87, 45, 1991.

51. **Roll, F. J., Alexander, A. M., Cua, D., Swanson, W., and Perez, H. D.,** Metabolism of ethanol by rat hepatocytes results in generation of a lipid chemotatic factor: studies using a cell-free system and role of oxygen-derived free radicals, *Arch. Biochem. Biophys.,* 287, 218, 1991.

52. **Curzio, M.,** Chemotactic activity of the lipid peroxidation products 4-hydroxynonenal and homologous hydroxyalkenals, *Biol. Chem. Hoppe-Seyler,* 367, 321, 1986.

53. **Shiratori, Y., Takada, H., Hai, K., Kiriyama, H., Nagura, T., Tanaka, M., Matsumoto, K., and Kamii, K.,** Generation of chemotactic factor by hepatocytes isolated from chronically ethanol-fed rats, *Dig. Dis. Sci.,* 37, 650, 1992.

54. **Shirley, M. A., Reidhead, C. T., and Murphy, R. C.,** Chemotactic LTB4 metabolites produced by hepatocytes in the presence of ethanol, *Biochem. Biophys. Res. Commun.,* 185, 604, 1992.

55. **Adams, D. H.,** Leukocyte adhesion molecules and alcoholic liver disease, *Alcohol Alcohol.,* 29, 249, 1994.
56. **Laine, L. and Weinstein, W. M.,** Histology of alcoholic hemorrhagic "gastritis": a prospective evaluation, *Gastroenterology,* 94, 1254, 1988.
57. **Beck, I. T. and Dinda, P. K.,** Acute exposure of small intestine to ethanol. Effects on morphology and function, *Dig. Dis. Sci.,* 26, 817, 1981.
58. **Albano, E., Tomasi, A., Goria-Gatti, L., Poli, G., Vannini, V., and Dianzani, M. U.,** Free radical metabolism of alcohols in rat liver microsomes, *Free Rad. Res. Commun.,* 3, 243, 1987.
59. **Reinke, L. A., Lai, E. K., DuBose, C. M., and McCay, P. B.,** Reactive free radical generation *in vivo* in heart and liver of ethanol-fed rats: correlation with radical formation *in vitro, Proc. Natl. Acad. Sci. U.S.A.,* 84, 9223, 1987.
60. **Albano, E., Tomasi, A., Goria-Gatti, L., and Dianzani, M. U.,** Spin trapping of free radical species produced during the microsomal metabolism of ethanol, *Chem. Biol. Interact.,* 65, 223, 1988.
61. **Reinke, L. A., Kotake, Y., McCay, P. B., and Janzen, E. G.,** Spin trapping studies of hepatic free radicals formed following the acute administration of ethanol to rats: *in vivo* detection of 1-hydroxyethyl radicals with PBN, *Free Rad. Biol. Med.,* 11, 31, 1991.
62. **Knecht, K. T., Bradfort, B. U., Mason, R. P., and Thurman, G. R.,** *In vivo* formation of free radical metabolite of ethanol, *Mol. Pharmacol.,* 38, 26, 1990.
63. **Knecht, K. T., Thurman, R. G., and Mason, P. R.,** Role of superoxide and trace transition metals in the production of α-hydroxyethyl radical from ethanol by microsomes from alcohol dehydrogenase-deficient deermice, *Arch. Biochem. Biophys.,* 303, 339, 1993.
64. **Albano, E., Tomasi, A., Goria-Gatti, L., Persson, J. O., Terelius, Y., Goria-Gatti, L., Ingelman-Sundberg, M., and Dianzani, M. U.,** Role of ethanol-inducible cytochrome P-450 (P450IIE1) in catalysing the free radical activation of aliphatic alcohols, *Biochem. Pharmacol.,* 41, 1895,1991.
65. **Albano, E., Tomasi, A., and Ingelman-Sundberg, M.,** ESR spin trapping of alcohol derived radicals in microsomes and reconstituted systems, *Methods Enzymol.* 233, 117, 1994.
66. **Albano, E., Parola, M., Comoglio, A., and Dianzani, M. U.,** Evidence for the covalent binding of hydroxyethyl radicals to rat liver microsomal proteins, *Alcohol Alcohol.,* 28, 453, 1993.
67. **Clot, P., Bellomo, G., Tabone, M., Aricò, S., and Albano, E.,** Detection of antibodies against proteins modified by hydroxyethyl free radicals in patients with alcoholic cirrhosis, *Gastroenterology,* 108, 201, 1995.
68. **Israel, Y., Hurwitz, E., Niemela, O., and Arnon, R.,** Monoclonal and polyclonal antibodies against acetaldehyde-containing epitopes in acetaldehyde-protein adducts, *Proc. Natl. Acad. Sci. U.S.A.,* 83, 7923, 1986.
69. **Worrall, S., De Jersey, J., Shanley, B. C., and Wilce, P. A.,** Ethanol induces the production of antibodies to acetaldehyde-modified epitopes in rats, *Alcohol Alcohol.,* 24, 217, 1989.
70. **Niemela, O., Klajner, F., Orrego, H., Vidinis, E., Blendis, L., and Israel, Y.,** Antibodies against acetaldehyde-modified protein epitopes in human alcoholics, *Hepatology,* 7, 1210, 1987.
71. **Koskinas, J., Kenna, J. G., Bird, G. L., Alexander, G. J. M., and Williams, R.,** Immunoglobulin A antibody to a 200-kilodalton cytosolic acetaldehyde adduct in alcoholic hepatitis, *Gastroenterology,* 103, 1860, 1992.
72. **McFarlane, I. G.,** Autoimmunity in liver disease, *Clin Sci.,* 67, 569–587, 1984.
73. **Albano, E., Clot, P., Comoglio, A., Dianzani, M. U., and Tomasi, A.,** Free radical activation of acetaldehyde and its role in protein alkylation, *FEBS Lett.,* 385, 65, 1994.
74. **Mizui, T. and Doteuchi, M.,** Lipid peroxidation: a possible role on gastric damage induced by ethanol in rats, *Life Sci.,* 38, 2163, 1986.
75. **Pihan, G., Regillo, C., and Szabo, S.,** Free radicals and lipid peroxidation in the ethanol- or aspirin-induced gastric mucosal injury, *Dig. Dis. Sci.,* 32, 1395, 1987.
76. **Evangelista, G. and Meli, A.,** Influence of antioxidants and radical scavengers on ethanol-induced gastric ulcer in rats, *Gen. Pharmacol.,* 16, 285, 1985.
77. **Mizui, T., Sato, H., Hirose, F., and Doteuchi, M.,** Effect of antiperoxidative drugs on gastric damage induced by ethanol in rats, *Life Sci.,* 41, 755, 1987.
78. **Terano, A., Hiraishi, H., Ota, S., Shiga, J., and Sugimoto, T.,** Role of oxygen-derived free radicals in ethanol-induced damage of rat stomach, *Gastroenterol. Jpn.,* 24, 488, 1989.
79. **Szelenyi, I. and Brune K.,** Possible role of oxygen free radicals in ethanol induced gastric mucosal damage, *Dig. Dis. Sci.,* 33, 865, 1988.
80. **Mutoh, H., Hiraishi, H., Ota, S., Ivey, K. J., Terano, A., and Sugimoto, T.,** Role of oxygen radicals in ethanol-induced damage to cultured gastric mucosal cells, *Am. J. Physiol.,* G603, 1990.
81. **Lin, R. T., Gentry, T. R., Ito, D., and Yokoyama, H.,** First pass metabolism of ethanol is predominantly gastric, *Alcoholism: Clin. Exp. Res.,* 17, 1228, 1994.
82. **Smith, S. M., Grisham, M. B., Manci, E. A., Granger, D. N., and Kvietys, P. R.,** Gastric mucosal injury in the rat. Role of iron and xanthine oxidase, *Gastroenterology,* 92, 950, 1987.
83. **Shaw, S., Herbert, V., Colman, N., and Jayalleke, E.,** Effect of ethanol-generated free radicals on gastric intrinsic factor and glutathione, *Alcohol,* 7, 153, 1990.
84. **Kvietys, P. R., Twohig, B., and Danzell, J.,** Ethanol-induced injury to rat gastric mucosa. Role of neutrophils and xanthine oxidase, *Gastroenterology,* 98, 909, 1990.

85. **Itoh, M. and Guth, P. H.,** Role of oxygen-derived free radicals in hemorrhagic shock-induced gastric lesions in rat, *Gastroenterology,* 88, 1167, 1985.

86. **Van der Vliet, A. and Bast, A.,** Role of oxygen species in intestinal diseases, *Free Rad. Biol. Med.,* 12, 49, 1992.

87. **Mennervik, B., Carlberg, I., and Larson, K.,** Glutathione: general review of mechanism of action, in *Glutathione. Chemical Biochemical and Medical Aspects,* Dolphin, D., Avramovic, O., and Poulson, R., Eds.,Wiley, New York, 1989, part A, 475.

88. **Victor, B. E., Schmidt, K. L., Smith, G. S., and Miller, T. A.,** Protection against ethanol injury in the canine stomach: role of mucosal glutathione, *Am. J. Physiol.,* 261, G966, 1991.

89. **Lauterburg, B. H., Davies, S., and Mitchell, J. R.,** Ethanol suppresses hepatic glutathione synthesis in rats *in vivo, J. Pharmacol. Exp. Ther.,* 203, 7, 1984.

90. **Speisky, H., MacDonald, A., Giles, G., Orrego, H., and Israel, Y.,** Increased loss and decreased synthesis of hepatic glutathione after acute ethanol intoxication, *Biochem. J.,* 225, 565, 1985.

91. **Loguercio, C., Romano, M., Di Sapio M., Nardi, G., Taranto, D., Grella, A., and Del Vecchio Blanco, C.,** Regional variations in total and nonprotein sulphydryl compounds in the human gastric mucosa and effect of ethanol, *Scand. J. Gastroenterol.,* 26, 1042, 1991.

92. **Loguercio, C., Taranto, D., Beneduce, F., Del Vecchio Blanco, C., De Vincentis, A. C., Nardi, G., and Romano, M.,** Glutathione prevents ethanol induced gastric mucosal damage and depletion of sulphydryl compounds in humans, *Gut,* 34, 161, 1993.

93. **Lavö, B., Colombel, J. F., Knutsson, L., and Hällgren, R.,** Acute exposure of small intestine to ethanol induces mucosal leakage and prostaglandin $E_2$ synthesis, *Gastroenterology,* 102, 468, 1992.

94. **Grogaard, B., Parks, D. A., Grangen, N., Mccord, J. M., and Forsberg, J. O.,** Effects of ischemia and oxygen radicals on mucosal albumin clearance in intestine, *Am. J. Physiol.,* 242, G448, 1982.

95. **Shimizu, M., Lasker, J. M., Tsutsumi, M., and Lieber, C. S.,** Immunohistochemical localization of ethanol-inducible P450IIE1 in the rat alimentary tract, *Gastroenterology,* 99, 1044, 1990.

96. **Hakkan, R., Ronis, M. J. J., and Badger, T. M.,** Effect of enteral nutrition and ethanol on cytochrome P-450 distribution in small intestine of male rats, *Gastroenterology,* 104, 1611, 1993.

97. **Seitz, H. M., Korsten, M. A., and Lieber, C. S.,** Ethanol oxidation by intestinal microsomes: increased activity after chronic ethanol administration, *Life Sci.,* 25, 1443, 1979.

98. **Grossrau, R., Federiks, W. M., and Van Noorden, C. J.,** Histochemistry of reactive oxygen-species (ROS) generating oxidases in cutaneous and mucus epithelial of laboratory rodents with special reference to xanthine oxidase, *Histochemistry,* 94, 539, 1990.

99. **Mufti, S. I., Eskelson, C. D., Odeleye, O. E., and Nachiappan, V.,** Alcohol-associated generation of oxygen free radicals and tumor promotion, *Alcohol Alcohol.,* 28, 621, 1993.

100. **Nachiappan, V., Mufti, S. I., and Eskelson, C. D.,** Ethanol mediated promotion of oral carcinogenesis in hamsters: association with lipid peroxidation, *Nutr. Cancer,* 20, 293, 1993.

101. **Troll, W. and Weisner, R.,** The role of oxygen radicals as possible mechanism of tumor promotion, *Annu. Rev. Pharmacol. Toxicol.,* 25, 509, 1985.

102. **Cerruti, P., Shah, G., Peskin, A., and Amstad, P.,** Molecular mechanisms of oxidant carcinogenesis, in *Free Radicals: From Basic Sciences to Medicine,* Poli, G., Albano, E., and Dianzani, M. U., Eds., Birkhäuser Verlag, Basel, 1993, 206.

103. **Rothman, K., Garfinkel, L., Keller, A. Z., Muir, C. S., and Schottenfeld, P.,** The proportion of cancer attributable to alcohol consumption, *Prev. Med.,* 9, 174, 1990.

# 5

# Endocrine Changes in Alcoholism With Special Reference to Gastrointestinal Hormones

Harry S. Ojeas, Richard F. Harty, and David Van Thiel

## CONTENTS

## 5.1   INTRODUCTION

Alcohol (ethanol) has profound effects on several organ systems. The mechanisms by which this drug exerts its potentially toxic effects have been enumerated or postulated in recent studies.[1] In many respects, the advances in our understanding of the actions of alcohol on a particular organ have occurred because investigators have been able to examine *in vitro* cells that have been exposed acutely or chronically to ethanol. These findings have then been applied to clinical situations to explain the pathophysiology of whole organ dysfunction.

When considering the effects of alcohol on the gastrointestinal endocrine system and the hormones it produces and secretes, it is helpful to define several terms and concepts. Examination of the alimentary tract reveals a number of morphologically distinct endocrine cells and enteric nerves that contain gastrointestinal peptides (hormones/neuropeptides) with regional distribution and varied function. Advances in the fields of gastrointestinal endocrinology and physiology have provided the realization that many, if not most, gastrointestinal peptides do not function solely as hormones. The term regulatory peptide has been widely used due to the fact that gastrointestinal peptides act in at least four distinct but not exclusive ways — as endocrine,

**TABLE 5.1   Peptides Extracted From the Gastrointestinal Tract Together With Their
Likely Role as Endocrine, Neurocrine, or Paracrine Substances**

| Endocrine | Neurocrine | Paracrine |
|---|---|---|
| Somatostatin[b] | Somatostatin[b] | Somatostatin[b] |
| Cholecystokinin (CCK)[a,b] | Cholecystokinin (CCK) | Peptide YY[b] |
| Gastrin[a] | Calcitonin gene-related peptide (CGRP) | |
| Secretin[a] | Gastrin-releasing peptide (GRP) | |
| Insulin[a] | Opioids | |
| Glucagon[a] | Substance P | |
| Enteroglucagon | Vasoactive intestinal polypeptide | |
| Pancreatic polypeptide[a] | Neuropeptide Y (NPY) | |
| Neurotensin[b] | Neurotensin[b] | |
| Motilin[a] | Peptide HM (PHM and PHI) | |
| Glucose-dependent insulinotropic | Pancreastatin | |
|   peptide (GIP)[a] | Galanin | |
| Peptide YY (PYY) | Motilin | |
| Urogastrone/epidermal factor | Peptide YY | |

[a]  Classical hormones with physiologic function.

[b]  Some peptides may serve multiple functions.

Modified from Taylor, I. L. and Mannon, P., Gastrointestinal hormones, in *Textbook of Gastroenterology*,
Vol. 1, Yamada, T., Ed., J. B. Lippincott, Philadelphia, 1991, 29. With permission.

paracrine, neurocrine, and autocrine substances.[2] In other words, peptides derived from gastrointestinal endocrine cells and nerves can exert their actions at a distant site (hormone), locally (paracrine), as a neuromodulator (neurocrine), or on themselves (autocrine). Table 5.1 lists several gastrointestinal peptides and their mechanisms of action. Certain peptides, such as somatostatin, have more than one type of action. The diversity of gastrointestinal peptide actions and their regional distribution makes any discussion of alcohol-induced changes on this system challenging.

Thus, this chapter will review pertinent clinical and experimental information that examines the causal relationships between alcohol effector substances and target cells within the gut–endocrine system. Studies in humans will be emphasized; however, in many instances, investigative studies will be presented which describe responses to either acute or chronic ethanol exposure performed either *in vivo* or *in vitro* using animal tissues and cells.

## 5.2   ESOPHAGUS

It is well known that both acute and chronic ethanol use by humans results in esophageal motor dysfunction.[3-6] However, it is not clear exactly how ethanol affects esophageal body peristalsis and/or lower esophageal sphincter (LES) function. Data exist to support a direct action of ethanol on smooth muscle with acute exposure and altered peripheral neurotransmitter release induced as a result of chronic ethanol use. Acute enteral alcohol administration to healthy volunteers has been shown to produce a reduction in the amplitude of esophageal peristaltic contractions. In addition, meal- and pentagastrin-stimulated LES pressures, but not resting tone, are reduced.[5] These changes generally tend to occur only with higher doses of ethanol. Conversely, withdrawal from chronic ethanol use has been associated with transient elevations in esophageal contraction amplitude and LES pressure. These findings are opposite to those observed with acute ethanol exposure.[6] The esophageal motor abnormalities that reportedly occur in chronic alcoholics are not uniformly observed in association with alcohol-induced peripheral neuropathy. Thus, their pathogenesis cannot be ascribed solely to an ethanol associated peripheral or autonomic neuropathy.

It is not possible to ascribe the effects of acute or chronic ethanol on esophageal motor function to any particular change in circulating gastrointestinal hormone levels or neurotransmitter alteration. Aside from a direct smooth muscle relaxing effect of acute ethanol exposure occurring at the level of the LES, it is reasonable to ask whether ethanol affects intrinsic inhibitory neurotransmission. Nonadrenergic noncholinergic (NANC) nerves are involved in the process of descending relaxation of the esophageal body and LES sphincter with swallowing. Until recently, vasoactive intestinal peptide (VIP), acting as a neuropeptide, has been thought to be the principal mediator of these NANC inhibitory events.[7] Recent data, however, suggest that nitric oxide may be the dominant inhibitory neurotransmitter substance in regulating esophageal smooth muscle function.[8] Pertinent to this discussion is the question of whether the release or action of these two neurotransmitter agents is affected by alcohol in such a way that either or both could account for the observed acute and chronic effects of ethanol exposure and use on esophageal motor function. Presently, studies reporting changes in the levels of either of these two substances in response to ethanol have not appeared in medical literature. Nonetheless, considerable data suggest that it is likely that ethanol exerts either its local or systemic effects on the esophagus at the level of the intrinsic neural control of esophageal smooth muscle function.

Sensory afferent nerves in the esophagus, as in the stomach (see below), respond to luminal stimuli by transmitting signals to the central nervous system.[9] In addition, peripheral sensory nerves exert local efferent function by releasing peptide and nonpeptide neurotransmitters including substance P, calcitonin gene-related peptide, VIP, and nitric oxide.[10,11] Recently, capsaicin-sensitive nerves have been shown to mediate esophageal mucosal protection against ethanol-induced injury in the cat.[12] The pathophysiologic role of sensory afferent nerves and transmitter substances such as VIP and NO in ethanol-induced changes in esophageal motor function have not yet been investigated.

In contrast, the role of cholinergic mechanisms acting via muscarinic receptors to maintain and increase lower esophageal sphincter tone has been studied.[13,14] A recent report by Pasricha et al.[15] on the effect of botulinum toxin, an inhibitor of acetylcholine release, in achalasia patients, has redirected attention to the importance of cholinergic nerves and acetylcholine in regulating esophageal motor and lower esophageal sphincteric function.[15] It has been postulated that chronic ethanol intake may increase esophageal pressures by suppressing cholinergic neurotransmission and subsequent upregulation of muscarinic receptors on esophageal smooth muscle.[16] Although studies in the cat did show an increased number of muscarinic receptors which could account for changes in LES pressure, a parallel increase in receptor sensitivity was not demonstrated. Hence, the changes observed were concluded to be secondary and not the primary cause of the alteration in LES function observed. However, the inhibitory NANC nerves and their transmitters act, in large part, to modulate cholinergic neurotransmission rather than to control directly esophageal and sphincteric muscle function.

## 5.3 STOMACH

Experimentally, it has been observed that intragastric ethanol, when administered at relatively high doses, causes both gastric mucosal and vascular injury with resultant mucosal ulceration and hemorrhage.[17,18] In contrast, either low-dose ethanol or other mild irritants exert a protective effect against certain forms of subsequent potential gastric injury.[19] The precise pathogenesis of these protective effects remains poorly understood, however. The following discussion will relate the effects of ethanol administration to those of recognized neuroendocrine events which are associated with either gastric injury or gastric protection.

Alcohol modulates both gastric acid secretion and gastrin release in humans. These changes in gastric exocrine and endocrine function depend on the concentration and type of alcoholic beverage consumed.

### 5.3.1 Gastric Acid Secretion

Ingestion of ethanol at concentrations ranging from 1 to 5% results in a modest stimulation of gastric acid secretion. On the other hand, higher concentrations of ethanol (6 to 40%) have either no effect or inhibit gastric acid secretion.[20] The reasons for these divergent effects of ethanol on gastric acid secretion are not fully understood, although cholinergic and histaminergic mechanisms have been proposed as being involved in their genesis.[21]

Gastric acid secretion stimulated by low concentrations of ethanol is prevented by both muscarinic and histamine receptor blockade.[21] Pirenzepine, an $M_1$ selective antagonist, and cimetidine, an $H_2$-receptor antagonist, are each capable of abolishing the acid secretory effect of low-dose ethanol. These data suggest that ethanol is capable of stimulating acetylcholine release from cholinergic neurons and histamine from enterochromaffin-like cells and mast cells in the lamina propria that subsequently enhances parietal cell secretion of acid. Higher concentrations of ethanol have an inhibitory effect on gastric acid secretion.[20] This effect may be more apparent than real since high-dose ethanol damages the gastric mucosa leading to increased mucosal permeability and hydrogen ion back diffusion reducing the absolute amount of acid recovered in the gastric lumen. Furthermore, ethanol-induced damage to the gastric mucosa increases the passive movement of bicarbonate from tissue into the lumen. Moreover, dose-dependent bimodal stimulatory and inhibitory effects of ethanol on synaptic transmission modulating acid secretion have been observed within the central nervous system.[22]

In contrast to pure ethanol, ingestion of certain distilled or fermented spirits exerts a stimulatory effect on gastric acid secretion.[23] Specifically, both beer and wine are strong stimulants of acid secretion.[24,25] Their effect is thought to be mediated, at least in part, by the nonalcoholic congener components of the alcoholic beverage such as divalent cations (calcium, magnesium), amino acids, or other nutrients — particularly nitrates and nitrites. Curiously, whiskey and cognac, which are distilled, have an inhibitory effect on acid secretion.[23]

### 5.3.2    Gastrin Release

In humans, pure ethanol when administered acutely does not result in antral gastrin release.[25,26] Both beer and wine, however, are potent stimulants of gastrin secretion. As with gastric acid secretion, distilled spirits such as whiskey and cognac do not release gastrin. Although the specific components of beer and wine which are responsible for this effect have not been elucidated, it is widely believed that the congener substance in these beverages rather than the ethanol *per se* are responsible for the observed gastric secretion. Further support for this hypothesis comes from the observation that in rodents, neither acute nor chronic ethanol treatment increases serum gastrin levels.[27]

### 5.3.3    Gastric Injury and Protection

#### 5.3.3.1    Acute Mucosal Events

Acute ethanol ingestion at concentrations above 6% causes gastric mucosal hyperemia, edema, and vascular congestion.[17,18] These responses are mediated by a marked increase in capillary hydrostatic pressure and resultant increase in permeability. A combined arteriolar vasodilation and venular vasoconstriction lead to further capillary disruption and eventually to submucosal hemorrhage. Additionally, direct contact between ethanol and gastric mucosa leads to a surface epithelial cell necrosis and release of cell-derived inflammatory mediators such as histamine and leukotrienes (e.g., $LTC_4$), which enhance the inflammatory process.[18] In support of this assertion, ethanol-induced hyperemia has been shown to be reduced markedly by both $H_1$ receptor antagonism and by selective lipoxygenase inhibitors.[18]

### 5.3.4    Gastrointestinal Peptides and Chemotransmitters

#### 5.3.4.1    Vasoactive Intestinal Peptide

Vasoactive intestinal peptide (VIP), a 28-amino acid peptide, is found in endocrine cells and in both extrinsic and intrinsic nerves of the gastrointestinal tract.[28] Karmeli and co-workers observed

**TABLE 5.2  Summary of Neuroendocrine and Chemotransmitter Substances Associated With Ethanol-Induced Gastric Injury or Cytoprotection**

| Factors | Action | Effect |
|---|---|---|
| Vasoactive intestinal peptide | Vasodilation; increase mast cell degranulation and leukotriene production | Injury |
| Substance P | Vasodilation; increase mast cell degranulation and leukotriene production | Injury |
| Somatostatin | Inhibit VIP and stimulate somatostatin release, substance P release; decrease mast cell degranulation and leukotriene production; gastric acid secretion | Cytoprotection |
| Calcitonin gene-related peptide | Vasodilation via nitric oxide | Cytoprotection |
| Endothelin-1 | Vasoconstriction | Injury |
| EGF, TGFα | Promote cell growth and proliferation; accelerate ulcer healing, inhibit gastric acid secretion | Cytoprotection |
| Prostaglandins | Increase mucus production, blood flow, bicarbonate secretion | Cytoprotection |
| Leukotrienes | Vasoconstriction; increase mucosal permeability | Injury |
| Nitric oxide | Vasodilation, derived from endothelium, nerves, and mast cells | Cytoprotection |
| Histamine | Vasodilation, released by mast cell degranulation | Injury |
| Adenosine | Vasodilation | ? |

in rats that mucosal VIP content is increased twofold as a result of intragastric ethanol administration.[29] In these same experiments, mucosal levels of substance P, a sensory neuropeptide, were found also to be increased in ethanol-treated animals. A possible role for endogenous VIP and substance P in ethanol-induced gastric injury was suggested further by studies in which both VIP and substance P antagonists significantly reduced the mucosal ulceration produced by ethanol. Furthermore, exogenous VIP augments the mucosal ulceration produced by absolute ethanol administration, but had no effect on lesser degrees of ulceration caused by ethanol at concentrations of 25 to 50%. In these studies, ethanol administration reduced systolic blood pressure by 40%, a process that independently could account for gastric mucosal injury. Nonetheless, these studies indicate that intraluminal ethanol at high concentration is associated with increased gastric mucosal levels of two potent vasoactive neuropeptides: VIP and substance P. Under these experimental conditions, both VIP and substance P may participate in the mucosal and capillary vascular injury induced by ethanol exposure. The specific roles of systemic and, more importantly, splanchnic hypotension in the pathogenesis of the observed gastric mucosal ulceration is also unclear. Nonetheless, taken together the data suggest that ethanol-administration produces a mucosal vascular injury which may be mediated, in part, by VIP and substance P.

## 5.3.4.2  Somatostatin

Somatostatin is an inhibitory regulatory peptide consisting of 14 amino acids which is found in endocrine cells (D cells) and nerves of the gastrointestinal tract.[30] Gastric somatostatin has important inhibitory paracrine actions that include the regulation of both gastrin release and gastric acid secretion.[31] In the rodent, the intragastric administration of absolute ethanol reduces gastric mucosal somatostatin levels by 38%.[32] On the other hand, the administration of exogenous somatostatin substantially reduces the gastric ulceration produced as a result of ethanol exposure. Exogenous somatostatin also reduced mucosal substance P and VIP levels and reduced leukotriene generation within gastric mucosa. The mechanisms by which ethanol increases VIP and reduces somatostatin secretion into tissue are uncertain. Previous studies have shown that VIP stimulates gastric somatostatin release.[31] The combined direct and indirect effects of ethanol on somatostatin release would be to reduce acid secretion. However, the potential neurotoxic and cytotoxic effects of different doses of ethanol as they relate to the stomach have not been examined systematically.

### 5.3.4.3 Calcitonin Gene-Related Peptide

Calcitonin gene-related peptide (CGRP) is a unique 37-amino acid neuropeptide which is located in extrinsic and intrinsic sensory nerves of the gastrointestinal tract.[33] Within the rodent stomach, CGRP is contained solely within primary sensory afferent nerves.[34] The majority (85%) of gastric CGRP is found in splanchnic nerves; the remaining 15% is found in vagal afferent fibers.[35] CGRP is a potent vasodilator and is thought to be involved in the mediation of acid-induced gastric mucosal hyperemia and increased blood flow.[36] In rats, ethanol-induced gastric mucosal ulceration is associated with a reduction in gastric CGRP content.[37] This fact suggests that mucosal ischemia may contribute to ethanol-induced gastric mucosal injury.

Capsaicin is an experimental agent which is able to excite peripheral sensory afferent nerves.[38] It has been used in this capacity to examine the role sensory nerves play in the control of gastric function. When administered intragastrically with ethanol to rats, capsaicin exerts a net protective effect on gastric mucosa.[39,40] This cytoprotective effect is thought to be due, at least in part, to an increased gastric mucosal blood flow mediated by capsaicin-sensitive afferent nerves coupled with CGRP release. Further studies have suggested that the nitric oxide released by CGRP may be involved in the observed capsaicin-mediated gastroprotection against ethanol.[41]

Somewhat paradoxically, low-dose ethanol has a measurable protective effect against higher-dose subsequent ethanol-induced gastric mucosal injury.[19] In preliminary studies, low concentrations of ethanol have been shown to potently stimulate CGRP release from gastric mucosal and submucosal sensory nerves.[42] In addition to its effect on gastric mucosal blood flow, CGRP also stimulates gastric somatostatin release, which in turn inhibits gastric acid secretion.[33] Thus, there are several potential pathways by which capsaicin-evoked CGRP release might exert a gastroprotective effect in response to ethanol exposure.

### 5.3.4.4 Endothelin

Endothelins include a group of related peptides with structural and functional similarities,[43] all of which belong to the larger endothelin family. Each is a 21-amino acid peptide having potent vasoconstrictor properties. Specific endothelin family members include endothelin-1, -2, -3, and vasoactive intestinal contractor (VIC) peptide. These agents are found in vascular endothelial cells as well as in other cell types. The role of endothelin-1 has been examined in ethanol-induced gastric injury.[44,45] High concentrations of intravascularly administered ethanol in the rabbit and intragastrically administered ethanol in the rat stimulate endothelin-1 release from gastric mucosal vessels leading to mucosal vasoconstriction and ischemia. These changes may be critical to the pathogenesis of ethanol-induced gastric mucosal injury at the level of the microcirculation. No studies have been performed to examine the interrelationships between the vasoconstricting actions of endothelin and the vasodilatory effects of either nitric oxide or CGRP in experimental models of the gastric mucosal injury produced as a result of ethanol exposure.

### 5.3.4.5 Growth Factors

Epidermal growth factor (EGF) and transforming growth factor $\alpha$ (TGF$\alpha$) share similar biological activities. Both stimulate DNA synthesis, promote cell growth and proliferation, protect the gastric mucosa against acute injury, and accelerate gastroduodenal ulcer healing.[46,47] Moreover, both agents act on a common receptor (EGFR) and inhibit gastric acid secretion. The adaptation of the gastric mucosa to chronic alcohol administration (50% v/v twice daily for 14 days) that occurs in the rat has been associated with increased mucosal proliferation and increased mucosal expression of EGF, TGF$\alpha$, and their common receptor.[48] The specific pathophysiologic mechanisms of EGF-associated cytoprotection have reportedly involved both prostaglandin synthesis and glutathione production.[49] Similar mechanisms are not reported to occur with TGFα exposure.[50]

### 5.3.4.6 Other Chemotransmitters

Several neural and nonneural substances which regulate gastric function are affected by ethanol. For example, a noncholinergic peptidergic vagal mechanism has been implicated in the exaggerated ethanol-induced gastric injury that occurs following vagotomy in rats.[51] Conversely, alpha and beta adrenergic mechanisms have been shown to protect against ethanol-mediated gastric mucosal damage.[52,53] The precise factors or mechanisms which confer gastric protection following adrenergic stimulation have not been identified specifically, but both nitric oxide and histamine of mast cell origin have been postulated as possible mediators.[21,22]

Adenosine is a product of metabolically active cells,[54] and is thought to be one of several putative mediators involved in the increase in gastric mucosal blood flow that occurs in association with stimulated gastric acid secretion.[55] The vasodilator action of adenosine is mediated by adenosine receptors ($A_1$, $A_2$) located in both endothelial and vascular smooth muscle.[56,57] In a canine model, adenosine contributed to ethanol-induced gastric vasodilation via an adenosine receptor mediated ($A_2$) process.[58] These and other studies suggest that vasoactive peptides and nonpeptide vasoactive substances, such as adenosine and nitric oxide, act together to maintain or alter gastric mucosal blood flow in response to various locally administered luminal stimuli.

In summary, the acute and chronic effects of ethanol to protect or injure the stomach involves several gut peptide and neurotransmitter substances. Since much of the literature in this area describes studies performed in experimental animals and not in humans, it is difficult to translate this information directly to a given clinical situation. Nonetheless, it is likely that, depending on the dose and duration of alcohol exposure, ethanol can evoke any of a wide variety of reactive responses in the gut endocrine system that are endocrine, paracrine, or neurocrine in nature. The specific mechanism of action depends on the neuropeptides and circumstances of the ethanol administration paradigm used. Nonetheless, in the presence of epithelial and vascular injury, cytoprotective mechanisms are exceeded and mucosal injury perpetuated by the elaboration of inflammatory mediators such as leukotrienes and histamine can occur.

## 5.4 SMALL INTESTINE AND COLON

Compared to the stomach, there have been relatively few reports of either acute or chronic mucosal injury occurring in the small bowel or colon in response to ethanol exposure. There has been some interest in the effects of ethanol on the proximal small intestine and as a result on the hormones secretin and cholecystokinin which are located predominantly in the proximal small bowel. In humans, ethanol ingestion stimulates secretin.[59] Subsequent studies, however, have shown that intraduodenal ethanol does not affect plasma secretin concentrations.[60,61] Thus, ethanol acts either indirectly to stimulate secretin release or alters the rate of acid being delivered to the duodenum. Furthermore, ingestion of alcohol by healthy subjects does not affect plasma levels of cholecystokinin (CCK) or pancreatic polypeptide.[62] Similarly, neither acute nor chronic administration of ethanol alters the CCK or enkephalin content of the proximal small intestine of the rat.[63] The effects of ethanol on secretion of trypsin-sensitive peptides which are involved in the negative feedback regulation of CCK secretion have not been examined. In rats, chronic ethanol administration is associated with increased circulating levels of enteroglucagon.[27] The mechanism accounting for this phenomenon and its clinical significance have not been determined.

The consequences of chronic ethanol administration on the interactions between vasoactive intestinal peptide (VIP) and enterocytes in the rat have been examined.[64] VIP binding to intestinal epithelial cells was decreased as was VIP-stimulated cyclic AMP production. A second study suggested that chronic ethanol consumption may alter the cellular events involved in receptor biosynthesis and processing.[65] Thus, ethanol-induced derangements in the ability of enterocytes to respond to gastrointestinal peptides may account, at least in part, for some of the impaired intestinal absorption and secretion that accompany acute or chronic alcohol ingestion in humans.

Although the colon and rectum contain abundant numbers of regulatory peptides, the effects of alcohol on the endocrine system of the large intestine have not been examined systematically.[66] Based on the effects of ethanol on the more proximal gastrointestinal tract, areas of potential interest for future studies should include the effect of ethanol on the function of the ileocecal valve. In particular, such studies might examine the effects of ethanol on the ability of ileal gut peptides to regulate proximal gastrointestinal motor function in response to lumen nutrients ("the ileal-brake").[67] Both the effects of luminal and probably more importantly blood alcohol levels will need to be studied. Other areas of interest would be an examination of the effect of alcohol on visceral pain perception and anorectal motility.

The effects of alcohol administration on hepatic function mediated by the effects of alcohol on hormonal function are even less well studied than those that examine luminal gastrointestinal tract function. Secretin increases bile flow by enhancing water and bicarbonate flow. Ethanol ingestion stimulates secretin secretion but not in its hormonal action. Thus, this effect on bile flow is probably limited to its effects locally in the small bowel to modulate duodenal bicarbonate content.

## 5.5   CONCLUSIONS

The effects of gastrointestinal hormones and neuropeptides are multiple. The specific action observed as a result of alcohol associated pertubation of the levels of these materials often depends more on the mechanism of this action either as a hormone, paracrine or autocrine effector molecule than on the identity of the specific molecule involved. The foregoing is an overview of the identifiable effects of alcohol and the consequences of alcohol exposure on these molecules.

## REFERENCES

1. **Rubin, E., Miller, K. W., and Roth, S. H.,** *Molecular and Cellular Mechanisms of Alcohol and Anesthetics*, New York Academy of Sciences, New York, 1991.
2. **Taylor, I. L. and Mannon. P.,** Gastrointestinal hormones, in *Textbook of Gastroenterology*, Yamada, T., Ed., J. B. Lippincott, New York, 1991, 24.
3. **Hogan, W. L., Viegas de Andrade, S. R., and Winship, D. H.,** Ethanol-induced acute esophageal motor dysfunction, *J. Appl. Physiol.*, 32, 755, 1972.
4. **Mayer, E. M., Garbowski, C. J., and Fisher, R. S.,** Effects of graded doses of alcohol upon esophageal motor function, *Gastroenterology*, 75, 1133, 1978.
5. **Winship, D. H., Catlisch, C. R., Zboralske, F. E., and Hogan, W. J.,** Deterioration of esophageal peristalsis in patients with alcoholic neuropathy, *Gastroenterology*, 55, 173, 1968.
6. **Keshavarzian, A., Iber, F. L., and Ferguson, Y.,** Esophageal manometry and radionuclide emptying in chronic alcoholics, *Gastroenterology*, 92, 651, 1987.
7. **Biancani, P., Walsh, J. H., and Beher, J.,** Vasoactive intestinal polypeptide: a neurotransmitter for lower esophageal sphincter relaxation, *J. Clin. Invest.*, 73, 963, 1984.
8. **Tottrup, A., Knudsen, M. A., and Gregersen, H.,** Nitric oxide mediating NANC inhibition in opossum lower esophageal sphincter, *Am. J. Physiol.* 260, G385, 1991.
9. **Grundy, D. and Richards W.,** Vagal and spinal afferent innervation: role in sensation and reflex regulation of upper gastrointestinal function, in *Basic and Clinical Aspects of Chronic Abdominal Pain*, Mayer, E. A. and Raybould, H. E., Eds., Elsevier, New York, 1993, 37.
10. **Buck, S. H. and Burks, T. F.,** The neuropharmacology of capsaicin: review of some recent observations, *Pharmacol. Rev.*, 38, 179, 1986.
11. **Holzer P.,** Local effector functions of capsaicin-sensitive sensory nerve endings, *Neuroscience*, 24, 739, 1988.
12. **Bass, B. L., Trad, K. S., Harmon, J. W., and Hakki, F. Z.,** Capsaicin-sensitive nerves mediate esophageal mucosal protection, *Surgery*, 100, 419, 1991.
13. **Rattan, S. and Goyal, R. K.,** Neural control of the lower esophageal sphincter: influence of the vagus nerves, *J. Clin. Invest.*, 54, 1119, 1974.

14. **Goyal, R. K. and Rattan, S.,** Neurohumoral, hormonal and drug receptors for the lower esophageal sphincter, *Gastroenterology*, 74, 598, 1978.

15. **Pasricha, P. J., Ravich, W. J., Hendrix, T. R., Sostre, S., Jones, B., and Kalloo, A. N.,** Treatment of achalasia with intrasphincteric injection of botulinum toxin, *Ann. Intern. Med.*, 121, 590, 1994.

16. **Keshavarzian, A., Gordon, J. H., Wilson, C., Urban, G., and Fields, J. Z.,** Chronic ethanol feeding produces a muscarinic receptor up-regulation, but not a muscarinic super-sensitivity in lower esophageal sphincter muscle, *J. Pharmacol. Exp. Ther.*, 260, 601, 1992.

17. **Laine, L. and Weinstein, W. M.,** Histology of alcoholic hemorrhagic "gastritis": a prospective evaluation, *Gastroenterology*, 94, 1254, 1988.

18. **Oates, P. J. and Hakkien, J. P.,** Studies on the mechanism of ethanol-induced gastric damage in rats, *Gastroenterology*, 94, 10, 1988.

19. **Robert, A., Nezamis, J. E., and Lancaster, C.,** Mild irritants prevent gastric necrosis through "adaptive cytoprotection" mediated by prostaglandins, *Am. J. Physiol.*, 245, G113, 1983.

20. **Singer, M. and Leffman, C.,** Alcohol and gastric acid secretion in humans: a short review, *Scand. J. Gastroenterol.*, 23 (Suppl. 146), 11, 1988.

21. **Singer, M. V., Calden, H., and Leffman, C.,** *Gastroenterology*, 86, A1254 (Abstr.), 1984.

22. **Carlen, P. L., Zhang, L., and Cullen, N.,** Cellular electrophysiological actions of ethanol on mammalian neurons in brain slices, *Ann. N.Y. Acad. Sci.*, 625, 17, 1991.

23. **Chari, S., Teyssen, S., and Singer, M. V.,** Alcohol and gastric acid in humans, *Gut*, 24, 843, 1993.

24. **Lenz, H. Z., Ferrari-Taylor, J., and Isenberg, J. I.,** Wine and five percent ethanol are potent stimulants of gastric acid secretion in humans, *Gastroenterology*, 85, 1082, 1983.

25. **Petersen, W. L., Barnett, C., and Walsh, J. H.,** Effect of intragastric infusion of ethanol and wine on serum gastrin concentration and gastric acid secretion, *Gastroenterology*, 91, 1390, 1986.

26. **Singer, M. V., Leffman, C., Eysselein, V. E., Calden, H., and Goebell, H.,** Action of ethanol and some alcoholic beverages on gastric acid secretion and release of gastrin in humans, *Gastroenterology*, 93, 1247, 1987.

27. **Siamanowski, U. A., Hubalek, K., Ghatei, M. A., Bloom, S. R., Polak, J. M., and Seitz, H. K.,** Effects of acute and chronic ethanol administration on the gastrointestinal hormones gastrin, neutroglucagon, pancreatic glucagon and peptide yy in the rat, *Digestion*, 42, 167, 1989.

28. **Dockray, G. J.,** Vasoactive intestinal polypeptide and related peptides, in *Gut Peptides: Biochemistry and Physiology*, Walsh, J. H. and Dockray, G. J., Eds., Raven Press, New York, 1994, 447.

29. **Karmeli, F., Eliakim, R., Okon, E., and Rachmilewitz, D.,** Role of vasoactive intestinal peptide (VIP) in pathogenesis of ethanol-induced gastric mucosal damage in rats, *Dig. Dis. Sci.*, 38, 1210, 1993.

30. **Chiba, T. and Yamada, T.,** Gut somatostatin, in *Gut Peptides: Biochemistry and Physiology*, Walsh, J. H. and Dockray, G. J., Eds., Raven Press, New York, 1994, 123.

31. **Schubert, M. L.,** The effects of vasoactive intestinal polypeptide on gastric acid secretion is predominantly mediated by somatostatin, *Gastroenterology*, 100, 1195, 1991.

32. **Karmeli, F., Eliakim, R., Okon, E., and Rachmilewitz, D.,** Somatostatin effectively prevents ethanol- and NSAID-induced gastric mucosal damage in rats, *Dig. Dis. Sci.*, 39, 615, 1994.

33. **Holzer, P.,** Calcitonin gene-related peptide, in *Gut Peptides: Biochemistry and Physiology*, Walsh, J. H. and Dockray, G. J., Eds., Raven Press, New York, 1994, 493.

34. **Lee, Y., Shiotani, Y., Hayashi, N., Kamada, T., Hillyard, C. J., Girgis, S. I., MacIntyre, I., and Tohyama, M.,** Distribution and origin of calcitonin gene-related peptide in rat stomach and duodenum: an immunohistochemical study, *J. Neur. Transmiss.*, 68, 1, 1987.

35. **Lee, Y., Takami, K., Kawai, Y., Girgis, S., Hillyard, C. J., MacIntyre, I., Emson, P. C., and Tohyama, M.,** Distribution of calcitonin gene-related peptide in the rat peripheral nervous system with reference to its coexistence with substance P, *Neuroscience*, 15, 1227, 1985.

36. **Li, D.-S., Raybould, H. E., Quintero, E., and Guth, P. H.,** Calcitonin gene-related peptide mediates the gastric hyperemic response to acid back-diffusion, *Gastroenterology*, 102, 1124, 1992.

37. **Evangelista, S.,** Gastric lesions induced by concentrated ethanol are associated with a decrease in gastric calcitonin gene-related peptide-like immunoreactivity in rats, *Scand. J. Gastroenterol.*, 28, 1112, 1993.

38. **Holzer, P.,** Capsaicin: cellular targets, mechanisms of action and selectivity for thin sensory neurons, *Pharmacol. Rev.*, 43, 143, 1991.

39. **Holzer, P. and Sametz, W.,** Gastric mucosal protection against ulcerogenic factors in the rat mediated by capsaicin-sensitive afferent neurons, *Gastroenterology*, 91, 975, 1986.

40. **Holzer, P. and Lippe, I. T.,** Stimulation of afferent nerve endings by intragastric capsaicin protects against ethanol-induced damage of gastric mucosa, *Neuroscience*, 27, 981, 1988.

41. **Lambrect, N., Burchert, M., Respondek, M., Muller, K.-M., and Peskar, B. M.,** Role of calcitonin gene-related peptide and nitric oxide in the gastroprotective effect of capsaicin in the rat, *Gastroenterology*, 104, 1371, 1993.

42. **Ren, J., Tuma, D. J., and Harty, R. F.,** Ethanol is a potent stimulant of acetylcholine and calcitonin gene-related peptide release from antral mucosal:submucosal fragments, *Gastroenterology*, 102, A752 (Abstr.), 1992.

43. **Ghatei, M. A., Takahaski, K., Kirkland, S. C., Jones, P. M., Perera, T., Wright, N. A., and Bloom, S. R.,** Endothelin, in *Gut Peptides: Biochemistry and Physiology*, Walsh, J. H. and Dockray, G. J., Eds., Raven Press, New York, 1994, 389.

44. **Masuda, E., Kawano, S., Nagano, K., Tsuji, S., Ishigami, Y., Tsujii, M., Haysashi, N., Fusamoto, H., and Kamada, T.,** Effect of intravascular ethanol on modulation of gastric mucosal integrity: possible role of endothelin-1, *Am. J. Physiol.*, 262, G785, 1992.

45. **Masuda, E., Kawano, S., Nagano, K., Tsuji, S., Takei, Y., Hayashi, N., Tsujii, M., Oshita, M., Michido, T., Kobayashi, I., Peng, H.-B., Fusamoto, H., and Kamada, T.,** Role of endogenous endothelin in pathogenesis of ethanol-induced gastric mucosal injury in rats, *Am. J. Physiol.*, 265, G474, 1993.

46. **Karnes, W. E., Jr.,** Epidermal growth factor and transforming growth factor -alpha, in *Gut Peptides: Biochemistry and Physiology*, Walsh, J. H. and Dockray, G. J., Eds., Raven Press, New York, 1994, 553.

47. **Brzozowski, T., Majka, J., Garlicki, J., Drozdowicz, D., and Konturek, S. J.,** Role of polyamines and prostaglandins in gastroprotective action of epidermal growth factor against ethanol injury, *J. Clin. Gastroenterol.*, 13(Suppl. 1), S98, 1991.

48. **Tarnowski, A., Lu, S.-Y., Stachura, J., and Sarfeh, I. J.,** Adaptation of gastric mucosa to chronic alcohol administration is associated with increased mucosal expression of growth factors and their receptors, *Scand. J. Gastroenterol.*, 27(Suppl. 193), 59, 1992.

49. **Konturek, P. K., Brzozowski, T., and Konturek, S. J.,** Role of epidermal growth factor, prostaglandin, and sulfhydryls in stress-induced gastric lesions, *Gastroenterology*, 99, 1607, 1990.

50. **Romano, M., Polk, W. H., and Coffey, R. J.,** Transforming growth factor alpha (TGF-alpha) protects rat gastric mucosa against ethanol injury — evaluation of mechanisms of action, *Gastroenterology*, 100, A149 (Abstr.), 1991.

51. **Ko, J. U. S., Cho, C., and Ogle, C.,** The vagus and its non-cholinergic mechanism in modulation of ethanol-induced gastric mucosal damage in rats, *J. Pharmacol.*, 46, 29, 1994.

52. **Howard, T., Passaro, E., and Guth, P. H.,** Isoproterenol prevents ethanol-induced microvascular stasis and deep histologic injury in rat gastric mucosa, *Dig. Dis. Sci.*, 38, 1201, 1993.

53. **Endoh, K., Kao, J., Baker, M., and Leung, F.,** Involvement of alpha adrenoreceptors in mechanism of intragastric nicotine production against ethanol injury in rat stomach, *Dig. Dis. Sci.*, 38, 713, 1993.

54. **Sawmiller, D. R. and Chou, C. C.,** Adenosine is a vasodilator in the intestinal mucosa, *Am. J. Physiol.*, 261, G9, 1991.

55. **Gerber, J. G. and Guth, P. H.,** Role of adenosine in the gastric blood flow response to pentagastrin in the rat, *J. Pharmacol. Exp. Ther.*, 251, 550, 1989.

56. **Proctor, K. G.,** Intestinal arteriolar responses to mucosal and serosal applications of adenosine analogues, *Circ. Res.*, 61, 187, 1987.

57. **Stiles, G. L.,** Adenosine receptors: structure, function and regulation, *Trends Pharmacol. Sci.*, 7, 486, 1986.

58. **Wood, J. G., Darnell, M. P., and Cheung, L. Y.,** Adenosine is a mediator of ethanol-induced gastric vasodilation in dogs, *Am. J. Physiol.*, 264, G664, 1993.

59. **Straus, E., Urbach, H.-J., and Yalow, R. S.,** Alcohol-stimulated secretion of immunoreactive secretin, *N. Engl. J. Med.* 293, 1031, 1975.

60. **Llanos, O. L., Swierczek, J. S., Teichmann, R. K., Rayford, P. L., and Thompson, J. C.,** Effect of alcohol on the release of secretin and pancreatic secretion, *Surgery*, 81, 661, 1977.

61. **Nishiwaki, H., Lee, K. Y., and Chey, W. Y.,** Effect of alcohol on plasma secretin concentration and pancreatic secretion in dogs, *Surgery*, 95, 85, 1984.

62. **Fried, G. M., Ogden, W. D., Zhu, X.-G., Greeley, G. H., Jr., and Thompson, J. C.,** Effect of alcohol on the release of cholecystokinin and pancreatic enzyme secretion, *Am. J. Surg.*, 147, 53, 1984.

63. **Ryder, S., Straus, E., Lieber, C. S., and Yalow, R. S.,** Cholecystokinin and enkephalin levels following ethanol administration in rats, *Peptides*, 2, 223, 1981.

64. **Jimenez, J., Celvo, J. R., Molinero, P., Goberna, R., and Guerrero, J. M.,** Chronic ethanol intake inhibits both the vasoactive intestinal peptide binding and the associated cyclic AMP production in rat enterocytes, *Gen. Pharmacol.*, 23, 607, 1992.

65. **Dalke, D. D., Sorrell, M. F., Casey, C. A., and Tuma, D. J.,** Chronic ethanol administration impairs receptor-mediated endocytosis of epidermal growth factor by rat hepatocytes, *Hepatology*, 12, 1085, 1990.

66. **Walsh, J. H. and Mayer, E. A.,** Gastrointestinal hormones, in *Gastrointestinal Disease: Pathophysiology, Diagnosis, and Management*, Sleissenger, M. H. and Fordtran, J. S., Eds., W. B. Saunders, Philadelphia, 1993, 18.

67. **Read, N. W., McFarlane, A., Kinsman, R. I., Bates, T. E., Blackhall, N. W., Farrar, G. B. J., Hall, J. C., Moss, G., Morris, A. P., O'Neil, B., Welch, I., Lee, Y., and Bloom, S. R.,** The effect of infusion of nutrient solutions into the ileum on gastrointestinal transit and plasma levels of neurotensin and enteroglucagon, *Gastroenterology*, 86, 274, 1984.

# 6

# The Physiology of Digestion, Absorption, and Metabolism in the Human Intestine

George K. Grimble

## CONTENTS

## 6.1    INTRODUCTION

Alcohol consumption has a special association with the process of digestion and absorption. Italian hospitality may include a Campari and soda before a meal (as a predigestive aid), while a good wine from Barolo provides a digestive aid and, perhaps a wine from the Friuli region would be a postdigestive aid when the dessert is served. No cultural commentary is required for this delightful thought, but a scientific commentary would suggest that excessive alcohol consumption has marked negative effects on nutrient assimilation. This author has noted that subjects who ingest alcohol the night before a jejunal perfusion (although asked not to) often have aberrant water and electrolyte absorption. This anecdotal impression is documented by jejunal perfusion studies which showed that 2% alcohol (equivalent to an oral dose of 40 g) coperfused with 3 mmol/l methionine inhibited absorption of the latter by nearly 60% in nonalcoholic and alcoholic subjects.[1] Recently, Pfeiffer and colleagues perfused the intestines of healthy volunteers with a hyperosmolar nutrient solution (with or without alcohol present) and found no inhibitory effect on nutrient uptake, although water and electrolyte secretion by the duodenum was impaired.[2] The ability of the mucosa to equilibrate with luminal contents plays a large part in uptake. This is especially true for $Na^+$-linked transport of glucose and alanine[3] which are inhibited by alcohol, but not for obvious reasons. In this study, passive diffusion of $Na^+$ across the mucosal membrane was increased, thus leading to a faster collapse of the $Na_{OUT}$:$Na_{IN}$ gradient with the consequence that transport velocities for $Na^+$-linked solutes were reduced.

Although there are several studies showing direct effects of alcohol on transport phenomena, it is unsafe to extrapolate this to the whole intestine and propose that muscle wasting in patients with alcoholic cirrhosis arises from persistent malabsorption. This has been proposed as a cause of muscle wasting in HIV-infected patients but does not seem to be the true cause. Reduced dietary intake and persistently increased energy requirements due to increased rates of whole-body protein degradation and amino acid oxidation[4] would be sufficient to explain a marked loss of skeletal muscle. This does not mean that alcohol has no adverse effects on intestinal function, but rather that malabsorption can only be demonstrated by increased fecal excretion of reducing sugars, fats, or nitrogen[5] and should not be assumed simply because there is persistent weight loss (see Chapter 11).

Neurological impairment of gastrointestinal function may also be evident in alcohol abusers. Patients with alcoholic cirrhosis have been shown to have longer mouth-to-cecum transit times ($154 \pm 29$ min) compared to patients with nonalcoholic cirrhosis or compared to normal subjects ($99 \pm 34$ min and $98 \pm 34$ min, respectively[6]). Increased transit may moderate the effects of impaired digestive and absorptive processes, merely by increasing the mucosal contact time with luminal nutrients. Certainly, malabsorption of fat and its appearance at the ileal mucosal surface provides a powerful signal for reducing small bowel motility and increasing transit times, the so-called "ileal-brake" which operates to maximize absorption.[7]

This chapter will therefore address the most significant features of digestion, absorption, and intestinal metabolism. An attempt will be made to describe the capacity of these processes and the limits of adaptation which are possible.

## 6.2    ABSORPTIVE CAPACITIES

### 6.2.1    Small Intestine

The capacity of the intestine has often been assumed to be several times greater than the normal dietary intake. The basic relationship in considering capacity is that between absorptive surface area and metabolic body-mass[8,9] since for species of similar body mass but different metabolic rate, increased absorptive area of the mammals is obtained by formation of villi and microvilli which multiply area fivefold over that of the lizards which achieve surface area increases through surface "folding" rather than villi.[8,10] The increase in absorptive area (fivefold) is reflected in higher rates of glucose uptake (sevenfold). Absorptive function is thus matched to metabolic mass but any excess, or "reserve capacity" or "safety margin," represents both an opportunity to capture nutrients and a metabolic burden since metabolic energy must be expended in synthesis and maintenance of the appropriate number of nutrient transporters. The mucosal surface is also a barrier between our internal and external environments with gut-associated lymphatic tissue representing the largest proportion of immune cells in the body. There is no good quantitative estimate of the proportion of whole-body protein synthesis this represents in humans, but in the rat it may be as much as 20%.[11] It is therefore costly to maintain "reserve capacity" which is greatly in excess of requirements.

One estimate has been obtained from mice which were made hyperphagic when transferred to a 6°C environment. The consequence of increased thermogenesis did not lead to marked alterations of digestive efficiency, but a slight adaptation was observed in absorptive capacity such that the safety margin was reduced from 220–300% to 60–90%.[12] In humans, this corresponds to a maximum intake of about 4500 to 7000 kcal/day. Indeed, in one ileal intubation study, nasoduodenal intakes of up to 6000 kcal/day were efficiently assimilated.[13]

This should be kept in mind when considering studies that show impairment of one or other aspect of absorptive function as a consequence of alcohol abuse. These impairments could be reduced pancreatic secretions, reductions in brush-border membrane hydrolases, or reductions in the kinetics of substrate uptake (*vide infra*). Few of these studies have addressed the question of whether such changes lead to clinically significant impairment of nutrient uptake. Because of the overlap between luminal and brush-border phases of digestion, the degree of impairment has to be profound before clinically significant malabsorption will occur. Malabsorption of some nutrients may occur but only if 90% impairment of organ function has occurred, e.g., exocrine pancreatic disease.[14-16] This may present as vitamin malabsorption and deficiency or as loose watery stools consequent on malabsorption of macronutrients and their fermentation by the colonic luminal microflora.[17] Notwithstanding this, malabsorption may occur if digestive and absorptive systems are overwhelmed by too high a luminal nutrient concentration for a sustained period. This "load" is defined as the product of the rate of administration of a nutrient and the resulting luminal concentration in relation to mouth-to-cecum transit time.

The relationship between rate and luminal concentration is exemplified by the assimilation of lactose and its hydrogenated derivative, lactitol. Because lactitol is not absorbed to any appreciable extent in the human small intestine, regardless of the oral load given, it will be rapidly fermented by luminal microflora[18] and at a dose high enough to elicit a laxative effect.[19] Lactose can be hydrolyzed by β-galactosidase to galactose and glucose which are absorbed; however, in lactase-deficient patients, a bolus of lactose will cause diarrhea,[20] whereas 24 h nasogastric infusion of lactose-containing enteral diets does not.[21] The difference can be explained by the fact that in alactasic patients brush-border β-galactosidase is never entirely absent but is insufficient to hydrolyze a lactose bolus (high load) within the orocecal transit time. During continuous infusion, load is low and residual β-galactosidase activity is not saturated by luminal concentration at that rate of delivery.

The relationship between load and transit is exemplified by the fact that ingestion of food *per se* slows transit quite markedly[22] thus increasing contact time between luminal contents and the mucosal surface. This is an economical mechanism for maintaining absorption, since the time available for absorption is load-sensitive and this obviates the need for rapid acute changes in transporter number in response to food intake.

## 6.2.2  Large Intestine

One of the most important functions of the colon is to salvage water and electrolytes. This process is often considered as a mucosal mechanism of the same type which exists in the small intestine,

**TABLE 6.1   Early Development of Colonic Activities Associated With the Microflora**

Mucin breakdown
Regulation of fecal trypsin activity
Conversion of bilirubin to urobilinogen
Cholesterol catabolism
Fermentation of malabsorbed carbohydrate and protein to organic acids including SCFA
Recycling of urea back into host amino acid metabolism

but in reality the process results from the action of two organs. The first is the colonic luminal microflora which have been termed an "organ within an organ." The second organ is the colon itself which comprises several functional compartments. The number of bacteria in the colon is several times greater than the number of cells in the human body, and comprises an organ which develops after birth, since the large bowel is initially sterile. Bacterial growth accompanies the establishment of six colonic characteristics which are described in Table 6.1.[23]

The microflora play no direct role in water and electrolyte salvage, but do this indirectly by hydrolyzing and fermenting malabsorbed nutrients (e.g., polysaccharides) to short-chain fatty acids (SCFA) which can be absorbed by the colonic mucosa, accompanied by water and electrolyte uptake. If the reserve capacity of the colon is exceeded, it is either because the rate of production of osmotically active solute exceeds the rate of uptake, or because the luminal water load is too large. The healthy colon has the capacity to hydrolyze, ferment, and absorb 70 to 80 g/day of lactitol, sorbitol, or lactulose before diarrhea ensues.[19,24] Impairment of colonic microflora function by antibiotics (e.g., ampicillin) reduces fermentation of oral doses of lactulose (which did not increase stool volume) to the point where inefficient fermentation and salvage lead to osmotic diarrhea.[25] With regard to fluid capacity, rapid intracolonic infusion of more than 500 ml of isotonic saline has been shown to provoke diarrhea in normal subjects,[26] and suggests an upper limit of fluid-absorbing capacity.

## 6.3   DIGESTION AND ABSORPTION IN THE SMALL INTESTINE

### 6.3.1   Protein

#### 6.3.1.1   Gastric Protein Digestion

The churning action of the stomach and gastric acid secretions will aid denaturation of food proteins, such that internal peptide bonds in previously stable protein structures are susceptible to hydrolysis by gastric pepsins. These enzymes do not have a particularly low pH optimum (approx. pH 4 to 5) but the effect of acid is to denature the protein, and also to protonate dicarboxylic acid side-chains, thus exposing more internal peptide bonds to pepsin hydrolysis. This compensates for the reduction in pepsin activity caused by the lower pH and constitutes a highly cooperative mechanism which will efficiently convert dietary protein to large soluble oligopeptides.[27] The soluble mixture of oligopeptides is the substrate for luminal digestion by pancreatic endo- and exopeptidases, whose pH optimum is much higher.

#### 6.3.1.2   Small Intestine Protein Digestion

The peptide-bond specificities of the three pancreatic endopeptidases and two pancreatic exopeptidases are cooperative, and will release large amounts of free amino acid and small peptides.[28,29] Because amino acids appear in blood so soon after a meal, it is likely that the jejunum is the major site of dietary protein assimilation.[30-32] Curiously, there is an increasing longitudinal gradient of specific activity of all major brush-border peptidases toward the ileum.[33-35] The functional differences in the ability of the jejunum and ileum to assimilate amino acids and dipeptides,[36] may result from differences in the source of amino acids absorbed at these two sites. It would not be unreasonable to propose that assimilation of endogenous proteins (i.e., from intestinal secretions, secreted plasma proteins, and desquamated cells) occurs at more distal sites although the distinction is not clear cut. Adibi and Mercer have shown that some electrophoretically identifiable bovine serum albumin protein will survive passage to the ileum 4 h after a meal of that protein.[37]

### 6.3.1.3   Large Intestine Protein Digestion

The colon is also a major site of assimilation of endogenously derived protein as has been suggested by the magnitude of stomal protein losses in ileostomy patients.[38] As discussed below, the luminal microflora of the colon have considerable capacity for digesting endogenous and dietary proteins *in vitro* and *in vivo*.[39-41] There is a cooperative interaction between protein fermentation (producing SCFA), isomeric SCFA, and copious amounts of $NH_4^+$ and carbohydrate fermentation which consumes $NH_4^+$.[40] This synergism will be discussed in more detail below (Section 6.3.6.2).

### 6.3.1.4   Free Amino Acid Transport

There are four major $Na^+$-dependent, group-specific, active transport systems in the brush-border membrane of the mammalian enterocyte: (1) monoamino, monocarboxylic (neutral amino acids), (2) glycine, proline, hydroxyproline, (3) dibasic amino acids and cystine, and (4) dicarboxylic (acidic) amino acids.[42,43] In addition, other transporters are present in the basolateral membrane which are also present in the plasma membrane of other tissues (Table 6.2).

### 6.3.1.5   Peptide Transport

Brush-border membrane hydrolysis of peptides and their uptake are closely related phenomena consistent with a dual mode of peptide-bound amino acid transport. A di- or tripeptide can be absorbed intact by a specific transporter (Table 6.2) and will be hydrolyzed intracellularly (Figure 6.1). Alternatively, constituent amino acids (or smaller peptide fragments) may be absorbed after brush-border membrane hydrolysis of the peptide. As indicated in Figure 6.1, there is also the possibility that di- and tripeptides which are resistant to brush-border and intracellular peptidases may translocate intact into the portal circulation to be hydrolyzed by blood or tissue peptidases.[44]

This transport system has unique characteristics (Table 6.2), namely that it is $H^+$-dependent,[45] and that it is stimulated by the low pH in the submucosal layer adjacent to the brush-border membrane.[46] It also has fairly wide tissue distribution, being present in the brush-border membrane of the small intestine and renal tubule[47] as well as the placental membrane.[48] In addition, cephalosporin antibiotics containing a peptide-bond share the same transport system.[49] A cDNA probe to this transporter (PepT1) showed that it is expressed in rabbit duodenum, jejunum, kidney, and, to a lesser extent, liver.[50] One puzzle in this work is that the colon only seems to express small amounts of the transporter. This would imply that little luminal peptide load is generated by the action of luminal microflora, even though significant amounts of protein are digested in the large bowel. If so, this would point to a marked difference between the colon and the rumen.[51]

The enterocyte basolateral membrane peptide transporter which has been described by Shirazi-Beechey and colleagues may be the same transport protein[52] expressed on the apical membrane. This would explain why basolateral membrane efflux of di- and tripeptides which have escaped intracellular hydrolysis can occur. In contrast, amino acids which have been absorbed as free L-amino acids or have been released by intracellular peptidase hydrolysis after uptake of the intact di/tripeptide can efflux from the basolateral membrane via transporters whose kinetic characteristics are sensitive to circulating amino acid concentrations.[53]

The substrate structural requirements of the peptide transporter have been defined by Daniel and colleagues from a study of renal brush-border membrane vesicles.[54] In some respects, the transporter is fastidious since it requires di- or tripeptides with a free terminal $\alpha$-$NH_2$ and COOH

**TABLE 6.2 Macronutrient Transporters in the Small Intestine**

| Transporter | Membrane location | | Coupling | | Typical substrates | Comments |
|---|---|---|---|---|---|---|
| | Brush border | Basolateral | Na$^+$ | H$^+$ | | |
| **Monosaccharides** | | | | | | |
| SGLT1 | Yes | No | Yes | No | Glucose/galactose | Main glucose/galactose transporter; unrelated to GLUT family; inducible by luminal glucose |
| System 2 | Yes | No | Yes | No | Glucose | Liver type, low affinity, high capacity; modulated by glycemia/diabetes |
| GLUT2 | No | Yes | No | No | Glucose/fructose | Brain type, moderate affinity/capacity; predominantly expressed in tissues with high glucose demand |
| GLUT3 | ? | ? | No | No | Glucose/galactose | |
| GLUT5 | Yes | No | No | No | Fructose | Intestine type, high abundance; high affinity for fructose, little for glucose |
| **Amino Acids** | | | | | | |
| NBB | Yes | No | Yes | No | Neutral AA | Also known as system B (see Reference 43) |
| IMINO | Yes | No | Yes | No | Imino acids | |
| PHE | Yes | No | Yes | No | Phe, Met | |
| β | Yes | No | Yes | No | β-ala | May be two types (ileum and jejunum) |
| X-G,A | Yes | (Yes) | Yes | No | Glu, Asp | High affinity, more than one Na$^+$ per amino acid transported |
| Y$^+$ | Yes | No | Yes | No | Lys, Cys, Arg, Orn | Electrogenic |
| y$^+$ | Yes | Yes | No | No | Lys, Cys, Arg, Orn | Electrogenic |
| L | Yes | Yes | No | No | Neutral, Cys | Not usually inducible |
| A | No | Yes | Yes | No | Short-chain polar | Inducible by starvation, hormones, and growth factors |
| ASC | No | Yes | Yes | No | Ala, Cys, Ser, Thr | Not usually inducible |
| asc | No | Yes | No | No | Ala, Cys, Ser, Thr | |
| N | No | Yes | Yes | No | Glx, His, Asx | |
| **Peptides** | | | | | | |
| Dipeptide | Yes | Yes | No | Yes | Di- and tripeptides | Unclear whether this is a single transporter or a family (cf. GLUT transporter) or whether the brush-border and basolateral transporters are the same. (See References 50 and 52.) |

Adapted from References 42, 43, 50, 52, and 103.

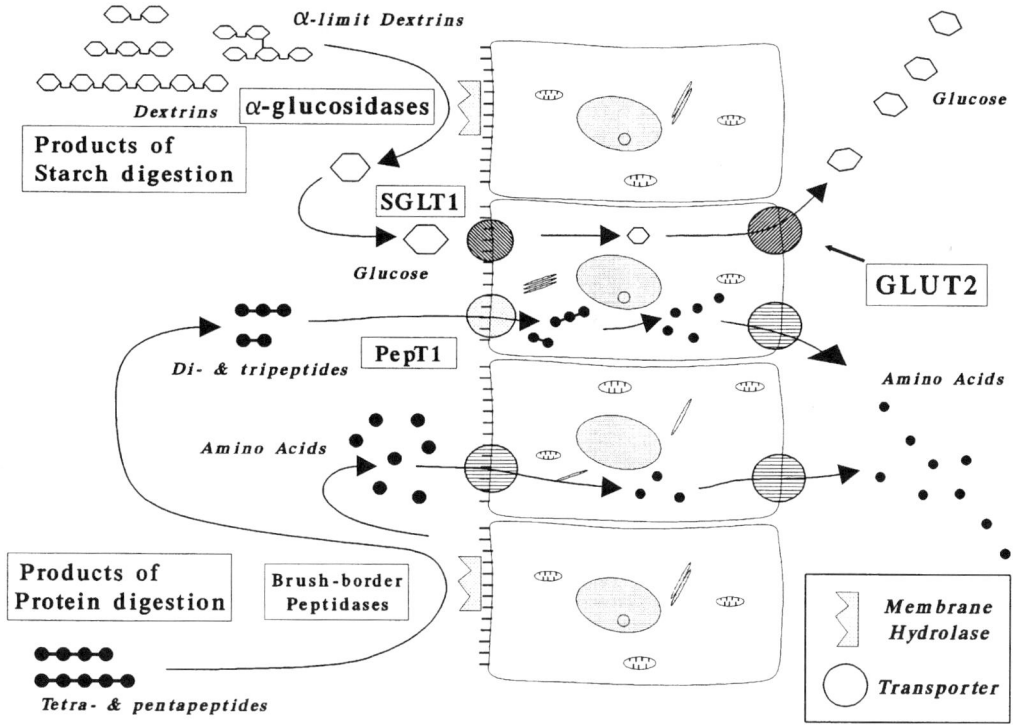

**FIGURE 6.1** Mechanisms of Amino Acid, Peptide, and Carbohydrate Uptake in the Small Intestine. An idealized view of the intestinal wall is shown. The major mechanisms of brush-border digestion of the products of luminal α-amylase hydrolysis of starch are shown at top left. The dual pathways of assimilation of the products of luminal protein hydrolysis by pancreatic proteases are shown at bottom left.

group, both being in the α-configuration. In other respects, the transporter is quite promiscuous and has a preference for a *trans-* rather than *cis*-peptide bond with L-amino acid isomers at both termini although hydrophobic D-amino acids are acceptable at the N-terminus.

Free L-amino acid transport often works "uphill" against a transmembrane concentration gradient, whereas di- and tripeptide uptake is "downhill" because the high activity of intracellular peptidases rapidly removes peptides from the intracellular compartment. Indeed, it has proved remarkably difficult to identify any intracellular pool of small peptides in tissues.[55] In contrast, the ratio of luminal:mucosal intracellular amino acids after a protein meal, is less than one for several amino acids, for which transport would have to be concentrative, or uphill.[37] A second consideration is that stimulation of $Na^+$ and water uptake by dipeptides is less strong than by amino acids[56] because transport of the latter is generally $Na^+$-dependent (Table 6.2). The author has observed that protein hydrolysates containing >70% di- and tripeptides had a rather weak effect on $Na^+$ and water uptake, in contrast to tetra- and pentapeptide preparations or free L-amino acids.[57] This is of considerable significance in design of oral rehydration solutions because it implies that solute cotransported with $Na^+$ should be proved to have a strong stoichiometric dependence on $Na^+$, as has been shown for glucose[58] and glutamine.[59] Dipeptides may not be good substrates in this respect.

### 6.3.1.6    Quantitative Importance of Peptide and Amino Acid Transport

Several lines of evidence suggest that peptide transport is regulated differently than that for L-amino acids. In early growth, dipeptide transport predominates over free L-amino transport[60,61] and is less sensitive to the effects of starvation,[62] which upregulate brush-border peptidase activity.[35,62] Sepsis downregulates amino acid transport,[63] but at present no data exists on comparative effects on peptide transport. In an attempt to disentangle possible proximate signals for amino acid and peptide transporter expression, Ferraris and colleagues fed isonitrogenous diets to rats, in which the nitrogen source was either whole protein, peptides (a protein hydrolysate), or the equivalent mixture of free L-amino acids.[64] Dipeptide transport was upregulated by all forms of dietary nitrogen, suggesting that induction of the peptide transporter does not necessarily rely on the presence of luminal peptides. In addition, L-amino acid transport was relatively unaffected by the form of nitrogen; however, there was slight downregulation of brush-border peptidase activity when L-amino acid diets were administered.[64] These data imply that peptide assimilation in the small intestine is strongly conserved when dietary amino acid supply is rate limiting to growth. In addition, they suggest that in the absence of protein intake, efficient assimilation of endogenous secretions is necessary.

In an attempt to define the relative capacities of amino acid and peptide transport, we have investigated the use of partial enzymic hydrolysates of protein. These materials are useful because they represent a mélange of peptides and free amino acids and thus model the contents of the jejunum after a protein meal. Estimates of absorptive capacity based on these materials are more realistic than if homopeptides of a single amino acid are used,[65] since these may not represent the generality of peptides. Human and animal intestinal-perfusion studies, have generally[66-70] shown that the rate of absorption of amino acid residues is both faster and more even when presented as partially hydrolyzed protein than as the equivalent free amino acid mixture. Although these findings suggest that peptide transport may have higher capacity, several factors are known to affect uptake. The starter protein, the enzymes used for hydrolysis, and the chain length of constituent peptides all affect amino acid residue uptake.[69-71] A small increase in the chain length of ovalbumin, casein, and whey hydrolysates from di- and tripeptides to tetra- and pentapeptides markedly reduced $\alpha$-NH$_2$ nitrogen uptake from these preparations.[57,72,73] Unlike the perfusion studies with glycine and glycine peptides,[65] we sometimes found no clear-cut difference in total nitrogen absorption from a di-/tripeptide hydrolysate or its equivalent free amino acid mixture. If the most significant mode of uptake from these hydrolysates were as peptides, then the most modest estimate of transport capacity for di- and tripeptides is that it is approximately 33 to 50% of that for total L-amino acid transport on a molar basis. The relatively high capacity of the peptide transporter can only be estimated from comparative studies of glycine and diglycine.[65] However, because postprandial jejunal contents after a protein meal comprise mainly small peptides and some amino acids,[74] it is likely that total peptide transport will be higher than that for L-amino acids.

In order to test this hypothesis, several groups have performed comparative feeding trials in which the amino acid composition of the diet was controlled, but the form (i.e., protein vs. L-amino acid mixture) was varied. Diets based on casein or the identical amino acid mixture produced equal growth rates in young, healthy rats.[75] Comparisons in healthy volunteers showed that regardless of the degree of hydrolysis of lactalbumin, nitrogen balance remained the same.[76] Similarly, in postsurgical patients[77] or short-bowel patients[78] receiving nasoenteral diets based on a protein hydrolysate or its equivalent free L-amino acids, there was no difference in whole-body protein turnover or nitrogen balance. Only one study has shown metabolic advantage for oral peptides over free L-amino acids. When rats were fed a diet as short intragastric infusions of 10 to 15 minutes twice daily,[79] animals receiving the protein hydrolysate diet achieved nitrogen retention values of nearly twice that of their amino acid controls. This may be due to the more rapid aminoacidemia which results from oral peptide feeding by bolus[31] and the consequent marked stimulation of insulin secretion.[80]

Although peptide diets are advocated in nasoenterally fed patients with "impaired gastrointestinal function," whole-protein or peptide diets have been shown to have equal nutritional efficacy.[81] Similar results have been obtained in patients with short bowel syndrome (60 to 150 cm of remaining jejunum)[82] and we were unable to observe any differences in N-balance, N-absorption, or $^{13}$C-leucine kinetics during 5-day feeding periods with a peptide diet or the

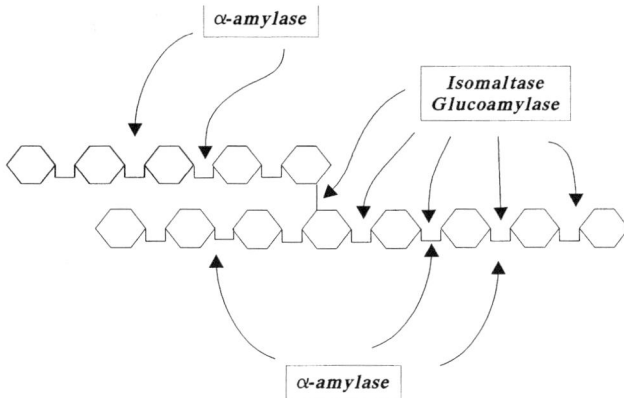

**FIGURE 6.2** Sites of Starch Hydrolysis by Luminal and Brush-Border α-Glucosidases. The branch point of starch is shown and the different glucosyl-bond specificities of intestinal α-glucosidases are indicated.

equivalent L-amino acid control diet, despite the shortness of the remaining small intestine (50- to 80-cm jejunum).[83] These data point to the capacity of the digestive and transport mechanisms of the remaining small bowel to adapt to adequate nutrient loads.[84,85]

In patients who had undergone total pancreatectomy, 91% of nitrogen from a lactalbumin hydrolysate-based diet was absorbed, compared to only 61% from a similar diet based on intact lactalbumin.[86] It was concluded that in the absence of measurable pancreatic luminal digestive activity, a significant amount of the products of gastric digestion (large oligopeptides) must have been hydrolyzed by brush-border peptidases to di- and tripeptides and L-amino acids which could be absorbed. This study therefore highlights the overlap between the different digestive systems of the intestine and provides an explanation as to why complete failure of one system will not lead to complete malabsorption. The second aspect of this study is that the positive longitudinal gradient of brush-border peptidases toward the ileum may result from the need for significant recapture of endogenous proteins[34,87] but is also an efficient safety net for dietary proteins.

## 6.3.2    Carbohydrate

As in the case of protein, carbohydrate assimilation proceeds by two phases of luminal (i.e., amylase) and brush-border digestion (by several α-glucosidases). The difference is that only monosaccharides are absorbed by identifiable transport processes, even though there may be passive permeation of small amounts of mono- and disaccharides across the mucosa.

### 6.3.2.1    Digestion and Absorption of Dietary Carbohydrate

The predominant site of dietary carbohydrate assimilation is the proximal small intestine, and approximately 75% of absorption occurs in the first 70 cm.[88] Luminal hydrolysis of starch is catalyzed by salivary and pancreatic α-amylase whose pH optimum of 7.0 corresponds to that of the lumen of the duodenum and upper jejunum.[89] Both enzymes are *endo*-glycosidases with a specificity for α-1,4 glucose linkages with two adjacent α-1,4 linkages, and will not hydrolyze lactose or sucrose (Figure 6.2). Thus, the end products of starch digestion are maltose, maltotriose, and the α-limit dextrins, with no free glucose release. The α-limit dextrins represent the branched structures which are either relatively resistant or absolutely resistant to α-amylase hydrolysis. The smallest which will be generated is a pentasaccharide comprising maltotriose linked by α-1,6 bond to maltose at the central glucose moiety. Further hydrolysis of this compound can only occur through the action of other brush-border α-glucosidases. The chain length of the linear, α-1,4 linked dextrins in the lumen after a starch meal depends on the extent to which α-amylase digestion has gone to completion, but probably ranges from 5 to 10 glucose units, similar to the chain length profile of maltodextrins used in enteral diets.

### 6.3.2.2    Membrane Digestion and the Brush-Border Oligosaccharidases

The final stage of starch (or dietary disaccharide) digestion is brush-border hydrolysis by several saccharidases to produce monosaccharides (Figure 6.1). These enzymes exist as multisubunit structures inserted into the brush-border membrane via a hydrophobic domain, while the hydrophilic domains contain the active site of the enzyme.[90-93] Several classifications have been applied to this group of enzymes (Table 6.3), but despite this, all are capable of hydrolyzing external α-1,4 glycosidic linkages at the nonreducing end of maltose, maltotriose, amylose, or amylopectin.[94,95] Maltases Ib, II, and perhaps III also have activity toward α-1,6 linkages, which exist in the amylopectin fraction of starch and in the branch points of the α-limit dextrins.[96] Sucrase-isomaltase is a hybrid enzyme with two activities. The isomaltase moiety has the ability to split α-1,6 linked glucose oligomers, albeit at a slower rate than α-1,4 linkages. The need for the second activity toward α-1,6 linkages is because about 8 to 10% of amylopectin is linked in this way. In contrast, the sucrase moiety has activity toward sucrose and toward the α-1,4 linkages in maltose.[96] Lactase or β-galactosidase exists as two forms in a dimeric structure, both of which can cleave lactose to glucose and galactose.[96]

Thus, hydrolysis of starch to glucose at the brush border utilizes all of the "maltases" of which sucrase-isomaltase is the most important (ca. 80% of total activity). The isomaltase moiety alone accounts for 50% of total activity, and Maltase II (glucoamylase) has considerable activity toward oligosaccharides.[97] These considerations help explain why starch assimilation can proceed after total pancreatectomy.

### 6.3.2.3    Rate-Limiting Steps in Carbohydrate Assimilation

There is little difference in the adult glycemic response to 50 g of glucose, maltose, a maltodextrin or starch,[98] suggesting the rapidity of action of luminal and brush-border hydrolyases. Even if an α-amylase inhibitor was coadministered with the meal at a level sufficient to completely inhibit luminal α-amylase, most of the starch intake was assimilated.[99] These data suggest that glucose polymer chain length has a slight effect on assimilation in the presence of normal pancreatic secretions and that brush-border saccharidase activity is high. In an attempt to dissociate luminal and brush-border activities, we varied the glucose polymer linkage from its usual form (α-1,4) to α-1,6 (dextran) and were able to show that it was almost completely assimilated by healthy volunteers.[100] Dextran is completely resistant to α-amylase digestion and it is likely that brush-border hydrolysis occurs via the isomaltase moiety of sucrase-isomaltase, as was suggested many years ago by Dahlqvist.[101,102] As in the case of luminal and brush-border protein digestion, the multiplicity of digestive systems ensures that carbohydrate assimilation is an extremely efficient process which is difficult to impair to any great extent.

### 6.3.2.4    Monosaccharide Transport

Glucose transport occurs via a $Na^+$-linked transporter SGLT1, a tetrameric protein with 73,000 Da subunits which is unrelated to the GLUT family of glucose transporters.[103] It is very closely related to the glucose transporter in the renal tubular brush-border membrane[104] and their kinetic and biochemical properties are reviewed elsewhere.[105] Expression of this transporter can be upregulated by luminal glucose concentrations, which is the nutrient load.[106] In contrast, uptake of fructose occurs by a distinct transporter, GLUT5 (Table 6.2), which provides a carrier-mediated system which is not inhibited by phloridzin or metabolic inhibitors.[107] A second component is electrogenic and can be inhibited by phloridzin, a specific inhibitor of the $Na^+$-glucose cotransporter.[108]

**TABLE 6.3  Membrane Digestion of Dietary Starch**

| Enzyme trivial name | Alternative name | Enzyme number | Substrate | Product | Comments | References |
|---|---|---|---|---|---|---|
| Sucrase | Maltase Ia | 3.2.1.48 | Sucrose | Glucose Fructose | Multienzyme complex, each subunit has high degree of sequence homology with acid $\alpha$-glucosidase (EC 3. 2. 1. 3) in liver and other tissues | 92, 93 |
| Isomaltase | Maltase Ib | 3.2.1.10 | Maltose $\alpha$-1,4/$\alpha$-1,6 linked oligomers | Glucose | | |
| Glucoamylase | Maltase II | 3.2.1.20 | Starch $\alpha$-1,4 >> $\alpha$-1,6 | Glucose | Multienzyme complex, may be similar enzymes but slightly different activities | 91, 94, 95 |
| Maltase | Maltase III | 3.2.1.20 | Maltose $\alpha$-1,4 linked oligomers | Glucose | | |
| **Other Membrane Saccharidases** | | | | | | |
| Lactase | $\beta$-D-galactosidase | 3.2.1.23 3.2.1.62 | Lactose | Glucose Galactose | Expression of this enzyme is genetically determined; can be induced by high intake of disaccharides, not monosaccharides | 20, 129, 253 |

This superfamily of glucose transporters (GLUT) is expressed in a tissue-specific fashion.[103] GLUT2, the liver type transporter (Table 6.2), is responsible for facilitated diffusion exit of glucose from the basolateral membrane of mucosal cells of the intestine and renal tubule, as well as uptake into liver cells.[109] This transporter and indeed the whole GLUT family are responsive to hormonal and substrate regulation. Thus, the density of GLUT2 on the basolateral membrane of intestinal cells is modulated by circulating glucose concentration, being upregulated in diabetes.[53] This may be a key control point for intracellular compartmentation of glucose and its uptake by the enterocyte since only a small fraction of the glucose is metabolized during passage through the absorptive cell.[110]

### 6.3.2.5    The Route of Mucosal Monosaccharide Uptake

There have been persistent claims that a significant proportion of glucose transport not only occurs via the tight-junction pathways ("solvent drag"), but that this process also controls peptide uptake.[111,112] This arose from the puzzle proposed by Pappenheimer and colleagues that luminal glucose concentrations were much higher than the $K_t$ of the sodium-linked glucose transporter (SGLT1; Table 6.2) and that another pathway of glucose uptake was necessary to explain the extra transport capacity required.[111] This reasoning is flawed for several reasons because, in reality, postprandial luminal glucose concentrations rarely exceed the $K_t$ of SGLT1[113] and during perfusion of the human small intestine with high glucose concentrations, Fordtran and colleagues could not detect any stimulation of net uptake of urea and passively absorbed sugar probes,[114] which should have occurred if Fisher's original proposal for "solvent drag" was correct.[115] Furthermore, one would expect that infants who lack the intestinal glucose/ galactose transporter would still absorb glucose via a mechanism of solvent drag. However, isolated segment jejunal perfusions in these children have failed to reveal any significant glucose uptake, even at high perfused concentrations of 100 mmol/l.[116] In addition, we have confirmed this in steady-state human jejunal perfusion studies in which enteral diets with different peptide profiles were used.[73] As seen in Figure 6.3, little free glucose was liberated by brush-border hydrolysis, which implies that rates of mucosal glucose liberation and uptake are well matched in humans.

In humans, the most significant mode of transmucosal passage of dietary carbohydrate is by specific monosaccharide transporters. This does not mean that di- and oligosaccharides cannot permeate the brush-border membrane (transcellular route) or pass through the tight-junction (paracellular route), but that the amount is small.[18] This phenomenon has been exploited as a useful noninvasive marker for increased intestinal permeability to sugar probes (e.g., lactulose, lactitol) in inflammatory illnesses, such as Crohn's disease.[117-120]

### 6.3.2.6    Absorption of Carbohydrates from Clinical Diets

We have expended considerable effort in defining the composition of the maltodextrins with chromatographic methods of increasing power.[121] Maltodextrins are widely used in enteral diets, in many weight-reducing and -increasing diets, and in sports formula diets for athletes. In their classic study of treatment of patients with ascites secondary to alcoholic cirrhosis, Fiaccadori and colleagues describe a branched-chain amino acid enriched diet which also contains these soluble maltodextrins.[122] Although maltodextrins can be defined by a single value for their dextrose equivalent (DE), this masks the fact that they are a very heterogeneous mixture of glucose polymers. This is shown for the base material used in one jejunal perfusion study (Figure 6.3). As a result, it is impossible to describe the material simply as "maltodextrin" without referring to its absorptive characteristics.

Despite the evidence of the *in vivo* studies described above, *in vitro*, glucose uptake by a rabbit jejunal preparations in an Ussing chamber was considerably faster from solutions of glucose than

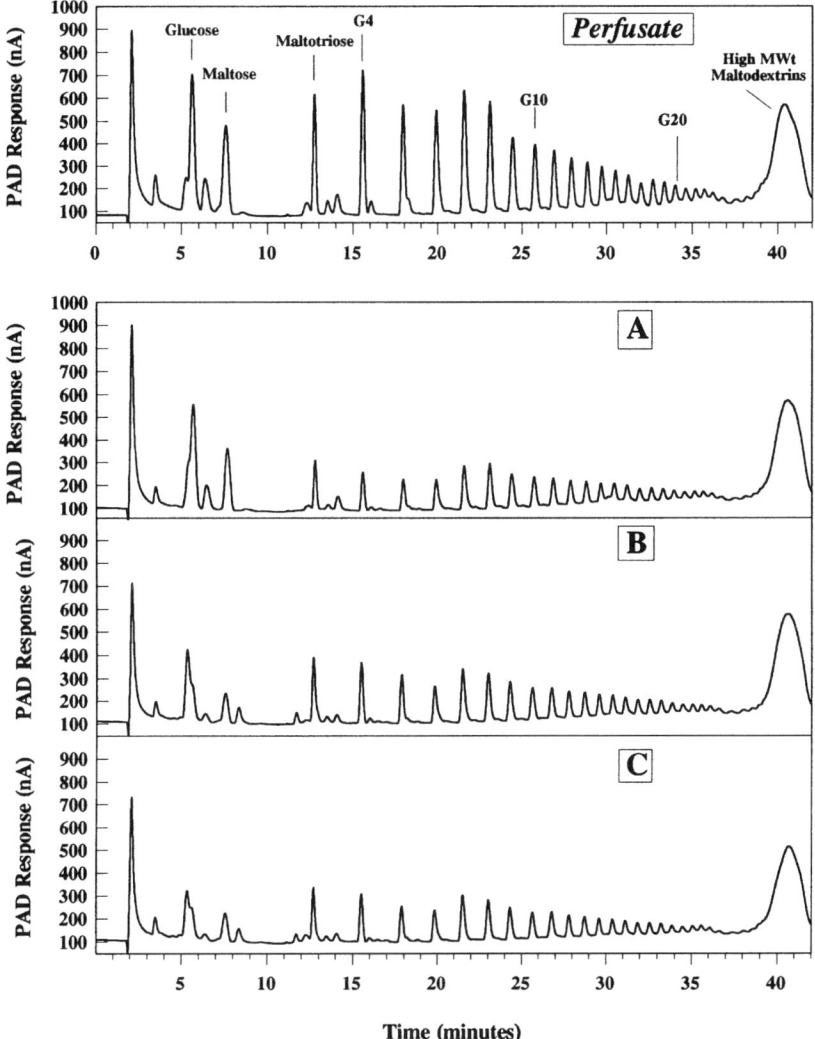

**FIGURE 6.3**   HPLC Analysis of Perfusates and Aspirates of Maltodextrins Perfused in the Human Jejunum. High-performance anion-exchange liquid chromatography (Carbopak PA-100, Pulsed Amperometric Detection) of maltodextrins in jejunal perfusate and aspirates, when coperfused with a short (B) or medium-chain whey hydrolysate (C), or its equivalent free L-amino acid mixture (A). (From Grimble et al., *Clin. Nutr.*, 13(Suppl.), 46, 1994.)

solutions of a short-chain maltodextrin (4 to 9 glucose units[123]). Although this suggests that brush-border hydrolysis is rate limiting to uptake (cf. peptide transport above), we have not observed the same in the perfused human jejunum with excluded pancreatic secretions. These studies were performed with fractionated maltodextrins having an average size range of <10 glucose units or >10 glucose units. In the absence of luminal α-amylase, lower MWt glucose polymers were assimilated more rapidly than higher MWt glucose polymers and seemed to be conferring a kinetic advantage on glucose uptake. An α-amylase hydrolysate of the low MWt glucose polymer fraction (<10 glucose molecules) conferred the expected kinetic advantage on glucose transport; the high MWt fraction (osmolality one fifth of the starting material) was surprisingly well absorbed even in the absence of α-amylase. In addition, the low MWt polymer was as rapidly assimilated as maltose and maltotriose, and more efficiently than equivalent concentrations of free glucose.[124-126] These data suggest that brush-border hydrolysis is a very active process, which is only rate limiting for high-molecular-weight polymers, if luminal pancreatic α-amylase is absent, as has also been confirmed by Kerzner and colleagues, who used a canine jejunal Thiry-Vella fistula model.[127] It is therefore more logical to use high-molecular-weight maltodextrins in clinical enteral diets since their energy content can be increased and diet osmolality reduced. In one diet (Tolerex, Sandoz) this concept has been utilized, with a subsequent lowering of osmolality from 830 to 630 mosmol/kg. Where digestive and absorptive function are both severely impaired, a low MWt maltodextrin could be used.

### 6.3.2.7    Sucrose and Enteral Nutrition

In patients with a very short small intestine which had not adapted, the remaining digestive and absorptive capacity of the mucosal surface may limit uptake of glucose from glucose polymer mixtures. Jejunal perfusion studies have shown that if glucose transport from glucose polymers is saturated, sugar absorption can be enhanced if the disaccharide sucrose is added.[128] This is because although sucrose and maltodextrin hydrolysis is by the same hybrid brush-border hydrolase, sucrase-isomaltase (Table 6.3), absorption of fructose occurs via GLUT5 and not SGLT1 (glucose/galactose carrier). Furthermore, both GLUT5 and sucrase activity can be induced by dietary sucrose.[107,129] The link between brush-border hydrolysis of sucrose and absorption of the monosaccharides fructose and glucose appears to confer a kinetic advantage on fructose uptake, since in one study 8 of 10 subjects malabsorbed 50 g of fructose, whereas none malabsorbed 100 g of sucrose.[130] Thus the addition of sucrose to enteral diets can further enhance carbohydrate uptake, quite apart from its beneficial taste properties.

### 6.3.3    Fat Absorption

The major dietary fats are triglycerides, cholesterol, and the fat-soluble vitamins. Triglycerides (TG) are fatty acid triesters of glycerol, which may contain long-chain fatty acids [C16 to C18; long-chain triglycerides (LCT)] or medium-chain fatty acids [C6 to C12; medium-chain triglycerides (MCT)], and inclusion of either in the fat source of enteral diets is related to the physiology of fat digestion and absorption.

### 6.3.3.1    Emulsification

If lipid absorption were based solely on the direct brush-border membrane uptake of TG, their water insolubility would severely limit the process, because of the droplet size of the TG emulsion and the limited permeability of fat droplets across the unstirred water layer. The efficiency of lipid assimilation is ensured by exogenous (e.g., bile acids) or endogenous (fatty acids, monoglycerides released *in situ*) chemical emulsifiers which produce small particles with high surface area/volume which aid enzyme hydrolysis. The actions of lingual lipase and gastric mechanical activity combine to provide some emulsification, with enzymic release of free fatty acid and diglyceride (DG).[131] Transfer of gastric contents, rich in fat, to the duodenum has two consequences: (1) $H^+$ stimulated secretin stimulates pancreatic water and $HCO_3^-$-secretion into the duodenum, raising the pH to 6 or 7; and (2) luminal free fatty acids in the duodenum stimulate cholecystokinin-pancreozymin (CCK-PZ) release by duodenal epithelial cells. This signals contraction of the gall bladder and release of bile acids into the intestinal lumen.

  The higher pH of the duodenal contents aids in further emulsification and facilitates the action of pancreatic lipase. At pH 6 or 7, bile salts are soluble in water, but above a certain concentration (critical micellar concentration) they will form pure bile salt micelles. Fatty acids, monoglycerides, and phospholipids interdigitate with this structure, forming mixed micelles with a hydrophobic core and hydrophilic outer surface. This has been reviewed in detail elsewhere.[132-135]

### 6.3.3.2    Enzyme Digestion

Pancreatic colipase binds tightly to the surface of mixed micelles and acts as electrostatic anchor for lipase which has considerable specificity for the 1,3 positions of TG. In addition to lingual and pancreatic lipase, a third and distinct mucosal acid-active intestinal lipase has been partially characterized and found in the villus tips in the proximal intestine,[136] which is the most mature population of enterocytes engaged in the absorption and transport of dietary lipid. Its binding to the brush-border involves heparin,[137] which allows fatty acids and monoglycerides to be generated in close proximity to the intestinal membrane prior to absorption.

### 6.3.3.3    Absorption

Osmotic and other pressures generated within the micelle by extensive TG hydrolysis cause budding of smaller micelles from the surface of these structures. The resulting smaller micelles are then available for uptake of MG and fatty acids at the microvilli surface. Lipolysis products are absorbed in the proximal intestine, whereas bile salts are absorbed at the distal ileum; as a result mixed micelles must dissociate.

The acidic microenvironment adjacent to the brush-border membrane is important in promoting lipid absorption since protonation of fatty acids allows their diffusion through the membrane.[138] Within the enterocyte, the higher intracellular pH results in their ionization, thus reducing the likelihood of back diffusion. Notwithstanding this, mucosal uptake of long-chain fatty acids is now known to occur as a result of binding to a specific intestinal membrane binding protein that is a member of a family of cytoplasmic hydrophobic ligand-binding proteins.[139,140] This intestinal fatty acid binding protein is thought to participate in the uptake, intracellular targeting, and metabolic processing of fatty acids within the intestinal epithelial cell.

Within the enterocyte, fatty acids are transferred by their specific cytoplasmic carrier proteins to the smooth endoplasmic reticulum for reesterification to TG.[133] These TG are transferred, along with cholesterol, phospholipids, and fat-soluble vitamins, to the Golgi apparatus, where they combine with apolipoproteins to form chylomicrons and very low density lipoproteins. The Golgi apparatus is transferred to the enterocyte lateral membrane and fuses with it. Subsequent rupture of the fused vesicle by exocytosis results in the release of lipid into the lymphatic system.

Although probably not of any clinical significance, not all the neutral lipid absorbed from the lumen of the intestine is destined for packaging and transport via the lymphatics in chylomicrons.[141,142] Experimental animal studies indicate that nearly half of neutral lipids may be transported out of the enterocytes via nonlymphatic pathways (presumably via the portal vein). These are postulated to require prior hydrolysis by a specific, nonpancreatic, alkaline-active lipase.

Medium-chain triglycerides appear to "short-circuit" some of these processes because they are more water soluble than LCT and may either be absorbed intact or undergo considerably more rapid lipase hydrolysis than LCT, with subsequent direct uptake of MG and fatty acid. There is no absolute requirement for mixed micelle formation with bile acids and, within the enterocyte, short- and medium-chain fatty acids are generally not reesterified to TG and incorporated into chylomicrons but may be released directly into the portal circulation where they bind to albumin.[133] These mechanisms are summarized in Table 6.4.

### 6.3.4    Water

Large amounts of water and electrolytes are handled by the normal human intestine during a 24-h period (Table 6.5). They comprise the small intestinal luminal intake of fluid of the diet and secretions from the salivary glands, stomach, pancreas, biliary tree, and intestinal mucosa, approximately 9 l in total. Of this about 1 to 5 l pass the ileocecal valve, with less than 200 ml escaping into the stool.[143] No specific active transport processes exist to absorb the water. The

**TABLE 6.4  Mechanisms Involved**
**in Assimilation of**
**Dietary Lipid**

Emulsification
Lipolysis
Micellar formation
Membrane transport
Intracellular triglyceride resynthesis
Chylomicron formation
Transfer into lymphatic system

intestinal mucosa acts as a semipermeable membrane through which water flows in either direction in response to differences in osmotic pressure. Thus, luminal nutrient digestion renders the bulk phase hypertonic and water moves from the intestinal fluid into the gut lumen[144]; nutrient absorption, however, renders it more hypotonic such that water is absorbed along with these solutes. In this way, the luminal contents are adjusted to near isotonicity throughout the small bowel.

Mucosal permeability varies along the length of the intestine, being highest in jejunum, intermediate in the ileum, and lowest in the colon.[144] Therefore, the jejunum effects the rapid equilibration of osmotic pressure gradients created by the digestion and absorption of nutrients. The lower permeability of the colonic mucosa prevents water from leaking back into the lumen when the mainly ionic solutes are actively absorbed, although this mechanism has specific properties.[145] Water has difficulty passing across the lipid membrane of the epithelial cells, and it is now clear that most of it passes between cells rather than through them.[146] Therefore, the differences in permeability throughout the intestine depend on the different permeabilities of the "tight" junctions between cells. The pores through which water passes in the jejunum have been calculated to be about twice the diameter of those in the ileum.[144] Thus, water absorption in the upper intestine is determined largely by absorption of nutrients; however, in the ileum, and particularly in the colon, the absorption of salt is the main driving force for water absorption and resulting dehydration of colonic contents.

### 6.3.5    Electrolytes

The gut has extremely efficient mechanisms for conserving $Na^+$ (Table 6.5). In the duodenum and upper jejunum, simple diffusion of sodium and chloride occurs down concentration gradients producing luminal concentrations similar to those in plasma. When a sodium chloride solution that is isotonic with plasma is perfused in the normal human jejunum, no net uptake of sodium or chloride ions occurs.[147] Sodium uptake is, however, stimulated in the presence of glucose,[148] amino acids, di- and tripeptides,[147] and bicarbonate ions[149] through the action of $Na^+$-nutrient cotransporters.[105] Bicarbonate is removed as $CO_2$ by reaction with actively secreted hydrogen

**TABLE 6.5  Water and Electrolyte Handling by the Intestine**

|                   | Water (ml) | Sodium (mmol) | Chloride (mmol) | Potassium (mmol) |
|-------------------|-----------|---------------|-----------------|------------------|
| Input             |           |               |                 |                  |
|   Diet            | 1500      | 150           | 150             | 80               |
|   Gut secretions  | 7500      | 1000          | 750             | 40               |
| Total             | 9000      | 1150          | 900             | 120              |
| Absorption        |           |               |                 |                  |
|   Small intestine | 7500      | 950           | 800             | 110              |
|   Colon           | 1350      | 195           | 97              | −3               |
| Output            | 150       | 5             | 3               | 1                |

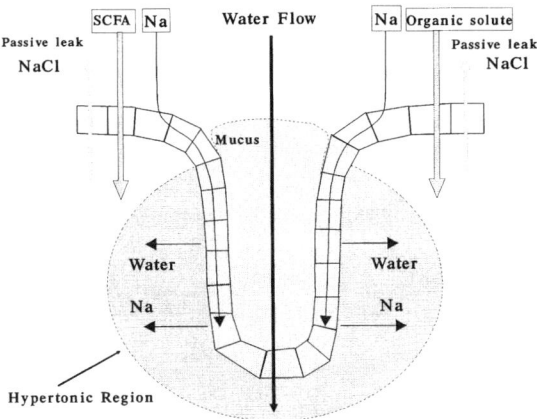

**FIGURE 6.4** Hypothetical Mechanism for Water and Electrolyte Uptake in the Colon. A cross section of one colonic crypt is shown. Substrate-stimulated Na$^+$ uptake is transferred by intercolonocyte movement to the submucosal region. This stimulates net water uptake against the countervailing force of the dehydrated fecal stream.

ions. Hydrogen ion is secreted by exchange with absorbed sodium on a specific cation exchange carrier. In addition to nutrient and bicarbonate-stimulated absorption in the jejunum, sodium and chloride ions are also thought to move in response to solvent drag (see above). A lower luminal nutrient concentration in the ileum results in the greater significance of active absorption processes, such as ion exchange of H$^+$ and Cl$^-$ for HCO$_3^-$.[146,150] The ileal mucosa is less permeable to ions than in the jejunum, so once absorbed only limited back diffusion occurs into the lumen.

In the colon 1.5 to 2.6 l of water are absorbed daily, compared to a reserve capacity of three to four times this amount. It is only when this absorptive capacity is overwhelmed, acutely, that diarrhea ensues.[26,143] Water absorption is determined mainly by absorption of Na$^+$, Cl$^-$, and SCFA.[151,152] There are marked differences between species in colonic water absorption which affects the water content of normal stool. As Naftalin and colleagues have suggested, pure mechanical contractile forces are not capable of dehydrating the fecal stream since the force necessary to reduce water content from 85 to <65% is equivalent to 5 to 10 atm. Clearly, some other osmotic mechanism operates to ensure efficient water salvage. Their suggestion is that water and Na$^+$ passage is differentiated between the crypt cells and adjacent colonocytes. Active uptake of Na$^+$ and its passage via cells to the base of the crypt (Figure 6.4) will produce a region of hyperosmolarity (>1000 mosm/kg) which is sufficient to provide the motive force for water passage from the colonic lumen and through the crypt lumen and crypt cells.[145,153] Na$^+$ and Cl$^-$, but not water, may then leak back into the colonic lumen via a passive route. Collapse of the crypt in response to these osmotic pressures is prevented by the mucus plug within the crypt.

Na$^+$ uptake by adjacent colonocytes may therefore be stimulated by uptake of solutes such as the SCFAs which are generated within the lumen by bacterial fermentation (see below). This system of necessity requires expenditure of metabolic energy to maintain the active transport of Na$^+$ against a concentration gradient, and any factor which inhibits this or stimulates passive permeation of Na$^+$ or Cl$^-$ back into the colonic lumen will result in impaired water uptake and diarrhea.[146]

### 6.3.6    Colonic Digestion and Absorption

#### 6.3.6.1    Development of Colonic Fermentation in Humans

The colonic luminal bacteria have been described as an organ-within-an-organ which develops slowly during the first 2 years of life in human infants[23] before establishment of a stable adult microflora.[154] Several characteristic luminal functions develop during this period, namely mucin breakdown, the regulation of fecal tryptic activity, the conversion of bilirubin to urobilinogen, cholesterol catabolism, and the generation of SCFA and other organic acids (Table 6.1). The rate of adaptation is driven by the pattern of fermentable substrates which enter the cecum and although carbohydrate fermentation is rapidly established, indicators of protein fermentation (*iso-* and *n*-valeric acids) are not complete until 16 months of life.[23] Acetate-producing bacteria are rapidly established and the resulting luminal "acetate-buffer" is strongly bacteriostatic for some gram negative bacteria. The adult pattern of colonic luminal metabolism requires development of a population of butyrate-producing bacteria at the expense of acetate production. This is essentially a reductive metabolic pathway which uses $H_2$ as substrate[155] as do nitrate and sulfate-reducing bacteria which are substrate inducible.[156,157] In addition, $CO_2$ reduction to $CH_4$ consumes $H_2$ and the significance of the methanogenic bacteria varies between individuals.[158]

### 6.3.6.2    Metabolism by Colonic Microflora

The relationship between bacteria and the colon is therefore truly symbiotic. The host makes a significant contribution to the growth of luminal bacteria by providing both fermentable carbohydrate (dietary sources, mucins) and nitrogen (urea, endogenous proteins, malabsorbed dietary protein) which act synergistically.[5,159] Establishment of this symbiosis may be retarded by antibiotic treatment in early life which allows the establishment of *clostridium difficile* colonies which may be detected by the presence of *iso*-caproic acid in fecal samples. Malabsorption of components of formula diet by infants, because of their strong buffering capacity, will tend to oppose establishment of an acetate buffer and thus allow establishment of coliform and streptococcal colonies. It is estimated that in adult humans, approximately 70 g/day of fermentable carbohydrate would be required to produce the bacterial mass of daily stool.[160]

### 6.3.6.3    Metabolism by the Colonocyte

Of the SCFAs, butyrate has the most pronounced effects on the epithelial cells of the cecum and colon.[161] It provides the function of a precursor for ketone production, which is not shared with acetate and propionate,[162,163] and of the possible metabolic fuels (e.g., glucose and glutamine) it appears to be preferentially used by colonocytes.[164] Butyrate promotes proliferation and differentiation of colonic epithelial crypt cells toward the mature, highly polarized form which express apical membrane hydrolases at the top of the crypt.[165-168] *In vivo* studies in rats have confirmed that it is the fermentation products of dietary fiber (i.e., SCFAs) and not its effects in lowering luminal pH[169] or the presence of bulk in the intestinal lumen which increases crypt-cell proliferation rates in the rat colon.[170,171] A recent study has shown that control of this may reside in the ability of butyrate to modulate plasmin activity directly. This enzyme is formed through activation of plasminogen by urokinase; plasmin is responsible for hydrolysis and remodeling of the basement membrane which attaches colonocytes. Thus, butyrate inhibits urokinase, but stimulates the urokinase inhibitor — plasminogen activator inhibitor 1. The effect occurs at the cellular level, in that mRNA levels were either up- or downregulated.[172] Thus, butyrate will alter the mobility and adhesion of colonocytes during their migration. Butyrate also appears to modulate the cell cycle at the level of gene transcription since it can downregulate N-*ras* oncogene expression and the proliferative potential of cultured human colon tumor cell lines.[166,173,174] In addition, butyrate added to the medium induces greater differentiation in terms of expression of surface hydrolases and glycosylated cell-surface components,[175] while reducing expression of surface tumor-specific antigens.[166]

A further unique feature of butyrate production by the colonic luminal microflora is that it provides for the unique polarity of uptake of butyrate of the colonocyte. Rombeau and colleagues have shown that healing of the colon in a rat model of surgical resection and reanastomosis was accelerated by luminal butyrate[176,177] but not by its intravenous administration.[178]

In contrast, acetate, the major SCFA produced by fermentation, has the most marked stimulatory effects on colonic blood flow.[179-181] In general, absorption of luminal nutrients is accompanied by increased regional blood flow to the intestine in health[182-184] and following injury.[185,186] It is difficult, however, to disentangle the contribution of direct metabolic trophism of the SCFAs and the consequences of regional stimulation of the intestine through increased blood flow.

### 6.3.6.4    SCFAs and Colonic Water and Electrolyte Uptake

Colonic (and jejunal) mucosal transport of SCFAs is accompanied by water and $Na^+$ uptake which appears to be mediated by two mechanisms. First, active uptake of unprotonated SCFAs and $Na^+$ occurs in exchange for $Cl^-$ and $H^+$, respectively. The second mode of uptake is probably by passive diffusion of protonated SCFA down a concentration gradient.[152,187,188] The latter may explain why inflammatory bowel disease reduces colonic uptake of other actively transported organic anions but has a lesser impact on SCFA uptake.[189] The capacity of the colonic luminal bacteria to ferment nonabsorbed disaccharides such as lactulose[24] and lactitol[19] and for the colon to absorb SCFAs is limited (approximately 80 g/day), and above this level of intake osmotic diarrhea will ensue. Thus, at lower levels of intake of fermentable carbohydrate, SCFAs, generated by luminal bacteria, aid the process of dehydrating the fecal stream and salvage 90% of the water and electrolytes which enter the colon from the small intestine (approx. 1350 ml/day).

### 6.3.6.5    Diarrhea

These considerations should therefore be kept in mind when considering the characteristics of diarrhea in patients with "malabsorption." Diarrhea is multifactorial but has the common mechanism of failure of the colon to efficiently salvage a normal or increased water and electrolyte load. Apart from infectious diarrhea, several other factors have been noted in enterally fed patients — a closely studied group. There is a close association with concurrent antibiotic therapy[21] but not the lactose content of enteral feeds or the rate of infusion[190] or the digestibility of the protein source.[191,192] In addition diarrhea may result from enteral diet malabsorption, aberrant small and large bowel motility, and an aberrant large bowel secretory response to the mode of nasoenteral feeding employed.

Antibiotic administration has been shown to elicit diarrheal symptoms in healthy volunteers consuming a 20 g dose of lactulose which had not previously altered stool output.[25] Antibiotics will inhibit many of the functions of the colonic luminal microflora and thus impair its function as an organ within an organ. Some antibiotics (most notably ampicillin, erythromycin, clindamycin, and metronidazole) will suppress indices of colonic bacterial fermentation, such as breath $H_2$ output,[25] acidification of the cecum,[193] urinary excretion of D-amino acids derived from colonic bacteria,[194] and *in vitro* production of SCFAs by fecal inoculates.[195] In addition, metronidazole therapy has been shown to be of significant clinical benefit in reducing the colonic production of SCFAs in children with inborn errors of methylmalonate and propionate metabolism.[196] It is likely that the effects of impaired microbial function are twofold: (1) reduced fermentation will reduce salvage of osmotically active colonic luminal nutrients and thus impair water uptake, and (2) impaired generation of SCFAs will lead to reduced water and electrolyte uptake.

A series of reports have demonstrated the link between carbohydrate malabsorption and impaired salvage in enterally fed postsurgical patients because a rise in breath $H_2$ concentrations preceded the onset of diarrhea by several hours.[197] This mechanism may be complex. Although antibiotics reduce colonic fermentation and breath $H_2$ production in the clinical setting[195] and would be expected to impair salvage of an increased colonic substrate load, some (e.g., erythromycin) can significantly shorten mouth to cecum transit time,[198] and may directly contribute to malabsorption resulting from increased motility.

As described above, nutrient assimilation in humans occurs predominantly in the upper small intestine. Severe impairment of gastric emptying or gastric atony is not uncommonly encountered in patients with neuropathy secondary to diabetes or alcohol misuse and in hospitalized patients with head injuries or abdominal trauma or sepsis resulting from penetrating wounds or surgery. This will reduce the efficiency with which food is homogenized by the stomach. Efficient absorption of nutrients from chyme in the upper small intestine requires a repetitive mixing action in which the mucosa dips into the chyme, minimizing the diffusion barrier to absorption. This movement is accompanied by villus contractions which aid blood and lymphatic flow to carry away the products of digestion and absorption. Interposed with these repetitive segmenting movements, there are erratic propulsive movements which rapidly propel chyme 10 to 30 cm distally and the segmenting process recommences.[199] Our understanding of how such complex patterns of motor activity are organized has advanced considerably in recent years, mainly as a result of improved monitoring techniques which allow the small intestinal and colonic motility patterns in the fasting and fed state to be measured in ambulant subjects.

In the fasting state[200] small intestinal motility is characterized by a period of inactivity (Phase I) followed by Phase II, a period of irregular spike activity lasting (like Phase I) for 30 to 40 min. Pressure activity increases steadily during the latter half of Phase II ushering in Phase III, during which there are intense repetitive high amplitude contractions. Phase III lasts for about 4 to 6 min of irregular activity (Phase IV), which then gives way to a new Phase I. The whole cycle of activity migrates down the upper small intestine at 4 to 6 cm/min, slowing distally to 1 to 2 cm/min in the terminal ileum. This migrating motor complex, referred to as the MMC, is thought to have the function of sweeping debris down the small intestine and does not occur until 4 to 6 h after a meal. The fasting pattern of motility is disrupted by feeding, and irregular activity is seen throughout the small intestine. It resembles that seen during Phase II of the MMC and hence is called "type II activity." Contraction frequency and speed are reduced by nutrients, thereby prolonging transit time.[201] The intestine appears able to discriminate between different nutrients since there are qualitative differences in motor response, fat generating particularly intense nonpropagating clustered contractions whose function is presumably to aid emulsification and hence absorption. In essence, therefore, the fasting function of the motility response is to propagate debris distally and the fed response is basically nonpropagative in type to aid digestion and absorption of nutrients.[202]

Where quantitative and qualitative nutrient supply is carefully controlled, as in enteral nutrition, it has been shown in humans and in dogs that a low rate of intragastric diet infusion (approx. 1.4 kcal/min) did not elicit the normal fed response, in that propagating MMCs were seen throughout diet infusion.[13,203] Intraduodenal infusion of the same and higher loads resulted in the normal switch from fasting to feeding motility in small bowel[13] and colon.[204] Thus, intragastric infusion of enteral diets elicits an "abnormal" small intestinal and colonic motility response which was shown in one experimental group of healthy volunteers to result in diarrhea. In addition, a series of *in vivo* colonic perfusion studies in normal human subjects showed that intragastric diet infusion caused a marked secretion of water (160 ml/h), $Na^+$, and $Cl^-$ in the ascending colon which could be reversed by cecal infusion of a mixture of SCFAs.[205] These results are intriguing because they show the importance of luminal SCFAs in the pathogenesis of colonic diarrhea. Therapeutic attempts to moderate diarrhea by increasing colonic SCFA production by use of fermentable fibers have been reviewed elsewhere.[206,207]

## 6.4   METABOLISM IN THE INTESTINE

### 6.4.1   Nutrition of the Mucosa — Luminal or Arterial?

If the mucosal cells of the small and large intestine derived their energy directly from absorbed substrates, this would result in a situation of "feast and famine," which would require a high level of spare capacity and adaptability for intracellular transport mechanisms (e.g., mitochondria). On logical grounds, it is more likely that the arterial supply provides the main source of nutrients. In the case of amino acids, intravenous infusions or jejunal luminal infusions of radiolabeled amino acids have been shown to lead to different rates of incorporation into mucosal protein. Even when these values were corrected for the specific radioactivity of each precursor pool (i.e., arterial blood or luminal fluid), the rate of incorporation from arterial supplies was still an order of magnitude higher.[208] Similar studies with radiolabeled glucose have suggested the same compartmentation of luminal and arterial supplies. During feeding, the proportion of luminal glucose which is transferred into the portal circulation is lower at high substrate loads, i.e., the process is saturable.[110] In the fasted state, arterial blood supplies all glucose for lactate production. This is an understandable functional compartmentation of substrate supply which is also exemplified by glutamine metabolism (see below). Windmueller showed a similar dependence of portal transfer on luminal concentration.[209] In other words the capacity of the mucosa to metabolize luminal glutamine was not unlimited or uncontrolled. There was a reciprocal relationship between metabolism of arterial and luminal glutamine sources but the effects were additive.[209] This interrelationship does not, however, appear to exist for the main luminal substrates generated in the cecum and colon. SCFAs have different effects when supplied to luminal and arterial faces of the mucosa. Chronic intracolonic infusion of SCFA was shown to increase the cellularity of the colonic mucosa and to increase the bursting strength of an anastomotic wound,[177] whereas chronic intravenous infusion of SCFA had little effect.[178] This is understandable since there are few other sources of butyrate generated in the body apart from the colonic lumen.[210]

### 6.4.2 Principal Substrates for Small Intestinal Metabolism

Four substrates have been investigated which have particular effects on the maintenance of mucosal barrier function. The SCFA have been described in detail above and can be truly described as "essential nutrients" because of the links between reduced luminal production and the onset of organ dysfunction, i.e., diarrhea.[211]

#### 6.4.2.1 Glutamine

Windmueller observed that luminal asparagine was quantitatively transferred to the portal circulation whereas luminal glutamine was extensively metabolized as was luminal glutamate.[209] This has been confirmed in organ balance studies in dogs[212,213] which showed that in the fasting state, intestinal glutamine consumption was $1.4 \pm 0.2$ μmol/kg/min compared to glucose consumption of $4.1 \pm 1.2$ μmol/kg/min. Glutamine consumption was further increased to $4.6 \pm 0.7$ μmol/kg/min by glutamine infusion, whereas glucose infusion elicited no marked increase in intestinal glucose oxidation.[212,213] These data clearly suggested that glutamine plays a major part in the metabolism of the intestine. An early suggestion by McKeehan was that high glutamine consumption ("glutaminolysis") was the hallmark of any cell type with high rates of proliferation.[214] His analysis showed that this was not for reasons of energy metabolism, since glycolysis could also meet the energy needs of these cells. Newsholme has provided an elegant metabolic dissection of the relative metabolic requirements of cells with rapid turnover (e.g., mucosal cells), with potential for rapid turnover (e.g., resting lymphocytes) or with high metabolic requirements but no need for rapid turnover (e.g., muscle, macrophages). Where high rates of glutamine consumption existed, it appeared not to be for energy production entirely.[215,216] Instead, Newsholme has proposed that high consumption provides control for other metabolic pathways which branch from the main pathway. Thus, glucose and glutamine metabolism also provide precursors for ribose (RNA, DNA) synthesis and for purine and pyrimidine (RNA, DNA) synthesis. If this is correct, then the role of glutamine is in maintenance of cell turnover rather than of energy production. Thus, it has a theoretical role in maintaining the mucosal barrier function of the gut, and of associated immune cells.

This chapter will not describe all of the clinical studies of glutamine supplementation which have been performed. These have been reviewed recently.[217] The most significant recent studies concern the effect of glutamine on gut barrier and transport function. In a pig model of infectious cryptosporidiosis and diarrhea,[59] it was noted that glutamine stimulated electroneutral and electrogenic Na$^+$ uptake, whereas glucose stimulated only electrogenic uptake via the SGLT-1 system (see above). This was linked to the process of active glutamine metabolism. The animal model which appears to be most sensitive to the effects of glutamine supplementation, the rat, has been used widely. Where barrier function was impaired by intravenous infusion of endotoxin, supplementation of the parenteral nutrition regime with glutamine led to improved nitrogen balance, but more importantly villus architecture was improved and the transmucosal movement of endotoxin into the portal supply was reduced.[218] Permeability of the rat intestine *in vivo* to sugar probes which resulted from parenteral nutrition was also reduced by glutamine supplementation.[219] This has been confirmed in the most recent clinical trial of critically ill patients who received intravenous nutrition supplemented with glutamine in dipeptide form.[220] It is therefore clear that glutamine is of great significance to intestinal metabolism.

### 6.4.2.2    Glutathione

The antioxidant effects of glutathione (GSH) are well documented[221] and in regard to gut barrier function, maintenance of intracellular GSH concentration may be important. This appears to be controlled by dietary intake (i.e., luminal sources), arterial supplies, and bile.[222] Undernutrition leads to reduction in gut GSH content,[222] whereas intravenous supply of the monoester has been shown to increase plasma concentrations as well as the liver intracellular concentration,[223] although intestinal levels were not measured. Glutamine supplementation has been shown to be an effective way to increase tissue GSH concentration. Preinfusion of glutamine for 24 h before intestinal ischemia and reperfusion injury has been shown to maintain intestinal intracellular GSH concentrations and to reduce peroxidative membrane damage.[224] It is likely that in the period after injury a further part of the acute-phase response may be increases in liver synthesis and output of GSH as an anti-oxidant measure.[225] This is impaired by undernutrition.[226]

### 6.4.2.3    Nucleotides

These have assumed greater significance in studies of intestinal metabolism because of the limited capacity of the small intestinal mucosa to synthesize purines and pyrimidines *de novo*.[227,228] In addition, they are present in milk,[229] and beneficial effects of formula-feed supplementation with nucleotides have been noted in one controlled study of infant diarrhea.[230] Histologically, the mucosal damage which occurs in the rat lactose/diarrhea model can be either completely (i.e., villus height) or partially reversed (abnormal mitochondrial structure) by adding nucleotides to the diet.[231] These and other data are reviewed elsewhere,[232] and they clearly point to a role for dietary nucleotides in maintaining gut barrier function, especially where nutrient intake is inadequate or there is preexisting malnutrition.

### 6.4.2.4    Arginine

Arginine is unusual because it is almost stoichiometrically converted to citrulline and ornithine during passage from lumen to portal blood.[233,234] The intestinal actions of arginine are in some sense indistinguishable from those of its metabolite, nitric oxide. Thus, induction of contractility in the rat small intestine after inhibition of nitric oxide synthesis by $N_G$-nitro-L-arginine-methyl ester (L-NAME), could be antagonized by arginine itself.[235] Luminal arginine is also a potent stimulator of water and electrolyte secretion — an action that occurs locally.[236] However, the role of nitric oxide production in this is unclear since inhibition of its synthesis by L-NAME increased the secretory effect of L-arginine.[237] Several studies have provided further evidence that this aspect of arginine metabolism is important for gut function. The ability of rats to survive burn injury and gavage with live bacteria was improved by dietary supplementation with arginine.[238] Indeed, pretreatment with L-NAME significantly increased mortality resulting from bacterial translocation across the intestine wall. This may partly stem from the ability of nitric oxide to maintain a permeability barrier, since *in vitro* L-NAME increases permeability to small ([51]Cr-EDTA) and large molecules (rhodamine-dextran, 17,200 Da MWt) by a process independent of macrophage function.[239] Ischemia/reperfusion injury is also potentiated by L-NAME, whereas the stimulation of nitric oxide production by addition of luminal arginine has been shown to reduce permeability to endotoxins.[240,241] These data strongly suggest a role for arginine in clinical diets as a protective agent against bacterial translocation across the gut barrier.[242] One trial has suggested this benefit[243] and the reader is directed to a metaanalysis of trials in critically ill patients who were provided with arginine-supplemented diets.[244]

### 6.4.2.5    Urea and Luminal Protein

Luminal production of $NH_3$ in the colon is a result of nitrogen recycling from urea by the action of colonic microbes. This $NH_3$ can be absorbed from the colon and thus can be incorporated into $\alpha$-$NH_2$ of amino acids via the transamination pathway. The nutritional significance of this pathway has been demonstrated by Jackson and colleagues, who observed that intravenously administered double-labeled urea (i.e., [15]N[15]N-urea) was excreted partly as [14]N[15]N-urea. This could have occurred only if plasma urea had permeated into the colonic lumen, that is, if it had been hydrolyzed to [15]$NH_3$ by urease from luminal bacteria and had then been reabsorbed as [15]$NH_3$ and entered the general $\alpha$-$NH_2$ nitrogen pool (via $\alpha$-ketoglutarate) to be combined finally with $\alpha$-[14]$NH_2$ in ureagenesis to form [14]N[15]N-urea.[245] The flux of urea nitrogen which this route represents is not inconsiderable, and has been estimated at 2.6 g N/d (of which 1.4 g N/d is recycled into amino acids) as compared to a daily urea production rate of 8.5 g N from 14 g N protein intake.[246] This significant contribution to blood $NH_4^+$ flux is additional to that derived from glutamine metabolism by the gastrointestinal tract[209,247] and from colonic fermentation of malabsorbed protein. Certainly, two early feeding studies in children suggested that addition of "nonspecific nitrogen" (in the form of urea) to diets with limiting protein content reversed the failure to maintain nitrogen balance.[248,249] Fermentation of carbon sources in the colonic lumen seems to alter this process.

As has been known for many years, lactulose is an effective agent in reversing hyperammonemia of colonic origin in patients with liver disease.[250] The two sources of nitrogen for colonic ammoniagenesis are urea (see above) and protein fermented by the colonic microflora.[159] One action of lactulose or lactitol is to provide sufficient carbon source for luminal bacteria to fix luminal $NH_3$ into bacterial protein.[251] A second action of these sugars is to provide a rapidly fermentable substrate which produces sufficient acetate to lower cecal and colonic pH.[40] This inhibits the class of bacteria responsible for protein fermentation and may also reduce formation of SCFA which are considered to be more toxic (*iso*-valerate and valerate). Oral intakes of lactitol or lactulose thus lead to increased fecal nitrogen output in pigs[252] or to patients with hepatic encephalopathy.[5] This represents a diversion of urea away from recycling, and a loss of protein, albeit a beneficial loss which would otherwise be salvaged by the large intestine.

## REFERENCES

1. **Israel, Y., Valenzuela, J. E., Salazar, I., and Ugarte, G.,** Alcohol and amino acid transport in the human small intestine, *J. Nutr.,* 98, 222, 1969.
2. **Pfeiffer, A., Schmidt, T., Vidon, N., and Kaess, H.,** Effect of ethanol on absorption of a nutrient solution in the upper human intestine, *Scand. J. Gastroenterol.,* 28, 515, 1993.
3. **O'Neill, B., Weber, F., Hornig, D., and Semenza, G.,** Ethanol selectively affects Na+-gradient dependent intestinal transport systems, *FEBS Lett.,* 194, 183, 1986.
4. **McCullough, A. J., Mullen, K. D., and Kalhan, S. C.,** Body cell mass and leucine metabolism in cirrhosis, *Gastroenterology,* 102, 1325, 1992.
5. **Mueller, K. J., Crosby, L. O., Oberlander, J. L., and Mullen, J. L.,** Estimation of fecal nitrogen in patients with liver disease, *J. Parent. Ent. Nutr.,* 7, 266, 1983.

6. **Huppe, D., Tonissen, R., Hofius, M., Kuntz, H. D., and May, B.,** Effect of chronic alcohol drinking and liver cirrhosis on oro-cecal transit time ($H_2$ breath test), *Z. Gastroenterol.,* 27, 624, 1989.

7. **Spiller, R. C., Trotman, I. F., Higgins, B. E., Ghatei, M. A., Grimble, G. K., Lee, Y. C., Bloom, S. R., Misiewicz, J. J., and Silk, D. B. A.,** The ileal brake — inhibition of jejunal motility after ileal fat perfusion in man, *Gut,* 25, 365, 1984.

8. **Karasov, W. H., Solberg, D. H., and Diamond, J. M.,** What transport adaptations enable mammals to absorb sugars and amino acids faster than reptiles?, *Am. J. Physiol.,* 249, G271, 1985.

9. **Martin, R. D., Chivers, D. J., MacLarnon, A. M., and Hladnik, C. M.,** Gastrointestinal allometry in primates and other mammals, in *Size and Scaling in Primate Biology,* Jungers, W. L., Ed., Plenum Press, New York, 1985, 61.

10. **Ferraris, R. P., Lee, P. P., and Diamond, J. M.,** Origin of regional and species differences in intestinal glucose uptake, *Am. J. Physiol.,* 257, G689, 1989.

11. **Preedy, V. R., Marway, J. S., Siddiq, T., Ansari, F. A., Hashim, I. A., and Peters, T. J.,** Gastrointestinal protein turnover and alcohol misuse, *Drug Alcohol Depend.,* 34, 1, 1993.

12. **Toloza, E. M., Lam, M., and Diamond, J.,** Nutrient extraction by cold-exposed mice: a test of digestive safety margins, *Am. J. Physiol.,* 261, G608, 1991.

13. **Raimundo, A. H., Rogers, J., Grimble, G., Cahill, E., and Silk, D. B. A.,** Colonic in-flow and small bowel motility during intraduodenal enteral nutrition, *Gut,* 29, A1469, 1988.

14. **Crane, C. W.,** Studies on the absorption of $^{15}N$ labelled yeast in normal subjects and patients with malabsorption, in *The Role of the Gastrointestinal Tract in Protein Metabolism,* Munro, H. N., Ed., F. A. Davis, Philadelphia, 1964, 333.

15. **DiMagno, E. P., Go, V. L. W., and Summerskill, W. H. J.,** Relations between pancreatic enzyme outputs and malabsorption in severe pancreatic insufficiency, *N. Engl. J. Med.,* 288, 813, 1973.

16. **Bronstein, M. N., Sokol, R. J., Abman, S. H., Chatfield, B. A., Hammond, K. B., Hambidge, K. M., Stall, C. D., and Accurso, F. J.,** Pancreatic insufficiency, growth, and nutrition in infants identified by newborn screening as having cystic fibrosis, *J. Pediatr.,* 120, 533, 1992.

17. **Hammer, H. F., Fine, K. D., Santa Ana, C. A., Porter, J. L., Schiller, L. R., and Fordtran, J. S.,** Carbohydrate malabsorption. Its measurement and its contribution to diarrhea, *J. Clin. Invest.,* 86, 1936, 1990.

18. **Grimble, G. K., Patil, D. H., and Silk, D. B. A.,** Assimilation of lactitol, an 'unabsorbed' disaccharide in the normal human colon, *Gut,* 29, 1666, 1988.

19. **Patil, D. H., Grimble, G. K., and Silk, D. B. A.,** Lactitol, a new hydrogenated lactose derivative: intestinal absorption and laxative threshold in normal human subjects, *Br. J. Nutr.,* 57, 195, 1987.

20. **O'Keefe, S. J. D., Adam, J. K., Cakata, E., and Epstein, S.,** Nutritional support of malnourished lactose intolerant African patients, *Gut,* 25, 942, 1984.

21. **Keohane, P. P., Attrill, H., Jones, B. J. M., Brown, B., Frost, P., and Silk, D. B. A.,** The roles of lactose and Clostridium difficile in the pathogenesis of enteral feeding associated diarrhea, *Clin. Nutr.,* 1, 259, 1983.

22. **Ladas, S. D., Latoufis, C., Giannopoulou, H., Hatziioannou, J., and Raptis, S. A.,** Reproducible lactulose hydrogen breath test as a measure of mouth-to-cecum transit time, *Dig. Dis. Sci.,* 34, 919, 1989.

23. **Midtvedt, A.-C. and Midtvedt, T.,** Production of short chain fatty acids by the intestinal microflora during the first 2 years of human life, *J. Pediatr. Gastroenterol. Nutr.,* 15, 395, 1992.

24. **Hammer, H. F., Santa Ana, C. A., Schiller, L. R., and Fordtran, J. S.,** Studies of osmotic diarrhea induced in normal subjects by ingestion of polyethylene glycol and lactulose, *J. Clin. Invest.,* 84, 1056, 1989.

25. **Rao, S. S., Edwards, C. A., Austen, C. J., Bruce, C., and Read, N. W.,** Impaired colonic fermentation of carbohydrate after ampicillin, *Gastroenterology,* 94, 928, 1988.

26. **Debongnie, J. C. and Phillips, S. F.,** Capacity of the human colon to absorb fluid, *Gastroenterology,* 74, 698, 1978.

27. **Foltmann, B.,** Pepsin, chymosin and their zymogens., in *Molecular and Cellular Basis of Digestion,* Desnuelle, P., Sjostrom, H., and Noren, O., Eds., Elsevier Science Publishers B. V., Amsterdam, 1986, 491.

28. **Desnuelle, P.,** Chemistry and enzymology of pancreatic endopeptidases, in *Molecular and Cellular Basis of Digestion,* Desnuelle, P., Sjostrom, H., and Noren, O., Eds., Elsevier Science Publishers B. V., Amsterdam, 1986, 195.

29. **Puigserver, A., Chapus, C., and Kerfelec, B.,** Pancreatic exopeptidases, in *Molecular and Cellular Basis of Digestion,* Desnuelle, P., Sjostrom, H., and Noren, O., Eds., Elsevier Science Publishers B. V., Amsterdam, 1986, 235.

30. **Craft, I. L., Geddes, D., Hyde, C. W., Wise, I. J., and Matthews, D. M.,** Absorption and malabsorption of glycine and glycine peptides in man, *Gut,* 9, 425, 1968.

31. **Silk, D. B. A., Chung, Y. C., Berger, K. L., Conley, K., Beigler, M., Sleisenger, M. H., Spiller, G. A., and Kim, Y. S.,** Comparison of oral feeding of peptide and amino acid meals to normal human subjects, *Gut,* 20, 291, 1979.

32. **Chung, Y. C., Kim, Y. S., Shadchehr, A., Garrido, A., MacGregor, I. L., and Sleisenger, M. H.,** Protein digestion and absorption in human small intestine, *Gastroenterology,* 76, 1415, 1979.

33. **Skovbjerg, H.,** Immunoelectrophoretic studies on human small intestinal brush border proteins — the longitudinal distribution of peptidases and disaccharidases, *Clin. Chim. Acta,* 112, 205, 1981.

34. **Triadou, N., Bataille, J., and Schmitz, J.,** Longitudinal study of the human intestinal brush border membrane proteins: distribution of the main disaccharidases and peptidases, *Gastroenterology,* 85, 1326, 1983.

35. **Tarvid, I.,** Effect of early postnatal long-term fasting on the development of peptide hydrolysis in chicks. *Comp. Biochem. Physiol. A.* 101, 161, 1992.

36. **Silk, D. B. A., Webb, J. P. W., Lane, A. E., Clark, M. L., and Dawson, A. M.,** Functional differentiation of human jejunum and ileum: a comparison of the handling of glucose, peptides and amino acids, *Gut,* 15, 444, 1974.

37. **Adibi, S. A. and Mercer, D. W.,** Protein digestion in human intestine as reflected in human mucosal and plasma amino acid concentrations after meals, *J. Clin. Invest.,* 52, 1586, 1973.

38. **Chacko, A. and Cummings, J. H.,** Nitrogen losses from the human small bowel: obligatory losses and the effect of physical form of food, *Gut,* 29, 809, 1988.

39. **Mortensen, P. B., Rasmussen, H. S., and Holtug, K.,** Lactulose detoxifies *in vitro* short-chain fatty acid production in colonic contents induced by blood: implications for hepatic coma, *Gastroenterology,* 94, 750, 1988.

40. **Mortensen, P. B., Holtug, K., Bonnen, H., and Clausen, M. R.,** The degradation of amino acids, proteins, and blood to short-chain fatty acids in colon is prevented by lactulose, *Gastroenterology,* 98, 353, 1990.

41. **MacFarlane, G. T., Cummings, J. H., and Allison, C.,** Protein degradation by human intestinal bacteria, *J. Gen. Microbiol.,* 132, 1647, 1986.

42. **Hirst, B. H.,** Dietary regulation of intestinal nutrient carriers, *Proc. Nutr. Soc.,* 52, 315, 1993.

43. **McGivan, J. D. and Pastor-Anglada, M.,** Regulatory and molecular aspects of mammalian amino acid transport, *Biochem. J.,* 299, 321, 1994.

44. **Gardner, M. L., Illingworth, K. M., Kelleher, J., and Wood, D.,** Intestinal absorption of the intact peptide carnosine in man, and comparison with intestinal permeability to lactulose, *J. Physiol.,* 439, 411, 1991.

45. **Ganapathy, V. and Leibach, F. K.,** Is intestinal transport energised by a proton gradient?, *Am. J. Physiol.,* 249, G153, 1985.

46. **Lucas, M. L., Schneider, W., Haberich, F. J., and Blair, J. A.,** Direct measurement by pH-microelectrode of the pH microclimate in rat proximal jejunum, *Proc. R. Soc. Lond.,* 192, 39, 1975.

47. **Ganapathy, V., Mendicino, J. F., and Leibach, F. H.,** Transport of glycyl-L-proline into intestinal and renal brush border vesicles from rabbit, *J. Biol. Chem.,* 256, 118, 1981.

48. **Ganapathy, M. E., Mahesh, V. B., Devoe, L. D., Leibach, F. H., and Ganapathy, V.,** Dipeptide transport in brush-border membrane vesicles isolated from normal term human placenta, *Am. J. Obstet. Gynecol.,* 153, 83, 1985.

49. **Okano, T., Inui, K. I., Takano, M., and Hori, R.,** $H^+$ gradient-dependent transport of aminocephalosporins in rat intestinal brush-border membrane vesicles, *Biochem. Pharmacol.,* 35, 1781, 1986.

50. **Fei, Y.-J., Kanal, Y., Nussberger, S., Ganapathy, V., Leibach, F. H., Romero, M. F., Singh, S. K., Boron, W. F., and Hediger, M. A.,** Expression cloning of a mammalian proton-coupled oligopeptide transporter, *Nature,* 368, 563, 1994.

51. **Wallace, R. J., McKain, N., and Broderick, G. A.,** Breakdown of different peptides by *Prevotella* (Bacteroides) ruminicola and mixed microorganisms from the sheep rumen, *Curr. Microbiol.,* 26, 333, 1993.

52. **Dyer, J., Beechey, R. B., Gorvel, J. P., Smith, R. T., Wootton, R., and Shirazi-Beechey, S. P.,** Glycyl-L-proline transport in rabbit enterocyte basolateral-membrane vesicles, *Biochem. J.,* 269, 565, 1990.

53. **Cheeseman, C.,** Role of intestinal basolateral membrane in absorption of nutrients, *Am. J. Physiol.,* 263, R482, 1992.

54. **Daniel, H., Morse, E. L., and Adibi, S. A.,** Determinants of substrate affinity for the oligopeptide/$H^+$ symporter in the renal brush border membrane, *J. Biol. Chem.,* 267, 9565, 1992.

55. **Botbol, V. and Scornik, O. A.,** Measurement of instant rates of protein degradation in the livers of intact mice by the accumulation of bestatin-induced peptides, *J. Biol. Chem.,* 266, 2151, 1991.

56. **Cook, G. C.,** Comparison of intestinal absorption rates of glycine and glycylglycine in man and the effect of glucose in the perfusing fluid, *Clin. Sci.,* 43, 443, 1972.

57. **Rees, R. G., Raimundo, A. H., Grimble, G. K., Hunjan, M. K., and Silk, D. B. A.,** Peptide based nitrogen source of enteral diets: studies with casein hydrolysates in man, *J. Parent. Ent. Nutr.,* 12 (Suppl), 21S, 1988.

58. **Wapnir, R. A., Litov, R. E., Zdanowicz, M. M., and Lifshitz, F.,** Improved water and sodium absorption from oral rehydration solutions based on rice syrup in a rat model of osmotic diarrhea, *J. Pediatr.,* 118, S53, 1991.

59. **Argenzio, R. A., Rhoads, J. M., Armstrong, M., and Gomez, G.,** Glutamine stimulates prostaglandin-sensitive $Na^+$-$H^+$ exchange in experimental porcine cryptosporidiosis, *Gastroenterology,* 106, 1418, 1994.

60. **Guandalini, S. and Rubino, A.,** Development of dipeptide transport in the intestinal mucosa of rabbits, *Pediatr. Res.,* 16, 99, 1982.

61. **Miller, P. M., Burston, D., Brueton, M. J., and Matthews, D. M.,** Kinetics of uptake of L-leucine and glycylsarcosine into normal and protein malnourished young rat jejunum, *Pediatr. Res.,* 18, 504, 1984.

62. **Vasquez, J. A., Morse, E. L., and Adibi, S. A.,** Effect of starvation on amino acid and peptide transport and peptide hydrolysis in humans, *Am. J. Physiol.,* 249, G563, 1985.

63. **Gardiner, K. and Barbul, A.,** Intestinal amino acid absorption during sepsis, *J. Parent. Ent. Nutr.,* 17, 277, 1993.

64. **Ferraris, R. P., Kwan, W. W., and Diamond, J.,** Regulatory signals for intestinal amino acid transporters and peptidases, *Am. J. Physiol.,* 255, G151, 1988.

65. **Adibi, S. A. and Morse, E. L.,** The number of glycine residues which limits intact absorption of glycine oligopeptides in human jejunum. *J. Clin. Invest.,* 60, 1008, 1977.

66. **Silk, D. B. A., Marrs, T. C., Addison, J. M., Burston, D., Clark, M. L., and Matthews, D. M.,** Absorption of amino acids from an amino acid mixture simulating casein and a tryptic hydrolysate of casein in man, *Clin. Sci. Mol. Med.,* 45, 715, 1973.

67. **Fairclough, P. D., Hegarty, J. E., Silk, D. B., and Clark, M. L.,** Comparison of the absorption of two protein hydrolysates and their effects on water and electrolyte movements in the human jejunum, *Gut,* 21, 829, 1980.

68. **Silk, D. B. A., Fairclough, P. D., Clark, M. L., Hegarty, J. E., Marrs, T. C., Addison, J. M., Burston, D., Clegg, K. M., and Matthews, D. M.,** Use of a peptide rather than free amino acid nitrogen source in chemically defined "elemental" diets, *J. Parent. Ent. Nutr.,* 4, 548, 1980.

69. **Grimble, G. K., Keohane, P., Higgins, B. E., Kaminski, M. V., and Silk, D. B. A.,** Effect of peptide chain-length on amino acid and nitrogen absorption from two lactalbumin hydrolysates in the normal human jejunum, *Clin. Sci.,* 71, 65, 1986.

70. **Keohane, P. P., Grimble, G. K., Brown, B., Spiller, R. C., and Silk, D. B. A.,** Influence of protein composition and hydrolysis method on intestinal absorption of protein in man, *Gut,* 26, 907, 1985.

71. **Friedrich, M., Noack, J., Proll, J., and Noack, R.,** Untersuchungen zur Absorption enzymatischer Proteinhydrolysate sowie aquimolarer Aminosauremischungen am perfundierten Dunndarm der Ratte (Absorption of enzymatic protein hydrolysates and equimolar amino acid mixtures in the perfused small intestine of the rat), *Biomed. Biochim. Acta,* 43, 117, 1984.

72. **Grimble, G. K., Rees, R. G., Keohane, P. P., Cartwright, T., Desreumaux, M., and Silk, D. B. A.,** The effect of peptide chain-length on absorption of egg-protein hydrolysates in the normal human jejunum, *Gastroenterology,* 92, 136, 1987.

73. **Grimble, G. K., Guilera Sarda, M., Sesay, H. F., Marrett, A. L., Kapadia, S. A., Bowling, T. E., and Silk, D. B. A.,** The influence of whey hydrolysate peptide chain length on nitrogen and carbohydrate absorption in the perfused human jejunum, *Clin. Nutr.,* 13 (Suppl), 46, 1994.

74. **Chen, M. L., Rogers, Q. R., and Harper, A. E.,** Observations on protein digestion *in vivo.* IV. Further observation of the gastrointestinal contents of rats fed different dietary proteins, *J. Nutr.,* 76, 235, 1962.

75. **Itoh, H., Kishi, T., and Chibata, I.,** Comparative effects of casein and amino acid mixture simulating casein on growth and food intake in rats, *J. Nutr.,* 103, 1709, 1973.

76. **Moriarty, K. J., Hegarty, J. E., Fairclough, P. D., Kelly, M. J., Clark, M. L., and Dawson, A. M.,** Relative nutritional value of whole protein, hydrolyzed protein and free amino acids in man, *Gut,* 26, 694, 1985.

77. **Velasco, N., Long, C. L., Nelson, K. M., and Blakemore, W. S.,** Whole-body protein kinetics in elective surgical patients receiving peptide or amino acid solutions, *Nutrition,* 7, 28, 1991.

78. **Grimble, G. K., Rees, R. G., Halliday, D., Ford, G. C., and Silk, D. B. A.,** Are enterally fed peptides better utilised than free amino acids in the short-bowel syndrome, *Clin. Nutr.,* 5 (Suppl), 50, 1986.

79. **Monchi, M., Vaugelade, P., Vaissade, P., and Rérat, A.,** Net protein utilisation after duodenal infusion of small peptides or free amino acids in growing rats, *Clin. Nutr.,* 10 (Suppl), 31, 1991.

80. **Monchi, M. and Rérat, A. A.,** Comparison of net protein utilization of milk protein mild enzymatic hydrolysates and free amino acid mixtures with a close pattern in the rat, *J. Parent. Ent. Nutr.,* 17, 355, 1993.

81. **Rees, R. G. P., Hare, W. R., Grimble, G. K., Frost, P. G., and Silk, D. B. A.,** Do patients with moderately impaired gastrointestinal function requiring enteral nutrition need a predigested nitrogen source? A prospective crossover controlled clinical trial, *Gut,* 33, 877, 1992.

82. **McIntyre, P. B., Fitchew, M., and Lennard-Jones, J. E.,** Patients with a high ileostomy do not need a special diet, *Gastroenterology,* 91, 25, 1986.

83. **Rees, R. G., Grimble, G., Halliday, D., Ford, C., and Silk, D. B. A.,** Influence of orally administered amino acids and peptides on protein turnover kinetics in the short-bowel syndrome, *Gut,* 28, A1397, 1987.

84. **Schmitz, J., Rey, F., Bresson, J. L., et al.,** Perfusion study of disaccharide absorption after extensive intestinal resection, in *Mechanisms of Intestinal Adaptation,* Robinson, J. W. L., Dowling, R. H., and Riecken, E. O., Eds., MTP Press, Lancaster, England, 1982, 413.

85. **Dowling, R. H.,** Small bowel adaptation and its regulation, *Scand. J. Gastroenterology,* 17 (Suppl 74), 53, 1982.

86. **Steinhardt, H. J., Wolf, A., Jakober, B., Schmuelling, R. M., Langer, K., Brandl, M., Fekl, W. E., and Adibi, S. A.,** Nitrogen absorption in pancreatectomised patients: protein versus protein hydrolysate as substrate, *J. Lab. Clin. Med.,* 113, 162, 1989.

87. **Buddington, R. K.,** Nutrition and ontogenetic development of the intestine, *Can. J. Physiol. Pharmacol.,* 72, 251, 1994.

88. **Johansson, C.,** Studies of gastrointestinal interactions: VII. Characteristics of the absorption pattern of sugar, fat and protein from composite meals in man: a quantitative study, *Scand. J. Gastroenterol.,* 10, 33, 1975.

89. **Meldrum, S. J., Watson, B. W., Riddle, H. C., Bown, R. L., and Sladen, G. E.,** pH profile of gut as measured by a radiotelemetry capsule, *Br. Med. J.,* 2, 104, 1972.

90. **Kenny, A. J. and Maroux, S.,** Topology of microvillar membrane hydrolases of kidney and intestine, *Physiol. Rev.,* 62, 91, 1982.

91. **Semenza, G.,** Anchoring and biosynthesis of stalked brush border membrane proteins: glycosidases and peptidases of enterocytes and renal tubuli, *Annu. Rev. Cell Biol.,* 2, 255, 1986.

92. **Hoefsloot, L. H., Hoogeveen Westerveld, M., Kroos, M. A., van Beeumen, J., Reuser, A. J., and Oostra, B. A.,** Primary structure and processing of lysosomal alpha-glucosidase; homology with the intestinal sucrase-isomaltase complex, *EMBO J.,* 7, 1697, 1988.

93. **Hoefsloot, L. H., Hoogeveen-Westerveld, M., Reuser, A. J. J., and Oostra, B. A.,** Characterization of the human lysosomal α-glucosidase gene, *Biochem. J.,* 272, 493, 1990.

94. **Sivakami, S. and Radhakrishnan, A. N.,** Kinetic studies on glucoamylase of rabbit small intestine, *Biochem. J.,* 153, 321, 1976.

95. **Pereira, B. and Sivakami, S.,** A comparison of the active site of maltase-glucoamylase from the brush-border of rabbit small intestine and kidney by chemical modification studies, *Biochem. J.,* 274, 349, 1991.

96. **Noren, O., Sjostrom, H., Danielsen, E. M., Cowell, G. M., and Skovbjerg, H.,** The enzymes of the enterocyte plasma membrane, in *Molecular and Cellular Basis of Digestion*, Desnuelle, P., Sjostrom, H., and Noren, O., Eds., Elsevier Science Publishers B. V., Amsterdam, 1986, 335.

97. **Gray, G. M.,** Carbohydrate digestion and absorption. Role of the small intestine, *N. Engl. J. Med.,* 292, 1225, 1975.

98. **Wahlqvist, M. L., Wilmshurst, E. G., Murton, C. R., and Richardson, E. N.,** The effect of chain length on glucose absorption and the related metabolic response, *Am. J. Clin. Nutr.,* 31, 1998, 1978.

99. **Layer, P., Sinmeister, A. R., and DiMagno, E. P.,** Effect of decreasing intraluminal amylase activity on starch digestion and post-prandial gastrointestinal functions in humans, *Gastroenterology,* 91, 41, 1986.

100. **Grimble, G. K., Collins, S., and Silk, D. B. A.,** *In vivo* and *in vitro* assimilation of orally administered dextran 40 KDa in man, *Proc. Nutr. Soc.,* 51, 120A, 1992.

101. **Dahlqvist, A.,** The location of carbohydrases in the digestive tract of the pig, *Biochem. J.,* 78, 282, 1961.

102. **Dahlqvist, A.,** Rat-intestinal dextranase: localization and relation to the other carbohydrases of the digestive tract, *Biochem. J.,* 86, 72, 1963.

103. **Gould, G. W. and Holman, G. D.,** The glucose transporter family: structure, function and tissue-specific expression, *Biochem. J.,* 295, 329, 1993.

104. **Pajor, A. M., Hirayama, B. A., and Wright, E. M.,** Molecular biology approaches to comparative study of Na(+)-glucose cotransport, *Am. J. Physiol.,* 263, R489, 1992.

105. **Stevens, B. R.,** Vertebrate intestine apical membrane mechanisms of organic nutrient transport, *Am. J. Physiol.,* 263, R458, 1992.

106. **Minami, H., Kim, J.-R., Tada, K., Takahashi, F., Miyamato, K.-I., Nakabou, Y., Sakai, K., and Hagihara, H.,** Inhibition of glucose absorption by phlorizin affects intestinal function in rats, *Gastroenterology,* 105, 692, 1993.

107. **Crouzoulon, G. and Korieh, A.,** Fructose transport by rat intestinal brush border membrane vesicles. Effect of high fructose diet followed by return to standard diet, *Comp. Biochem. Physiol. A,* 100, 175, 1991.

108. **Milla, P. J., Oyesiku, J. E. J., Mullet, D. P. R., and Harries, J. T.,** Fructose absorption and the effects of other monosaccharides on its absorption in the rat jejunum *in vivo, Gut,* 18, A425, 1977.

109. **Thorens, B., Cheng, Z. Q., Brown, D., and Lodish, H. F.,** Liver glucose transporter: a basolateral protein in hepatocytes and intestine and kidney cells, *Am. J. Physiol.,* 259, C279, 1990.

110. **Fernandez Lopez, J. A., Casado, J., Argiles, J. M., and Alemany, M.,** Intestinal handling of a glucose gavage by the rat, *Mol. Cell. Biochem.,* 113, 43, 1992.

111. **Pappenheimer, J. R.,** Paracellular intestinal absorption of glucose, creatinine, and mannitol in normal animals: relation to body size, *Am. J. Physiol.,* 259, G290, 1990.

112. **Atisook, K. and Madara, J. L.,** An oligopeptide permeates intestinal tight junctions at glucose-elicited dilatations. Implications for oligopeptide absorption, *Gastroenterology,* 100, 719, 1991.

113. **Ferraris, R. P., Yasharpour, S., Lloyd, K. C. K., Mirzayan, R., and Diamond, J. M.,** Luminal glucose concentrations in the gut under normal conditions, *Am. J. Physiol.,* 259, G822, 1990.

114. **Fine, K. D., Santa Ana, C. A., Porter, J. L., and Fordtran, J. S.,** Effect of D-glucose on intestinal permeability and its passive absorption in human small intestine *in vivo, Gastroenterology,* 105, 1117, 1993.

115. **Fisher, R. B. and Parsons, D. S.,** Glucose absorption from surviving rat small intestine, *J. Physiol.,* 110, 281, 1949.

116. **Fairclough, P. D., Clark, M. L., Dawson, A. M., Silk, D. B., Milla, P. J., and Harries, J. T.,** Absorption of glucose and maltose in congenital glucose-galactose malabsorption, *Pediatr. Res.,* 12, 1112, 1978.

117. **Maxton, D. G., Bjarnason, I., Reynolds, A. P., Catt, S. D., Peters, T. J., and Menzies, I. S.,** Lactulose, $^{51}$Cr-labelled ethylenediaminetetra-acetate, L-rhamnose and polyethyleneglycol 400 (corrected) as probe markers for assessment *in vivo* of human intestinal permeability [published erratum appears in *Clin. Sci.,* 1986 Dec;71(6):following xxi]. *Clin. Sci.* 71, 71, 1986.

118. **Maxton, D. G., Catt, S. D., and Menzies, I. S.,** Combined assessment of intestinal disaccharidases in congenital asucrasia by differential urinary disaccharide excretion. *J. Clin. Pathol..* 43, 406, 1990.

119. **Katz, K. D., Hollander, D., Vadheim, C. M., McElree, C., Delahunty, T., Dadufalza, V. D., Krugliak, P., and Rotter, J. I.,** Intestinal permeability in patients with Crohn's disease and their healthy relatives, *Gastroenterology*, 97, 927, 1989.

120. **Travis, S. and Menzies, I.,** Intestinal permeability: functional assessment and significance, *Clin. Sci.*, 82, 471, 1992.

121. **Grimble, G. K.,** Ion chromatography in clinical research: a neglected technique?, *Analyt. Proc.*, 29, 468, 1992.

122. **Fiaccadori, F., Elia, G. F., Missale, G., Pizzaferri, P., and Pedretti, G.,** Nitrogen balance in the assessment of cirrhotic patients, *Ital. J. Gastroenterol.*, 25, 336, 1993.

123. **Heitlinger, L. A., Sloan, H. R., DeVore, D. R., Lee, P.-C., Lebenthal, E., and Duffey, M. E.,** Transport of glucose polymer-derived glucose by rabbit jejunum, *Gastroenterology*, 102, 443, 1992.

124. **Jones, B. J. M., Brown, B. E., Spiller, R. C., and Silk, D. B. A.,** Energy dense enteral feeds — the use of high molecular weight glucose polymers, *J. Parent. Ent. Nutr.*, 5, 567, 1981.

125. **Jones, B. J. M., Brown, B. E., Loran, J. S., Kennedy, J. F., Stead, J. A., and Silk, D. B. A.,** Glucose absorption from starch hydrolysates in the human jejunum, *Gut*, 24, 1152, 1984.

126. **Jones, B. J. M., Higgins, B. E., and Silk, D. B. A.,** Glucose absorption from maltotriose and glucose oligomers in the human jejunum. *Clin. Sci.* 72, 409, 1987.

127. **Kerzner, B., Sloan, H. R., Haase, G., McClung, H. J., and Ailabouni, A. H.,** The jejunal absorption of glucose oligomers in the absence of pancreatic enzymes, *Pediatr. Res.*, 15, 250, 1981.

128. **Spiller, R. C., Jones, B. J. M., and Silk, D. B. A.,** Jejunal water and electrolyte absorption from two proprietary enteral feeds in man: importance of sodium content, *Gut*, 28, 681, 1986.

129. **Samulitis-dos Santos, B. K., Goda, T., and Koldovsky, O.,** Dietary-induced increases of disaccharidase activities in rat jejunum, *Br. J. Nutr.*, 67, 267, 1992.

130. **Rumessen, J. J. and Gudmand Hoyer, E.,** Absorption capacity of fructose in healthy adults. Comparison with sucrose and its constituent monosaccharides, *Gut*, 27, 1161, 1986.

131. **Hamosh, M., Klaeveman, H. L., Wolf, R. D., and Scow, R. D.,** Pharyngeal lipase and digestion of dietary triglyceride in man, *J. Clin. Invest.*, 55, 908, 1975.

132. **Gluckman, R. M.,** Fat absorption and malabsorption, in *Clinics in Gastroenterology, Number 2*, Vol. 12, Sleisenger, M. H., Ed., W. B. Saunders, London, 1983, 323.

133. **Stremmel, W.,** Intestinal absorption of fat and fat-soluble vitamins, in *Clinical Nutrition and Metabolic Research*, Dietze, G., Grunert, A., and Wolfram, G., Eds., Karger, Basel, Munich, 1986, 118.

134. **Hauton, J. C.,** A quantitative dynamic concept of the role of bile in fat digestion, in *Molecular and Cellular Basis of Digestion*, Desnuelle, P., Sjostrom, H., and Noren, O., Eds., Elsevier Science Publishers B. V., Amsterdam, 1986, 147.

135. **Caspary, W. F.,** Physiology and pathophysiology of intestinal absorption, *Am. J. Clin. Nutr.*, 55 (Suppl), 299S, 1992.

136. **Rao, R. H. and Mansbach, C. M., II,** Acid lipase in rat intestinal mucosa: physiological parameters. *Biochim. Biophys. Acta* 1043, 273, 1990.

137. **Bonner, M. S., Gulick, T., Riley, D. J. S., Spilburg, C. A., and Lange, L. G.,** Heparin-modulated binding and pancreatic lipase and uptake of hydrolyzed triglycerides in the intestine, *J. Biol. Chem.*, 264, 20261, 1989.

138. **Shiau, Y.,** Mechanism of intestinal fatty acid uptake in the rat: the role of an acidic environment, *J. Physiol.*, 421, 463, 1990.

139. **Sacchettini, J. C., Gordon, J. I., and Banaszak, L. J.,** Refined apoprotein of rat intestinal fatty acid binding protein produced in Escherichia coli, *Proc. Natl. Acad. Sci. U.S.A.*, 86, 7736, 1989.

140. **Iseki, S. and Kondo, H.,** Light microscopic localization of HFABP proteins mRNA in jejunal epithelia in rats using *in situ* hybridization, immunohistochemical, and autoradiographic techniques, *J. Histochem. Cytochem.*, 38, 111, 1990.

141. **Mansbach, C. M., II, Arnold, A., and Cox, M. A.,** Factors influencing triacylglycerol delivery into mesenteric lymph, *Am. J. Physiol.*, 249, G642, 1985.

142. **Tipton, A. D., Frase, S., and Mansbach, C. M., II,** Isolation and characterisation of a mucosal triacylglycerol pool undergoing hydrolysis, *Am. J. Physiol.*, 257, G871, 1989.

143. **Phillips, S. F. and Giller, J.,** The contribution of the colon to electrolyte and water conservation in man, *J. Lab. Clin. Med.*, 81, 733, 1973.

144. **Fordtran, J. S., Rector, F. C., Jr., Ewton, M. F., Soter, N., and Kinney, J.,** Permeability characteristics of the human small intestine, *J. Clin. Invest.* 44, 1935, 1965.

145. **McKie, A. T., Goecke, I. A., and Naftalin, R. J.,** Comparison of fluid absorption by bovine and ovine descending colon *in vitro*, *Am. J. Physiol.*, 261, G433, 1991.

146. **Turnberg, L.,** Cellular basis of diarrhea. The Croonian lecture 1989, *J. R. Coll. Physicians Lond.*, 25, 53, 1991.

147. **Silk, D. B. A., Fairclough, P. D., Park, N. J., Lane, A. E., Webb, J. P. W., Clark, M. L., and Dawson, A. M.,** A study of relations between the absorption of amino acids, dipeptides, water and electrolytes in the normal human jejunum, *Clin. Sci. Mol. Med.*, 49, 401, 1975.

148. **Sladen, G. E. and Dawson, A. M.,** Inter-relationship between the absorption of glucose, sodium and water by the normal human jejunum, *Clin. Sci.*, 36, 119, 1969.

149. **Sladen, G. E. and Dawson, A. M.,** Effect of bicarbonate on sodium absorption by the human jejunum, *Nature,* 218, 267, 1968.

150. **Turnberg, L. A., Bieberdorf, F. A., Morawski, S. G., and Fordtran, J. S.,** Inter-relationships of chloride bicarbonate sodium and hydrogen transport in the human ileum, *J. Clin. Invest.,* 49, 557, 1970.

151. **Devroede, G. J. and Phillips, S. F.,** Conservation of sodium, chloride and water by the human colon, *Gastroenterology,* 56, 101, 1969.

152. **Ruppin, H., Bar-Meir, S., Soergel, K. H., Wood, C. M., and Schmitt, M. G.,** Absorption of short chain fatty acids by the colon, *Gastroenterology,* 78, 1500, 1980.

153. **Bleakman, D. and Naftalin, R. J.,** Hypertonic fluid absorption from rabbit descending colon *in vitro, Am. J. Physiol.,* 258, G377, 1990.

154. **Weaver, G. A., Krause, J. A., Miller, T. L., and Wolin, M. J.,** Constancy of glucose and starch fermentations by two different human fecal microbial communities, *Gut,* 30, 19, 1989.

155. **Grimble, G. K.,** Fibre, fermentation, flora and flatus, *Gut,* 30, 6, 1989.

156. **Gibson, G. R., Cummings, J. H., and MacFarlane, G. T.,** Use of a three-stage continuous culture system to study the effect of mucin on dissimilatory sulphate reduction and methanogenesis by mixed populations of human gut bacteria, *Appl. Environ. Microbiol.,* 54, 2750, 1988.

157. **Gibson, G. R., MacFarlane, G. T., and Cummings, J. H.,** Occurrence of sulphate-reducing bacteria in human faeces and the relationship of dissimilatory sulphate reduction to methanogenesis in the large gut, *J. Appl. Bacteriol.,* 65, 103, 1988.

158. **Flourié, B., Pellier, P., Florent, CH., Marteau, P., Pochart, P., and Rambaud, J.-C.,** Site and substrates for methane production in human colon, *Am. J. Physiol.,* 260, G752, 1991.

159. **Mortensen, P. B., Clausen, M. R., Bonnen, H., Hove, H., and Holtug, K.,** Colonic fermentation of Ispaghula, wheat bran, glucose and albumin to short-chain fatty acids and ammonia evaluated *in vitro* in 50 subjects, *J. Parent. Ent. Nutr.,* 16, 433, 1992.

160. **Smith, C. J. and Bryant, M. P.,** Introduction to metabolic activities of intestinal bacteria, *Am. J. Clin. Nutr.,* 32, 149, 1979.

161. **Scheppach, W.,** Effects of short chain fatty acids on gut morphology and function, *Gut,* 35 (Suppl 1), S35, 1994.

162. **Windmueller, H. G. and Spaeth, A. E.,** Identification of ketone bodies and glutamine as the major respiratory fuels *in vivo* for postabsorptive rat small intestine, *J. Biol. Chem.,* 253, 69, 1978.

163. **Henning, S. J. and Hird, F. J. R.,** Concentrations and metabolism of volatile fatty acids in the fermentative organs of two species of kangaroo and the guinea-pig, *Br. J. Nutr.,* 24, 145, 1970.

164. **Roediger, W. E. W.,** Role of anaerobic bacteria in the metabolic welfare of the colonic mucosa in man, *Gut,* 21, 793, 1980.

165. **Young, G. P. and Gibson, P.,** Contrasting effects of butyrate on proliferation and differentitation of normal and neoplastic cells, in *Short Chain Fatty Acids: Metabolism and Clinical Importance. Report of 10th Ross Conference on Medical Research,* Roche, A. F., Ed., Ross Laboratories, Columbus, Ohio, 1991, 50.

166. **Niles, R. M., Wilhelm, S. A., Thomas, P., and Zamcheck, N.,** The effect of sodium butyrate and retinoic acid on growth and CEA production in a series of human colorectal tumor cell lines representing different states of differentiation, *Cancer Invest.,* 6, 39, 1988.

167. **Scheppach, W., Bartram, P., Richter, A., Richter, F., Liepold, H., Dusel, G., Hofstetter, G., Ruthlein, J., and Kasper, H.,** Effect of short-chain fatty acids on the human colonic mucosa *in vitro, J. Parent. Ent. Nutr.,* 16, 43, 1992.

168. **Sakata, T.,** Stimulatory effect of short-chain fatty acids on epithelial cell proliferation in the rat intestine: a possible explanation for trophic effects of fermentable fibre, gut microbes and luminal trophic factors, *Br. J. Nutr.* 58, 95, 1987.

169. **Lupton, J. R., Coder, D. M., and Jacobs, L. R.,** Influence of luminal pH on rat large bowel epithelial cell cycle, *Am. J. Physiol.,* 249, G382, 1985.

170. **Goodlad, R. A., Lenton, W., Ghatei, M. A., Adrian, T. E., Bloom, S. R., and Wright, N. A.,** Effects of an elemental diet, inert bulk and different types of dietary fibre on the response of the intestinal epithelium to refeeding in the rat and relationship to plasma gastrin, enteroglucagon and PYY concentrations, *Gut,* 28, 171, 1987.

171. **Goodlad, R. A., Ratcliffe, B., Fordham, J. P., and Wright, N. A.,** Does dietary fibre stimulate intestinal epithelial cell proliferation in germ free rats?, *Gut,* 30, 820, 1989.

172. **Gibson, P. R., Rosella, O., Rosella, G., and Young, G. P.,** Butyrate is a potent inhibitor of urokinase secretion by normal colonic epithelium *in vitro, Gastroenterology,* 107, 410, 1994.

173. **Kruh, J., Defer, N., and Tichonicky, L.,** Molecular and cellular effects of sodium butyrate. In: *Short Chain Fatty Acids: Metabolism and Clinical Importance. Report of the 10th Ross Conference on Medical Research,* Roche, A. F., Ed., Ross Laboratories, Columbus, Ohio, 1991, 45.

174. **Tanaka, Y., Bush, K. K., Klauck, T. M., and Higgins, P. J.,** Enhancement of butyrate-induced differentiation of HT-29 human colon carcinoma cells by 1,25-dihydroxyvitamin D3, *Biochem. Pharmacol.,* 38, 3859, 1989.

175. **Siddiqui, B. and Kim, Y. S.,** Effects of sodium butyrate, dimethyl sulfoxide, and retinoic acid on glycolipids of human rectal adenocarcinoma cells, *Cancer Res.,* 44, 1648, 1984.

176. **Rolandelli, R. H., Koruda, M. J., Settle, R. G., and Rombeau, J. L.,** Effects of intraluminal infusion of short-chain fatty acids on the healing of colonic anastomoses in the rat, *Surgery,* 100, 198, 1986.

177. **Kripke, S. A., Fox, A. D., Berman, J. M., Settle, R. G., and Rombeau, J. L.,** Stimulation of intestinal mucosal growth with intracolonic infusion of short-chain fatty acids, *J. Parent. Ent. Nutr.,* 13, 109, 1989.

178. **Koruda, M. J., Rolandelli, R. H., Settle, R. G., Zimmaro, D. M., and Rombeau, J. L.,** Effect of parenteral nutrition supplemented with short-chain fatty acids on adaptation to massive small bowel resection, *Gastroenterology,* 95, 715, 1988.

179. **Remesy, C. and Demigne, C.,** Specific effects of fermentable carbohydrates on blood urea flux and ammonia absorption in the rat cecum, *J. Nutr.,* 119, 560, 1989.

180. **Mortensen, F. V., Nielsen, H., Mulvany, M. J., and Hessov, I.,** Short chain fatty acids dilate isolated human colonic resistance arteries, *Gut,* 31, 1391, 1990.

181. **Kvietys, P. R. and Granger, D. N.,** Effect of volatile fatty acids on blood flow and oxygen uptake by the dog colon, *Gastroenterology,* 80, 962, 1981.

182. **Crissinger, K. D. and Burney, D. L.,** Influence of luminal nutrient composition on hemodynamics and oxygenation in developing intestine, *Am. J. Physiol.,* 263, G254, 1992.

183. **Buckley, N. M. and Frasier, I. D.,** Regional circulatory responses to intestinal work in developing swine, *Am. J. Physiol.,* 258, H1119, 1990.

184. **Qamar, M. I., Read, A. E., and Mountford, R.,** Increased superior mesenteric artery blood flow after glucose but not lactulose ingestion, *Q. J. Med.,* 60, 893, 1986.

185. **Flynn, W. J. J., Gosche, J. R., and Garrison, R. N.,** Intestinal blood flow is restored with glutamine or glucose suffusion after hemorrhage, *J. Surg. Res.,* 52, 499, 1992.

186. **Lang, C. H., Obih, J. C., Bagby, G. J., Bagwell, J. N., and Spitzer, J. J.,** Increased glucose uptake by intestinal mucosa and muscularis in hypermetabolic sepsis, *Am. J. Physiol.,* 261, G287, 1991.

187. **Binder, H. J. and Mehta, P.,** Short-chain fatty acids stimulate active sodium chloride absorption *in vitro* in the rat distal colon, *Gastroenterology,* 96, 989, 1989.

188. **Watson, A. J. M., Elliott, E. J., Rolston, D. D. K., Borodo, M. M., Farthing, M. J. G., and Fairclough, P. D.,** Acetate absorption in the normal and secreting rat jejunum, *Gut,* 31, 170, 1990.

189. **Vernia, P., Gnaedinger, A., Hauck, W., and Breuer, R. I.,** Organic anions and the diarrhea of inflammatory bowel disease, *Dig. Dis. Sci.,* 33, 1353, 1988.

190. **Rees, R. G. P., Keohane, P. P., Grimble, G. K., Frost, P. G., Attrill, H., and Silk, D. B. A.,** Tolerance of elemental diet administered without starter regimen, *Br. Med. J.,* 290, 1869, 1985.

191. **Mowatt-Larssen, C. A., Brown, R. O., Wojtysiak, S. L., and Kudsk, K. A.,** Comparison of tolerance and nutritional outcome between a peptide and a standard enteral formula in critically ill, hypoalbuminemic patients, *J. Parent. Ent. Nutr.,* 16, 20, 1992.

192. **Kemen, M., Homann, H.-H., Mumme, A., and Zumtobel, V.,** Is intact protein superior for post-operative enteral nutrition than hydrolyzed protein?, *Clin. Nutr.,* 10 (Suppl), 37, 1991.

193. **Patil, D. H., Westaby, D., Mahida, Y. R., Palmer, K. R., Rees, R., Clark, M. L., Dawson, A. M., and Silk, D. B. A.,** Comparative modes of action of lactitol and lactulose in the treatment of hepatic encephalopathy, *Gut,* 28, 255, 1987.

194. **Konno, R., Niwa, A., and Yasumura, Y.,** Intestinal bacterial origin of D-alanine in urine of mutant mice lacking D-amino-acid oxidase, *Biochem. J.,* 268, 263, 1990.

195. **Clausen, M. R., Bonnen, H., Tvede, M., and Mortensen, P. B.,** Colonic fermentation to short-chain fatty acids is decreased in antibiotic-associated diarrhea, *Gastroenterology,* 101, 1497, 1991.

196. **Thompson, G. N., Chalmers, R. A., Walter, J. H., Bresson, J. L., Lyonnet, S. L., Reed, P. J., Saudubray, J. M., Leonard, J. V., and Halliday, D.,** The use of metronidazole in management of methylmalonic and propionic acidaemias, *Eur. J. Pediatr.,* 149, 792, 1990.

197. **Homann, H.-H., Kemen, M., Mumme, A., Bauer, K. H., and Zumtobel, V.,** The role of carbohydrate malabsorption in the pathogenesis of diarrhea during postoperative enteral nutrition, *J. Clin. Nutr. Gastroenterol.,* 7, 54, 1992.

198. **Lehtola, J., Jauhonen, P., Kesaniemi, A., Wikberg, R., and Gordin, A.,** Effect of erythromycin on the oro-caecal transit time in man, *Eur. J. Clin. Pharmacol.,* 39, 555, 1990.

199. **Cannon, W. B.,** The movements of the intestines studied by means of the roentgen rays, *Am. J. Physiol.,* 6, 251, 1902.

200. **Szurszewiski, J. J.,** A migrating electrical complex of canine small intestine, *Am. J. Physiol.,* 217, 1757, 1969.

201. **Schemann, M. and Ehrlein, H. J.,** Post prandial patterns of canine jejunal motility and transit of luminal contents, *Gastroenterology,* 90, 991, 1986.

202. **Silk, D. B. A. and Spiller, R. C.,** The small intestine, in *Scientific Foundations of Surgery,* Kyle, J. and Carey, L. C., Eds., Heineman Medical Books, Oxford, 1989, 409.

203. **Ehrlein, H. J., Schmid, H. R., and Feinle, C.,** Recording of intestinal motility is a useful control of enteral nutrition, *Clin. Nutr.,* 11 (Suppl), 62, 1992.

204. **Raimundo, A. H., Jameson, J. S., Rogers, J., and Silk, D. B. A.,** The effect of enteral nutrition on distal colonic motility, *Gastroenterology,* 102 (4 Pt 2), A573, 1992.

205. **Bowling, T. E., Raimundo, A. H., Grimble, G. K., and Silk, D. B. A.,** Reversal by short-chain fatty acids of colonic fluid secretion induced by enteral feeding, *Lancet,* 342, 1266, 1993.

206. **Silk, D. B. A.,** Progress report: fibre and enteral nutrition, *Gut,* 30, 246, 1989.

207. **Silk, D. B. A.,** Fibre and enteral nutrition, *Clin. Nutr.,* 12 (Suppl 1), S106, 1993.

208. **Egan, C. J. and Rennie, M. J.,** Protein synthesis in rat jejunum: precursor pools and adaptation to protein/energy restriction, *Clin. Nutr.,* 5 (Suppl), 68, 1986.

209. **Windmueller, H. G.,** Glutamine utilization by the small intestine, *Adv. Enzymol.,* 53, 201, 1982.

210. **Sbaï, D., Narcy, C., Thompson, G. N., Mariotti, A., Poggi, F., Saudubray, J. M., and Bresson, J. L.,** Contribution of odd-chain fatty acid oxidation to propionate production in disorders of propionate metabolism, *Am. J. Clin. Nutr.,* 59, 1332, 1994.

211. **Grimble, G. K.,** Essential and conditionally-essential nutrients in clinical nutrition, *Nutr. Res. Rev.,* 6, 97, 1993.

212. **Souba, W. W. and Wilmore, D. W.,** Postoperative alterations of arteriovenous exchange of amino acids across the gastrointestinal tract, *Surgery,* 94, 342, 1983.

213. **Souba, W. W., Scott, T. E., and Wilmore, D. W.,** Intestinal consumption of intravenously administered fuels, *J. Parent. Ent. Nutr.,* 9, 18, 1985.

214. **McKeehan, W. L.,** Glycolysis, glutaminolysis and cell proliferation, *Cell Biol. Int. Rep.,* 6, 635, 1982.

215. **Newsholme, E. A., Crabtree, B., and Ardawi, M. S. M.,** Glutamine metabolism in lymphocytes: its biochemical, physiological and clinical importance, *Q. J. Exp. Physiol.,* 70, 473, 1985.

216. **Newsholme, E. A. and Carrié, A.-L.,** Quantitative aspects of glucose and glutamine metabolism by intestinal cells, *Gut,* 35 (Suppl 1), S13, 1994.

217. **Payne-James, J. J. and Grimble, G. K.,** The present status of glutamine, *Curr. Opin. Gastroenterol.,* 11, 161, 1995.

218. **Chen, K., Okuma, T., Okamura, K., Torigoe, Y., and Miyauchi, Y.,** Glutamine-supplemented parenteral nutrition improves gut mucosa integrity and function in endotoxaemic rats, *J. Parent. Ent. Nutr.,* 18, 167, 1994.

219. **Li, J., Langkamp-Henken, B., Suzuki, K., and Stahlgren, L. H.,** Glutamine prevents parenteral nutrition-induced increases in intestinal permeability, *J. Parent. Ent. Nutr.,* 18, 303, 1994.

220. **Tremel, H., Kienle, B., Weilemann, L. S., Stehle, P., and Fürst, P.,** Glutamine dipeptide-supplemented parenteral nutrition maintains intestinal function in the critically ill, *Gastroenterology,* 107, 1595, 1994.

221. **Halliwell, B. and Chirico, S.,** Lipid peroxidation: its mechanism, measurement and significance, *Am. J. Clin. Nutr.,* 57 (Suppl), 715S, 1993.

222. **Kelly, F. J.,** Glutathione content of the small intestine: regulation and function, *Br. J. Nutr.,* 69, 589, 1993.

223. **Robinson, M. K., Ahn, M. S., Rounds, J. D., Cook, J. A., Jacobs, D. O., and Wilmore, D. W.,** Parenteral glutathione monoester enhances tissue antioxidant stores, *J. Parent. Ent. Nutr.,* 16, 413, 1992.

224. **Harward, T. R. S., Coe, D., Souba, W. W., Klingman, N., and Seeger, J. M.,** Glutamine preserves gut glutathione levels during intestinal ischaemia/reperfusion, *J. Surg. Res.,* 56, 351, 1994.

225. **Austgen, T. R., Chen, M. K., Flynn, T. C., and Souba, W. W.,** The effects of endotoxin on the splanchnic metabolism of glutamine and related substrates, *J. Trauma,* 31, 742, 1991.

226. **Grimble, R. F., Jackson, A. A., Persaud, C., Wride, M. J., Delers, F., and Engler, R.,** Cysteine and glycine supplementation modulate the metabolic response to tumor necrosis factor alpha in rats fed a low protein diet, *J. Nutr.,* 122, 2066, 1992.

227. **Leleiko, N. S., Bronstein, A. D., and Munro, H. N.,** Effect of dietary purines on *de novo* synthesis of purine nucleotides in the small intestinal mucosa, *Pediatr. Res.,* 13, 403, 1979.

228. **Leleiko, N. S., Bronstein, A. D., Baliga, B. S., and Munro, H. N.,** *De novo* purine nucleotide synthesis in the rat small and large intestine: effect of dietary protein and purines, *J. Pediatr. Gastroenterol. Nutr.,* 2, 313, 1983.

229. **Janas, L. and Picciano, M.,** The nucleotide profile of human milk, *Pediatr. Res.,* 16, 659, 1982.

230. **Brunser, O., Espinoza, J., Araya, M., Cruchet, S., and Gil, A.,** Effect of dietary nucleotide supplementation on diarrheal disease in infants, *Acta Pediatr.,* 83, 188, 1994.

231. **Bueno, J., Torres, M., Almendros, A., Carmona, R., Nuñez, M. C., Rios, A., and Gil, A.,** Effect of dietary nucleotides on small intestinal repair after diarrhea. Histological and ultrastructural changes, *Gut,* 35, 926, 1994.

232. **Grimble, G. K.,** Dietary nucleotides and gut mucosal defence, *Gut,* 35 (Suppl), S46, 1994.

233. **Blachier, F., Darcy Vrillon, B., Sener, A., Duee, P. H., and Malaisse, W. J.,** Arginine metabolism in rat enterocytes, *Biochim. Biophys. Acta,* 1092, 304, 1991.

234. **Rérat, A., Simoes-Nuñes, C., Mendy, F., and Roger, L.,** Amino acid absorption and production of pancreatic hormones in non-anaesthetised pigs after duodenal infusions of a milk enzymic hydrolysate or of free amino acids, *Br. J. Nutr.,* 60, 121, 1988.

235. **Calignano, A., Whittle, B. J., Di Rosa, M., and Moncada, S.,** Involvement of endogenous nitric oxide in the regulation of rat intestinal motility *in vivo, Eur. J. Pharmacol.,* 229, 273, 1992.

236. **Hegarty, J. E., Fairclough, P. D., Clark, M. L., and Dawson, A. M.,** Jejunal water and electrolyte secretion induced by L-arginine in man, *Gut,* 22, 108, 1981.

237. **Mourad, F. H., Andre, E. A., O'Donnell, L. J. D., Clark, M. L., and Farthing, M. J. G.,** Does L-arginine induce intestinal water secretion through formation of nitric oxide?, *Gut,* 34 (Suppl. 4), S60, 1993.

238. **Gianotti, L., Alexander, J. W., Pyles, T., and Fukushima, R.,** Arginine-supplemented diets improve survival in gut-derived sepsis and peritonitis by modulating bacterial clearance: the role of nitric oxide, *Ann. Surg.,* 217, 644, 1993.

239. **Kubes, P.,** Nitric oxide modulates epithelial permeability in the feline small intestine, *Am. J. Physiol.,* 262, G1138, 1992.

240. **Kubes, P.,** Ischemia-reperfusion in feline small intestine: a role for nitric oxide, *Am. J. Physiol.,* 264, G143, 1993.

241. **Boughton Smith, N. K., Deakin, A. M., and Whittle, B. J.,** Actions of nitric oxide on the acute gastrointestinal damage induced by PAF in the rat, *Agents Actions,* Special Suppl., C3, 1992.

242. **Cynober, L.,** Can arginine and ornithine support gut functions?, *Gut,* 35 (Suppl 1), S42, 1994.

243. **Daly, J. M., Lieberman, M. D., Goldfine, J., Shou, J., Weintraub, F., Rosato, E. F., and Lavin, P.,** Enteral nutrition with supplemental arginine, RNA and omega-3 fatty acids in patients after operation: immunologic, metabolic, and clinical outcome, *Surgery,* 112, 56, 1992.

244. **Heyland, D. K., Cook, D. J., and Guyatt, G. H.,** Does the formulation of enteral feeding products influence infectious morbidity and mortality rates in the critically ill patient? A critical review of the evidence, *Crit. Care Med.,* 22, 1192, 1994.

245. **Hibbert, J. M., Forrester, T., and Jackson, A. A.,** Urea kinetics: comparison of oral and intravenous dose regimens, *Eur. J. Clin. Nutr.,* 46, 405, 1992.

246. **Moran, B. J. and Jackson, A. A.,** $^{15}$N-urea metabolism in the functioning human colon: luminal hydrolysis and mucosal permeability, *Gut,* 31, 454, 1990.

247. **Souba, W. W.,** Intestinal glutamine metabolism and nutrition, *J. Nutr. Biochem.,* 4, 2, 1993.

248. **Kies, C.,** Nonspecific nitrogen in the nutrition of human beings, *Fed. Proc.,* 31, 1172, 1972.

249. **Snyderman, S. E., Holt, L. E., Jr., Dancis, J., Roitman, E., Boyer, A., and Balis, M. E.,** "Unessential" nitrogen: a limiting factor for human growth, *J. Nutr.,* 78, 57, 1962.

250. **Morgan, M. Y.,** The treatment of chronic hepatic encephalopathy, *Hepatogastroenterology,* 38, 377, 1991.

251. **Weber, F. L. J., Banwell, J. G., Fresard, K. M., and Cummings, J. H.,** Nitrogen in fecal bacterial, fiber, and soluble fractions of patients with cirrhosis: effects of lactulose and lactulose plus neomycin, *J. Lab. Clin. Med.,* 110, 259, 1987.

252. **Bird, S. P., Hewitt, D., Ratcliffe, B., and Gurr, M. I.,** Effects of lactulose and lactitol on protein digestion and metabolism in conventional and germ free animal models: relevance of the results to their use in the treatment of portosystemic encephalopathy, *Gut,* 31, 1403, 1990.

253. **Collins, A. J., James, P. S., and Smith, M. W.,** Sugar-dependent selective induction of mouse jejunal disaccharidase activities, *J. Physiol.,* 419, 157, 1989.

# 7

# The Effects of Ethanol on Salivary Glands

Gordon B. Proctor and Deepak K. Shori

## CONTENTS

## 7.1 INTRODUCTION

Salivas are secreted into the mouth by three pairs of major salivary glands and many minor glands and contain mixtures of ions, proteins, and glycoproteins which are necessary for maintaining oral homeostasis, exerting many effects on hard and soft tissues. Salivas must influence oral disease processes such as those which have been shown clearly to be associated with chronic ethanol consumption, although the mechanisms of such influences are ill-defined. Likewise, it is not clear if a causative relationship exists between ethanol-induced changes in salivary gland secretion and ethanol-associated oral disease.

This chapter reviews the literature concerning the effects of ethanol on salivary gland function. Much of the literature is mainly concerned with parotid gland secretion, probably because the effects of ethanol abuse usually are clinically most evident here. Also in human experimental studies parotid saliva can be more easily collected than those from other salivary glands. Before consideration is given to the mechanism(s) by which ethanol might be affecting salivary gland function, and in order to evaluate the experimental evidence it is necessary to understand the physiological mechanisms involved in salivary secretion.

## 7.2 THE PHYSIOLOGY OF SALIVARY SECRETION

The main control of salivary secretion is exerted by nerves; the glands have a rich supply from both divisions of the autonomic nervous system. If one sections the autonomic nerve supply to salivary glands, secretion ceases almost entirely.[1] The main afferent nerve-mediated stimuli for salivary secretion are mastication and taste (Figure 7.1), which are mediated through specific receptors.[2] In the absence of mastication and taste there is a neurally mediated "resting" flow of

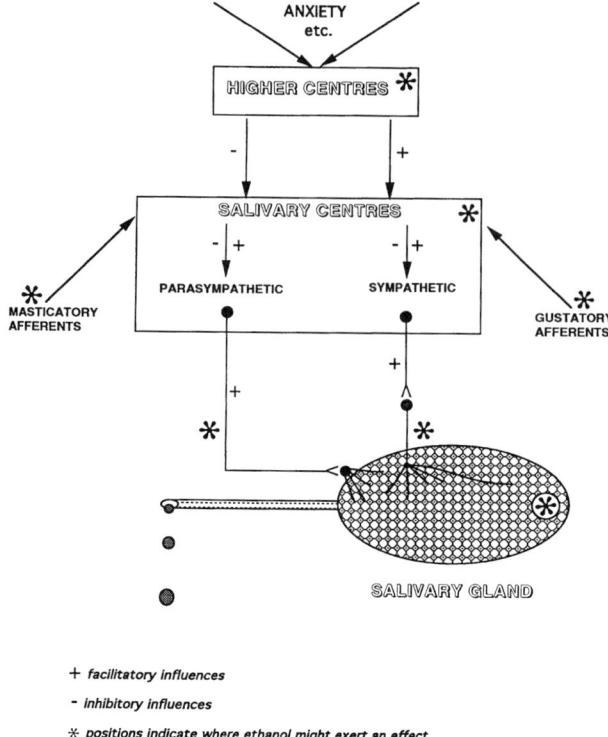

**FIGURE 7.1**   Chart of nerve pathways involved in reflex secretion of saliva and the possible sites of ethanol action. The parasympathetic and sympathetic nerves represent the efferent arms of the reflexes.

saliva which is all but abolished during sleep.[3,4] Salivary flow can also be reflexly evoked by the actions of chemicals (e.g., ethanol) on free nerve endings in the oral mucosa.[5] The major salivary glands appear to show different dependencies on mastication and taste; submandibular and sublingual salivary flow is higher than parotid flow under resting conditions and less dependent on mastication.[3] Parotid flow shows a relatively greater increase on stimulation and appears to heavily depend on masticatory stimuli as demonstrated by the atrophy which occurs when animals are maintained on a liquid diet.[6] The atrophy is accompanied by a reduced parotid flow which has also been observed in humans maintained on a liquid diet.[6,7] The submandibular and sublingual glands do not show as great an atrophy under similar conditions.[6]

In parotid glands of different species, secretion evoked by mastication is mediated primarily by efferent parasympathetic nerves and those from gustatory stimuli primarily by efferent sympathetic nerves.[8,9] It is important, however, to realize that during reflex salivary secretion the parasympathetic and sympathetic efferent nerve supplies to salivary glands are activated simultaneously and interact with each other in a positive way often producing augmented effects.[10] In studies of human reflex salivary secretion a citric acid stimulus is frequently used to evoke secretion because it stimulates a large flow of saliva.[3] Apart from whole saliva, parotid saliva has been the most frequently studied as it can be easily collected using a suction device fitted over the ductal orifice on the buccal mucosa.[3] Submandibular saliva in contrast, requires collection devices molded to the individual's mouth which makes a study of patient populations much more difficult.[3] As indicated in Figure 7.1 the higher centers of the brain can influence nerve traffic to the gland. This is best illustrated by the dry mouth experienced in moments of high anxiety, for example, when speaking in public. This effect can be attributed to the higher centers of the brain inhibiting the salivary centers.[11]

The neurotransmitters released from nerves act on a variety of receptors and secretion can be evoked by a number of autonomimetics and blocked by specific antagonists.[2] Those referred to later in the chapter in animal studies of salivary secretion are the cholinergic agonists methacholine and pilocarpine, the muscarinic receptor blocker atropine, the β-adrenergic agonist isoprenaline and the β-blocker propranolol. Such studies in animal models and humans have demonstrated that fluid secretion is evoked principally by parasympathetic nerve stimulation and para-sympathomimetics and can be largely blocked by atropine. Protein secretion appears to depend more on sympathetically mediated stimuli and β-adrenoceptor agonists and can be blocked by β-adrenoceptor blocking drugs such as propranolol or more specific β1 receptor antagonists (e.g., atenolol).

The autonomic innervation of salivary glands exerts a long-term influence on their function. In general, cutting the parasympathetic nerve supply to the parotid or submandibular glands leads to a glandular atrophy[1] with a decrease in weight of up to 40% in the case of the rat.[12] Cutting the sympathetic nerve supply has a more variable effect[1] but in the case of the rat parotid gland can decrease weight up to 28%.[13] If the postganglionic nerve supply is lost in such experiments, then the gland becomes supersensitive to autonomimetics.[1] Increased nerve traffic has the opposite effect to denervation and can cause glandular hypertrophy/ hyperplasia. This is seen in rats maintained on a bulk diet and most strikingly following chronic treatment with β-adrenoceptor agonists such as isoprenaline.[14]

There are hormonal influences on salivary glands but these are mostly long term. An exception is aldosterone, which can alter the sodium and potassium concentrations of saliva entering the mouth by affecting the reuptake of sodium and its exchange for potassium.[15] Destruction or removal of different endocrine glands has been shown to affect rat salivary glands. The effects of diabetes, adrenalectomy, and thyroidectomy can be reversed by administration of insulin,[16] glucocorticoids, and thyroid hormone, respectively.[17] Administration of thyroid hormone to normal rats increases salivary flow while glucocorticoid and insulin have a less obvious effect. Each of these hormones, however, regulates the synthesis of some secretory proteins and alters the protein composition of salivas.[17]

The fluid and protein components of saliva are produced mainly by cells present in acini which form end pieces on the ductal system of the gland. As this primary saliva, the ionic composition of which resembles extracellular fluid, travels through the ductal tree its ionic composition but not its volume, is altered, so that the final secretion delivered into the mouth is hypotonic and relatively potassium rich. The extent of these alterations in ionic composition is inversely proportional to flow rate of saliva.[15]

## 7.3 EFFECTS OF ETHANOL ON HUMAN SALIVARY GLANDS

### 7.3.1 Sialadenosis and Neuropathy

The most obvious clinical manifestation of the effects of ethanol on salivary glands is a bilateral swelling termed sialadenosis or sialosis.[18-20] Parotid sialadenosis is not only seen in chronic alcoholism but may accompany a number of systemic diseases such as malnutrition or bulimia. The swelling is usually not painful but is sufficient to give the patient a "hamster-like" appearance. It is often associated with hormonal disturbances, for example, hypothyroidism, diabetes, or changes in sex hormones.[19,21] In chronic alcoholism it is most frequently encountered in those with liver cirrhosis (45 to 80% of patients), and less frequently in noncirrhotic alcoholics (10%).[19,22]

Sialographical and histological examinations are useful in diagnosing sialadenosis allowing inflammatory conditions to be excluded. When radiopaque material is injected into the parotid duct the ductal system takes on a normal or thread-like appearance which contrasts with the dilated ductal tree characteristic of recurrent parotitis.[19] In the late stages of sialadenosis sialography reveals a typical picture described as a "tree-in-bloom," caused by the swollen acini compressing the proximal ductal system. The enlarged acinar cells which give rise to the sialographic picture are clearly visible in histological material taken by aspiration cytology. Seifert et al.[21] describes three histological appearances of sialadenosis: (1) a granular form in which acinar cytoplasm is packed with granules; (2) a honeycomb pattern in which the cytoplasm is vacuolated; and (3) a mixed form demonstrating both of the above features. Ultrastructurally, there is conspicuous myoepithelial cell degeneration and lesions of the sympathetic nerves within the gland including a loss of neurosecretory granules, swelling of axoplasm, and axolysis.[23] Thus there is a characteristic triad of acinar hypertrophy, myoepithelial cell, and neural degeneration in sialadenosis.[21] There may be some association between the histological appearance and the underlying clinical cause; for example, experimentally induced sialadenosis shows acinar hypertrophy while acinar edema and fatty infiltration are often associated with alcoholic sialadenosis.[24] In the absence of sialadenosis stereological analysis of salivary glands from chronic alcoholics showed fatty infiltration without acinar cell enlargement.[25] Similar qualitative observations have been made by others.[26,27] Submandibular sialadenosis is less frequently observed although the increased fatty infiltration of submandibular glands seen in stereological analysis of necropsy material suggests that the glands are affected by chronic alcoholism.[25]

It is possible that raised levels of serum salivary type amylase seen in alcoholic cirrhosis[28-30] are associated with sialadenosis[31] as is apparently seen in sialadenosis due to bulimia.[32] It is likely, however, that other sources of salivary type amylase, possibly even the liver itself, may be contributing to serum amylase under such circumstances.[33,34]

Given the physiology of salivary gland function and the intimate association with nerves described earlier there are a number of ways in which ethanol may conceivably have an effect on salivary gland function and secretion (Figure 7.1). Most of the studies on humans and animals described below have considered the direct effect of ethanol on the secretory cells. However, the neural influences on salivation extend to the higher centers in the brain which can influence events.[11] Thus ethanol might possibly affect salivary secretion indirectly through its action on the CNS. Ethanol may affect afferent or efferent nerve pathways; sensory motor and autonomic neuropathies can be diagnosed by testing for reductions in nerve conduction and changes in cardiovascular responses to standing.[35] Such neuropathies are frequently seen in liver disease induced by ethanol or otherwise and there have been descriptions in the literature of autonomic cardiac neuropathies associated with an increased mortality rate.[36-38] Ethanol-induced autonomic neuropathy, like diabetic autonomic neuropathy, could influence events in salivary glands.[39,40] Seifert et al. have hypothesized that autonomic dysfunction and neuropathy are the most important factors in the etiology of sialadenosis. Circumstantial evidence for this is persuasive since neuropathies are frequently seen in diseases leading to sialadenosis, for example, diabetes, alcoholism, and vitamin deficiencies.[21] In a study of 30 cases of sialadenosis in patients with different underlying diseases (e.g., diabetes, liver cirrhosis, etc.) Donath and Seifert in 1975 found abnormal nerve terminals showing signs of degeneration.[23] There are similarities in the histological picture presented in some human sialadenoses and the experimental sialadenosis which can be induced in laboratory animals by manipulating the autonomic innervation (see below).

## 7.3.2    Ethanol and Salivary Secretion

The acute effects of ethanol on salivary function have been little studied in human subjects. Ethanol can stimulate a moderate flow of parotid saliva possibly due to an irritant effect.[41] Following a large dose of ethanol (0.8 g/kg) producing a peak circulating level of $92 \pm 13$ mg%, parotid salivary flow was reduced by approximately 50% compared to flow before dosage and was accompanied by reductions in protein and amylase outputs. This effect was exerted for approximately 90 min following dosage.[42]

Different studies have produced some varying results on the chronic effects of ethanol on salivary secretion. Dutta et al.[43] stimulated parotid secretion in a group of 24 alcoholic males without evidence of malnutrition or cirrhosis of the liver. Salivary flow rate was reduced by more than 70% and it appeared that the amylase concentration was also reduced. Although the concentrations of protein and epidermal growth factor (EGF) were not altered, the reduced salivary flow resulted in significantly lowered output of each of the proteins measured. The bioactivity of EGF in saliva was greatly reduced even though the concentration of immunoreactive EGF was not decreased. The effects of ethanol consumption on flow rate were found to be reversible in this study because after 7 days of abstinence mean salivary flow rate had significantly increased and was no longer different from the mean in control subjects. An earlier study by Dutta et al.[26] focused on a group of alcoholic cirrhotic patients who were compared with alcoholic noncirrhotic and normal control groups. In this study, patients had been sober for at least 4 weeks before parotid saliva collection. Consistent with the reversible effects on flow rate described above there was no significant difference between flow rates in the alcoholic and normal control groups, but alcoholic cirrhotic patients had both reduced basal and stimulated parotid salivary flow rates compared to normal controls and noncirrhotic patients. This gave rise to changes in the ionic composition and output of proteins into saliva. Thus the bicarbonate concentration and pH of saliva were reduced as were the sodium and chloride concentrations. These changes probably arose as a result of the normal modification by salivary ductal cells of a reduced volume of primary saliva being produced by acinar cells (see above).

These more recent studies by Dutta's group should be compared with earlier studies by other groups. Abelson et al.[22] examined 18 alcoholic cirrhotic patients many of whom showed evidence of parotid enlargement and found significant increases in lemon candy–stimulated parotid flow rate, protein, and amylase concentration. The salivary concentrations of sodium and potassium suggested hyperfunction of ductal cells, which the authors speculated may have been due to increases in circulating aldosterone in these patients as a result of liver cirrhosis. The authors described the increase in flow rate and protein secretion as "indicative of acinar hypertrophy" associated with sialadenosis. Durr et al.[44] found no change in citric acid stimulated parotid flow in a group of 12 alcoholic cirrhotic patients compared to controls. Similarly Scott et al.[45] found no differences in citric acid stimulated parotid salivary flow rate in a small group of noncirrhotic alcoholic patients. However, in spite of the small sample size ($n = 7$), there was a significant, threefold increase in resting flow rate compared to normal controls which was accompanied by changes in ionic and protein composition. Rausch and Gorlin[19] refer to their own studies as indicating that salivary flow is generally reduced in parotid sialadenosis, regardless of the underlying cause, with a concomitant increase in the potassium concentration and a reduction in the sodium concentration.

Overall, therefore, the above results appear to be contradictory. It is difficult to resolve how such variation has come about; possibly the selection of patients and diagnostic parameters for cirrhosis have varied. Circulating levels of ethanol should not have been elevated as patients were required not to drink prior to the studies and usually circulating levels of ethanol were assessed. The stimulation (citric acid as a solution or in candy) and collection of saliva were carefully controlled. The latter is important as there are a number of variables, for example, time of day or time of last meal, which can influence salivary flow.[46]

## 7.4  EXPERIMENTAL STUDIES ON ANIMAL SALIVARY GLANDS

Animal studies provide an opportunity to take a more controlled look at the effects of ethanol on salivary function and to examine possible mechanisms by which these effects are exerted. Acute intragastric doses of ethanol decrease parotid salivary flow evoked from anesthetized rats by pilocarpine at a time when the level of ethanol in blood is elevated[47]; this is similar to the response described in humans[42] (see above). Proctor et al.[48,49] investigated the acute effects of ethanol on protein synthesis in the major salivary glands. Rats were given intraperitoneal injections of ethanol and protein synthesis was measured using phenylalanine in the flooding dose technique[50] 2.5 h later when the level of ethanol in blood was still elevated.[51] Protein synthesis was reduced by approximately 40% in parotid, submandibular, and sublingual glands. Similar reductions in protein synthesis have been measured in skeletal muscle[52] and other tissues[53] following acute ethanol injection. The reduced parotid protein synthesis would appear to coincide with the reduced parotid secretory response following acute ethanol.[47] It was interesting that protein synthesis in all three glands should have been similarly affected. Protein synthesis in the sublingual gland unlike the other glands is high under resting conditions and does not increase in response to refeeding; this is likely to be related to the fact that this gland secretes spontaneously in the absence of external stimuli.[54] Thus, the uniform effects of acute ethanol suggest that it must be affecting some aspect of secretory cell function in addition to any effect on the autonomic innervation. Given the importance of salivary mucin in the oral cavity (see later) and the effects of ethanol on gastric mucin, Slomiany et al.[55] investigated the influence of ethanol on the synthesis of submandibular mucin, specifically the posttranslational sulfation of mucin *in vitro*. Reduction in submandibular glandular sulforyltransferase activity was found to be proportional to ethanol concentration. This effect could be physiologically relevant as inhibition of sulforyltransferase activity was approximately 40% at an ethanol concentration equivalent to its isoosmotic concentration (1.7%). Although the influence of decreased sulfation on specific functions of mucin is unclear, it might be that less sulfated mucins are less hydrated and therefore do not have the same gel-forming characteristics which appear to be functionally important.[56] It is clear therefore from these experiments that ethanol acutely affects salivary gland function and it appears that all of the major salivary glands are affected.

The mechanism by which ethanol exerts its acute affects is not clear. Impaired prostaglandin ($PGE_2$, $PGF_{2a}$, and 6-keto-$PGF_{1a}$) production and increased prostaglandin ($PGF_2$) receptor binding by submandibular and sublingual cells *in vitro* in the presence of ethanol was cited as a possible mechanism by which ethanol influences salivary secretion.[57,58] However, since prostaglandins appear not to play a significant role in the control of secretion as found with submandibular acini,[59] it is unlikely that inhibition of prostaglandin synthesis or changes in affinity of receptors can account for the observed inhibition of salivary secretion by acute doses of ethanol. The effects of ethanol on membrane lipid composition have been much studied.[60,61] Acute ethanol reduces $Na^+$, $K^+$ ATPase activity in cultured hepatocytes while chronic ethanol adminstration has been found to have the opposite effect on membranes of central neurons.[62,63] If membranes of salivary secretory cells are similarly affected by ethanol, then this may influence secretion which has been shown to depend on the activity of large amounts of the $Na^+$, $K^+$ ATPase present in the basolateral membrane.[15] Recently, acute ethanol has been found to reduce polyphosphoinositide (PI) metabolism in mouse brain leading to decreased levels of the second messenger inositol 1,4,5-triphosphate.[64] The latter is a particularly important second messenger in salivary fluid secretion being generated following occupation of muscarinic cholinergic receptors and leading to rises in intracellular calcium,[2] and acute ethanol exposure has been shown to lead to a decreased uptake of calcium.[65] Thus if ethanol affects salivary glands similarly, this might be responsible for the decreased fluid secretion observed following acute exposure to ethanol.

Scott and Berry[66,67] have shown that rats given intragastric ethanol for periods of 30 or 100 days secrete significantly greater volumes of parotid saliva over a 5-min period in response to both pilocarpine (mainly a cholinergic agonist) or isoprenaline (a β-adrenergic agonist) administered during anesthesia. However, subsequent collections of saliva over a 25-min period did not show significant changes. This difference between short initial and longer subsequent collections remains unexplained. Following dosage of rats for 30 days with ethanol the same group found that there was an increase in salivary sodium concentration and a decrease in potassium concentration in initial saliva samples which suggested a normal flow-dependent ductal modification of saliva (see earlier). After 100 days of ethanol, the changes in sodium and potassium suggested ductal transport of these ions was greater than expected. Protein concentrations tended to be decreased significantly in the 100-day study, although the amylase concentration was maintained. Stereological analysis of parotid gland morphology revealed no changes in glandular acinar structure. However, there was an increased vascular component of the glands which led the authors to conclude that increased glandular blood flow may have been responsible for increased salivary flow. Given the very large doses of secretogogues used in these studies it is likely that maximal flow rates were being elicited which may have been limited by gland vascularity. Perec et al.[68] examined a number of aspects of the effects of ethanol on parotid and submandibular secretion. In this study 32% (v/v) ethanol was given as the sole source of fluid for 12 weeks. This type of model has been criticized as it might lead to dehydration which can also affect salivary secretion.[67] In the study by Perec et al., however, a more physiological examination of salivary secretion was carried out as threshold doses and dose–response curves for methacholine- and noradrenaline-evoked secretion were determined as opposed to responses to huge, supramaximal doses of secretogogues.[68] Doses of methacholine (cholinergic agonist) tenfold higher than controls were required to elicit both submandibular and parotid secretion and dose–response curves were shifted to the right by tenfold. Response curves to noradrenaline were also shifted to the right though to a lesser extent than with methacholine.

Morphological evidence of gland atrophy and fatty infiltration have been found in studies in which rats have been given an ethanol-containing diet over a 3 month period.[69] These changes were accompanied by decreases in parotid salivary flow rate, amylase, and protein concentrations along with the changes in sodium and potassium expected for decreased flow rate, in response to pilocarpine stimulation under anesthesia. The major problem with these studies is the liquid, ethanol-containing diet given to the rats. As mentioned, parotid function is heavily dependent on masticatory stimuli and liquid diet leads to parotid atrophy with decreases in salivary flow rate. A morphological study of parotid glands following 12 months of ethanol administered in drinking water revealed only slight fatty infiltration. The main findings in this study were cellular pleomorphism and oncocytic metaplasia reminiscent of the cellular changes previously seen in senile rats.[70]

Little experimental work appears to have been done on the effects of ethanol on the autonomic innervation of laboratory animals. As mentioned, sialadenosis can be experimentally induced in the rat by increased autonomic nerve traffic as seen when animals are maintained on a bulk (cellulose-rich) diet, or by chronic administration of β-adrenoceptor agonists. There is a wealth of literature on the hyperplasia/hypertrophy and increased gene expression associated with the latter.[14,71] Under these conditions of increased protein synthesis the experimental gland becomes packed with electron-lucent granules, in contrast to the normal electron-dense appearance, a changed histological picture which looks similar to that seen in some forms of human sialadenosis.[21] Perec et al.[68] assessed not only the thresholds of salivary gland responses to autonomimetics in chronically dosed ethanol-treated rats but also the levels of choline acetyltransferase and noradrenaline. These were used as indices of parasympathetic and sympathetic nerve activity respectively and were both found to be increased in parotid and submandibular glands following 12 weeks of ethanol delivered in drinking water. The increased nerve activity was associated with a decreased responsiveness of the salivary secretory cells (see above) but it remains unresolved as to which of these — increased nerve activity or decreased cellular responsiveness — developed first. Recently, the effect of heavy ethanol exposure on the structure of autonomic nerves was assessed.[72] Degenerative changes and vacuolation were found to be more prevalent in parasympathetic than sympathetic ganglia and although some recovery was noted following withdrawal of ethanol the number of vacuolated nerves remained elevated.

## 7.5 MALNUTRITION AND SALIVARY FUNCTION

Malnutrition or malabsorption and in particular protein malnourishment can give rise to sialadenosis[19,73] and are therefore likely to be a factor in the sialadenosis seen in patients with alcoholic cirrhosis, given that the latter is associated with malnutrition.[74] Not surprisingly there appear to have been few studies on the effects of malnutrition on salivary gland function in humans.[17,75] Experimental studies in rats indicate that the stimulated flow of whole saliva and its protein concentration are reduced in protein deficient rats.[17] Vitamin and mineral deficiencies are frequently associated with chronic alcoholism particularly in association with liver cirrhosis.[76,77] Experimental studies have been performed in rats in which deficiencies of some vitamins and minerals have been found to alter salivary secretion; for example, vitamin D deficiency has been found to reduce parotid salivary flow rates without affecting protein outputs.[78] It may be that vitamin D exerts a direct effect on calcium mobilization within salivary secretory cells as indicated by *in vitro* studies on calcium-ATPase activity and other calcium associated proteins.[79] Certainly fluid and protein secretion from salivary cells is profoundly dependent on extracellular and intracellular calcium levels.[2] Vitamin A deficiency reduced both flow rate and protein secretion and was found to induce changes in protein composition compared to controls.[80] Vitamin A deficiency in alcoholism can result from an underlying zinc deficiency, which is a common finding in chronic and acute alcohol abuse.[76] Zinc deficiency has been shown to affect the parotid gland, causing reductions in weight, cell number, and RNA content.[81] The flow, protein output, and protein composition of saliva are all altered in zinc deficiency.[81] Many of these changes appear to result from a self-imposed reduction in caloric intake which accompanies zinc deficiency.

## 7.6    ORAL HOMEOSTASIS AND THE EFFECTS OF ETHANOL

The clinical relevance of ethanol-induced changes in salivary gland secretion is not clear. However, saliva is important for maintaining oral homeostasis, exerting many effects on hard and soft surfaces,[82] some of which are described below. A graphic illustration of the importance of saliva to the hard and soft tissues of the mouth can be gained by considering the effects of its absence. In patients with extreme oral dryness, mucosal soreness and ulceration are common and are accompanied by rapidly progressing dental caries.[83]

The main buffering capacity of saliva is provided by bicarbonate while hydrogen phosphates provide a residual buffering effect.[84] Buffering has long been recognized as important in increasing plaque pH and preventing caries.[84] However, it appears that saliva also plays an important role in returning esophageal pH to normal following an acid bolus.[85] Mucin secreted by submandibular, sublingual, and minor salivary glands has several important roles in the oral cavity.[56] It covers epithelial surfaces, functioning as a lubricant and a permeability barrier preventing dessication and tissue damage. Along with some other glycoprotein components of saliva, mucin modulates bacterial adhesion to hard and soft surfaces and bacterial aggregation and clearance from the mouth.[56] Saliva has an antimicrobial activity based predominantly on secretory Ig A[86] and on the peroxidase system.[87] The latter is a combination of salivary peroxidase and thiocyanate which generates antibacterial hypothiocyanate in the presence of hydrogen peroxide. This same system is responsible for reducing the toxic effects of hydrogen peroxide, superoxide, and hydroxyl radicals.[88] Various peptide growth modulating factors are known to be present in saliva.[89] Probably the best characterized is epidermal growth factor (EGF),[90] which plays an important role in modulating the proliferation of epithelial layers in the gastrointestinal tract, promoting wound-healing,[91] and inhibiting gastric acid secretion.[92]

Given that acute ingestion of ethanol reduces salivary secretion, it is important to know how deleterious effects exerted by ethanol on other tissues might be modulated or prevented by saliva. A clear association exists between ethanol consumption and cancer of the mouth, pharynx, and esophagus.[93] Chronic alcohol consumption appears also to be associated with chronic ulceration, gingivitis, and periodontitis.[27] A reduction in buccal mucosal thickness has been described in chronic alcoholism and is associated with shrinkage of maturational epithelial layers accompanied by hypertrophy of the progenitor epithelial layer.[94] It is unclear whether these deleterious effects result from a direct action of ethanol on the oral structures, from an indirect effect, or as a result of accompanying problems such as vitamin B deficiency and malnourishment. The latter study on buccal mucosal thinning appeared to be carefully controlled and suggested a direct action of ethanol. EGF likely exerts an effect on the growth of the buccal mucosa as EGF receptors have been identified in buccal epithelial cells.[95] Saliva can reduce the concentration of ethanol acting on epithelial surfaces by having a diluting effect. The latter might be enhanced by the salivary secretion stimulated by ethanol.[41] The buffering function of saliva may be particularly important to those suffering from reflux esophagitis, a common condition in alcoholism.[43] Thus the harmful effect of ethanol may be greater if salivary secretion is reduced.

The effects of chronic alcoholism on mucin secretion and mucin secreting glands (submandibular, sublingual, and mucin glands) have not been well studied. However, the acute effect of ethanol in altering the posttranslational processing of mucin[55] and in reducing the rates of protein synthesis in the major salivary glands[48] has been discussed above. Given the protective function of mucin, any changes in its properties or in the amounts in which it is secreted may have deleterious effects, making the epithelia more vulnerable to physical and chemical insult, not least by ethanol itself. Similarly, given the importance of EGF to wound healing and epithelial proliferation, its reduced secretion might play a role in ethanol-induced disease conditions. In addition, ethanol has been found to decrease the binding of EGF to buccal mucosal cell membrane preparations and to decrease EGF-stimulated buccal cell protein synthesis apparently through alterations in the EGF receptor molecule.[96] The function of EGF in relation to the gastric mucosa has been much studied. EGF plays an important role in protecting the stomach mucosa by inhibiting parietal cell acid secretion[92] and by its trophic influence on the mucosa.[91] It appears from studies in which submandibular sialadenectomized rats have been compared to intact controls that saliva plays a role in protecting the gastric mucosa against ethanol-induced damage and that this effect of saliva can be attributed to EGF.[97] A recent study showed that the healing of oral ulcers was not affected by sialadenectomy.[98] There may well be other complicating factors, however, for example, infection, which may make an assessment of the effects of EGF on oral ulceration more difficult.

## 7.7   CONCLUSION

Consumption of ethanol affects salivary function in the short term by reducing salivary secretion and secretory protein synthesis. The mechanism by which acute ethanol exerts an effect is not certain but may possibly be through inositol phosphate metabolism and calcium mobilization and/or Na+, K+ ATPase activity. Chronic consumption of ethanol clearly affects salivary glands as can be seen by the occurrence of sialadenosis. Animal studies indicate that malnourishment and vitamin/mineral deficiencies present in alcoholic cirrhosis are likely to affect salivary function. However, the chronic effects of ethanol abuse on salivary gland function both in the presence and absence of sialadenosis and/ or liver cirrhosis remain unclear; this therefore requires further investigation. Given the contradictory evidence from studies of chronic alcoholics reviewed earlier, it would seem appropriate to carry out more controlled studies in animal models using physiological stimuli of salivary gland function to assess the functions of both the secretory cell and its autonomic innervation. In such animal studies it is important to select the correct model of chronic ethanol administration. The pros and cons of different models of administration have been reviewed[99] but for studies of parotid function the liquid diet model would seem inappropriate due to the resulting glandular atrophy.

Very frequent consumption of ethanol and the acute reduction in salivation which results may be sufficient to have a deleterious effect on the maintainence of oral homeostasis by the many important constituents of saliva. It is not clear how an ethanol-induced reduction in the influence of saliva might affect the oral disease associated with ethanol abuse.

# REFERENCES

1. **Emmelin, N.,** Salivary glands: secretory mechanisms, in *Scientific Foundations of Gastroenterology,* Sircus, W. and Smith, A. N., Eds., W. Heineman, London, 1981, 219.
2. **Baum B. J.,** Neurotransmitter control of secretion, *J. Dent. Res.,* 66, 628, 1987.
3. **Kerr, A. C.,** The physiological regulation of salivary secretions in man: a study on the responses of human salivary glands to reflex stimulation, in *Monographs in Oral Biology,* Vol. 1, Pergamon Press, Oxford, 1961, chaps. 9 and 24.
4. **Schneyer, L. H., Pigman, W., Hanahan, L. B., and Gilmore, R.W.,** Rate of flow of human parotid, sublingual and submaxillary secretions during sleep, *J. Dent. Res.,* 35, 109, 1956.
5. **Linden, R. W. A.,** Taste, *Br. Dent. J.,* 243, 175, 1993.
6. **Hall, H. D. and Schneyer, C. A.,** Salivary gland atrophy in rat induced by liquid diet, *Proc. Soc. Exp. Biol. Med.,* 117, 789, 1964.
7. **Menard, T., Bloomquist, D., Izutsu, K., Johnson, D., Kauffman, D., and Keller, P.,** Parotid salivary changes following orthognathic surgery, *J. Dent. Res.,* 64, 326, 1985.
8. **Gjörstrup, P.,** Parotid secretion of fluid and amylase in rabbits during feeding, *J. Physiol.,* 309, 101, 1980.
9. **Ikawa, M., Hector, M. P., and Proctor, G. B.,** Parotid protein secretion from the rabbit during feeding, *Exp. Physiol.,* 76, 717, 1991.
10. **Emmelin, N.,** Nerve interactions in salivary glands, *J. Dent. Res.,* 66, 509, 1987.
11. **Garrett, J. R.,** The proper role of nerves in salivary secretion: a review, *J. Dent. Res.,* 66, 387, 1987.
12. **Proctor, G. B., Asking, B., and Garrett, J. R.,** Effects of parasympathectomy on protein composition of sympathetically evoked parotid saliva in rats, *Comp. Biochem. Physiol.,* 97A, 335, 1990.
13. **Proctor, G. B. and Asking, B.,** A comparison between changes in rat parotid protein composition 1 and 12 weeks following surgical sympathectomy, *Q. J. Exp. Physiol.,* 74, 835, 1989.
14. **Selye, H., Veilleux, R., and Cantin, M.,** Excessive stimulation of salivary gland growth by isoproterenol, *Science,* 133, 44, 1961.
15. **Young, J. A., Cook, D. I., Vanlenner, E. W., and Roberts, M.,** Secretion of the major salivary gland, in *Physiology of the Gastrointestinal Tract,* Johnson, L. R., Ed., Raven Press, New York, 1987, 773.
16. **Anderson, L. C.,** Parotid gland function in streptozotocin-diabetic rats, *J. Dent. Res.,* 66, 425, 1987.
17. **Johnson, D. A.,** Regulation of salivary glands and their secretions by masticatory, nutritional, and hormonal factors, in *The Salivary System,* Sreebny, L. M., Ed., CRC Press, Boca Raton, FL, 1987, chap. 7.
18. **Mandel, L. and Baurmash, H.,** Parotid enlargement due to alcoholism, *J. Am. Dent. Assoc.,* 82, 369, 1971.
19. **Rausch, S. and Gorlin, R. J.,** Diseases of salivary glands, in *Thoma's Oral Pathology,* 6th ed., Gorlin, R. J. and Goldman, H. M., Eds., Mosby, St. Louis, 1970, chap. 22.
20. **Wolfe, S. J., Summerskill, W. H. J., and Davidson, C. S.,** Parotid swelling, alcoholism and cirrhosis, *N. Engl. J. Med.,* 256, 491, 1957.
21. **Seifert, G., Miehlke, A., Haubrich, J., and Chilla, R.,** *Diseases of Salivary Glands,* Georg Thieme Verlag, New York, 1986, 78.
22. **Abelson, D. C., Mandel, I. D., and Karmiol, M.,** Salivary studies in alcoholic cirrhosis, Oral Surg., 41, 188, 1976.
23. **Donath, K. and Seifert, G.,** Ultrastructural studies of the parotid glands in sialadenosis, *Virchows Arch. Pathol. Anat.,* 365, 119, 1975.
24. **Mason, D. K. and Chisholm, D. M.,** *Salivary Glands in Health and Disease,* W. B. Saunders, London, 1975, chap. 12.
25. **Scott, J., Burns, J., and Flower, E. A.,** Histological analysis of parotid and submandibular glands in chronic alcohol abuse: a necropsy study, *J. Clin. Pathol.,* 41, 837, 1988.
26. **Dutta, S. K., Dukehart, M., Narang, A., and Latham, P. S.,** Functional and structural changes in parotid glands in alcoholic cirrhotic patients, *Gastroenterology,* 96, 510, 1989.
27. **Larato, D. C.,** Oral tissue changes in the chronic alcoholic, *J. Periodontol.,* 43, 772, 1972.
28. **MacGregor, I. A. and Zakim, D.,** A cause of hyperamylasemia associated with chronic liver disease, *Gastroenterology,* 72, 519, 1977.
29. **Dutta, S. K., Douglass, W., Smalls, U. A., Nipper, H. C., and Levitt, M. D.,** Prevalence and nature of hyperamylasemia in acute alcoholism, *Dig. Dis. Sci.,* 26, 136, 1981.
30. **Barros, F. P., Espinheira, R., Geada, H., and Carneiro de Moura, M.,** Hyperamylasemia with abnormal isoamylase distribution in patients with liver diseases, *Am. J. Gastroenterol.,* 81, 261, 1986.
31. **Deenmamode, J. M., Sherwood, R. A., Sherman, D. I. N., and Peters, T. J.,** Total pancreatic and salivary serum iso-amylase activities in alcohol misusers in relapse and remission in alcoholic liver disease, *Clin. Chim. Acta,* 223, 169, 1993.
32. **Kronvall, P., Fahy, T. A., Isaksson, A., Theander, S., and Russell, G. F.,** The clinical relevance of salivary amylase monitoring in bulimia nervosa, *Biol. Psychiatry,* 32, 156, 1992.
33. **Warshaw, A. L. and Lee, K.-H.,** Characteristic alteration of serum isoenzymes of amylase in diseases of liver, pancreas, salivary gland, lung, and genitalia, *J. Surg. Res.,* 22, 362, 1977.
34. **Proctor, G. B., Asking, B., and Garrett, J. R.,** Serum amylase of non-parotid and non-pancreatic origin increases on feeding in rats and may originate from the liver, *Comp. Biochem. Physiol.,* 98B, 631, 1991.

35. **Ewing, D. J. and Clarke, B. F.,** Diabetic autonomic neuropathy: present insights and future prospects, *Diabetes Care*, 9, 648, 1986.

36. **Hendrickse, M. T., Thuluvath, P. J., and Triger, D. R.,** Natural history of autonomic neuropathy in chronic liver disease, *Lancet*, 339, 1462, 1992.

37. **Matikainen, E., Juntunen, J., and Salmi, T.,** Autonomic dysfunction in long-standing alcoholism, *Alcohol Alcohol.*, 21, 69, 1986.

38. **Mills, K. R., Ward, K., Martin, F., and Peters, T. J.,** Peripheral neuropathy and myopathy in chronic alcoholism, *Alcohol Alcohol.*, 21, 357, 1986.

39. **Lamey, J., Fisher, B. M., and Frier, B. M.,** The effect of diabetes and autonomic neuropathy on parotid and salivary flow in man, *Diabetic Med.*, 3, 537, 1986.

40. **Anderson, L. C., Garrett, J. R., Thulin, A., and Proctor, G. B.,** Effects of Streptozotocin-induced diabetes on sympathetic and parasypmpathetic stimulation of parotid salivary gland function in rats, *Diabetes*, 38, 1381, 1989.

41. **Martin, S. and Pangborn, M.,** Human parotid secretion in response to ethyl alcohol, *J. Dent. Res.*, 50, 485, 1971.

42. **Dutta, S. K., Parasher, V., and Smalls, U.,** Evidence for marked suppression of parotid saliva secretion and altered composition following a single dose of ethanol ingestion in man, *Gastroenterology*, 86, 1065, 1984.

43. **Dutta, S. K., Orestes, M., Vengulekar, S., and Kwo, P.,** Ethanol and human saliva: effect of chronic alcoholism on flow rate, composition, and epidermal growth factor, *Am. J. Gastroenterol.*, 87, 350, 1992.

44. **Durr, H. K., Bode, J. C., and Gieseking, R.,** Changes in exocrine function of the parotid gland and pancreas in patients with liver cirrhosis and chronic alcoholism, *Verh. Dtsch. Ges. Inn. Med.*, 81, 1322, 1975.

45. **Scott, J. and Baxter, P.,** Salivary flow rate, protein and electrolyte concentrations in chronic alcoholic patients, *J. Biol. Buccale*, 16, 215, 1988.

46. **Söderling, E.,** Collection of saliva, in *Human Saliva: Clinical Chemistry and Microbiology*, Vol. 1, Tenovuo, J. O., Ed., CRC Press, Boca Raton, FL, 1989, chap. 1.

47. **Scott, J., Berry, M. R., and Woods, K.,** Effects of acute ethanol administration on stimulated parotid secretion in the rat, *Alcoholism: Clin. Exp. Res.*, 13, 560, 1989.

48. **Proctor, G. B., Shori, D. K., and Preedy, V. R.,** Protein synthesis in the major salivary glands of the rat and the effects of re-feeding and acute ethanol injection, *Arch. Oral Biol.*, 38, 971, 1993.

49. **Shori, D. K., Proctor, G. B., Teare, J., and Preedy, V. R.,** Indices of protein synthesis and RNA translating activities in the major salivary glands of rat and comparison to synthetic rates in liver, *Biochem. Soc. Trans.*, 22, 182S, 1994.

50. **Garlick, P. J., McNurlan, M. A., and Preedy, V. R.,** A rapid and convenient technique for measuring the rate of protein synthesis in tissues by injection of $^3$H-phenylalanine, *Biochem. J.*, 192, 719, 1980.

51. **Marway, J. S., Keating, J. W., Reeves, J., Salisbury, J. S., and Preedy, V. R.,** Seromuscular and mucosal protein synthesis in various anatomical regions of the rat gastrointestinal tract and their response to acute ethanol toxicity, *Eur. J. Gastroenterol. Hepatol.*, 5, 27, 1993.

52. **Preedy, V. R., Siddiq, T., Cook, E., Black, D., Palmer, T. N., and Peters, T. J.,** Alcohol and protein turnover, in *Alcoholism: A Molecular Perspective*, Palmer, T. N., Ed., Plenum Press, New York, 1991, 253.

53. **Tiernan, J. M. and Ward, L. C.,** Acute effects of ethanol in protein synthesis in the rat, *Alcohol Alcohol.*, 21, 171, 1986.

54. **Ohlin, P. and Perec, C.,** Salivary secretion of the major sublingual gland of rats, *Experentia*, 21, 408, 1965.

55. **Slomiany, B. L., Liau, Y. H., Zalesna, G., and Slomiany, A.,** Effect of ethanol on the *in vitro* sulfation of salivary mucin, *Alcoholism: Clin. Exp. Res.*, 12, 774, 1988.

56. **Tabak, L. A., Levine, M. J., Mandel, I. D., and Ellison, S. A.,** Role of salivary mucins in the protection of the oral cavity, *J. Oral Pathol.*, 11, 1, 1982.

57. **Wu-Wang, C.-Y., Wang, S.-L., Lim, C., Slomiany, A., and Slomiany, B. L.,** Impairment of ethanol of prostaglandin production in rat salivary glands, *Arch. Oral Biol.*, 36, 9, 1991.

58. **Wu-Wang, C.-Y., Wang, S.-L., Lim, C., Slomiany, A., and Slomiany, B. L.,** Effect of ethanol on prostaglandin $E_2$ receptor in rat submandibular salivary glands, *Arch. Oral Biol.*, 37, 869, 1992.

59. **Bradbury, N. A. and MacPherson, M. A.,** Actions of prostaglandin $E_2$ and $F_2$ alpha on release of $^{14}$C-labelled mucins from rat submandibular salivary acini *in vitro*, *Arch. Oral Biol.*, 32, 719, 1987.

60. **Sun, G. Y. and Sun, A. Y.,** Ethanol and membrane lipids, *Alcoholism: Clin. Exp. Res.*, 9, 164, 1985.

61. **Taraschi, T. F., Ellingson, J. S., Wu-Sun, A., and Rubin, E.,** Rats withdrawn from ethanol rapidly re-acquire membrane tolerance after resumption of ethanol feeding, *Biochim. Biophys. Acta*, 1021, 51, 1990.

62. **McCall, D., Henderson, G. I., Gray, P., and Schenker, S.,** Ethanol effects on active $Na^+$ and $K^+$ transport in cultured fetal rat hepatocytes, *Biochem. Pharmacol.*, 38, 2593, 1989.

63. **Sun, G. Y. and Sun, A. Y.,** Chronic ethanol administration induced an increase in phosphatidylserine in guinea pig synaptic plasma membranes, *Biochem. Biophys. Res. Commun.*, 113, 262, 1983.

64. **Lin, T. A., Navidi, M., James, W., Lin, T. N., and Sun, G. Y.,** Effects of acute ethanol administration on polyphosphoinositide turnover and levels of inositol 1,4,5-trisphosphate in mouse cerebrum and cerebellum, *Alcoholism: Clin. Exp. Res.*, 17, 401, 1993.

65. **Ghandi, C. R. and Ross, D. H.,** Influence of ethanol on calcium, inositol phospholipids and intracellular signalling mechanisms, *Experentia*, 45, 407, 1989.

66. **Berry, M. R. and Scott, J.,** Functional and structural adaption of the parotid gland to medium-term chronic ethanol exposure in the rat, *Alcohol Alcohol.*, 25, 523, 1990.
67. **Scott, J. and Berry, M. R.,** The effect of chronic ethanol administration on stimulated parotid secretion in the rat, *Alcohol Alcohol.*, 24, 145, 1989.
68. **Perec, C. J., Celener, D., and Tiscornia, O. M.,** Effects of chronic ethanol administration on the autonomic innervation of salivary glands, pancreas and heart, *Am. J. Gastroenterol.*, 72, 46, 1979.
69. **Maier, H., Seitz, H. K., Mayer, B., Adler, D., Mall, G., and Born, I. A.,** Lipomatous atrophy of the parotid gland after chronic ethanol consumption, *Laryngorhinootologie*, 69, 600, 1990.
70. **Banderas, J. A., Gaitan, L. A., Portilla, J., and Aguirre, A.,** Effects of chronic ethanol consumption on the rat parotid gland, *Arch. Oral Biol.*, 37, 69, 1992.
71. **Mehansho, H., Ann, D. K., Butler, L. G., Rogler, J., and Carlson, D. M.,** Induction of proline-rich proteins in hamster salivary glands by isoproterenol treatment and an unusual growth inhibition by tannins, *J. Biol. Chem.*, 262, 12344, 1987.
72. **Jaatinen, P., Kiianmaa, K., Lahtivirta, S., and Hervonen, A.,** Ethanol-induced vacuolation in the peripheral nervous system, *J. Auton. Nerv. Syst.*, 46, 107, 1994.
73. **Buchner, A. and Sreebny, L. M.,** Effect of prolonged food reduction on the rat parotid gland and exocrine pancreas, *J. Nutr.*, 100, 655, 1970.
74. **Morgan, M. Y.,** Alcohol and nutrition, *Br. Med. Bull.*, 38, 21, 1982.
75. **Mandel, I. D.,** Sialochemistry in diseases and clinical situations affecting salivary glands, *CRC Crit. Rev. Clin. Lab. Sci.*, 12, 321, 1980.
76. **Hoyumpa, A. M.,** Mechanisms of vitamin deficiencies in alcoholism, *Alcohol Clin. Exp. Res.*, 10, 573, 1986.
77. **Pitts, T. O. and van Thiel, D. H.,** Disorders of divalent ions and vitamin D metabolism in chronic alcoholism, *Recent Dev. Alcohol*, 4, 357, 1986.
78. **Glijer, B., Peterfy, C., and Tenehouse, A.,** The effect of vitamin D deficiency on the secretion of rat parotid gland *in vivo*, *J. Physiol.*, 363, 323, 1985.
79. **Hayakawa, M., Aoki, H., Terao, N., Abiko, M., and Takiguchi, H.,** Vitamin D-mediated decrease in $Ca^{2+}$ pump activity in the rat parotid gland, *Int. J. Biochem.*, 15, 1175, 1983.
80. **Anzano, M. A., Lamb, A. J., and Olson, J. A.,** Impaired salivary gland secretory function following the induction of rapid, synchronous vitamin A deficiency in rats, *J. Nutr.*, 111, 496, 1981.
81. **Alvarez, O. and Johnson, D. A.,** Effects of zinc deficiency on the rat parotid gland, *J. Oral Pathol.*, 10, 430, 1981.
82. **Mandel, I. D.,** The functions of saliva, *J. Dent. Res.*, 66, 623, 1987.
83. **Mason, D. K. and Chisholm, D. M.,** *Salivary Glands in Health and Disease*, W. B. Saunders, London, 1975, chap. 10.
84. **Birkhed, D. and Heintze, U.,** Salivary secretion rate, buffer capacity, and pH, in *Human Saliva: Clinical Chemistry and Microbiology*, Vol. 1, Tenovuo, J. O., Ed., CRC Press, Boca Raton, FL, 1989, chap. 2.
85. **Helm, J. F., Dodds, W. J., Hogan, W. J., Soergel, K. H., Egide, M. S., and Wood, C. M.,** Acid neutralizing capacity of human saliva, *Gastroenterology*, 83, 69, 1982.
86. **Ørstavik, D. and Brandtzaeg, P.,** Secretion of parotid Ig A in relation to gingival inflammation and dental caries experience in man, *Archs. Oral Biol.*, 20, 701, 1975.
87. **Pruitt, K. M.,** The salivary peroxidase system: thermodynamic, kinetic and antibacterial properties, *J. Oral Pathol.*, 16, 417, 1987.
88. **Carlsson, J.,** Salivary peroxidase: an important defense against oxygen toxicity, *J. Oral Pathol.*, 16, 412, 1987.
89. **Barka, T.,** Biologically active polypeptides in the submandibular glands, *J. Histochem. Cytochem.*, 28, 836, 1980.
90. **Cohen, S.,** Epidermal growth factor, *J. Invest. Dermatol.*, 59, 13, 1972.
91. **Baldwin, G. S. and Whitehead, R. H.,** Gut hormones, growth and malignancy, *Baillieres Clin. Endocrinol. Metab.*, 1, 185, 1994.
92. **Ostrowski, J., Wojciechowski, K., Konturek, S. J., and Butruk, E.,** Inhibitory effect of EGF on secretory response of rat parietal cells is associated with an induction of ODC, *Am. J. Physiol.*, 264, C1428, 1993.
93. **MacSween, R. N. M.,** Alcohol and cancer, *Br. Med. Bull.* 38, 31, 1982.
94. **Valentine, J. A., Scott, J., West, C. R., and St. Hill, C. A.,** A histological analysis of the early effects of alcohol and tobacco usage on human lingual epithelium, *J. Oral Pathol.*, 14, 654, 1985.
95. **Wang, S. L., Milles, M., Wu-Wang, C. Y., Liu, J., Slomiany, A., and Slomiany, B. L.,** Identification of epidermal growth factor receptor in human buccal mucosa, *Arch. Oral Biol.*, 35, 823, 1990.
96. **Wang, S. L., Wu-Wang, C. Y., Slomiany, A., and Slomiany, B. L.,** Effect of acute ethanol treatment on epidermal growth factor receptor in the rat stomach, *Alcohol*, 11, 11, 1994.
97. **Leitch, G. J.,** Role of the salivary glands in protecting the stomach against ethanol, *Alcohol Alcohol.*, 20, 305, 1985.
98. **Konturek, S. J., Pytkopolonczyk, J., Brzozowski, T., Bielanski, W., and Majka, J.,** Healing of oral and gastric ulcers — effects of blood flow, epidermal growth factor and sensory innervation, *Eur. J. Gastroenterol. Hepatol.*, 5, S 45, 1993.
99. **Keane, B. and Leonard, B.E.,** Rodent models of alcoholism: a review, *Alcohol Alcohol.*, 24, 299, 1989.

# 8

# Gastric Cytoprotection and Adaptation to Ethanol

Stanisław J. Konturek, Jerzy Stachura, and Jan W. Konturek

## CONTENTS

## 8.1 INTRODUCTION

The gastrointestinal tract, particularly the stomach, is constantly exposed to various irritants and aggressive factors of endogenous origin such as gastric acid, pepsins, lipases, and bile as well as ingested elements including ethanol, certain drugs (e.g., nonsteroidal antiinflammatory drugs [NSAID]), and bacteria (e.g., *Helicobacter pylori*). Any other tissue would rapidly disintegrate if exposed to such a variety of irritants that bathe the lining of the stomach. The gastric mucosa exhibits, however, remarkable chemical resistance properties, so-called gastric "mucosal barrier," representing a very sophisticated multicomponent defense system that is set against the continuous threat of autodigestion and permits the mucosal tissue to reside comfortably in contact with highly corrosive substances.[1] These defenses comprise a rapidly regenerating epithelium that is protected from gastric luminal irritants by a continuous mucus–alkali sheet and phospholipid surfactant layer. The control element of this gastric mucosal defense system, which is also pivotal to mucosal restitution and healing processes, is adequate mucosal blood flow that maintains tissue integrity, provides nutrients and oxygen, and protects the mucosa by removing noxious substances from the gastric lumen.[2]

    Stomach exposed to repeated insults of hostile environment has the ability for quick adaptation to survive the challenge of everyday life and to withstand the action of various irritants. This

0-8493-2480-7/96/$0.00+$.50
© 1996 by CRC Press, Inc.

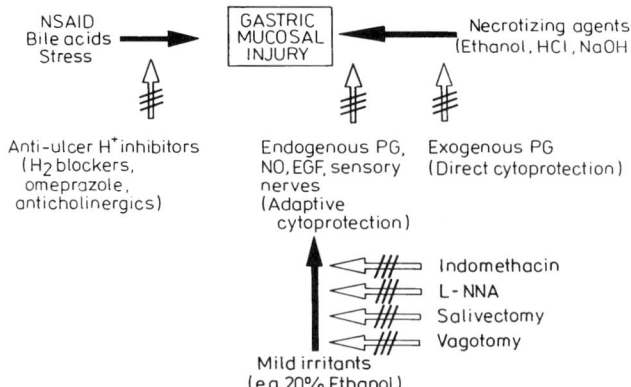

**FIGURE 8.1**  Diagrammatic representation of direct and adaptive cytoprotection. Direct cytoprotection can be achieved by pretreatment with prostaglandins. Adaptive cytoprotection induced by "mild irritants" such as 20% ethanol can be prevented by pretreatment with indomethacin, blockers of NO synthase (e.g., L-NNA), salivectomy, or vagotomy. The decrease of gastric acidity prevents the formation of gastric ulcerations by acid-dependent irritants such as NSAID, bile salts, or stress but does not influence the damage induced by necrotizing substances.

adaptation occurs in response to the action on the mucosa of various "mild" irritants (e.g., 20% ethanol) and includes the protection against necrosis that occurs when the stomach is exposed to very strong irritants such as 100% ethanol. This short-lived mucosal response called "adaptive" cytoprotection[3] is accompanied by increased mucosal blood flow probably due to excessive local production of prostaglandins,[3,4] growth factors[5] and nitric oxide,[6] and excitation of afferent sensory nerves[7] (Figure 8.1).

Repeated exposures to strong irritants result in a gradual attenuation of the mucosal lesions despite successive insults. This increased mucosal resistance or reduced susceptibility to damage in response to repeated injuries is called gastric adaptation.[8] Unlike adaptive cytoprotection which develops quickly but is a transient effect of mild irritants, the gastric adaptation develops slowly and is a long-term effect mediated by increased mucosal cell proliferation probably due to overexpression of growth factors such as epidermal growth factor (EGF) and transforming growth factor alpha (TGFα) and their receptors in the adapted mucosa.[8,9]

## 8.2    ETHANOL IN THE STOMACH: ABSORPTION AND METABOLISM

The influence of ethanol on gastric secretion and mucosal integrity depends on its volume, concentration, and ingested form. Pure ethanol present in the stomach in low concentration (<5% v/v) is a mild stimulant of gastric acid secretion and fails to affect mucosal morphology; however, alcoholic beverages with low ethanol content such as beer or wine are strong stimulants of gastric acid secretion and strong releasers of gastrin. This powerful gastric stimulatory action depends not on the presence of ethanol but of thermostable, probably peptic and amino acid, compounds.[10] Beverages with a higher ethanol content (whisky, gin, cognac) do not stimulate gastric acid or gastrin release but they do cause multiple bleeding erosions mostly present in the oxyntic portion of the gastric mucosa. The standard ethanol test to induce acute gastric lesions in humans uses 50% ethanol in a volume of 100 ml sprayed over the mucosa during the endoscopy.[11] It induces numerous hemorrhagic lesions as observed endoscopically and is used as a model to evaluate the gastroprotective activity of tested drugs, e.g., sucralfate or PGE$_2$.[11]

Ethanol present in gastric lumen appears to act directly on the gastric mucosa in which it is metabolized by separate class IV alcohol dehydrogenase (ADH) closely related to class I classical (liver) ADH.[12] The activity of this enzyme depends on the patient's age and sex. Below the age of 50, women have enzyme activity much lower than men, but this difference disappears after age 50.[13] Due to relatively high gastric mucosal activity of ADH, oral consumption of alcohol results in much lower blood alcohol concentration than does the same dose administered intravenously. This lowered blood concentration of alcohol can be attributed to significant "first-pass metabolism" of this substance during absorption in the stomach.[14]

Absorption of ethanol from the stomach depends mainly on its diffusion and is fastest when strong drinks are taken on an empty stomach. Dilute beverages such as beer (3 to 5%) or wine (12%) are absorbed more slowly than distilled spirits containing 40 to 60% ethanol per volume.[15] The intake of ethanol with food also slows absorption because food dilutes the ethanol and delays gastric emptying into the duodenum, where the absorption is even faster than from the stomach. Blood ethanol concentrations after ethanol intake in the fasting state usually peak after 1 to 2 h and these concentrations could be several times lower if food is taken with ethanol.

## 8.3    PATHOMORPHOLOGY OF ACUTE GASTRIC MUCOSAL INJURY BY ETHANOL

### 8.3.1    Functional Anatomy of Gastric Mucosa

There are five anatomical gastric regions: cardia, fundus, body (corpus), antrum, and pylorus. The cardiac gastric mucosa occupies a small area at the esophagogastric junction. Mucoid cardiac glands are arranged in acinar structures but they rapidly convert into oxyntic glands.[16]

Fundus and corpus mucosa in humans consist of the test tube-like oxyntic glands draining into gastric pits. Oxyntic glands contain parietal cells secreting hydrochloric acid and intrinsic factor, chief cells producing pepsinogens and endocrine cells (most common are enterochromaffin-like cells) whose functions are still only partially elucidated. Regenerative zone occupies the neck area of oxyntic glands and consists of poorly differentiated mucus cells which differentiate and migrate at the same time. Cells migrating upward differentiate mostly into surface mucus cells (some also into parietal cells which are lost during migration before they reach pit area).[16] Surface epithelium has a short life span. Cells migrating downward differentiate mostly into parietal, chief, and endocrine cells. All of them are characterized by a long life span. Cellular migration (and completed differentiation) within the gland requires an intact glandular basal membrane. Cells migrate by extending pseudopodia attached to basal membrane. Damage to the basal membrane affects the process of rapid restitution of surface epithelium.

Gradually (through the intermediate zone), oxyntic mucosa converts into the antral mucosa extending to the pylorus. Antral glands are lined with mucus cells and endocrine cells, especially gastrin-producing G cells and somatostatin-producing D cells.[17]

The gastric luminal surface and gastric pits are lined with surface mucus cells which are tall columnar, with apical portion filled with mucus granules. Mucus released from these cells along with cytomembrane-derived phospholipids (forming a hydrophobic layer) are essential for the mucosal defense barrier against digestive forces and various irritants present in the gastric lumen. Surface epithelial cells shed at the rate of half a million cells per minute. Some surface epithelial cells could be also lost by the process of apoptosis (a silent genetically programmed cell death distinct from necrosis).[18] Lost cells are replaced by new cells from the glandular neck area. It usually takes 2 to 3 days to replace the whole population of surface epithelial cells.[16,19] In case of massive denudation of surface epithelium the process of restitution is very rapid and effective. Within 15 min, migrating cells cover more than 90% of the mucosal surface.

Gastric glands are separated from the surrounding connective tissue (lamina propria) by the basal membrane which is crucial for epithelial-mesenchymal cooperation. In addition to connective tissue, there is a mucosal blood and nerve supply. Gastric mucosa blood supply comes from submucosa. Arteries branch into smaller arteries and arterioles.[1,2] Arterioles reach muscularis mucosae. Further on, microvessels are formed by capillaries which penetrate (with numerous interconnections) the mucosa between glands, then turn back and as postcapillary venules drain into collecting veins again reaching the submucosa. In smaller curvature in the antral area, another blood

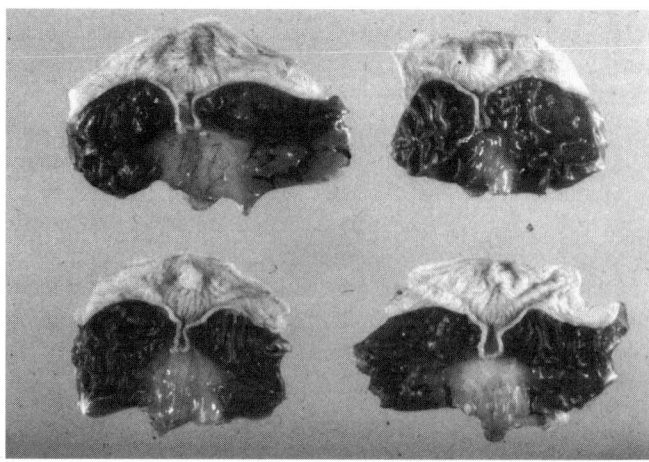

**FIGURE 8.2**  Macroscopic appearance of the intact rat stomach (upper left), stomach exposed for 15 min to 1.5 ml of 100% ethanol alone (upper right), stomach pretreated with 1 ml 20% ethanol followed 30 min later by 1.5 100% ethanol (lower left), and stomach pretreated with dimethyl-PGE$_2$ (10 µg/kg i.g.) followed 30 min later by 1.5 ml 100% ethanol (lower right).

supply exists by arteries penetrating the entire gastric wall from the serosal surface. These end arteries are considered to be responsible (ischemia) for the common gastric ulcer localization in this region.[20] Arteriolar and venous constrictions or dilations in submucosa are essential for the mucosal blood distribution and are crucial for gastric mucosal injury and repair.[1,2,20]

Gastric mucosa and submucosa are closely applied to the muscular layers. They are responsible for the gastric motility. Gastric mucosa is applied to the deeper wall layers in such a way that it forms a system of folds. The top of the folds is directly exposed to injurious agents, while the thicker mucus "cap" separates gastric mucosa between folds. This is reflected by localization of gastric mucosal lesions after injury, for example, ethanol-induced injury.

### 8.3.2   Morphology of an Acute Alcohol-Induced Injury to the Gastric Mucosa

A trace amount of alcohol is not harmful to the gastric mucosa or gastric mucosal cells. Also *in vitro*, ethanol acting on separated gastric gland cells in concentrations up to 2% ethanol does not decrease the cell viability. With increased alcohol concentration the number of nonviable cells increases. *In vivo*, a substantial damage to the gastric mucosa is produced by more than 20% ethanol. Desquamation of surface epithelium, dilation of gastric glands, swelling of parietal cells and congestion (or stasis), and edema of lamina propria and submucosa are observed with increased intensity along with ethanol concentration. Denudation of the gastric mucosal surface by desquamating surface epithelium is common in any kind of acute gastric injury.[21,22] In ethanol-induced injury, desquamation of gastric surface epithelium in large sheets separating from the underlying basal membrane is characteristic, while tight junctions still keep desquamating cells together. Concomitant mucus release causes the formation of thick mucosal cap with numerous sheets of mucus cells and separate mucus cells floating in the mucus cap. By viability test, a proportion of floating cells are still alive. One can wonder whether some of them could "seed back" the mucosal surface contributing to the rapid repair.

In more concentrated ethanol (more than 50%), massive congestion, stasis, and extravasation of red blood cells accompanies formerly described morphological events. This could be a tiny petechia in the superficial lamina propria, a larger subepithelial hemorrhage, or even massive hemorrhagic necrosis involving the entire thickness of the gastric mucosa. These hemorrhagic necrotic lesions are usually irregularly linear and most common at the top of mucosal folds (Figure 8.2). In the rat, the oxyntic area is more affected and there are longitudinal, linear

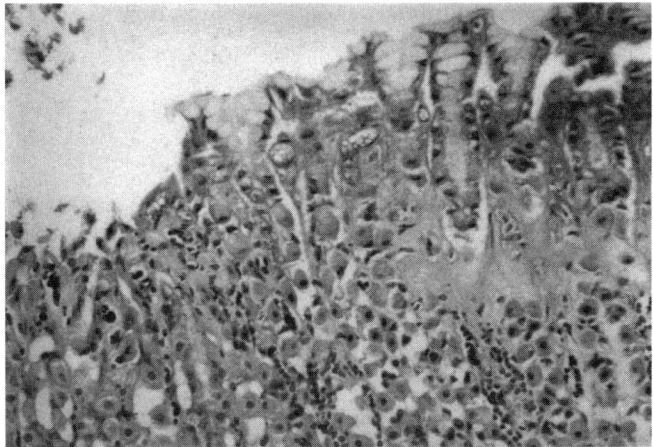

**FIGURE 8.3** Rat gastric oxyntic mucosa 15 min after intragastric instillation of 1.5 ml 100% ethanol. Nonprotected mucosa shows early hemorrhagic necrosis. (Hematoxylin-eosin; original magnification ×260.)

hemorrhagic necrotic lesions, reflecting the distribution of mucosal folds. In most severe cases (in the rat 1 h after 1 to 2 ml of 100% ethanol intragastrically), there is a confluent massive hemorrhagic necrosis involving most of the gastric mucosa.

Concentrated ethanol in experimental animals causes damage to the whole exposed surface epithelium and some mucosal microvessels within a few minutes. Deep hemorrhagic lesions in experiments could be seen as early as 5 to 15 min after ethanol (Figure 8.3). These early hemorrhagic lesions will progress within the first 3 h to full hemorrhagic necrosis penetrating to the muscularis mucosae and separated from the surrounding nonnecrotic mucosa by the polymorphonuclears, as usual at the necrotic border. Microcirculation in the gastric mucosa is crucial for both development and prevention of ethanol-induced damage.[1,2,20,23,24]

Such a massive hemorrhagic necrosis in humans is not observed. Hemorrhagic necrosis in humans is also observed at the top of mucosal folds. The surface of denuded human gastric mucosa from the epithelium and superficial lamina propria shows edema and petechiae (Figure 8.4). Superficial subepithelial hemorrhagic lesions may also be present (Figure 8.5). Some

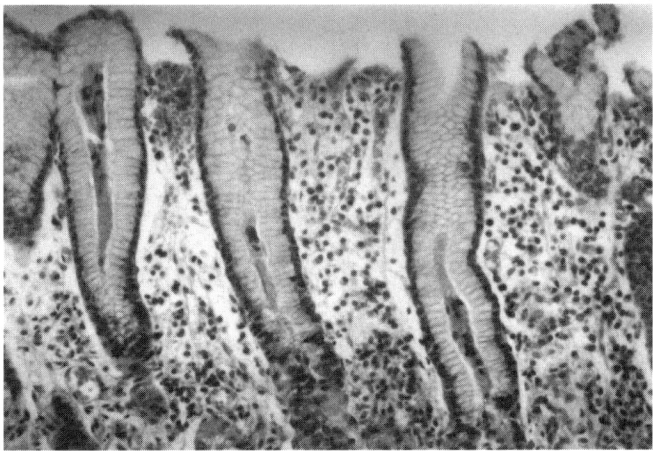

**FIGURE 8.4** Human gastric mucosa 15 min after instillation of 50% ethanol. Surface is denuded of surface epithelium. Superficial lamina propria shows edema and petechiae. (Hematoxylin-eosin; original magnification ×400.)

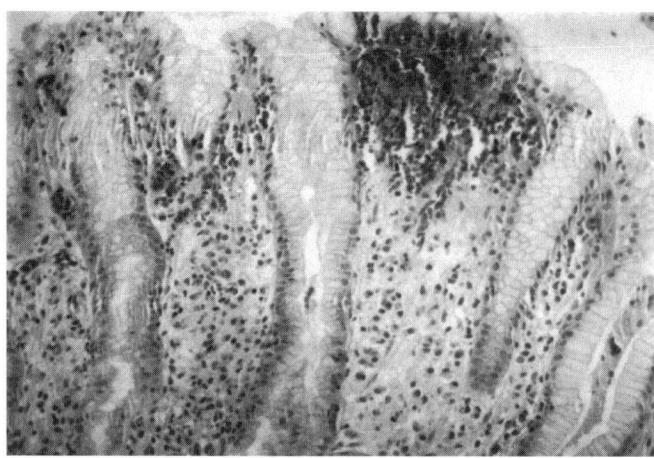

**FIGURE 8.5**  Human gastric mucosa 15 min after instillation of 50% ethanol. Superficial subepithelial hemorrhagic lesions are present. (Hematoxylin-eosin; original magnification ×400.)

necrotic tissue is already "fixed" by concentrated ethanol. Direct exposure of the human gastric mucosa to 40% ethanol applied as spray during endoscopy produces extensive exfoliation of the surface cells and disruption of the microvessels combined with an extravasation of erythrocytes as early as 1 min after ethanol administration.[11,18] These ultrastructural changes were seen in the interfoveolar areas and only occasionally were extended to the neck areas. Aggregation of platelets combined with activated neutrophils on the injured endothelium leads to thrombus formation and impairs oxygen and nutrient transport, resulting in focal ischemia.

When 100% ethanol is administered to the stomach for 1 min and then removed, only the surface is damaged.[21,22] Almost the entire surface (over 90%) is denuded. This does not involve the destruction of basal lamina or glandular regenerative zone (neck area). This superficial damage is very efficiently and rapidly repaired within 15 min (most of the mucosa is within this short period again covered with glandular neck and pit cells migrating upward in the process of rapid repair). This does not involve cell proliferation. The cell cycle for gastric mucosal cells is 16 to 21 h. Rapid repair of the superficial injury is achieved long before this time. Cell proliferation follows rapid repair and possibly contributes to the process of gastric adaptation to repeated injuries. Deeper hemorrhagic necrotic lesions which occupy half of the mucosal thickness heal within 2 to 3 days. Necrotic lesions reaching muscularis mucosae need 5 to 7 days for healing. During this time, necrotic tissue is disintegrated (24 h), becomes homogeneous, mixed with leukocytes, and eventually erosions are depurated (48 h). In addition to glandular regeneration, there is also a regeneration of adjacent lamina propria. In this more chronic process of regeneration spouting of new microvessels from collecting veins is crucial. Newly formed microvessels are responsible for improved blood supply and allow the whole process of regeneration of the necrotic area.[23,24]

## 8.4   DIRECT AND ADAPTIVE CYTOPROTECTION AGAINST ETHANOL INJURY

### 8.4.1   Direct Cytoprotection

Gastric mucosa is permanently exposed to the irritant effects of digestive juices, bacteria and their toxins, ingested food, beverages, and drugs. In the mucosa with decreased defense mechanisms, such irritants may result in the formation of acute mucosal erosions or ulcerations, whereas the protected mucosa — for example, by pretreatment with prostaglandins — does not develop deep

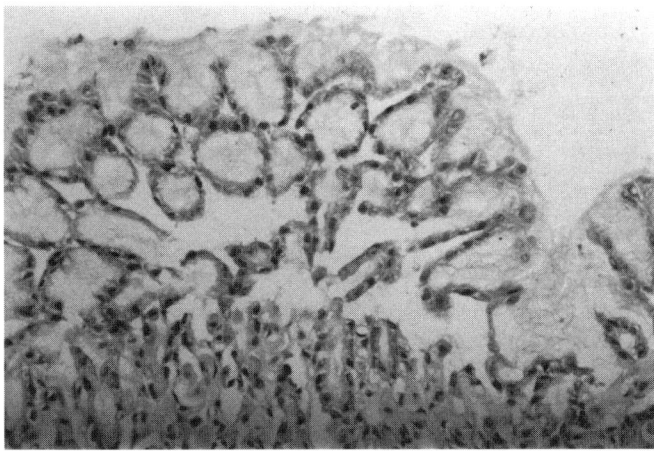

**FIGURE 8.6** Rat gastric oxyntic mucosa 15 min after intragastric instillation of 1 ml 96% ethanol in an animal pretreated with dimethyl-PGE$_2$ 5 μg/kg 30 min prior to medication. No hemorrhagic necrosis was observed but there was a massive desquamation of surface epithelium. (Hematoxylin-eosin; original magnification ×260.)

hemorrhagic necrosis when exposed to concentrated ethanol, strong acids or bases, or even boiling water.[3,25,26] Such "protected" mucosa exposed to absolute ethanol looks grossly normal (see Figure 8.2) with only minor swelling but without hemorrhagic necrotic lesions. By histology, gastric mucosa within 15 to 30 min after ethanol becomes swollen and denuded of surface epithelium (Figures 8.6 and 8.7). The submucosa is also swollen, but no deep hemorrhagic necrosis is observed. By ultrastructure, some damage to most superficial capillary profiles is also observed, but there is no vascular necrosis comparable to that in response to absolute ethanol in "nonprotected" animals.[27] It is of interest that the penetration of [14]C-labeled ethanol into the mucosa protected by PG is similar to that in nonprotected mucosa, yet, the extent of mucosal damage is remarkably reduced by PG (Figure 8.8). Within 3 h, hemorrhagic necrotic lesions are much better delineated from nonnecrotic mucosa, while the surface of nonnecrotic mucosa has been reepithelialized.[27-29] It should be emphasized that the rapid repair of nonnecrotic mucosa is

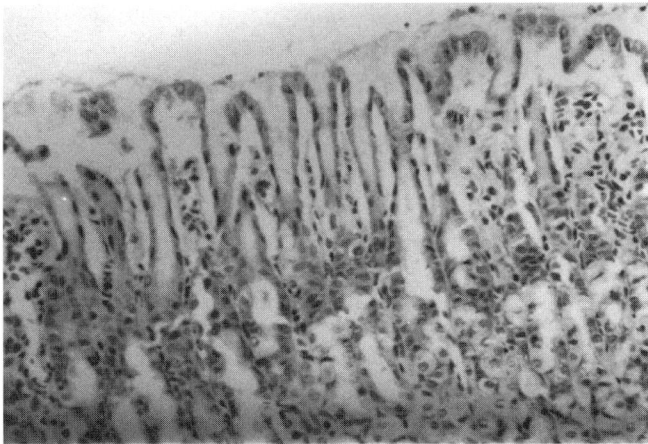

**FIGURE 8.7** Rat gastric oxyntic mucosa 1 h after intragastric instillation of 1 ml 96% ethanol in animal pretreated with dimethyl-PGE$_2$ 30 min prior to ethanol instillation. Mucosa is heavily swollen but most of the surface is already restituted. (Hematoxylin-eosin; original magnification ×260.)

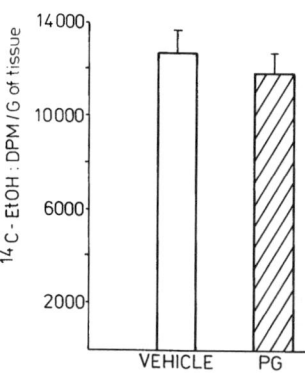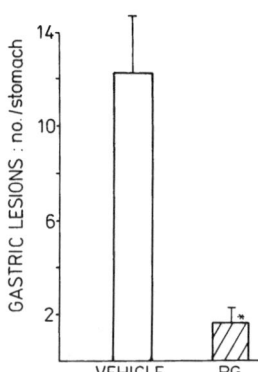

**FIGURE 8.8**   The content of [14]C-labeled ethanol in the rat oxyntic mucosa of vehicle and $PGE_2$-treated stomach and then exposed to 1.5 ml of 100% ethanol (left) and the number of gastric lesions induced by 100% ethanol in these animals (right).

not perfect. Reepithelialized mucosa is flat and interfoveolar cristae are not yet formed. In addition, this new epithelium is cubic, noncolumnar, with much fewer mucus granules. In spite of this, the most important part of repair of nonnecrotic mucosa has already occurred. Within 24 h, nonnecrotic mucosa looks, by morphology, entirely normal.

The protection of gastric mucosa obtained by the administration of exogenous PG is called "direct cytoprotection." Although PG are potent inhibitors of gastric acid secretion, their protective influence on gastric mucosa appears to be unrelated to their antisecretory action, because it has been observed with virtually all PG tested, including those that do not affect gastric acid secretion. Many PG possessing antisecretory properties still protect the mucosa even when given in nonantisecretory doses. Robert et al.[26] showed that PG with known antisecretory action given in a dose less than 1% of the threshold gastric inhibitory dose protect the gastric mucosa against various necrotizing agents. PG have also been shown to protect the intestinal mucosa against indomethacin-induced ulcerations or against ethanol-induced damage of colonic mucosa (intestinoprotection), and this effect has nothing to do with the gastric acid inhibition since it occurred in the nonacid environment of the gut.[25] Although PG are effective against various types of irritants, the cytoprotection was best described in rats with ethanol-induced damage. As mentioned, this protection does not include the entire mucosa. Topical irritants such as ethanol cause widespread destruction and massive desquamation of surface epithelial cells, and PG do not prevent this immediate topical damage,[27-29] but retain the integrity of remaining layers of mucosa. The mucosa denuded by ethanol gastric surface is very efficiently repaired by the process of rapid restitution.[28,29] For these reasons, the term "cytoprotection" has been criticized,[30] and its original definition had to be changed. It now refers more specifically to the prevention of deeper necrotic and hemorrhagic lesions. It is better understood now that massive desquamation of gastric surface epithelium is a physiological phenomenon and may occur even after food intake. The rapid restitution of repair of the mucosa that follows food intake is probably mediated, at least in part, by the release of enterohormones such as gastrin and cholecystokinin, which show prodigious capability of protecting the mucosa from damage by various irritants including ethanol.[31]

An immediate consequence of the destruction of much of the surface epithelium by topical irritants is the process of rapid healing and restitution which has been recognized recently.[28-30] If the microvascular supply of the deeper part of the mucosa is intact and the basal membrane is preserved, there is a rapid cell migration from the gastric pits along this membrane, so that within a few minutes a new surface epithelium is formed by locomotion and maturation of preserved gland cells.[32] A gelatinous layer composed of mucus, lysed cells, and mucosal proteinaceous exudate forms a protective cover of the healing mucosa, so-called "mucoid cap," to provide a

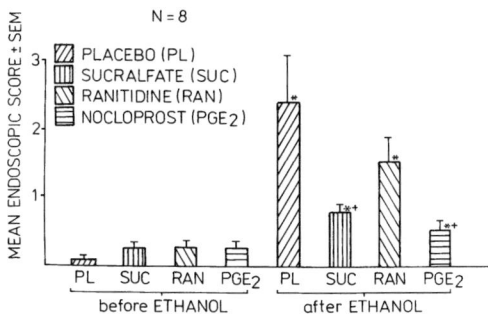

**FIGURE 8.9**  Endoscopic score of acute gastric lesions 5 to 10 min before (left) and 30 min after (right) intragastric spray of 50% ethanol in eight healthy humans pretreated with placebo (vehicle), sucralfate (1.0 g/day t.i.d.), ranitidine (150 mg/day, b.i.d.) or nocloprost, a stable $PGE_2$ analog (100 μg t.i.d.).

favorable environment for rapid epithelial restitution.[33] Removal of this mucoid cap mechanically or by mucolytic agents inhibits this rapid mucosal repair.

In humans, topical application of ethanol does not cause such massive hemorrhagic necrosis as observed in rats given 1 to 2 ml of 100% ethanol. Following spray of 50% ethanol through endoscope directly on the mucosa, almost immediate endoscopic changes occur and they include mucosal opacification, extensive hyperemia, and the appearance of individual hemorrhagic lesions usually located at the top of the congested mucosal folds. These lesions become progressively extensive with time. Histologically, an extensive disruption and exfoliation of the large surface epithelium are observed. In the unprotected mucosa, deeper mucosal lesions, such as subepithelial hemorrhages and deep hemorrhagic erosions with necrosis of glandular cells, are present. For quantitative evaluation of the mucosal injury by ethanol, the endoscopic grading scale has been applied from zero (normal mucosa) to five (more than ten hemorrhagic lesions or a large area of confluent hemorrhage[11]). Pretreatment with stable $PGE_2$-analog such as nocloprost in a dose (100 μg) that does not affect gastric acid secretion prevented the development of acute mucosal lesions. Similar effects were obtained with the pretreatment with sucralfate (1.0 g),[11] but administration of ranitidine in a dose (150 mg) that inhibits gastric acid secretion failed to affect the formation of acute gastric lesions in humans (Figure 8.9).

The process of restitution is rapid in rats but relatively slower in humans because of the greater distance between the gland openings in the human stomach. It is reduced at lower pH (below pH 3.0) possibly due to the inactivation of basic fibroblast growth factor (bFGF) that stimulates the cell migration from the intact gastric pits and to restore the surface epithelium.[34] Restitution of surface epithelium is a prompt autonomous process, but it does not suffice to prevent the production by ethanol of hemorrhagic erosions if the underlying mucosal vascular supply is destroyed. Exposure of the mucosa to ethanol and other necrotizing agents (without addition of PG) results in vasocongestion, stasis, and thrombus formation in the subepithelial microvasculature. PG appear to maintain the microvascular integrity (vasoprotection) and reduce the underlying vasocongestion to preserve the capability of the epithelial cells to migrate from intact gastric pits and to restore the surface epithelium.[28,29,32,35]

The vascular effects of PG seem to play an important role in direct cytoprotection[23,24,36,37] and the elimination of the mucosal factors that compromise the vascular supply appears to be as effective in cytoprotection as administration of PG. The importance of vascular factor in cytoprotection is supported by the fact that PG failed to protect the *in vitro* gastric mucosa against various types of damage.[38] On the other hand, cytoprotection by PG was observed *in vitro* in isolated gastric mucosal cells or whole gastric glands. Such isolated cells or glands suspended in nutrient medium deteriorate slowly and eventually die. This deterioration could be delayed by cytoprotective agents such as prostaglandins. In addition, these isolated cells or glands could be protected against damage by ethanol or other damaging agents when prostaglandins are given

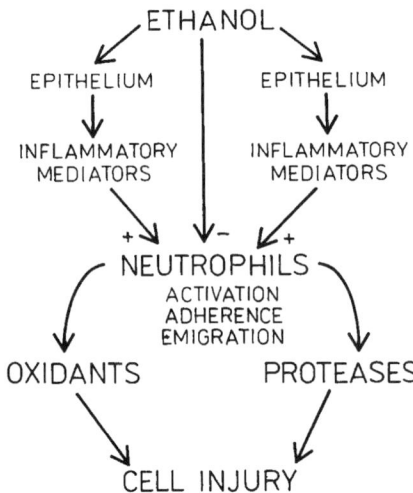

**FIGURE 8.10** Gastric mucosal lesions, blood neutrophil activation, mucosal infiltration by neutrophils and the release of inflammatory mediators as well as tissue oxidants and injurious proteases.

prior to or together with the damaging agent. Protected cells retain most of their normal morphology and ultrastructure, are viable in dye exclusion tests, and do not "leak" some enzymes.[39]

Neutrophils have been also implicated in the pathogenesis of ethanol-induced gastropathy by the process of migration, adherence to endothelial cells, and release of procoagulants and inflammatory modulators. Neutrophil activation could account for the reduced mucosal perfusion[40] (Figure 8.10). The adherence of neutrophils to the endothelium is mediated by special glycoprotein adhesion molecules[41] and occurs within minutes after administration of ethanol. This may be the source of the increased synthesis of other mediators such as endothelins and leukotrienes and the release of injurious oxidants and proteases.[40] PG protect the gastric mucosa from ethanol-induced ulcerations, at least in part, through the inhibitory effect on neutrophil activation.[40] PG of E and I series have been shown to inhibit the adherence, chemotaxis, and secretion of neutrophils in response to various secretogogues. Prostacyclin ($PGI_2$) derived from the endothelium may be a physiological modulator of neutrophil function and its inhibition by ethanol may contribute to the leukocyte adherence and the synthesis of leukotrienes after acute mucosal injury.

### 8.4.2   Adaptive Cytoprotection

Gastroprotection can be induced not only by exogenous PG but also by the application of various mild irritants to the mucosa.[3,4] Oral administration of 10 to 20% ethanol, 5% NaCl, or 5 m$M$ taurocholate prevented massive mucosal damage caused by necrotizing substances such as 100% ethanol, 25% NaCl, 80 m$M$ taurocholate, 0.6 $M$ HCl, and 0.2 $M$ NaOH. These mild irritants prevented macroscopic mucosal lesions provoked by necrotizing agents, and these effects resembled those induced by PG.[3] The phenomenon has been called "adaptive" cytoprotection because it was later demonstrated to be mediated by endogenous release of PG by gastric mucosa. The supporting evidence was obtained first by pretreating animals with indomethacin (to block mucosal generation of PG),[3,4] which resulted in a partial reversal of the protection afforded by mild irritants. Such treatment failed to prevent the protective effect of exogenous PG. More direct evidence of PG involvement in the adaptive cytoprotection has been obtained by using bioassay or radioimmunoassay of mucosal PG. Mild irritants were found to increase the mucosal capability to generate PG[3,4] while reducing the formation of acute gastric lesions induced by necrotizing

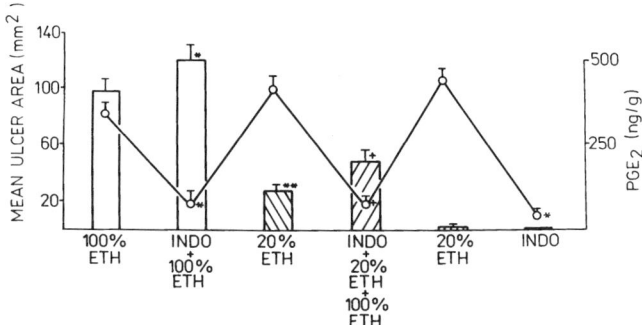

**FIGURE 8.11** Pretreatment of rats with 20% ethanol prevents the formation of acute gastric lesions induced in rats by 100% ethanol and this "adaptive cytoprotection" can be reversed, in part, by the pretreatment with indomethacin (5 mg/kg i.p.) given 90 min before administration of 20% ethanol. Indomethacin by itself almost completely abolished the generation of $PGE_2$ (open circles) in gastric mucosa but did not cause any macroscopic mucosal damage (columns).

agents. Indomethacin, which reversed cytoprotection, abolished the mucosal generation of PG and the protective effects of mild irritants (Figure 8.11).[4,30]

Although adaptive cytoprotection is believed to be mediated mainly by endogenous PG, recent studies have provided evidence that this phenomenon may be explained in other ways. Wallace and Whittle[33] and Wallace[42] proposed that mild irritants cause injury to surface epithelial cells, resulting in the formation of a protective layer of alkaline mucoid debris that mitigates the effects of further insult of luminal irritants and enhances the rapid repair or restitution of surface epithelium. As the role of endogenous PG in adaptive cytoprotection has been questioned,[43] it is possible that nonprostaglandin components may be implicated in this protection. It is likely that the physical irritation of surface epithelial cells enhances the mucus-alkaline secretion and increases the thickness of the protective layer to dissipate physically as well as increases water secretion that dilutes the necrotizing agent when applied as the second challenge to the mucosa.[44]

The protection against ethanol injury was also demonstrated after the pretreatment of gastric mucosa with arachidonic acid.[45] It was shown that arachidonic acid–induced protection is mediated via local increase in PG biosynthesis because indomethacin prevented the protective effects of arachidonic acid and abolished the accompanying increase in luminal release of PG. To some extent the arachidonic acid–induced protection was similar to that provoked by mild irritants because this acid, like mild irritants, caused increased mucosal exfoliation and partial disruption of the gastric mucosal surface epithelium which occurred after exposure to ethanol. Arachidonic acid protected and preserved the mucosal proliferative zone and, like PG, stimulated the migration of the gland cells from the protected zone, resulting in a prompt restoration of surface epithelium and resumption of its barrier and transport functions.

Adaptive cytoprotection as induced by mild irritating effect of one substance such as 20% ethanol prevents the formation of acute lesion caused by high necrotizing concentration of the same substance (e.g., 100% ethanol) and this could be called "homocytoprotection" or by different strong irritant such as 0.6 $M$ HCl ("cross-cytoprotection").[25]

The adaptive cytoprotection induced by hypertonic saline was shown to be accompanied by a marked increase in the mucosal blood flow.[46,47] This hyperemia and accompanying decrease in mucosal damage was not affected by the inhibition of nitric oxide (NO) synthase, the blockade of $H_1$ receptors, or the ablation of capsaicin-sensitive afferent nerves but was abolished by the suppression of cyclooxygenase with indomethacin, confirming the earlier concept of the involvement of endogenous PG in this protective hyperemia.[3,4]

Although the adaptive cytoprotection by hypertonic saline does not seem to be mediated by NO, recent evidence indicates that other forms of this protection, such as induced by 20% ethanol,

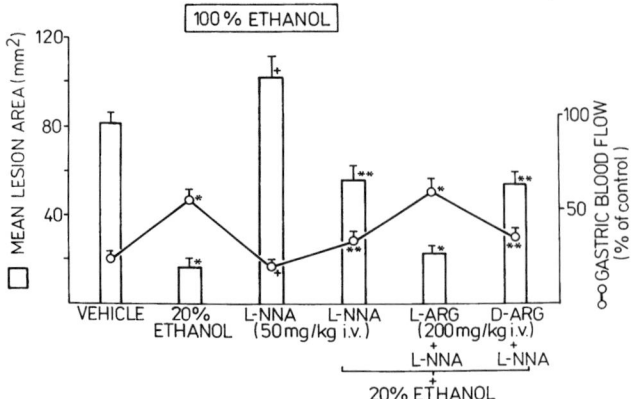

**FIGURE 8.12** Pretreatment with L-nitro-L-arginine (L-NNA) prevents the "adaptive" protection and increase in mucosal blood flow (measured by laser Doppler flowmetry) caused by 20% ethanol given 30 min before 100% ethanol. The addition of L-arginine but not D-arginine restored in part the protection by 20% ethanol against the damage by 100% ethanol.[6]

may be mediated, at least in part, by this compound (Figure 8.12).[6,51] Nitrovasodilators, such as nitroglycerin or sodium nitroprusside, that act by releasing NO have been shown to protect the gastric mucosa against acute damage by ethanol or acid and this effect was attributed to the potent vasorelaxant action of NO.[6,48] Other studies demonstrated that NO acts as a prime mediator of functional vasodilation and a close interaction between PG, NO, and sensory neuropeptides has been proposed in the regulation of gastric mucosal integrity.[49,50] Selective inhibition of NO synthase by the pretreatment with L-NMMA or L-NNA was found to augment acute mucosal injury induced by indomethacin and by inactivation of afferent nerves with capsaicin.[49,50] In rats with capsaicin applied topically on the mucosa to stimulate the release of sensory neuropeptides such as calcitonin gene-related peptide (CGRP), a marked increase in gastric mucosal blood flow and a marked protection against the damage by various noxious agents have been observed.[51] This capsaicin-induced protection can be significantly reduced by the pretreatment with either L-NMMA or by indomethacin, suggesting that both NO and PG are implicated in this process. Since the activation of neutrophils is known to contribute to the mucosal injury,[40] it is likely that NO and PG inhibit this activation and microvascular injury (Figure 8.13).

The major properties of adaptive cytoprotection are that (1) it is associated with gastric hyperemia and increased PG biosynthesis, (2) it is a short-lasting phenomenon and disappears after about 1.5 to 2 h, (3) its common initial cause is the damage of the mucosal cells exposed to mild irritants, and (4) it may serve in a short-term adaptation of the stomach to withstand the damaging action of strong irritants.

### 8.4.3    Cytoprotection by Antiulcer Drugs

Several drugs widely used in peptic ulcer disease appear to exert both beneficial effects on ulcer healing and preventive effects against acute mucosal damage induced, for instance, by absolute ethanol or acidified aspirin. These include sucralfate,[6] colloidal bismuth preparation,[52] and antacids.[48] CBS, sucralfate, and antacids appear to precipitate or polymerize at the mucosal surface to form a viscous gel onto the gastroduodenal epithelium through mild irritation of the mucosa and subsequent stimulation of mucosal release of PG as well as an increase in gastric mucosal blood flow probably mediated by endogenous nitric oxide. The involvement of endogenous PG in the protective activity of aluminum-containing antacids has been questioned and attributed, in part, to the release by these drugs, especially at lower pH, of an activated form of hexa-aquoaluminum cation which exerts protective properties.[53] It is not clear how this cation could activate the mucosal protective mechanisms but the stimulation of the biosynthesis of NO could be a reasonable explanation.[48]

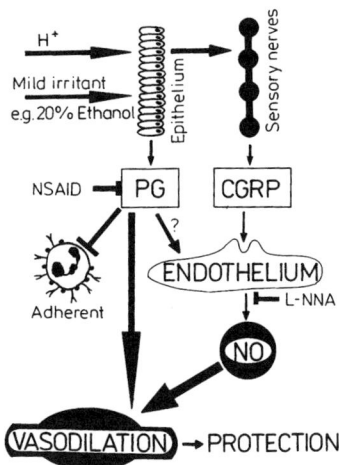

**FIGURE 8.13** Diagrammatic representation of cytoprotection induced by topical mild irritants such as 20% ethanol that involves the stimulation of sensory nerves, the release of CGRP, NO, and PG enhancing the mucosal blood flow and preventing the activation of neutrophils.

## 8.5 GASTRIC ADAPTATION TO REPEATED INSULTS OF TOPICAL IRRITANTS

### 8.5.1 Gastric Adaptation to Aspirin-Like Agents

It is well established that aspirin and other NSAID are ulcerogenic in animals and humans and their effects are dose dependent.[54] The pathogenesis of NSAID gastropathy is poorly understood but it has been causally linked to the direct damage of the mucosa as well as to the inhibition of PG biosynthesis.[54,55] The vascular etiology for NSAID gastropathy has recently been proposed by demonstration of the ability of these drugs to cause vascular endothelial damage, the activation of neutrophils, and the formation of thrombi occluding gastric microvasculature and leading to the mucosal damage.[56]

An interesting and practically important discovery related to the gastric damage induced by NSAID is an increase in mucosal tolerance or adaptation to the ulcerogenic action of these drugs that develops with their more prolonged administration. Attenuation of mucosal damage has been first demonstrated in rats[57] and then confirmed in humans.[58] The mechanism of gastric adaptation is not known. One hypothesis assumes that NSAID cause a widespread initial injury that is followed by the adaptation of the mucosa with an increased ability to tolerate further insult without significant injury. Animal experimentation indicates that the initial damage of surface epithelium is necessary for the gastric adaptation to occur on continued exposure to NSAID.[59] Our recent studies in rats confirmed that repeated insults of acidified ASA results in the attenuation of deep hemorrhagic lesions with the continuation of the ASA treatment.[60] This gastric adaptation was accompanied by gastric hyperemia and the enhancement of expression of EGF and cell proliferation in the gastric mucosa, especially in the regeneration area. Neither the inhibition of NO synthase by nitro-L-arginine nor the ablation of afferent sensory nerves affected the adaptation of the mucosa to aspirin. The fact that the adapting mucosa exhibits remarkable regenerative changes and increased expression of EGF and its receptors suggests that EGF may be involved in the mechanism of mucosal adaptation. Wright et al.[61] reported that EGF may be secreted in the area of gastrointestinal ulcerations from novel cell lines. It is likely that gastric mucosa respond to ASA-induced lesions by excessive local production of EGF that initiates cell proliferation and mucosal repair. Such acute mucosal damage could also cause an increase in the expression of TGFα[62] that could participate in mucosal repair and adaptation of the mucosa to the continued

ASA treatment. One has also to consider that the regenerating gastric surface epithelial cells are more resistant to noxious agents simply by being in a different stage of the cell cycle.

### 8.5.2 Gastric Adaptation to Ethanol and Other Necrotizing Substances

Chronic administration of 50% ethanol was reported to be significantly less toxic in animals given ethanol repeatedly than in rats receiving ethanol only once. Robert et al.[63] reported that oral administration of another strong irritant such as 0.2 $M$ NaOH to fasted rats produced initially widespread mucosal necrosis hemorrhages and edema, but with repeated challenge using that necrotizing solution every other day the lesions became less severe as the number of treatments increased. Similar gastric adaptation was observed when hypertonic NaCl (2 mol/l) was applied chronically into the stomach.[64]

It has been well documented that chronic (4 week) intragastric administration of ethanol in rats produces adaptation of the gastric mucosa to subsequent challenge with acute dose of 50% ethanol.[65] Rats which received 4-week daily treatment with 1 ml of 50% ethanol showed 3.5-fold reduction in the formation of gross hemorrhagic necrosis produced by acute dose of 3.5 ml of 50% ethanol as compared to animals treated with vehicle saline and then exposed to acute dose of 50% ethanol. In another study[9] chronic administration of ethanol (1 ml 50% ethanol twice daily for 2 weeks) significantly increased the extent of gastric mucus and proliferative cell zones and the number of proliferating cells as measured by DNA synthesis and bromodeoxyuridine uptake (Figures 8.14 and 8.15). Furthermore, there was remarkable increase in the expression of EGF and TGFα and their receptors in the mucosa (Figure 8.16). It was concluded similarly, as in adaptation to ASA, that repeated exposures to ethanol result in the increased cell proliferation probably due to overexpression of growth factors and their receptors in the gastric mucosa.

The mechanisms of mucosal adaptation to alcohol are unknown but in other systems they are related to the changes in cell membranes.[66] Because the receptors for EGF and TGFα are located in the plasma membrane and operate through the activation of protein kinases, it was proposed that chronic administration of ethanol results in the increase of expression of these receptors leading to increased cell proliferation and mucosal repair.[9] In studies by Robert et al.,[63] repeated exposure to 0.2 $M$ NaOH also resulted in remarkable regeneration at the gland neck suggesting the enhanced cell proliferation but the possible implication of growth factors in these morphological changes has not been explored. Instead, the generation of PG by the mucosa adapting to 0.2 $M$ NaOH was greatly augmented and the pretreatment with indomethacin abolished the rise in PG biosynthesis and partially reversed the gastric adaptation. These results have been explained by the fact that endogenous PG may contribute to the gastric adaptation to necrotizing solution of NaOH. In recent studies by Lacy et al.,[64] the repeated insults of ethanol or chronic treatments with mild irritants resulted in the appearance of superficial mucosal injury and enhanced the resistance of the gastric mucosa to the damage by necrotizing substances. In the studies with adaptation to aspirin we also found that the mucosa, which is adapted to this ulcerogen, is more resistant to the damage by strong irritants such as absolute ethanol, acidified taurocholate, or stress.[67] This has been checked on rats adapted by 6-day treatment with acidified ASA and then by the challenge with one of the necrotizing substances such as absolute ethanol, acidified 100 m$M$ taurocholate, or 25% NaCl given intragastrically in a volume of 1.5 ml. In nonadapted rats such necrotizing substances produced severe gastric mucosal damage accompanied by the fall in gastric blood flow and the decrease in luminal EGF and mucosal expression of EGF and TGFα. In contrast, in adapted animals, a significant reduction in the lesion area and the enhancement of mucosal blood flow were observed. Moreover, this increased resistance of the mucosa to the formation of acute lesions was associated with the overexpression of EGF and TGFα and their receptors in the mucosa.[8,67] A number of studies with gastric adaptation[8] to injurious agents such as ethanol, aspirin, or stress, underlie the increased mucosal regeneration of the adapted mucosa. An increase in cell proliferation (as determined by morphology,

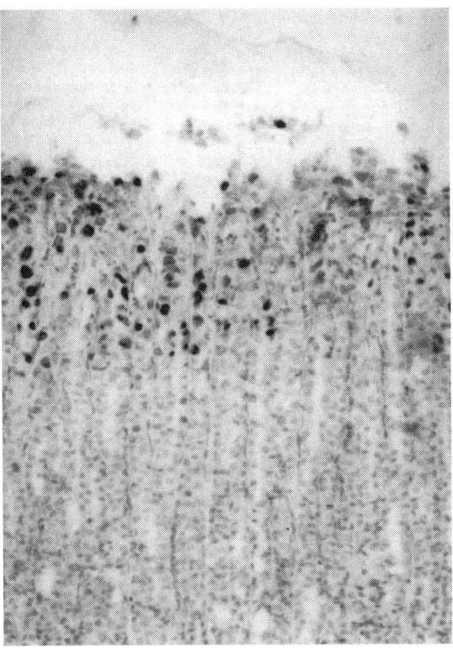

**FIGURE 8.14** Rat gastric oxyntic mucosa 1 h after second daily exposure to 96% ethanol. Bromodeoxyuridine given 100 mg/kg 1.5 h prior to killing. No massive hemorrhagic necrosis was observed. Numerous surface, foveolar, and neck cells incorporated bromodeoxyuridine. (BSA method; original magnification ×260.)

bromodeoxyuridine uptake, proliferating cell antigen expression, and DNA synthesis) was probably due to the increased expression of growth factors and their receptors in the adapted mucosa.

### 8.5.3 Chronic Ethanol Abuse in Men

This topic commonly assumed the presence of repeated gastric mucosal injury and recurrent acute gastritis.[68] There is, however, no direct evidence to support this notion. Chronic gastritis is

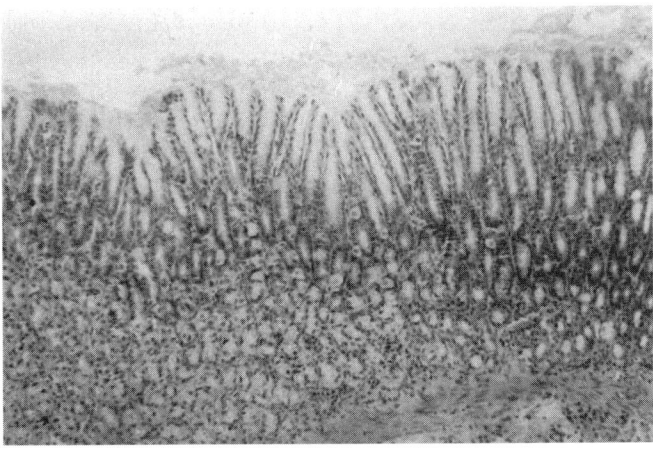

**FIGURE 8.15** Rat gastric mucosa 4 days after daily intragastric instillation of 96% ethanol. Increased regeneration is present with elongated *foveolae* and thickened neck regenerative zone. (Hematoxylin-eosin; original magnification ×150.)

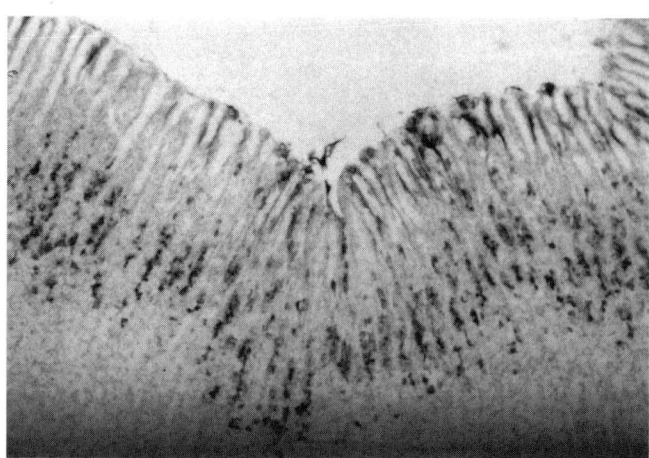

**FIGURE 8.16** Rat gastric mucosa 4 days after daily intragastric instillation of 96% ethanol. Regenerating gastric mucosa shows increased expression of epidermal growth factor receptor in the entire regenerating neck, foveolar, and surface area. (BSA method; original magnification ×150.)

reported in chronic alcoholism from 10 to 70%.[69] An improvement in chronic gastritis was noticed in 12 alcoholics following abstinence lasting up to 9 months.[70] On the other hand, Brown et al.[71] reported that chronic gastritis is not any higher in patients with alcoholic cirrhosis than in healthy controls. There is no doubt that acute ethanol abuse damages the human gastric mucosa including hemorrhagic erosions after intake of highly concentrated ethanol but these lesions heal rapidly. There is also no direct evidence that "chemical" gastritis can be hostile to infection by *Helicobacter pylori*, the most common etiological factor of gastritis.[72] In addition, chronic gastritis in alcoholics could be caused by other factors such as improper diet, malabsorption, bile reflux, etc. Chronic alcoholism is not associated with hyperplastic or hypertrophic changes in the gastric mucosa.

## 8.6   SUMMARY AND CONCLUSIONS

Cytoprotection induced by ethanol is a complex phenomenon in which cellular and tissue (especially microcirculation and nerve supply) mechanisms amplify, leading to the very effective and impressive phenomenon. Superficial damage occurring in protected gastric mucosa is rapidly repaired by the migration and restitution of surface epithelial cells. This rapid process is shorter than the cell cycle and does not involve cellular division which follows after repair has been completed. Gastric adaptation to repeated injurious episodes is connected with local growth factors leading to rapid repair and regeneration of the injured mucosa including DNA synthesis and mitoses. This results in the increased resistance of regenerating epithelium to repeated injury and is associated with increased expression of EGF and TGFα and their receptors, the maintenance of the gastric blood flow and improvement of gastric mucosal integrity. These adaptive mucosal changes are transient and regress after discontinuation of injurious episodes.

## REFERENCES

1. **Oates, P. J.,** Gastric blood flow and mucosal defense, in *Gastric Cytoprotection. A Clinicians Guide*, Hollander, D. and Tarnawski, A. S., Eds., Plenum Medical Book Company, New York, 1989, chap. 7.
2. **Tepperman, B. L. and Jacobson, E. D.,** Circulatory factors in gastric mucosal defense and repair, in *Physiology of the Gastrointestinal Tract*, Johnson, L. R., Ed., Raven Press, New York, 1994, 1331.
3. **Robert, A., Nezamis, J. T., Davies, J. P., Field, S. A., and Hanchar, A. J.,** Mild irritant prevent gastric necrosis through "adaptive cytoprotection" mediated by prostaglandins, *Am. J. Physiol.*, 245, G113, 1983.

4. **Konturek, S. J., Brzozowski, T., Piastucki, I., Radecki, T., and Dembinska-Kiec, A.,** Role of locally generated prostaglandins in adaptive gastric cytoprotection, *Dig. Dis. Sci.*, 27, 967, 1982.

5. **Tepperman, B. L., Soper, B. D., and Morris, G. P.,** Effect of sialoadenectomy on adaptive cytoprotection in the rat, *Gastroenterology*, 97, 123, 1989.

6. **Konturek, S. J., Brzozowski, T., Majka, J., Szlachcic, A., and Czarnobilski, K.,** Nitric oxide in gastroprotection by sucralfate, mild irritant and nocloprost. Role of mucosal blood flow, *Dig. Dis. Sci.*, 39, 593, 1994.

7. **Matsumoto, J., Veshima, K., Takeuchi, K., and Okabe, S.,** Capsaicin-sensitive afferent neurons in adaptive responses of the rat stomach induced by a mild irritant, *Jpn. J. Pharmacol.*, 55, 181, 1991.

8. **Konturek, S. J. and Konturek, J. W.,** Gastric adaptation. Basic and clinical aspects, *Digestion*, 55, 131, 1994.

9. **Tarnawski, A., Lu, S. Y., Stachura, J., and Sarfeh, I. J.,** Adaptation of gastric mucosa to chronic alcohol administration is associated with increased mucosal expression of growth factors and their receptors, *Scand. J. Gastroenterol.*, 193 (Suppl.), 59, 1992.

10. **Chari, S., Teyssen, S., and Singer, M. U.,** Alcohol and gastric acid secretion in humans, *Gut*, 34, 843, 1993.

11. **Konturek, S. J., Mach, T., Konturek, J. W., Bogdal, J., and Stachura, J.,** Comparison of sucralfate and ranitidine in gastroprotection against alcohol in humans, *Am. J. Med.*, 86, 55, 1989.

12. **Pares, X., Cederlung, E., Moreno, A., Helmquist, L., Farres, J., and Jornvall, H.,** Mammalian class IV alcohol dehydrogenase (stomach alcohol dehydrogenase); structure, origin and correlation with enzymology, *Proc. Natl. Acad. Sci. U.S.A.*, 91, 1893, 1994.

13. **Seitz, H. K., Egerer, G., Simanowski, V. A., Waldherr, R., Eckey, R., Agarwal, D. P., Gredde, H. W., and Warthburg, J. P.,** Human gastric alcoholic dehydrogenase activity: effect of age, sex and alcoholism, *Gut*, 34, 1433, 1933.

14. **Lim, R. T., Gentry, R. T., Ito, D., Tokoyama, H., Baraona, E., and Lieber, G. S.,** First-pass metabolism of ethanol is predominantly gastric, *Alcoholism: Clin. Exp. Res.*, 17, 1337, 1993.

15. **Goldstein, D. B.,** *Pharmacology of Alcohol,* Oxford University Press, New York, 1983, 3.

16. **Stachura, J.,** Pathomorphology of gastric mucosal injury, in *Gastric Cytoprotection. A Clinicians Guide,* Hollander, D. and Tarnawski, A., Eds., Plenum Press, New York, 1989, 33.

17. **Solcia, E., Capella, C., Buffa, R., Usellini, L., Fiocca, R., and Sessa, T.,** Endocrine cells in the digestive system, in *Physiology of the Gastrointestinal Tract,* Johnson, L. R., Ed., Raven Press, New York, 1987, 111.

18. **Stachura, J., Tarnawski, A., and Dabros, W.,** Apoptosis: genetically programmed physiologic cell loss in normal gastric oxyntic mucosa and in mucosa of grossly healed gastric ulcer, *J. Clin. Gastroenterol.*, 17, S70, 1993.

19. **Johnson, L. R. and McCormack, S. A.,** Regulation of gastrointestinal mucosal growth, in *Physiology of the Gastrointestinal Tract,* Johnson, L. R., Ed., Raven Press, New York, 1994, 611.

20. **Piasecki, C.,** Evidence for an infarctive pathogenesis of acute and chronic gastroduodenal ulceration, *J. Physiol. Pharmacol.*, 43, 99, 1992.

21. **Ito, S. and Lacy, E. R.,** Morphology of rat gastric mucosal damage. Defense and restitution in the presence of luminal ethanol, *Gastroenterology*, 88, 250, 1985.

22. **Lacy, E. R.,** Gastric mucosal resistance to a repeated ethanol insult, *Scand. J. Gastroenterol.*, 20 (Suppl. 1), 63, 1985.

23. **Tarnawski, A., Stachura, J., Hollander, D., Sarfeh, I. J., and Bogdal, J.,** Cellular aspects of alcohol-induced injury of the human gastric mucosa. Focus on the mucosal microvessels, *J. Clin. Gastroenterol.*, 10 (Suppl. 1), 553, 1988.

24. **Tarnawski, A., Stachura, J., Gergely, H., and Hollander, D.,** Microvascular endothelium — a major target for alcohol injury of the human gastric mucosa. Histochemical and ultrastructural study, *J. Clin. Gastroenterol.*, 10 (Suppl. 1), 553, 1988.

25. **Robert, A.,** Cytoprotection by prostaglandins, *Gastroenterology*, 77, 761, 1979.

26. **Robert, A., Nezamis, J. E., Lancaster, C., and Hanchar, A. J.,** Cytoprotection by prostaglandins in rats. Prevention of gastric necrosis produced by alcohol, HCl, NaOH, hypertonic NaCl and thermal injury, *Gastroenterology*, 77, 433, 1979.

27. **Lacy, E. R. and Ito, S.,** Microscopic analysis of ethanol damage to rat gastric mucosa after treatment with prostaglandin, *Gastroenterology*, 83, 619, 1982.

28. **Lacy, E. R. and Ito, S.,** Rapid epithelial restitution of the rat gastric mucosa after ethanol injury, *Lab. Invest.*, 51, 573, 1984.

29. **Ito, S., Lacy, E. R., Rutten, M. J., Critchlow, J., and Silen, W.,** Rapid repair of injured gastric mucosa, *Scand. J. Gastroenterol.*, 19 (Suppl. 101), 87, 1984.

30. **Konturek, S. J.,** Mechanisms of gastroprotection, *Scand. J. Gastroenterol.*, 25 (Suppl. 174), 15, 1990.

31. **Konturek, S. J., Brzozowski, T., Drozdowicz, D., and Pytko, J.,** Gastroprotection by cholecystokinin (CCK) against ethanol damage. Role of CCK-A and CCK-B receptors and nitric oxide (NO), *Gastroenterology*, 106, 4, A110, 1994.

32. **Tarnawski, A., Hollander, D., Stachura, J., Krause, W. J., and Gergely, H.,** Prostaglandin protection of the gastric mucosa against alcohol injury — a dynamic tile-related process. Role of muscular proliferative zone, *Gastroenterology*, 88, 334, 1985.

33. **Wallace, J. L. and Whittle, B. J.,** Role of mucus in the repair of gastric epithelial damage in the rat. Inhibition of epithelial recovery by mucolytic agents, *Gastroenterology,* 91, 603, 1986.

34. **Paimela, H., Goddard, P. J., Carter, K., Khakee, R., McNeil, P. L., Ito, S., and Silen, W.,** Restitution of frog gastric mucosa *in vitro*: effect of basic fibroblast growth factor, *Gastroenterology,* 104, 1337, 1993.

35. **Wallace, J. C. and Whittle, B. J. R.,** Acceleration of recovery of gastric epithelial integrity by 16,16-dimethyl prostaglandin E$_2$, *Br. J. Pharmacol.,* 86, 838, 1985.

36. **Guth, P. H., Paulsen, G., and Nagata, H.,** Histological and microcirculatory changes in alcohol-induced gastric lesions in rats: effect of prostaglandin cytoprotection, *Gastroenterology,* 87, 1083, 1984.

37. **Leung, F. W., Robert, A., and Guth, P. H.,** Gastric mucosal blood flow in rats after administration of 16,16-dimethyl prostaglandin E$_2$ at a cytoprotective dose, *Gastroenterology,* 88, 1948, 1985.

38. **Rowe, P. H., Starlinger, M. J., Kasdon, E., Marrone, G., and Silen, W.,** Effect of simulated systemic administration of aspirin, salicylate and indomethacin on amphibian gastric mucosa, *Gastroenterology,* 90, 559, 1986.

39. **Tarnawski, A., Brzozowski, T., Sarfeh, I. J., Krause, W. J., Ulich, T. R., Gergely, H., and Hollander, D.,** Prostaglandin protection of human isolated gastric glands. Evidence for direct cellular action of prostaglandin, *J. Clin. Invest.,* 81, 1091, 1988.

40. **Kvietys, P. R., Twohig, B., Danzell, J., and Specian, D. N.,** Ethanol-induced injury to the rat gastric mucosa. Role of neutrophils and xantine oxidase-derived radicals, *Gastroenterology,* 98, 909, 1990.

41. **Wallace, J. E., Arfors, K.-E., and McNight, G. W.,** A monoclonal antibody against the CD18 leukocyte adhesion molecule prevents indomethacin-induced gastric damage in the rabbit, *Gastroenterology,* 100, 878, 1991.

42. **Wallace, J. L.,** Increased resistance of the rat gastric mucosa to hemorrhagic damage after exposure to an irritant. Role of "mucoid cap" and prostaglandin synthesis, *Gastroenterology,* 94, 22, 1988.

43. **Hawkey, C. J., Kemp, R. T., Walt, R. P., Bhaskar, N. K., Davies, J., and Filipowicz, B.,** Evidence that adaptive cytoprotection in rats is not mediated by prostaglandins, *Gastroenterology,* 94, 948, 1988.

44. **Philan, G. and Szabo, S.,** Dimethyl PGE$_2$ and thiosulfate increase gastric mucosal penetration of hypertonic NaCl and increase net transmucosal water flux, *Gastroenterology,* 94, A354, 1988.

45. **Tarnawski, A., Hollander, D., Stachura, J., and Krause, W.,** Arachidonic acid protection of gastric mucosa against alcohol injury: sequential analysis of morphologic and functional changes, *J. Lab. Clin. Med.,* 102, 340, 1983.

46. **Svanes, K., Gislason, H., Guttu, K., Herfjord, J. K., Fevang, J., and Gronbech, J. E.,** Role of blood flow in adaptive protection of the cat gastric mucosa, *Gastroenterology,* 100, 1249, 1991.

47. **Endo, K., Kao, J., Bomek, M. J., and Leung, F. W.,** Mechanism of gastric hyperemia induced by intragastric hypertonic saline in rats, *Gastroenterology,* 104, 114, 1993.

48. **Konturek, S. J., Brzozowski, T., Majka, J., Szlachcic, A., Nauert, Ch., and Slomiany, B.,** Nitric oxide in gastroprotection by aluminum-containing antacids, *Eur. J. Pharmacol.,* 229, 155, 1992.

49. **Whittle, B. J. R., Lopez-Belmonte, J., and Moncada, S.,** Regulation of gastric mucosal integrity by endogenous nitric oxide; interactions with prostanoids and sensory neuropeptides in the rat, *Br. J. Pharmacol.,* 99, 607, 1990.

50. **Whittle, B. J. R.,** Nitric oxide in gastrointestinal physiology and pathology, in *Physiology of the Gastrointestinal Tract,* Johnson, L. R., Ed., Raven Press, New York, 1994, 267.

51. **Brzozowski, T., Drozdowicz, D., Szlachcic, A., Pytko-Polonczyk, J., Majka, J., and Konturek, S. J.,** Role of nitric oxide and prostaglandins in gastroprotection induced by capsaicin and papaverine, *Digestion,* 54, 24, 1993.

52. **Konturek, S. J., Radecki, T., Piastucki, I., Brzozowski, T., and Drozdowicz, D.,** Gastroprotection by colloidal bismuth subcitrate (De-Nol) and sucralfate. Role of endogenous prostaglandins, *Gut,* 28, 201, 1987.

53. **Konturek, S. J., Brzozowski, T., Marks, N. J., Miederer, S., Peskar, B. M., Preclik, G., and Weberg, R.,** Antacids and mucosal protection, *Eur. J. Gastroenterol. Hepatol.,* 4, 954, 1992.

54. **Konturek, S. J., Piastucki, I., Brzozowski, T., Dembinska-Kiec, A., and Gryglewski, R.,** Role of prostaglandins in the formation of apirin-induced gastric ulcers, *Gastroenterology,* 80, 4, 1981.

55. **Rainford, K. D. and Willis, C.,** Relationship of gastric mucosal damage induced in pigs by antiinflammatory drugs to their effect on prostaglandin production, *Dig. Dis. Sci.,* 27, 624, 1992.

56. **Wallace, J. L.,** Non-steroidal anti-inflammatory drug gastropathy and cytoprotection. Pathogenesis and mechanisms re-examined, *Scand. J. Gastroenterol.,* 27 (Suppl. 192), 3, 1992.

57. **St. John, D. J. B., Yeomans, N. D., McDermott, F. T., and de Boer, W. G. R. M.,** Adaptation of the gastric mucosal to repeated administration of aspirin in the rat, *Am. J. Dig. Dis.,* 18, 881, 1973.

58. **Graham, D. Y., Smith, J. L., and Dobbs, S. M.,** Gastric adaptation occurs with aspirin administration in man, *Am. J. Dig. Dis.,* 28, 1, 1983.

59. **Robert, A., Lancaster, C., Olafsson, A. S., Gilberston-Beadling, S., and Zhang, W.,** Gastric adaptation to the ulcerogenic effect of aspirin, *Gastroenterology,* 1, 73, 1991.

60. **Konturek, S. J., Brzozowski, T., Konturek, J. W., and Domschke, W.,** Role of prostaglandins, sensory nerves, nitric oxide and growth factors in gastric adaptation to topical irritants, *J. Physiol. Pharmacol.,* 44 (Suppl. 2), 69, 1993.

61. **Wright, N. A., Pike, C., and Elia, G.,** Induction of an epithelial growth factor-secreting lineage by mucosal ulceration in human gastrointestinal stem cells, *Nature,* 343, 82, 1990.

62. **Polk, W. H., Dempsey, P. J., Russel, W. E., Brown, P. I., Beauchamp, R. D., Bernard, J. A., and Coffey, R. J.,** Increased production of transforming growth factor alpha following acute gastric injury, *Gastroenterology,* 102, 1467, 1992.

63. **Robert, A., Lancaster, C., Olafson, A. S., and Zhang, W.,** Gastric adaptation of repeated administrations of a necrotizing agent, in *Mechanisms of Injury Protection and Repair of the Upper Gastrointestinal Tract,* Garner, A. and O'Brien, P. G., Eds., Chichester, Wiley, 1991, 357.

64. **Lacy, E. K., Cowart, K. S., and Hund, P.,** Effects of chronic superficial injury on the rat gastric mucosa, *Gastroenterology,* 103, 1179, 1992.

65. **Ivey, K. J., Tarnawski, A., and Stachura, J.,** The induction of gastric mucosal tolerance to alcohol by chronic administration, *J. Lab. Clin. Med.,* 96, 922, 1980.

66. **Goldstein, D. B.,** Ethanol-induced adaptation in biological membranes, *Ann. N.Y. Acad. Sci.,* 492, 103, 1987.

67. **Brzozowski, T., Drozdowicz, D., Stachura, J., and Konturek, S. J.,** Gastric mucosa adapted to aspirin (ASA) or stress is more resistant to the damage induced by strong irritants, *Gastroenterology,* 106, A58, 1994.

68. **Morson, B. C. and Dawson, I. M. P.,** *Gastrointestinal Pathology,* Blackwell Science Publishers, Oxford, 1990, 94.

69. **Whitehead, R.,** *Mucosal Biopsy of the Gastrointestinal Tract,* W. B. Saunders, Philadelphia, 1990, 84.

70. **Dinoso, V. P., Jr., Chey, W. Y., and Braverman, S. P.,** Gastric secretion and gastric mucosal morphology in chronic alcoholics, *Arch. Intern. Med.,* 130, 715, 1972.

71. **Brown, R. C., Hardy, G. J., and Temperly, J. M.,** Gastritis and cirrhosis: no association, *J. Clin. Pathol.,* 34, 744, 1981.

72. **Quinn, C. M., Bjarnason, I., and Price, A. B.,** Gastritis in patients on non-steroidal anti-inflammatory drugs, *Histopathology,* 23, 341, 1993.

# 9

## Alcoholic Pancreatitis

I. D. Norton and J. S. Wilson

## CONTENTS

## 9.1   INTRODUCTION

Alcoholic pancreatitis is an important complication of alcohol abuse, occurring in up to 5% of heavy drinkers.[1] It is generally a chronic disorder, resulting in significant mortality and a morbidity characterized by malabsorption, malnutrition, abdominal pain, diabetes, and the frequent need for surgery. Unemployment and narcotic addiction are frequent social sequelae. In severely affected patients, financial costs have been estimated to approximate that of liver transplantation (R. Strong, personal communication). Research into the pathogenesis of this disorder has been hampered by the lack of a suitable animal model. Nonetheless, a number of metabolic effects of ethanol on the pancreas which may render the gland susceptible to injury have recently been described.

Management of the patient with alcoholic pancreatitis comprises support of acute episodes of inflammation and the treatment of chronic pain and the complications of pancreatic failure (exocrine and endocrine).

## 9.2   HISTORY

Recognition of ethanol as an etiological factor for pancreatic damage is attributed to Friedreich who, in 1878, described a chronic interstitial pancreatitis which he termed the "Drunkard's Pancreas."[2] Acute hemorrhagic pancreatitis was first described in association with alcohol abuse in 1889 by Reginald Fitz.[3] The relative frequency of ethanol as a cause of pancreatitis is said to have increased in Western society during the twentieth century. This trend has been particularly noticeable in the U.K.[4,5] and Germany[6] and probably relates to increasing per capita consumption of ethanol in these societies since World War II. In Britain, the number of admissions to hospital for alcoholic pancreatitis has increased from 11.1 per million admissions in 1964 to 32.4 per million admissions in 1984.[5] This correlates with increased annual ethanol consumption over the same period, which rose from 4.9 to 7.7 l per capita. More accurate detection of alcohol abuse may have also contributed to the increasing frequency of the diagnosis of alcoholic pancreatitis.

## 9.3   CLASSIFICATION

Pancreatitis is generally classified as either "acute" or "chronic." The older terms "acute relapsing" and "chronic relapsing" were of little benefit to the clinician and are no longer used.

Acute pancreatitis typically presents with constant abdominal pain and raised serum levels of pancreatic enzymes due to inflammation of the gland. The disease ranges from a mild, self-limiting disorder to severe (often lethal) necrotizing pancreatitis. In patients surviving acute pancreatitis, complete recovery of pancreatic function is the rule. This distinguishes it from chronic pancreatitis, where ongoing inflammation causes irreversible morphological changes, often with chronic pain and loss of pancreatic exocrine and endocrine function.

The distinction between acute and chronic pancreatitis is often difficult in the initial stages: acute pancreatitis can recur, and chronic pancreatitis often presents initially as an acute episode, clinically and biochemically indistinct from "acute" pancreatitis. This rarely causes clinical difficulty in the management of the patient, as a flare of chronic pancreatitis is managed in a similar manner as acute pancreatitis.

Alcoholic pancreatitis is usually classified as an example of chronic pancreatitis which may present acutely. Although the patient may initially appear to have discrete episodes of pancreatitis (often precipitated by an alcoholic binge) with complete recovery between attacks, there is evidence that patients with alcoholic pancreatitis may have irreversible pathological changes and radiological evidence of chronic pancreatitis present at the time of the first attack.[7,8] Furthermore, pancreatic fibrosis has been described at post-mortem examination in alcoholics without a history of clinical pancreatitis.[9] Therefore, patients presenting with an acute episode of pancreatic inflammation related to alcohol abuse should be considered as having acute exacerbations of chronic pancreatitis. Recently, however, this view has been challenged. There is increasing evidence that chronic pancreatitis may result from recurrent clinical and subclinical necroinflammatory episodes. A large prospective Swiss study[10] concluded that chronic changes of alcoholic pancreatitis were likely to occur in patients with recurrent episodes of acute inflammation, and suggested that these acute episodes lead to chronic changes. This notion is supported by an autopsy study of 247 cases of fatal alcoholic pancreatitis in which 53% of specimens had no evidence of chronic changes.[11] Further support comes from animal studies where repeated acute experimental pancreatitis led to changes similar to those seen in chronic pancreatitis (atrophy, fibrosis, and fatty infiltration).[12] Given the above evidence, it is possible that a rigid distinction between acute and chronic pancreatitis may have hampered our understanding of the pathogenesis of alcoholic pancreatitis.

## 9.4    INCIDENCE

The incidence of pancreatitis associated with ethanol abuse varies widely between countries and in different studies in the same country. For example, the association of ethanol with acute episodes of pancreatitis has been reported to vary in the U.S. between 5[13] and 90%.[14] These variations are likely to be due to differences in the study populations and the accuracy of identification of alcohol abuse. Approximately 40 to 50% of episodes of acute pancreatic inflammation in Western countries are due to ethanol.

## 9.5    CLINICAL FEATURES

The majority of patients are males between 20 and 50 years of age[15] (mean age 38.7 years at clinical onset[16]). The predominance of males is probably a reflection of the increased incidence of ethanol abuse among men as females appear to be more susceptible to the pancreatotoxic effects of ethanol, with a shorter mean time between onset of heavy drinking and development of pancreatitis.[17] Alcoholic pancreatitis rarely, if ever, follows a single alcoholic debauch,[18] though episodes of acute inflammation often follow a bout of heavy drinking.[19]

The disease usually presents with acute episodes of abdominal pain. With continued alcohol abuse, the attacks become more frequent and pain may be constant. Intractable pain often leads to narcotic addiction. Less commonly, the condition is painless throughout, and the patient presents with pancreatic failure (steatorrhea, diabetes).

Surgery is often performed in an attempt to relieve pain or for complications such as pseudocysts and abscesses. Side-to-side pancreaticojejunostomy (Puestow procedure) totally or substantially relieves pain in more than 70% of patients.[20] Unfortunately, only 30 to 50% of patients are suitable for this procedure.[18] Although the mechanism of the pain is poorly understood, it may relate to duct obstruction leading to intraductal hypertension[21] and/or elevated pancreatic tissue interstitial fluid pressure.[22]

Patients who abstain from ethanol tend to suffer less pain,[23] but studies suggest that parenchymal destruction proceeds in spite of cessation of alcohol.[23,24] The rate of progression, however, is significantly less in those patients who abstain compared to those who continue to drink.[25] There is some evidence that pain tends to subside with time as exocrine pancreatic function declines.[26]

Pancreatic insufficiency usually develops 6 to 8 years after the first episode of pain.[27] Patients tend to become emaciated in the later stages of the disease and die within 5 to 10 years of diagnosis. Death is usually due to pancreatitis, its complications, or ethanol-induced damage to other organs.

## 9.6    PATHOLOGY

Our knowledge about the histological changes in this disease has generally been acquired by examination of operative or post-mortem specimens, and as such, may overrepresent advanced forms of the disease. The histological changes are nonspecific. Even pancreatic calcification, which is commonly found, is not pathognomonic.

An acute episode is accompanied by edema and inflammatory cell infiltrate, and in severe cases, necrosis and hemorrhage. Peripancreatic inflammation may also be present. Pseudocysts may develop over the ensuing weeks. (A pseudocyst is a persistent, localized collection of necrotic tissue and pancreatic secretions surrounded by a rim of fibrous tissue. The cavity is lined by granulation tissue, as opposed to a true cyst, which has an epithelial lining.) Abscesses may

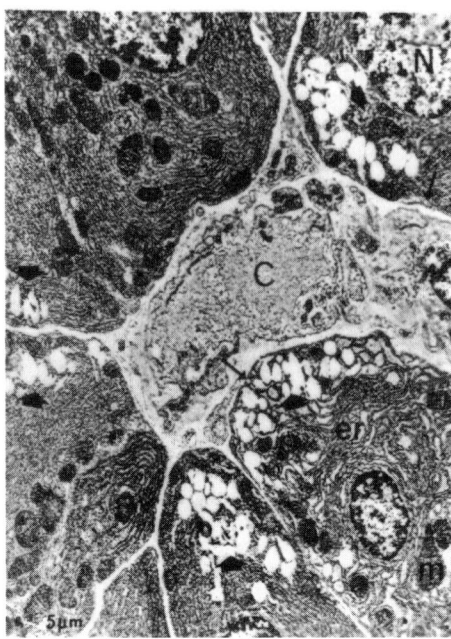

**FIGURE 9.1**  Electron micrograph showing acinar tissue of a rat fed ethanol. Capillary (C) is surrounded by acinar cells containing nuclei (N), mitochondria (m), and endoplasmic reticulum (er). Numerous fat droplets (large arrows) are seen in these cells near the capillary. Pinocytic vesicles (small arrows) are also present. (Original magnification: ×6700.)

arise from either necrotic tissue or infection in a pseudocyst. Infective complications carry a high mortality even with surgical debridement.

The chronically affected gland appears fibrosed and atrophic. The main pancreatic duct and secondary ducts contain strictures with dilatation of the duct system proximally. Intraductal proteinaceous deposits are a characteristic (but not pathognomonic) finding. Intrapancreatic retention cysts may also be present. These alterations to the ductal system lead to a characteristic appearance at endoscopic pancreatography. Microscopically, islets of Langerhans tend to be preserved until late in the process.

Ultrastructural changes have been reported within acinar cells of alcoholics in the absence of pancreatitis (fat droplet accumulation, mitochondrial distortion, and hyperplasia of endoplasmic reticulum).[28-30] Similar changes have been described in animals fed ethanol (Figure 1).[31] One study demonstrated a correlation between alcoholism and interstitial pancreatitis at autopsy.[32]

## 9.7    PATHOGENESIS

The pathogenesis of alcoholic pancreatitis has not been elucidated, mainly because of the lack of a suitable animal model of this disorder and practical difficulties in obtaining pancreatic tissue from patients during various phases of the disease.

Research into the pathogenesis of this condition has generally followed two directions: (1) at the clinical level, since only a minority of alcoholics develop pancreatitis, there has been a search for possible predisposing factors; and (2) at the experimental level, the constant effects of ethanol on the pancreas which may predispose to, or initiate, damage have been studied.

### 9.7.1    Factors Influencing Individual Susceptibility

Despite a great deal of research in this area, no predisposing factors to alcoholic pancreatitis have been clearly identified (see Table 9.1). The essential comparison in studies into the susceptibility

**TABLE 9.1   Predisposing Factors**

Heredity
HLA serotype
Alpha$_1$-antitrypsin phenotype
Blood group antigens
Smoking
Lipid intolerance/hypertriglyceridemia
Cystic fibrosis genotype
Type of beverage ingested
Pattern of alcohol consumption
Diet

*Note:* This table summarizes the factors which have been previously studied in an attempt to identify a subgroup of heavy drinkers at risk of developing alcoholic pancreatitis. There is no convincing evidence that any of these factors predispose individuals to pancreatitis.

to alcoholic pancreatitis must be between alcoholic patients with pancreatitis and alcoholics without pancreatitis, so that the only variable between the index and control groups is the presence or absence of pancreatitis.

The following lists some of the predisposing factors to alcoholic pancreatitis which have been investigated.

### 9.7.1.1   Heredity

#### *9.7.1.1.1   HLA Serotype*

A genetic predisposition to alcoholic pancreatitis has been suggested by reports of increased incidences in this condition of HLA antigens B40,[33] Aw23,[34] Aw24,[34] B13,[35] and Bw39.[36] Only the last study incorporated an alcoholic control group, thus eliminating the presence of alcoholism as an additional variable. In this study, the incidence of HLA Bw49 was increased in patients with alcoholic pancreatitis (odds ratio: 3:4). However, given the fact that only 14% of patients with alcoholic pancreatitis manifested the HLA Bw39 serotype, the significance of this finding is uncertain.

#### *9.7.1.1.2   Alpha$_1$-Antitrypsin Phenotype*

Alpha$_1$-antitrypsin is the major protease inhibitor of serum. It is possible that a less effective phenotype may predispose the pancreas to damage by proteases such as trypsin. Studies examining the relationship of alpha$_1$-antitrypsin phenotype to alcoholic pancreatitis have provided conflicting results.[37,38] However, most of these studies were poorly designed, utilizing the general population as a control group. Only one recent study has used alcoholics without pancreatitis as the control group, and in this study there was no association between alcoholic pancreatitis and either particular alpha$_1$-antitrypsin phenotypes or total serum levels of the inhibitor.[39]

#### *9.7.1.1.3   Blood Group Antigens*

Blood groups O[40] and Lewis a- b-[40,41] have reportedly occurred more frequently in patients with alcoholic pancreatitis, but these results have not been corroborated by other studies.[42,43]

### 9.7.1.2   Smoking

There is evidence that smoking (and nicotine exposure) may play a role in pancreatic damage. Smoking has been shown to inhibit pancreatic secretion *in vivo*[44] and *in vitro*[45] while high dose nicotine has been shown to increase pancreatic enzyme synthesis.[46] Nicotine exposure has also been associated with pancreatic acinar vacuole formation and nuclear pyknosis in rats.[47,48]

Several studies have reported an association between smoking and alcoholic pancreatitis.[49,50] There is a correlation, however, between smoking and ethanol abuse *per se*, so that the high incidence of smoking in patients with alcoholic pancreatitis may reflect their heavy ethanol consumption rather than a direct association with pancreatic disease. A recent study comparing patients with alcoholic pancreatitis with an alcoholic control group failed to demonstrate a link between smoking and alcoholic pancreatitis.[51]

### 9.7.1.3    Lipid Intolerance and Hypertriglyceridemia

Hypertriglyceridemia is a well-established cause of pancreatitis.[52] Furthermore, chronic ethanol consumption is associated with both fasting and postprandial hypertriglyceridemia which are thought to result from increased hepatic production of lipoproteins. Therefore, it has been hypothesized that ethanol-induced hypertriglyceridemia may be a significant cause of pancreatitis in alcoholics.

Some studies have suggested that postprandial hypertriglyceridemia (assessed by a tolerance test) may be associated with pancreatitis more commonly than previously recognized. Guzman et al.[53] reported impaired oral lipid tolerance in subjects with previous pancreatitis (mostly gallstone induced). Serum triglyceride levels after an oral lipid load rose to higher levels in patients with previous pancreatitis than in controls. Subsequent investigations by this group demonstrated a delay in the clearance of chylomicron remnants from the blood in those patients with impaired lipid tolerance.[54] Delayed lipid clearance in pancreatitis patients has also been reported following an intravenous lipid tolerance test.[55] In contrast, others have reported normal clearance of intravenous fat in patients with hyperlipemic pancreatitis.[56] Recently, however, a comprehensive study by Haber et al.[57] showed no difference in oral lipid tolerance between patients with alcoholic pancreatitis and alcoholics without pancreatitis. This suggests that hypertriglyceridemia is unlikely to be the link between alcohol abuse and the development of pancreatitis.

### 9.7.1.4    Cystic Fibrosis Genotype

The cystic fibrosis transmembrane conductance regulator (CFTR) gene codes for an epithelial chloride channel which spans the apical membrane of exocrine ductal cells. This gene has recently been located and sequenced and its protein product characterized.[58,59] In the homozygote state, abnormalities of this protein lead to impaired chloride transport and clinical cystic fibrosis. There is some evidence that heterozygosity for CF causes subclinical changes in exocrine secretion.[60] It is theoretically possible that heterozygosity for an abnormal CFTR could lead to viscid pancreatic secretions predisposing to small duct obstruction with subsequent pancreatic injury in the presence of excess alcohol consumption. However, a recent study has failed to demonstrate a link between heterozygosity for various CFTR mutations ($\Delta$F-508, G551D, and G542X) and alcoholic pancreatitis.[61]

### 9.7.1.5    Type of Alcoholic Beverage Ingested

Some studies have reported an increased incidence of alcoholic pancreatitis among patients who consumed predominantly beer,[62,63] wine,[64] or spirits.[64] However, these findings probably reflect the predominant drinking habits of the populations being studied. Wilson et al.[65] could find no difference in the type of alcoholic beverage ingested when patients with alcoholic pancreatitis were compared to an alcoholic control group.

### 9.7.1.6    Pattern of Alcohol Consumption

It is a common clinical perception that binge drinking occurs more commonly in patients with alcoholic pancreatitis. However, literature on whether the drinking pattern of ethanol affects the risk of developing alcoholic pancreatitis is conflicting.[62,65] When this was examined in a controlled fashion, there was no difference between the drinking patterns of alcoholics with pancreatitis and alcoholics without pancreatitis.[65] Nonetheless, binge drinking is associated with the precipitation of acute attacks of pancreatic inflammation.

### 9.7.1.7. Diet

The traditional view has been that poor nutrition is an etiological factor in alcoholic pancreatitis. Malnutrition is a well-known association of alcoholism and can be associated with alterations in pancreatic structure and function. Pancreatic hyposecretion in alcoholics in the U.S. has been associated with malnutrition.[66] In addition, protein deficient human infants in Hungary following World War II were noted to have decreased pancreatic exocrine function and acinar cell atrophy at autopsy.[67] Furthermore, in animal models, experimental protein deficiency has been shown to result in pancreatic atrophy and decreased digestive enzyme activity,[68] as well as exacerbating some of the pancreatotoxic effects of experimental ethanol administration.[69] Finally, it is of interest to note that malnutrition is associated with chronic calcific pancreatitis in parts of Africa, India, and Southeast Asia (so called "tropical pancreatitis").[70]

In contrast to malnutrition, there is evidence to suggest that a *high* caloric intake predisposes to alcoholic pancreatitis. Increases in dietary fat and protein have intensified experimental pancreatitis in animals.[71] This could be due to increased enzyme synthesis and thus an increased propensity for autodigestion, since the pancreas demonstrates dietary adaptation by increasing its content of digestive enzymes in response to the composition of the diet.[72,73] In accord with this view is the finding of Durbec and Sarles that patients with alcoholic pancreatitis tend to consume more fat and protein than age and sex matched controls.[74] However, this study used nonalcoholic controls rather than alcoholics without pancreatitis. Another study found that patients with alcoholic pancreatitis consume more fat than patients with alcoholic cirrhosis (without pancreatitis).[75] Unfortunately, the alcoholic controls in this latter study were on average 13 years older than those with pancreatitis and this difference may have accounted for the dietary differences. Wilson et al.[65] compared dietary intake of patients with alcoholic pancreatitis and a control group with alcoholic cirrhosis. When adjusted for differences in age and sex using multiple regression analysis, there was no difference in dietary composition in the two groups. In fact, both groups were well nourished and had a nonethanol caloric intake comparable to that of the normal population.

## 9.7.2    Constant Effects of Ethanol on the Pancreas

These include the effects of ethanol on the pancreas (either parenchyma or ductal system) which may render the gland susceptible to injury.

### 9.7.2.1    Role of Pancreatic Digestive Enzymes

The pancreas is the major digestive organ of the body. It functions as an "enzyme factory." Each acinar cell synthesizes up to $10^7$ enzyme molecules per day, resulting in the gland delivering 6 to 20 g of digestive enzyme per day to the duodenum. In health, the gland is protected from enzyme-induced injury by synthesizing many of these digestive enzymes as inactive precursors, by segregating digestive enzymes from other components of the cell, and by intracellular protease inhibitors.

Given the central role of the acinar cell in digestive enzyme production and the potential of activated enzymes for tissue injury, it seems reasonable to implicate activated digestive enzymes in pancreatic injury. Active digestive enzymes (including proteases and lipase[76] and phospholipase $A_2$[77]) have been shown to produce necrosis when instilled into the pancreatic duct. Similarly, the injection of elastase into the pancreatic interstitium results in injury, particularly to intrapancreatic blood vessels.[78] Active digestive enzymes have been identified in ascitic fluid,[79,80] pancreatic juice,[81] and pancreatic tissue[82] in both clinical and experimental pancreatitis. Furthermore, protease inhibitors have been shown to reduce the severity of experimental pancreatitis.[83,84]

Several animal models of acute pancreatitis (hyperstimulation with the CCK analog caerulein,[85] main pancreatic duct obstruction,[86,87] and the choline deficient/ethionine supplemented diet model[88]) have highlighted the potential importance of digestive enzyme activation by lysosomal hydrolases in pancreatitis. In this regard, the lysosomal enzyme cathepsin B is known to be capable of activating trypsinogen to trypsin.[89] Trypsin thus activated, as well as disrupting enzymes and structural proteins within the pancreas, can activate other inactive enzyme precursors, thereby initiating a digestive enzyme cascade.

### 9.7.2.2   Pathogenetic Theories

Currently, the main theories concerning the pathogenesis of alcoholic pancreatitis are (1) sphincteric theories, (2) protein plug theory, and (3) direct acinar cell toxicity theories.

Theories on the pathogenesis of alcoholic pancreatitis originally focused on altered motility of the sphincter of Oddi induced by ethanol. This focus was inspired by Opie's observations regarding the pathogenesis of gallstone pancreatitis.[90] In the 1970s, due mainly to the work of Sarles and co-workers, focus shifted to the effects of ethanol on the small ducts, in particular, the precipitation of protein within the ducts. Over the past 10 years, research has centered on the effects of ethanol or its metabolites on the acinar cell. Each of these theories will now be dealt with in detail.

#### *9.7.2.2.1   Sphincteric Theories*

Several different theories postulate a central role for sphincter of Oddi dysfunction in the pathogenesis of alcoholic pancreatitis. Each of these theories depends on altered motility (spasm or relaxation) of the sphincter of Oddi in response to ethanol administration.

*9.7.2.2.1.1  Biliary-Pancreatic Reflux.*   This theory, as applied to the pathogenesis of alcoholic pancreatitis, proposes that ethanol-induced spasm of the sphincter of Oddi creates a common channel between the common bile duct and pancreatic duct, enabling bile to reflux into the pancreatic duct and initiate pancreatitis. The theoretical requirements for biliary-pancreatic reflux to cause pancreatitis are:

- *The presence of a common pancreaticobiliary channel in the ampulla of Vater via which bile can reflux from the biliary tree into the main pancreatic duct.* This common channel is present in between 50 and 90% of the population.[91,92] It has been demonstrated, however, that alcoholic pancreatitis can occur in the absence of a common channel. Indeed, a common channel has reportedly been absent in the majority of patients with alcoholic pancreatitis.[93] Furthermore, the components of the sphincter which surround both ducts have been demonstrated to function as a single unit in the cat;[95] hence, sphincter contraction would most likely impede both flow out of the common bile duct as well as reflux into the main pancreatic duct.
- *Biliary pressure in excess of pancreatic pressure.* Pancreatic duct pressure generally exceeds common duct pressure in both experimental animal models[94-97] and humans.[98,99] It has been demonstrated, however, that biliary pressure may intermittently exceed pancreatic pressure, particularly during maneuvers such as coughing, straining, and vomiting.[100]
- *The capability of bile to initiate pancreatitis.* Early investigators induced pancreatitis in animals by injecting bile into the pancreatic duct.[90,101] However, the bile was generally injected under high pressure and volume. Diversion of the entire bile flow at normal pressure through the pancreatic duct of experimental animals does not result in pancreatitis.[102,103]

Potentially toxic constituents of bile include reactive hepatic metabolites, bile salts, lysolecithin, and enterokinase. When injected into the pancreatic duct, bile from ethanol-fed rats induces more severe pancreatitis than control bile or control bile with ethanol added to it.[104,105] Braganza[106] has proposed that reactive products of ethanol metabolism in the liver may be excreted in the bile, then reflux into the pancreatic duct and initiate pancreatitis.

Bile salts have been shown to induce pancreatitis when injected into the pancreatic duct[107] or pancreatic interstitium.[108] Physiological concentrations of bile salts injected into the cat pancreatic duct have resulted in injury to pancreatic duct epithelium with increased permeability to macromolecules.[109]

Lysolecithin is a potent detergent which is toxic to pancreatic membranes.[110,111] Lysolecithin may be formed from lecithin in the pancreatic duct via the action of phospholipase $A_2$. Theoretically, this is possible following the reflux of bile into the pancreatic duct and activation of digestive enzymes by enterokinase, which is present in bile via an enterohepatic circulation.[112]

*9.7.2.2.1.2 Duodenopancreatic Reflux.*   This theory postulates that damage occurs via reflux of duodenal juice (containing enterokinase) into the pancreatic duct. This would result in intraglandular activation of digestive enzymes. Support for this theory comes from the work of Viceconte,[113] who demonstrated via an endoscopic manometric technique that human sphincter of Oddi resistance decreased in response to ethanol administration (via both decreased basal tone as well as frequency and amplitude of phasic contractions). In contrast, the work of Pirola and Davis[114-116] has demonstrated that acute ethanol administration to humans causes increased resistance to flow at the choledochoduodenal junction, suggesting a "spasmogenic" effect of ethanol on the sphincter.

*9.7.2.2.1.3 Sphincteric Obstruction.*   This theory proposes that ethanol increases pancreatic duct pressure by simultaneously inducing sphincter of Oddi spasm as well as increasing pancreatic secretion.

Ligation of the main pancreatic duct (usually in the presence of stimulation of secretion) has caused experimental pancreatitis in a number of animal models.[117-119] Ductal rupture and extravasation of pancreatic juice into the parenchyma has been reported at ductal pressures achieved with stimulation *in vivo*.[119] The effect of ductal obstruction without stimulation, however, has varied in different animal models. Obstruction without stimulation in the rat[120] results in pancreatic atrophy with little inflammation. In contrast, ligation of the opossum pancreatic duct without pancreatic stimulation results in acute necrotizing pancreatitis.[121]

Ductal hypertension has been shown to result in colocalization of lysosomal and digestive enzymes within the acinar cell,[86,122] thereby possibly initiating pancreatitis intracellularly by trypsinogen activation (via cathepsin B[123] or autoactivation in an acidic environment[124]).

Over the years, much research has focused on the effect of ethanol on pancreatic secretion and this will be reviewed here. The assumption in this direction of research is that altered pancreatic secretion plays a role in the pathogenesis of alcoholic pancreatitis. This notion is implied in the "sphincteric obstruction theory" of alcoholic pancreatitis (*vide supra*) and several recently developed models of acute pancreatitis.[125]

Experiments determining the effect of ethanol on pancreatic secretion have varied in a number of respects:

    a. The species studied — human, rat, guinea pig, rabbit.
    b. The mode of ethanol administration — oral (intragastric) or intravenous.
    c. Whether or not gastric acid has been diverted from the intestine.
    d. The secretory state of the pancreas during the study — resting or stimulated.
    e. Whether ethanol was administered acutely or chronically.
    f. Whether an *in vivo* or *in vitro* study was performed.
    g. The conscious state of the animal at the time of the study.

For the purposes of this review, the effects of acute ethanol administration on pancreatic secretion will be discussed first followed by the effects of chronic administration.

The effect of acute oral (or intragastric) ethanol administration appears to be species dependent. An acute intragastric dose of ethanol increases basal pancreatic secretion in the rat[126] and dog.[127] Traditionally, this response has been thought to be mediated by stimulation of gastric acid release which can be produced by intravenous as well as oral ethanol.[128,129] Gastric acid in turn stimulates secretion of secretin from the duodenal mucosa.[130] Ethanol also stimulates the gastric antrum to release gastrin which stimulates pancreatic secretion.[131] However, this traditional view of the stimulatory effect of ethanol has been challenged. Rendering rats achlorhydric with cimetidine has not abolished the effect of intragastric ethanol on pancreatic secretion.[130] In addition, oral alcohol has been reported to cause a prompt rise (within 5 min) in serum secretin in human subjects — an effect thought to be due to a direct release of secretin by ethanol,[132] but this finding has not been corroborated by other researchers in human subjects, dogs, or cats.[133,134] Therefore, the exact mechanism whereby oral ethanol administration stimulates pancreatic secretion in experimental animals remains unknown.

The recent work by Hajnal et al.[135] has suggested that oral ethanol inhibits pancreatic secretion in humans. In this study, patients received a test meal with or without different alcoholic beverages. Pancreatic output was assessed by constant duodenal aspiration. However, as juice was obtained from the duodenum, ethanol-induced spasm of the sphincter of Oddi could have impeded pancreatic flow,[114-116] thus accounting for the results.

Ethanol also exerts a direct influence on pancreatic secretion but the type of effect appears to depend on the secretory state of the gland, i.e., resting or stimulated. Acute ethanol administration inhibits pancreatic secretion in glands which are stimulated by secretagogues. This has been demonstrated following intravenous ethanol administration in dogs[136] and rats[137] as well as isolated guinea pig acinar cells.[138] Ethanol and acetaldehyde have been shown to inhibit pancreatic secretion *in vitro*, but only at high concentrations which are not observed *in vivo*.[139,140] The mechanism of this phenomenon is unknown, but may result from direct cellular toxicity of ethanol and/or its metabolites or stimulation of secretion of an inhibitory hormone. In humans, intravenous ethanol administration has been reported to depress pancreatic secretion,[141] but as with the Hajnal study (*vide supra*), this effect may be explained by effects of ethanol on the sphincter of Oddi.

The mechanism of the direct inhibitory effect of ethanol on stimulated pancreatic secretion is unknown. The work of Uhlemann et al.[138] with isolated guinea pig acinar cells has indicated that ethanol does not interfere with secretagogue binding but rather enhances adenylate cyclase activity and c-AMP production in response to secretagogues. The effect is abolished in dogs by vagotomy,[142] atropine,[143] and ganglion blockade,[142] indicating that it may be vagally mediated.

The direct effect of ethanol on pancreatic basal secretion is more controversial. Intravenous ethanol has been reported to stimulate basal secretion in the rat,[137] but to cause inhibition in the rabbit.[144] Species differences and differences in the conscious state of the animals may account for this discrepancy. The effect of ethanol on basal pancreatic secretion has also been studied *in vitro* with reports of both stimulation[143] and inhibition[140] with rabbit pancreas and of stimulation using isolated guinea pig acinar cells.[138] However, these *in vitro* studies have utilized concentrations of ethanol far in excess of what would be found during intoxication. Using more physiological doses, Valenzuela et al.[145] have demonstrated no effects of *in vitro* ethanol on pigeon pancreas enzyme release.

Examination of pure pancreatic juice collected endoscopically from alcoholic human subjects without pancreatic insufficiency or pancreatitis has revealed an increased output of enzymes,[146,147] together with an increased trypsinogen:trypsin inhibitor ratio following pancreatic stimulation.[147] Such a situation of increased enzyme output in the presence of a relative deficiency of trypsin inhibitor could conceivably contribute to the susceptibility of the gland to injury.

Several investigators have examined the effect of chronic ethanol administration on basal *and* stimulated pancreatic secretion in experimental animals.[148-152] Most of these studies have been characterized by a failure to strictly match caloric intake in ethanol-fed and control animals and their findings therefore cannot be interpreted with precision. A study by Singh[153] utilizing isocaloric diets found that chronic ethanol administration led to increased basal, but not stimulated secretion of amylase, trypsinogen and lipase *in vitro*.

From the foregoing review, the following facts emerge concerning the effect of ethanol on human pancreatic secretion: (1) acute ethanol administration probably inhibits pancreatic secretion but the mechanism of this effect is not resolved; and (2) alcoholics without evidence of pancreatic damage secrete a pancreatic juice with increased concentrations of digestive enzymes and an increased trypsinogen:trypsin inhibitor ratio.

### 9.7.2.2.2    Protein Plug Theory

This theory, originally proposed by Sarles,[154,155] proposes that ethanol consumption leads to pancreatitis via precipitation of secreted protein within the pancreatic ducts. Obstruction of the ducts leads to acinar inflammation, atrophy, and fibrosis. In addition, the plugs may cause inflammatory lesions in adjacent pancreatic ductal walls with secondary damage to acini.[156] A problem with this theory is that it has not been convincingly demonstrated that the formation of ductal plugs *precedes* acinar damage. Hence, it is debated that the protein plugs may result from events in the acinar cell, rather than cause them. Regardless of whether intraductal protein plugs are an initiating event in pancreatitis or a consequence of pancreatic inflammation, they are a prominent pathological feature and may help propagate pancreatic injury once initiated.

Several factors may contribute to intraductal plug formation. Ethanol consumption increases the total protein concentration of pancreatic juice in humans.[157] Recent studies suggest that alterations in two secretory proteins (lactoferrin, and in particular lithostathine) may favor plug formation.

Lactoferrin is an iron binding protein which may facilitate the precipitation of protein plugs by binding to acidic proteins.[158] Lactoferrin is increased in the pancreatic juice of patients with alcoholic pancreatitis.[159] However, whether this observed increase in lactoferrin precedes pancreatitis, or is secondary to pancreatic injury is debatable. Furthermore, studies examining lactoferrin levels in the pancreatic juice of alcoholics without pancreatitis have provided conflicting results.[160,161]

A novel pancreatic secretory protein, initially called "pancreatic stone protein" and later "lithostathine," has been recently described. It was initially identified as a major component of ductal plugs.[162] It is now known to be a normal component of pancreatic juice, accounting for 5 to 10% of total pancreatic secretory protein. Lithostathine is a 144 amino acid protein. The active region of the protein is the N-terminal 11 amino acids. Cleavage of this peptide from the protein leads to the formation of a 133-amino acid insoluble protein (lithostathine $S_1$). Two properties of lithostathine give it relevance to the protein plug theory:

a. Inhibition of $CaCO_3$ crystallization. Normal pancreatic juice is supersaturated with calcium carbonate ($CaCO_3$).[163] Native lithostathine inhibits $CaCO_3$ crystallization *in vitro*[164] and probably serves as a physiological inhibitor of calcium carbonate crystallization. Similar proteins are also excreted by the urinary tract, presumably with the same function.

b. Spontaneous precipitation. The tendency of lithostathine to form precipitates has been highlighted by studies on pancreatic juice obtained at endoscopic pancreatography.[165] This is due to hydrolysis of the Arg-Ile bond at position 11-12, yielding the insoluble 133-amino acid $S_1$ form of lithostathine. This occurs in pancreatic juice of normal patients, but occurs with increasing frequency in alcoholics and those with established pancreatitis. Significantly, trypsin is capable of cleaving the protein at this site, suggesting a possible role for active proteolytic enzymes in the generation of lithostathine $S_1$.

The physical property of lithostathine maintaining $CaCO_3$ in solution in pancreatic juice may be important in the development of pancreatic calcification. Reduced levels of lithostathine in the pancreatic juice of patients with chronic pancreatitis have been detected by Sarles et al.,[166] but this has not been confirmed by Schmiegel et al.[167] Reduced levels of lithostathine may favor

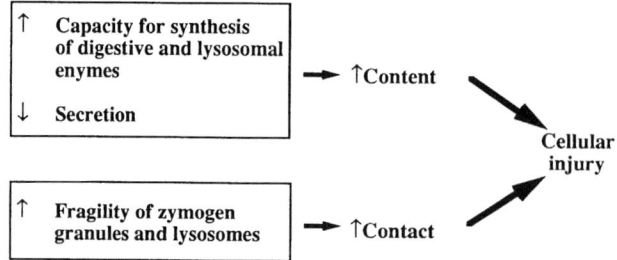

**FIGURE 9.2**  Proposed mechanism of direct cellular toxicity. Ethanol increases the pancreatic content of digestive enzymes and the lysosomal enzyme cathepsin B. This occurs via increased enzyme synthesis, and, in the case of digestive enzymes, possibly also via inhibition of secretion. In addition, ethanol increases the fragility of lysosomal and zymogen membranes, thus potentiating intracellular contact between digestive and lysosomal enzymes. This "colocalization" has been identified as an early event in experimental pancreatitis.

precipitation of calcium salts, facilitating stone formation. In this regard, it is interesting to note that pancreatic messenger RNA levels for lithostathine are reduced in patients with chronic pancreatitis.[168]

The effect of experimental ethanol administration on gene expression of lithostathine in the pancreas has attracted the attention of several groups, but the results of these studies have been conflicting. On one hand, Dagorn concluded that chronic ethanol administration had no effect on messenger RNA levels for lithostathine.[169] However, under conditions of strict nutritional control, using Lieber-DeCarli diets, Apte and co-workers have recently shown that lithostathine mRNA levels are increased by both chronic ethanol administration and protein deficiency — two conditions associated with chronic pancreatitis.[170]

### 9.7.2.2.3  *Direct Toxicity of Ethanol Theories*

Mainly as a result of the work by Steer and Meldolesi,[171] attention has recently focused on the effects of ethanol or its metabolites on the acinar cell. Currently there are two major theories concerning this direct toxicity. Common to both theories is the hypothesis that the initiating event of alcoholic pancreatitis occurs within the acinar cell.

*9.7.2.2.3.1 Intracellular Autodigestion.*  This theory postulates that the initiating event of alcoholic pancreatitis is colocalization of digestive enzymes within the acinar cell with subsequent activation of trypsinogen either by cathepsin B or autoactivation at an acidic pH. Though intracellular activation of digestive enzymes has not been demonstrated after chronic ethanol administration, there is substantial evidence from animal models that ethanol consumption leads to changes within the acinar cell which provide a primed setting for digestive enzyme activation (Figure 9.2).

It has recently been reported that rats chronically fed ethanol exhibit increased pancreatic lysosomal fragility.[172] Furthermore, this effect is probably mediated by fatty acid ethyl esters and cholesteryl esters, substances which accumulate in the pancreas following consumption of ethanol,[173,174] and have been shown to be capable of increasing the fragility of pancreatic lysosomes *in vitro*.[174,175] Interestingly, neither ethanol nor acetaldehyde (a product of ethanol metabolism) had any effect on lysosomal fragility *in vitro*.[174]

Similar to the effect of ethanol on lysosomes, chronic ethanol consumption has been shown to increase the fragility of rat pancreatic zymogen granules.[176] The mechanism of this effect is unknown.

Chronic consumption of ethanol in rats has been shown to increase pancreatic tissue levels of trypsinogen,[177] chymotrypsinogen,[177] lipase,[178] and the lysosomal enzyme cathepsin B.[179] Recent work has demonstrated that these ethanol-induced increases are associated with increases in the corresponding messenger RNA levels for these enzymes. In addition, for each enzyme studied there was a close correlation between the increase in mRNA levels and the increase in the

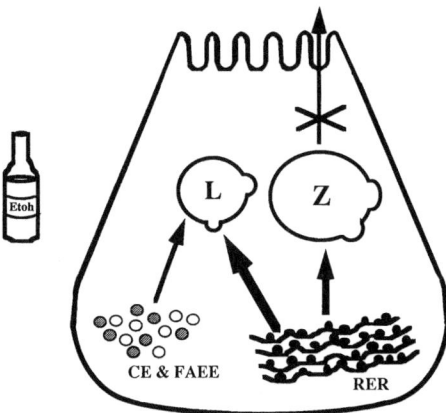

**FIGURE 9.3**  "The Drinker's Pancreas."

corresponding protein product, suggesting that the observed ethanol-induced increases in pancreatic enzyme levels are regulated predominantly at the mRNA level.[180] Another possible mechanism whereby ethanol may increase digestive enzyme content is via inhibition of secretion of digestive enzymes. This topic is discussed in more detail in the section dealing with the effect of ethanol on pancreatic secretion (*vide supra*).

The studies described above have led to the concept of "The Drinker's Pancreas" (see Figure 9.3), an organ in which there is both increased content of digestive and lysosomal enzymes and the potential for contact between these enzymes (via increased organelle fragility). These alterations in rat pancreas occur in the absence of overt cellular injury suggesting that one or more trigger factors may be required to initiate autodigestion in this primed setting. Such putative trigger factors are as yet unknown.

*9.7.2.2.3.2 Oxidant Stress Theory.* Braganza and co-workers[181] have hypothesized that the metabolism of xenobiotics within the acinar cell results in the formation of reactive oxygen species which subsequently damage the cell.

Under conditions of low to moderate ethanol intake, ethanol is primarily oxidized to acetaldehyde via alcohol dehydrogenase. At higher levels of ethanol consumption, another microsomal enzyme system is induced which becomes a major pathway of ethanol metabolism in heavy drinkers. Originally termed the microsomal ethanol oxidizing system (MEOS), it is now clear that this is almost entirely due to a single form of cytochrome P-450 (CYP) termed CYP2E1[182] ("cytochrome P-450" is actually a superfamily of over 300 enzymes, of which CYP2E1 is one). In the process of catalyzing the oxidation of ethanol to acetaldehyde, CYP2E1 generates toxic oxygen species such as hydrogen peroxide and hydroxyl radicals. Usually, these compounds are rapidly metabolized by enzymes or inactivated by free radical scavengers.

The oxidant stress theory proposes that under conditions of heavy ethanol intake and subsequent CYP2E1 induction within the acinar cell these protective mechanisms become saturated and fail, leading to oxidant damage within the acinar cell. Although there is no direct evidence that these events occur within the acinar cell, several indirect lines of evidence support this theory's plausibility:

- Although the vast majority of CYP2E1 activity is within the liver, it has been identified in many other parts of the gastrointestinal tract.[183] Following chronic ethanol administration to rats, induction of CYP2E1 has been demonstrated in many tissues, but to date pancreatic tissue has not been assessed in this regard. However, in a human study, the levels of two other CYPs (3A1 and 1A2) were elevated in pancreatic acinar cells of patients with chronic pancreatitis (the etiology of chronic pancreatitis in these patients was not specified).[184]

- Products of reactive oxygen species (free radical oxidation products) such as diene conjugates and 9 *cis*,11 *trans* linoleic acid have been found in increased quantity in the duodenal juice of patients with both acute and chronic pancreatitis.[185]
- Increased pancreatic tissue levels of free radicals have been observed in animal models of experimental pancreatitis.[186,187] The significance of this finding is questioned, since free radical generation is a nonspecific response to tissue injury.
- Antioxidant therapy (with allopurinol and superoxide dismutase) has been shown to ameliorate acute experimental pancreatitis.[188] Furthermore, antioxidants have reportedly been of value in the treatment of both acute and chronic pancreatitis in uncontrolled clinical trials.[189,190]

## 9.8   SUMMARY

Alcoholic pancreatitis is a relatively frequent and potentially lethal complication of ethanol abuse. Ethanol has many effects on the pancreas which may predispose the gland to digestive enzyme-induced injury, although the mechanisms by which ethanol (or its metabolites) causes pancreatic injury remain largely unknown. While activated digestive enzymes are undoubtedly involved in the inflammatory process, the initiating event has yet to be identified. Studies of sphincteric function in response to ethanol provide conflicting results, and it is increasingly unlikely that sphincteric dysfunction plays a significant role in most patients. While pancreatic duct damage and lithiasis are prominent in advanced cases, their role in the early stages of the process remains unproved.

The long-term complications of alcoholic pancreatitis are exocrine and endocrine pancreatic failure, chronic pain, and frequent narcotic addiction. These complications occur more rapidly in patients who continue to drink. Other than abstention, there are no specific measures to prevent, reverse, or slow the disease process. Management of the patient with alcoholic pancreatitis is essentially supportive, both in the acute and chronic phases of the illness. Significant improvement in the management of these patients will hopefully occur as the pathogenesis of the disorder becomes more clear.

## REFERENCES

1. **Steinberg, W. and Tenner, S.,** Acute pancreatitis, *N. Engl. J. Med.,* 330, 1198, 1994.
2. **Friedreich, N.,** Disease of the pancreas, in *Cyclopedia of the Practice of Medicine,* Ziemssen, H., Ed., William Wood, New York, 1878, 549.
3. **Fitz, R. H.,** Acute pancreatitis, *Med. Rec.,* 35, 197, 1889.
4. **Pollock, A. V.,** Acute pancreatitis. Analysis of 100 patients, *Br. Med. J.,* 1, 6, 1959.
5. **Trapnell, J. E. and Duncan, E. H. L.,** Patterns in incidence of acute pancreatitis, *Br. Med. J.,* 2, 179, 1975.
6. **Bocker, W. and Seifert, G.,** Zur pathologie der alkohol — pankreatitis. Haufigkeit, Klassification, Pathogenese, *Dtsch. Med. Wochenschr.,* 97, 803, 1972.
7. **Strum, W. B. and Spiro, H. M.,** Chronic pancreatitis, *Ann. Intern. Med.,* 74, 264, 1971.
8. **Howard, J. M. and Ehrlich, E. W.,** The etiology of pancreatitis. A review of clinical experience, *Ann. Surg.,* 152, 135, 1960.
9. **Pitchumoni, C. S., Glasser, M., Saran, R. M., Panchacharam, P., and Thelmo, W.,** Pancreatic fibrosis in chronic alcoholics and nonalcoholics without clinical pancreatitis, *Am. J. Gastroenterol.,* 79, 382, 1984.
10. **Ammann, R. W. and Muellhaupt, B.,** Progression of alcoholic acute to chronic pancreatitis, *Gut,* 35, 552, 1974.
11. **Brenner, I. G., Savage, W. T., Pantoja, J. L., and Renner, V. J.,** Death due to acute pancreatitis, *Dig. Dis. Sci.,* 30, 1005, 1985.
12. **Niederau, C., Ferrell, L. D., Liddle, R. A., and Grendell, J. H.,** Biochemical, secretory and morphological effects of repetitive experimental acute pancreatitis, *Gastroenterology,* 90, 1565A, 1986.
13. **Thal, A. P., Perry, J. F., and Egner, W. A.,** Clinical and morphological study of forty-two cases of fatal acute pancreatitis, *Surg. Gynecol. Obstet.,* 105, 191, 1957.
14. **Albo, R., Silen, W., and Goldman, L.,** A critical analysis of acute pancreatitis, *Arch. Surg.,* 86, 1032, 1963.
15. **Wilson, J. S. and Pirola, R. C.,** Pathogenesis of acute pancreatitis, *Aust. N.Z. J. Med.,* 13, 307, 1983.
16. **Sarles, H., Sarles, J. C., Camatte, R., Muratore, R., Gaini, M., Guien, C., Pastor, J., and Le Roy, F.,** Observations of 205 confirmed cases of acute pancreatitis, *Gut,* 6, 545, 1965.

17. **Durbec, J. P. and Sarles, H.,** Multicentre study of the epidemiology of pancreatic diseases. Relationship between the relative risk of developing chronic pancreatitis and alcohol, protein and lipid consumption, *Digestion,* 18, 337, 1978.

18. **Bode, J. C.,** in *Topics in Gastroenterology, No. 12,* Jewell, D. P. and Gibson, P. R., Eds., Blackwell Scientific, Oxford, 1985, 39.

19. **Phillps, A. M.,** Chronic pancreatitis — pathogenesis and clinical features, *Arch. Intern. Med.,* 93, 337, 1954.

20. **Warshaw, A. L.,** Pain in chronic pancreatitis. Patients, patience and the impatient surgeon, *Gastroenterology,* 86, 987, 1984.

21. **Bradley, E. L., III,** Pancreatic duct pressure in chronic pancreatitis, *Am. J. Surg.,* 144, 313, 1982.

22. **Ebbehoj, N., Borley, L., Bulow, J., Rasmussen, S. G., Madsen, P., Matzen, P., and Owre, A.,** Pancreatic tissue fluid pressure in chronic pancreatitis. Relation to pain, morphology and function, *Scand. J. Gastroenterol.,* 25, 1046, 1990.

23. **Strum, W. B. and Spiro, H. M.,** Chronic pancreatitis, *Ann. Intern. Med.,* 74, 264, 1971.

24. **Nagata, A., Homma, T., Tamai, K., Ueno, K., Shimakura, K., Oguchi, H., Furuta, S., and Oda, M.,** A study of chronic pancreatitis by serial endoscopic pancreatography, *Gastroenterology,* 81, 884, 1981.

25. **Gullo, L., Barbara, L., and Labo, G.,** Effect of cessation of alcohol use on the course of pancreatic dysfunction in alcoholic pancreatitis, *Gastroenterology,* 95, 1063, 1988.

26. **Ammann, R. W., Akovbiantz, F., Largiader, F., and Scueler, G.,** Course and outcome of chronic pancreatitis. Longitudinal study of a mixed medical-surgical series of 245 patients, *Gastroenterology,* 86, 820, 1984.

27. **Kalthoff, L., Layer, P., Clain, J. E., and DiMagno, E. P.,** The course of alcoholic and non alcoholic chronic pancreatitis, *Dig. Dis. Sci.,* 29, 953, 1984.

28. **Dreiling, D. A. and Bordalo, O.,** A toxic metabolic hypothesis of pathogenesis of alcoholic pancreatitis, *Alcoholism: Clin. Exp. Res.,* 1, 293, 1977.

29. **Bordalo, O., Noronha, M., and Dreiling, D. A.,** Functional and morphological studies of the effect of alcohol on the pancreatic parenchyma, *Mt. Sinai J. Med.,* 44, 481, 1977.

30. **Sarles, H., Lebreuil, G., and Tasso, F.,** A comparison of alcoholic pancreatitis in rat and in man, *Gut,* 12, 377, 1971.

31. **Wilson, J. S., Colley, P. W., Sosula, L., Pirola, R. C., Chapman, B. A., and Somer, J. B.,** Alcohol causes a fatty pancreas. A rat model of ethanol-induced pancreatic steatosis, *Alcoholism: Clin. Exp. Res.,* 6, 117, 1982.

32. **Czernobilsky, B. and Mikat, K. W.,** The diagnostic significance of interstitial pancreatitis found at autopsy, *Am. J. Clin. Pathol.,* 41, 33, 1964.

33. **Gosselin, M., Fauchet, R., Genetet, B., and Gastard, J.,** Les antigenes HLA dans la pancreatitechronique alcoholique, *Gastroenterol. Clin. Biol.,* 2, 883, 1978.

34. **Dani, R., Antunes, L. J., Rocha, W. M., and Nogueira, C. E.,** HLA Aw 23 and Aw24 associated with chronic calcifying pancreatitis, *Arch. Gastroenterol.,* 15, 163, 1978.

35. **Gullo, L., Tabacchi, P. L., Corazza, G. R., Calanca, F., Canpione, O., and Labo, G.,** HLA B13 and chronic calcific pancreatitis, *Dig. Dis. Sci.,* 27, 214, 1982.

36. **Wilson, J. S., Gossat, D., Tait, A., Rouse, S., Juan, X. J., and Pirola, R. C.,** Evidence for an inherited predisposition to alcoholic pancreatitis. A controlled HLA typing study, *Dig. Dis. Sci.,* 29, 727, 1984.

37. **Novis, B. H., Bank, S., Young, G. O., and Marks, I. N.,** Chronic pancreatitis and alpha$_1$-antitrypsin, *Lancet,* 2, 748, 1975.

38. **Braxel, C., Versieck, J., Lemey, G., Vanballenberghe, L., and Barbier, F.,** Alpha$_1$-antitrypsin in pancreatitis, *Digestion,* 23, 93, 1982.

39. **Haber, P. S., Wilson, J. S., McGarity, B. H., Hall, W., Thomas, M. C., and Pirola, R. C.,** Alpha$_1$-antitrypsin phenotypes and alcoholic pancreatitis, *Gut,* 32, 945, 1991.

40. **Marks, I. N., Bank, S., duTroit, A., Keraan, M. M., Krut, L. H., Mann, J., and Edelstein, I.,** Genetic and nutritional factors in calcific pancreatitis, in *4th World Congress of Gastroenterology. Advance Abstracts,* Riis, P., Ed., The Danish Gastroenterological Association, Copenhagen, 1970, 220.

41. **Moshal, M. G.,** A study of chronic pancreatitis in Natal, *Digestion,* 9, 438, 1973.

42. **Stigendal, L., Olssen, R., Rydberg, L., and Samuelsson, B. O. E.,** Blood group Lewis phenotype on erythrocytes and in saliva in alcoholic pancreatitis and chronic liver disease, *J. Clin. Pathol.,* 37, 778, 1984.

43. **Anderson, R. J. L., Dyer, P. A., Donnai, D., Klouda, P. T., Jennison, R., and Braganza, J. M.,** Chronic pancreatitis, HLA and autoimmunity, *Int. J. Pancreatol.,* 3, 83, 1988.

44. **Bynum, T. E., Solomon, T. E., Johnson, L. R., and Jacobsen, E. D.,** Inhibition of pancreatic secretion in man by cigarette smoking, *Gut,* 13, 36, 1972.

45. **Konturek, S. J., Soloman, T. E., McCreight, W. G., Johnson, L. R., and Jacobson, E. D.,** Effects of nicotine on gastrointestinal secretion, *Gastroenterology,* 60, 1098, 1971.

46. **Majumdar, A. P. N., Davis, G. A., Dubick, M. A., and Geokas, M. C.,** Nicotine stimulation of protein secretion from isolated pancreatic acini, *Am. J. Physiol.,* 250, G598, 1985.

47. **Chowdhury, P., Hosotani, R., Chang, L., and Rayford, P. L.,** Metabolic and pathologic effects of nicotine on gastrointestinal tract and pancreas of rats, *Pancreas,* 5, 222, 1990.

48. **Lau, P. P., Dubick, M. A., Yu, G. S. M., Morrill, P. R., and Geokas, M. C.,** Dynamic changes of pancreatic structure and function in rats treated chronically with nicotine, *Toxicol. Appl. Pharmacol.,* 104, 457, 1990.

49. **Yen, S., Hsieh, C. C., and MacMahon, B.,** Consumption of alcohol and tobacco and other risk factors for pancreatitis, *Am. J. Epidemiol.,* 116, 407, 1982.

50. **Bourliere, M., Barthet, M., Berthezene, P. Durbec, J. P., and Sarles, H.,** Is tobacco a risk factor for chronic pancreatitis and alcoholic cirrhosis?, *Gut,* 32, 1392, 1991.

51. **Haber, P. S., Wilson, J. S., and Pirola, R. C.,** Smoking and alcoholic pancreatitis, *Pancreas,* 8, 568, 1993.

52. **Dickson, A. P., O'Neill, J., and Irmie, C. W.,** Hyperlipidaemia, alcohol abuse and acute pancreatitis, *Br. J. Surg.,* 71, 685, 1984.

53. **Guzman, S., Nervi, F., Llanos, O., Leon, P., and Valdivieso, V.,** Impaired lipid clearance in patients with previous acute pancreatitis, *Gut,* 28, 888, 1985.

54. **Rollan, A., Guzman, S., Pimental, F., and Nervi, F.,** Catabolism of chylomicron remnants in patients with previous acute pancreatitis, *Gastroenterology,* 98, 1649, 1990.

55. **Durrington, P. N., Twentyman, O. P., Braganza, J. M., and Miller, J. P.,** Hypertriglyceridemia and abnormalities of triglyceride catabolism persisting after pancreatitis, *Int. J. Pancreatol.,* 1, 195, 1986.

56. **Buch, A., Buch, J., Carlson, A., and Schmit, A.,** Hyperlipidaemia and pancreatitis, *World J. Surg.,* 4, 307, 1980.

57. **Haber, P. S., Wilson, J. S., Apte, M. V., and Pirola, R. C.,** Lipid intolerance does not account for susceptibility to alcoholic and gall stone pancreatitis, *Gastroenterology,* 106, 742, 1993.

58. **Riordan, J. R., Rommens, J., Kerem, B. S., Alon, N., Rozmahler, R., Grzelczak, Z., Zielenski, J., Lok, S., Plavsic, N., Chou, J. L., Drumm, M. L., Iannuzzi, M. C., Collins, F. C., and Tsui, L. C.,** Identification of the cystic fibrosis gene: cloning and characterisation of complementary DNA, *Science,* 245, 1066, 1989.

59. **Kerem, B. S., Rommens, J. M., Buchanan, J. A., Markiewicz, D., Cox, T. K., Chakravarti, A., Buchwald, M., and Tsui, L. C.,** Identification of the cystic fibrosis gene: genetic analysis, *Science,* 245, 1073, 1989.

60. **Behm, J. K., Hagiwara, G., Lewiston, N. J., Quinton, P. M., and Wine, J. J.,** Hyposecretion of β-adrenergically induced sweating in cystic fibrosis heterozygotes, *Pediatr. Res.,* 22, 271, 1987.

61. **Norton, I. D., Apte, M. V., Dixon, H., Trent, R. J., Pirola, R. C., and Wilson, J. S.,** Heterozygosity for cystic fibrosis ΔF-508 mutation does not predispose alcoholics to pancreatitis, *J. Gastroenterol. Hepatol.,* 9, A89 1994.

62. **Kager, L., Lindberg, S., and Agren, G.,** Alcohol consumption and acute pancreatitis in men, *Scand. J. Gastroenterol.,* 15 (Suppl.), 1, 1972.

63. **McEntee, G. P., Gillen, P., and Peel, A. L. G.,** Alcohol induced pancreatitis: social and surgical aspects, *Br. J. Surg.,* 74, 402, 1987.

64. **Gastrard, J., Joubaud, F., Farbos, T., Loussouarn, J., Marian, J., Pannier, M., Renaudet, F., Valdazo, R., and Gosselin, M.,** Etiology and course of primary chronic pancreatitis in Western France, *Digestion,* 9, 416, 1973.

65. **Wilson, J. S., Bernstein, L., McDonald, C., Tait, A., McNeil, D., and Pirola, R. C.,** Diet and drinking habits in relation to the development of alcoholic pancreatitis, *Gut,* 26, 882, 1985.

66. **Mezey, E., Jow, E., Slaven, R. E., and Tobon, F.,** Pancreatic function and intestinal absorption in chronic alcoholism, *Gastroenterology,* 59, 657, 1970.

67. **Veghelyi, P. V., Kemeny, T. T., Pozsonyi, J., and Sos, J.,** Dietary lesions of the pancreas, *Am. J. Dis. Child,* 79, 658, 1950.

68. **Bucko, A., Kopec, Z., and Babala, J.,** Effect of starvation on the function and morphology of rat pancreas, *Nutr. Dicta,* 10, 266, 1968.

69. **Wilson, J. S., Korsten, M. A., Leo, M. A., and Lieber, C. S.,** Combined effects of protein deficiency and chronic ethanol consumption on rat pancreas, *Dig. Dis. Sci.,* 33, 1250, 1988.

70. **Pitchumoni, C. S.,** Pancreas in primary malnutrition disorders, *Am. J. Clin. Nutr.,* 26, 374, 1973.

71. **Maki, T., Kakizaki, G., Sato, T., Saito, Y., Suda, Y., Onuma, T., and Hayasaka, N.,** Effect of diet on experimental pancreatitis in rat, *Tohoku J. Exp. Med.,* 92, 301, 1967.

72. **Grossman, M. I., Greengard, H., and Ivy, A. C.,** The effect of dietary composition on pancreatic enzymes, *Am. J. Physiol.,* 138, 676, 1943.

73. **Deschodt-Lanckman, M., Robberecht, P., Camus, J., and Christophe, J.,** Short-term adaptation of pancreatic hydrolases to nutritional and physiological stimuli in adult rats, *Biochemie,* 53, 789, 1971.

74. **Durbec, J. P. and Sarles, H.,** Multicentre survey of the etiology of pancreatic diseases: relationship between the relative risk of developing chronic pancreatitis and alcohol, protein and lipid consumption, *Digestion,* 18, 337, 1978.

75. **Pitchumoni, C. S., Sonnenshein, M., Candido, F. M., Panchacharam, P., and Cooperman, J. M.,** Nutrition in the pathogenesis of alcoholic pancreatitis, *Am. J. Clin. Nutr.,* 33, 631, 1980.

76. **Anderson, M. C., Needleman, S. B., Gramatica, L., Toronto, I. R., and Briggs, D. R.,** Further inquiry into the pathogenesis of acute pancreatitis, *Arch. Surg.,* 99, 185, 1969.

77. **Schmidt, H. and Crutzfeldt, W.,** The possible role of phospholipase $A_2$ in the pathogenesis of acute pancreatitis, *Scand. J. Gastroenterol.,* 4, 39, 1969.

78. **Geokas, M. C.,** The role of elastase in acute pancreatitis. III. The destructive capacity of elastase on pancreatic tissue *in vitro* and *in vivo, Arch. Pathol.,* 86, 135, 1968.

79. **Ohlsson, K.,** Experimental pancreatitis in the dog. Demonstration of trypsin in ascitic fluid, lymph and plasma, *Scand. J. Gastroenterol.,* 8, 129, 1973.

80. **Dubick, M. A., Mayer, D., Majumdar, A. P. N., Mar, G., McMahon, M. J., and Geokas, M. C.,** Biochemical studies in peritoneal fluid from patients with acute pancreatitis. Relationship to etiology, *Dig. Dis. Sci.,* 32, 305, 1987.

81. **Geokas, M. C. and Rinderknecht, H. L.,** Free proteolytic enzymes in pancreatic juice of patients with acute pancreatitis, *Dig. Dis.,* 19, 591, 1974.

82. **Yamaguchi, H., Kimura, T., Mimura, K., and Nawata, H.,** Activation of proteases in caerulein induced pancreatitis, *Pancreas,* 4, 565, 1989.

83. **Lankisch, P. G., Pohl, U., Goke, B., Otto, J., Wereszczynska-Siemiatkowska, U., Grone, H.-J., and Rahlf, G.,** Effect of FOY-305 (camostate) on severe acute pancreatitis in two experimental animal models, *Gastroenterology,* 96, 193, 1989.

84. **Ono, H., Hayakawa, T., Kondo, T., Shibata, T., Kitagawa, M., Sakai, Y., Kiriyama, S., and Sobajima, H.,** Prevention of experimental acute pancreatitis by intraduodenal trypsin inhibitor in rat, *Dig. Dis. Sci.,* 35, 787, 1990.

85. **Lampel, M. and Kern, H. F.,** Acute interstitial pancreatitis in the rat induced by excessive doses of a pancreatic secretagogue, *Virch. Arch.,* 373, 97, 1977.

86. **Saluja, A., Saluja, M., Villa, A., Leli, U., Rutledge, P., Meldolesi, J., and Steer, M.,** Pancreatic duct obstruction in rabbits causes digestive zymogen and lysosomal enzyme co-localisation, *J. Clin. Invest.,* 84, 1260, 1989.

87. **Ohshio, G., Saluja, A., and Steer, M.,** Effects of short term pancreatic obstruction in rats, *Gastroenterology,* 100, 196, 1991.

88. **Lombardi, B., Ester, L. W., and Longnecker, D. S.,** Acute hemorrhagic pancreatitis (massive necrosis) with fat necrosis induced in mice by DL-ethionine fed with a choline deficient diet, *Am. J. Pathol.,* 79, 465, 1975.

89. **Greenbaum, L. M., Hirschkowitz, A., and Shoichet, I.,** The activation of trypsinogen by cathepsin B, *J. Biol. Chem.,* 234, 2885, 1959.

90. **Opie, E. L.,** The aetiology of acute hemorrhagic pancreatitis, *Johns Hopkins Hosp. Bull.,* 12, 182, 1901.

91. **Sterling, J. A.,** The common channel for bile and pancreatic ducts, *Surg. Gynecol. Obstet.,* 98, 420, 1954.

92. **Hand, B. H.,** An anatomical study of the choledochoduodenal area, *Br. J. Surg.,* 50, 486, 1963.

93. **McCutcheon, A. D.,** Aetiological factors in pancreatitis, *Lancet,* 1, 710, 1962.

94. **Yatto, R. P. and Siegal, J. H.,** The role of pancreaticobiliary anatomy in the etiology of alcoholic pancreatitis, *J. Clin. Gastroenterol.,* 6, 419, 1984.

95. **Thune, A., Friman, S., Conradi, N., and Svanvik, J.,** Functional and morphological relationships between the feline main pancreatic and bile duct sphincters, *Gastroenterology,* 98, 758, 1990.

96. **Parry, E. W., Hallenbeck, G. A., and Grindlay, J. H.,** Pressures in the pancreatic and common bile ducts, *Arch. Surg.,* 70, 757, 1955.

97. **Menguy, R. B., Hallenbeck, G. A., Bollman, J. L., and Grindlay, J. H.,** Intraductal pressures and sphincteric resistance in canine pancreatic and biliary ducts after various stimuli, *Surg. Gynecol. Obstet.,* 106, 306, 1958.

98. **Csendes, A., Kruse, A., Funch-Jenson, P., Oster, M. J., Ornsholt, J., and Amdrup, E.,** Pressure measurements in the biliary and pancreatic duct systems in controls and in patients with gallstones, previous cholecystectomy, or common bile duct stones, *Gastroenterology,* 77, 1203, 1979.

99. **Carre-Locke, D. L. and Gregg, J. A.,** Endoscopic manometry of pancreatic and biliary sphincter zones in man: basal results in healthy volunteers, *Dig. Dis. Sci.,* 26, 7, 1981.

100. **Anderson, M. C. and Hagstrom, W. J.,** A comparison of pancreatic and biliary pressures recorded simultaneously in man, *Can. J. Surg.,* 5, 461, 1962.

101. **Archibald, E.,** The experimental production of pancreatitis in animals as a result of the resistance of the common duct sphincter, *Surg. Gynecol. Obstet.,* 28, 529, 1919.

102. **Whitrock, R. M., Hine, D., Crane, J., and McCorkle, H. J.,** The effect of bile flow through the pancreas, *Surgery,* 38, 122, 1955.

103. **White, T. T. and MaGee, D. F.,** Perfusion of the dog pancreas with bile without production of pancreatitis, *Ann. Surg.,* 151, 245, 1960.

104. **Gamklou, R. and Edlund, Y.,** Acute alcoholic pancreatitis in the rat, *Scand. J. Gastroenterol.,* 1, 75, 1966.

105. **Jalovaara, P. and Apaja, M.,** Alcohol and acute pancreatitis: an experimental study in the rat, *Scand. J. Gastroenterol.,* 13, 703, 1978.

106. **Braganza, J. M.,** Pancreatic disease: a casualty of hepatic detoxification?, *Lancet,* 2, 1000, 1983.

107. **Anderson, M. C., van Hagen, F., Method, H. L., and Mehn, W. H.,** An evaluation of the use of bile, bile salts and trypsin in the production of experimental pancreatitis, *Surg. Gynecol. Obstet.,* 107, 693, 1958.

108. **Bawnik, J. B., Orda, R., and Wiznitzer, T.,** Acute necrotizing pancreatitis: an experimental model, *Dig. Dis.,* 19, 1143, 1974.

109. **Farmer, R. C., Tweedie, J., Maslin, S., Reber, H. A., Adler, G., and Kern, H.,** Effects of bile salts on permeability and morphology of main pancreatic duct in cats, *Dig. Dis. Sci.,* 29, 740, 1974.

110. **Cotran, R. J. and Majno, G.,** A light and electron microscopic analysis of vascular injury, *Ann. N.Y. Acad. Sci.,* 116, 750, 1964.

111. **Poncelet, P. and Thomson, A. G.,** Action of bile phospholipids on the pancreas, *Am. J. Surg.,* 123, 196, 1972.

112. **Grant, D.,** Acute necrotising pancreatitis — a role for enterokinase, *Int. J. Pancreatol.,* 1,167, 1986.

113. **Viceconte, G.,** Effect of ethanol on the sphincter of Oddi: an endoscopic manometric study, *Gut,* 24, 20, 1983.

114. **Pirola, R. C. and Davis, A. E.,** Effects of intravenous alcohol on motility of the duodenum and the sphincter of Oddi, *Aust. Ann. Med.,* 19, 24, 1970.

115. **Davis, A. E. and Pirola, R. C.,** The effects of ethyl alcohol on exocrine pancreatic function, *Med. J. Aust.,* 2, 757, 1966.

116. **Pirola, R. C. and Davis, A. E.,** Effect of pressure on the integrity of the duct-acinar system of the pancreas, *Gut,* 11, 69, 1970.

117. **Wangenstein, O. H., Leven, N. L., and Manson, M. H.,** Acute pancreatitis (pancreatic necrosis). An experimental and clinical study with special reference to the biliary tract factor, *Arch. Surg.,* 23, 47, 1931.

118. **Lium, R. and Maddock, S.,** Etiology of acute pancreatitis. An experimental study, *Surgery,* 24, 593, 1948.

119. **Menguy, R. B., Hallenbeck, G. A., Bollman, G. L., and Grindlay, J. H.,** Ductal and vascular factors in etiology of experimentally induced acute pancreatitis, *Arch. Surg.,* 74, 881, 1957.

120. **Graves, A. J., Holmquist, D. R. G., and Githens, S.,** Effect of duct obstruction on histology and on activities of γ-glutamyl transferase, adenosine triphosphate alkaline phosphatase and amylase in the rat pancreas, *Dig. Dis. Sci.,* 31, 1254, 1986.

121. **Lerch, M. M., Saluja, A. K., Dawra, R., Ramarao, P., Saluja, M., and Steer, M. L.,** Acute necrotising pancreatitis in the opossum: earliest morphological changes involve acinar cells, *Gastroenterology,* 103, 205, 1992.

122. **Saluja, A., Hashimoto, S., Saluja, M., Powers, R. E., Meldolesi, J., and Steer, M. L.,** Subcellular redistribution of lysosomal enzymes during caerulein-induced pancreatitis, *Am. J. Physiol.,* 253, G508, 1987.

123. **Greenbaum, L. M. and Hirschkowitz, A.,** Endogenous cathepsin activates trypsinogen in extracts of dog pancreas, *Proc. Soc. Exp. Biol. Med.,* 107, 74, 1961.

124. **Niederau, C. and Grendell, J. H.,** Intracellular vacuoles in experimental acute pancreatitis in rats and mice are an acidified compartment, *J. Clin. Invest.,* 81, 229, 1988.

125. **Bettinger, J. R. and Grendell, J. H.,** Intracellular events in the pathogenesis of acute pancreatitis, *Pancreas,* 6, S2, 1991.

126. **Korsten, M. A., Hodes, S. F., Saeli, J. F., Seitz, H. K., and Lieber, C. S.,** Effects of ethanol on pancreatic secretion: roles of gastric acid and exogenous secretin, *Gastroenterology,* 76, 1175, 1979.

127. **Walton, B., Schapiro, H., and Woodward, E. R.,** The effect of alcohol on pancreatic secretion, *Surg. Forum,* II, 365, 1960.

128. **Newman, H. W. and Mehrtens, H. G.,** Effect of intravenous injection of ethyl alcohol on gastric secretion in man, *Proc. Soc. Exp. Biol. Med.,* 30, 145, 1932.

129. **Woodward, E. R., Robertson, C., Ruttenberg, H. D., and Schapiro, H.,** Alcohol as a gastric secretory stimulant, *Gastroenterology,* 32, 727, 1957.

130. **Bayliss, W. M. and Starling, E. H.,** The mechanism of pancreatic secretion, *J. Physiol.,* 28, 325, 1902.

131. **Schapiro, H., Wruble, L. D., Estes, A. W., and Britt, L. G.,** Pancreatic secretion stimulated by the action of alcohol on the gastric antrum, *Am. J. Dig. Dis.,* 13, 536, 1968.

132. **Straus, E., Urbach, H. J., and Yaloe, R. S.,** Alcohol-stimulated secretion of immunoreactive secretin, *N. Engl. J. Med.,* 293, 1031, 1975.

133. **Llanos, O. L., Swierczek, J. S., Teichmann, R. K., Rayford, P. L., and Thompson, J. C.,** Effect of alcohol on the release of secretin and pancreatic secretion, *Surgery,* 81, 661, 1977.

134. **Fahrenkrug, J. and Schraffalitsky de Muckadell, O. B.,** Plasma secretin concentration in man: effect of intraduodenal glucose, fat, amino acids, ethanol, HCl or ingestion after a meal, *Eur. J. Clin. Invest.,* 201, 1977.

135. **Hajnal, F., Flores, M. C., Radley, S., and Valenzuela, J. E.,** Effect of alcohol and alcoholic beverages on meal stimulated pancreatic secretion in humans, *Gastroenterology,* 98, 191, 1990.

136. **Bayer, M., Rudick, J., Lieber, C. S., and Janowitz, H. D.,** Inhibitory effect of ethanol on canine exocrine pancreatic secretion, *Gastroenterology,* 63, 619, 1972.

137. **Korsten, M. A., Seitz, H., Hodes, S. F., Klingenstein, J., and Lieber, C. S.,** Effect of intravenous ethanol on pancreatic secretion in the conscious rat, *Dig. Dis. Sci.,* 26, 790, 1981.

138. **Uhlemann, E. R., Robberecht, P., and Gardner, J. D.,** Effects of ethanol on the actions of VIP and secretin on acinar cells from guinea pig pancreas, *Gastroenterology,* 76, 917, 1979.

139. **Lewin, M. D., Wong, A., Deveney, C. W., and Sankaran, H.,** Reversible acetaldehyde inhibition of A23187-stimulated amylase secretion from isolated rat pancreatic acini, *FEBS Lett.,* 184, 259, 1985.

140. **Steer, M. L., Glaser, G., and Manabe, T.,** Direct effects of ethanol on exocrine secretion from the *in vitro* rabbit pancreas, *Dig. Dis. Sci.,* 24, 769, 1979.

141. **Valenzuela, J. E., Salinas, J., and Petermann, M.,** Effect of ethanol on pancreatic secretion, *Gastroenterology,* 56, 1203, 1969.

142. **Tiscornia, O. M., Hage, G., Palasciano, G., Brasca, A. P., Deveau, M. A., and Sarles, H.,** The effects of pentolinium and vagotomy on the inhibition of canine exocrine pancreatic secretion by intravenous ethanol, *Biomedicine,* 18, 159, 1973.

143. **Tiscornia, O. M., Gullo, L., and Sarles, H.,** The inhibition of canine exocrine pancreatic secretion by intravenous ethanol, *Digestion,* 9, 231, 1973.

144. **Solomon, N., Solomon, T. E., Jacobson, E. D., and Shanbour, L. L.,** Direct effects of alcohol on *in vivo* and *in vitro* exocrine pancreatic secretion and metabolism, *Dig. Dis.,* 19, 253, 1974.

145. **Valenzuela, J. E., Salinas, J., and Petermann, M.,** Effect of ethanol on pancreatic enzyme secretion, *Gastroenterology,* 67, 991, 1975.

146. **Sahel, J. and Sarles, H.,** Modifications of pure human pancreatic juice induced by chronic alcohol consumption, *Dig. Dis. Sci.,* 24, 897, 1979.

147. **Renner, I. G., Rindernecht, H., Valenzuela, J. E., and Douglas, A. P.,** Studies of pure pancreatic secretions in chronic alcoholic subjects without pancreatic insufficiency, *Scand. J. Gastroenterol.,* 15, 241, 1980.

148. **Sarles, H., Tiscornia, O., Palasciano, G., Brasca, A., Hage, G., Devaux, M. A., and Gullo, L.,** Effects of chronic intragastric ethanol administration on canine exocrine pancreatic secretion, *Scand. J. Gastroenterol.,* 8, 85, 1973.

149. **Tiscornia, O. M., Palasciano, G., and Sarles, H.,** Effect of chronic ethanol administration on canine exocrine pancreatic secretion, *Digestion,* 11, 172, 1974.

150. **Huttenen, R., Huttenen, P., and Jalovaara, P.,** Effect of chronic intragastric alcohol ingestion on the pancreatic secretion of the rat, *Scand. J. Gastroenterol.,* 11, 103, 1976.

151. **Noel-Jorand, M. C., Colomb, E., Astier, J. P., and Sarles, H.,** Pancreatic basal secretion in alcohol-fed and normal dogs, *Dig. Dis. Sci.,* 26, 783, 1981.

152. **Schmidt, D. N. and Pandol, S. J.,** Differing effects of ethanol on *in vitro* stimulated pancreatic enzyme secretion in ethanol fed and control rats, *Pancreas,* 5, 27, 1990.

153. **Singh, M.,** Effect of chronic ethanol feeding on pancreatic enzyme secretion in rats *in vitro, Dig. Dis. Sci.,* 28, 117, 1983.

154. **Sarles, H.,** Alcoholism and pancreatitis, *Scand. J. Gastroenterol.,* 6, 193, 1971.

155. **Sarles, H.,** Chronic calcifying pancreatitis — chronic alcoholic pancreatitis, *Gastroenterology,* 66, 604, 1974.

156. **Nakamura, K., Sarles, H., and Payan, H.,** Three dimensional reconstruction of the pancreatic ducts in chronic pancreatitis, *Gastroenterology,* 62, 942, 1972.

157. **Renner, I. G., Rindernecht, H., Valenzuela, J. E., and Douglas, A. P.,** Studies of pure pancreatic secretions in patients with acute pancreatitis: the possible role of proteolytic enzymes in pathogenesis, *Gastroenterology,* 5, 1090, 1978.

158. **Hekman, A.,** Association of lactoferrin with other proteins as demonstrated by changes in electrophoretic mobility, *Biochim. Biophys. Acta,* 251, 380, 1971.

159. **Colomb, E., Estevenon, J. P., Figarella, C., Guy, O., and Sarles, H.,** Characterisation of an additional protein in pancreatic juice of men with chronic calcifying pancreatitis: identification to lactoferrin, *Biochim. Biophys. Acta,* 342, 306, 1974.

160. **Brugge, W. R. and Burke, C. A.,** Lactoferrin secretion in alcoholic pancreatic disease, *Dig. Dis. Sci.,* 33, 178, 1988.

161. **Multigner, L., Figarello, C., Sahel, J., and Sarles, H.,** Lactoferrin and albumin in human pancreatic juice: a valuable test for diagnosis in pancreatic diseases, *Dig. Dis. Sci.,* 25, 173, 1980.

162. **De Caro, A., Bonicel, J. J., Rouimi, P., De Caro, J. D., Sarles, H., and Rovery, M.,** Complete amino acid sequence of an immunoreactive form of human pancreatic stone protein isolated from pancreatic juice, *Eur. J. Biochem.,* 168, 201, 1987.

163. **Moore, E. W. and Verine, H. J.,** Pathogenesis of pancreatic and biliary $CaCO_3$ lithiasis: the solubility product (Ksp) of calcite determined with the $Ca^{++}$ electrode, *J. Lab. Clin. Med.,* 106, 611, 1985.

164. **Multigner, L., De Caro, A., Lombardo, D., Campese, D., and Sarles, H.,** Pancreatic stone protein, a phospholipid which inhibits calcium carbonate precipitation from human pancreatic juice, *Biochem. Biophys. Res. Commun.,* 110, 69, 1983.

165. **Guy, O., Roble-Diaz, G., Aldrich, Z., Sahel, J., and Sarles, H.,** Protein content of precipitates present in pancreatic juice of alcoholic subjects and patients with chronic calcific pancreatitis, *Gastroenterology,* 84, 102, 1983.

166. **Multigner, L., Sarles, H., Lombardo, D., and De Caro, A.,** Pancreatic stone protein II. Implication in stone formation during the course of chronic calcifying pancreatitis, *Gastroenterology,* 89, 387, 1985.

167. **Schmiegel, W.-H., Burchert, M., Kaltoff, H., Thiele, H.-G., Butzow, G., Klose, G., and Greten, H.,** Pancreatic stone protein in serum of patients with pancreatitis, *Lancet,* 2, 686, 1986.

168. **Giorgi, D., Bernard, J. P., Rouquier, S., Iovanna, J., Sarles, H., and Dagorn, J. C.,** Pancreatic stone protein messenger RNA: nucleotide sequence and expression in chronic calcifying pancreatitis, *J. Clin. Invest.,* 84, 100, 1989.

169. **Dagorn, J. C.,** Lithostathine, in *The Pancreas: Biology, Pathobiology and Disease,* Go, V. L. W., DiMagno, E. P., Gardner, J. D., Lebenthal, E., Reber, H. A., and Scheele, G. A., Eds., Raven Press, New York, 1993, 253.

170. **Apte, M. V., Wilson, J. S., McCaughan, G. W., Norton, I. D., and Pirola, R. C.,** Ethanol and dietary protein deficiency increase gene expression of pancreatic lithostathine, *J. Gastroenterol. Hepatol.,* 9, A93, 1994.

171. **Steer, M. L. and Meldolesi, J.,** The cell biology of experimental pancreatitis, *N. Engl. J. Med.,* 316, 144, 1987.

172. **Wilson, J. S., Korsten, M. A., Apte, M. V., Thomas, M. C., Haber, P. S., and Pirola, R. C.,** Both ethanol and protein deficiency increase the fragility of pancreatic lysosomes, *J. Lab. Clin. Med.,* 115, 749, 1990.

173. **Laposata, E. A. and Lange, L. G.,** Presence of nonoxidative ethanol metabolism in human organs commonly damaged by ethanol abuse, *Science,* 231, 497, 1986.

174. **Wilson, J. S., Apte, M. V., Thomas, M. C., Haber, P. S., and Pirola, R. C.,** Effects of ethanol, acetaldehyde and cholesteryl esters on pancreatic lysosomes, *Gut,* 33, 1099, 1992.

175. **Haber, P. S., Wilson, J. S., Apte, M. V., and Pirola, R. C.,** Fatty acid ethyl esters increase rat pancreatic lysosomal fragility, *J. Lab. Clin. Med.,* 121, 759, 1993.

176. **Haber, P. S., Wilson, J. S., Apte, M. V., Korsten, M. A., and Pirola, R. C.,** Chronic ethanol consumption increases the fragility of rat pancreatic zymogen granules, *Gut,* 35, 1474, 1995.

177. **Singh, M.,** Effect of chronic ethanol feeding on pancreatic enzyme secretion in rats *in vitro, Dig. Dis. Sci.,* 28, 117, 1983.

178. **Ponnappa, B. C., Hoek, J. B., Jubinsyi, L., and Rubin, E.,** Ethanol withdrawal stimulates protein synthesis in rat pancreatic lobules, *Biochem. Biophys. Acta,* 1036, 107, 1990.

179. **Wilson, J. S., Korsten, M. A., Apte, M. V., Thomas, M. C., Haber, P. S., and Pirola, R. C.,** Both ethanol and protein deficiency increase the fragility of pancreatic lysosomes, *J. Lab. Clin. Med.,* 115, 749, 1990.

180. **Apte, M., Wilson, J. S., McCaughan, G. W., Korsten, M. A., Haber, P. S., Norton, I. D., and Pirola, R. C.,** Ethanol induced alterations in gene expression correlate with glandular content of pancreatic enzymes, *J. Lab. Clin. Med.,* 125, 634, 1995.

181. **Uden, S., Acheson, D. W. K., Reeves, J., Worthington, M. V., Hunt, L. P., Brown, S., and Braganza, J. M.,** Antioxidants, enzyme induction and chronic pancreatitis, *Eur. J. Clin. Nutr.,* 42, 561, 1988.

182. **Lieber, C. S.,** Biochemical and molecular basis of alcohol induced injury to liver and other tissues, *N. Engl. J. Med.,* 319, 1639, 1988.

183. **Shimizu, M., Lasker, J. M., Tsutsumi, M., and Lieber, C. S.,** Immunohistochemical localisation of ethanol-inducible P450IIE1 in the rat alimentary tract, *Gastroenterology,* 99, 1044, 1990.

184. **Foster, J. R., Idle, J. R., Hardwick, J. P., Bars, R., Scott, P., and Braganza, J. M.,** Induction of drug metabolising enzymes in human pancreatic cancer and chronic pancreatitis, *J. Pathol.,* 169, 457, 1993.

185. **Guyan, P. M., Uden, S., and Braganza, J. M.,** Heightened free radical activity in pancreatitis, *Free Rad. Biol. Med.,* 8, 347, 1990.

186. **Nonaka, A., Monabe, T., Asano, N., Kyogoku, T., Imanishi, K., Tamura, K., and Tobe, T.,** Direct ESR measurement of free radicals in mouse pancreatic lesions, *Int. J. Pancreatol.,* 5, 203, 1989.

187. **Gough, D. B., Boyle, B., Joyce, W. P., Delaney, C. P., McGeeney, K. F., Gorey, T. F., and Fitzpatrick, J. M.,** Free radical inhibition and serial chemiluminescence in evolving experimental pancreatitis, *Br. J. Surg.,* 77, 1256, 1990.

188. **Schoenberg, M. H., Buchler, M., Younes, Y., Kirchmayr, R., Bruckner, U. B., and Beger, H. G.,** Effect of antioxidant treatment in rats with acute hemorrhagic pancreatitis, *Dig. Dis. Sci.,* 39, 1034, 1994.

189. **Whitely, G. S. W., Kienle, A. P. B., McCloy, R. F., and Braganza, J. M.,** Long-term pain relief without surgery in chronic pancreatitis: value of antioxidant therapy, *Gastroenterology,* A343, 1993.

190. **Whitely, G. S. W., Scott, P. D., Sharer, N. M., Schofield, D., Taylor, P., McCloy, R. F., and Braganza, J. M.,** Combined antioxidant and surgical approach to extensive hemorrhagic pancreatic necrosis, *Gastroenterology,* A343, 1993.

# 10

## Small Bowel Injury by Ethanol

Ivan T. Beck

## CONTENTS

## ABBREVIATIONS

ARG = L-arginine; BBM = Brush-border membrane; BLM = Basolateral membrane; BM = Basement membrane; BSA = bovine serum albumin; CL = Circulating leukocyte; [51]Cr-EDTA = [51]Cr - ethylene diamine tetra acetic acid; END = Endothelial cell; EP = Epithelial cell; ETH = Ethanol; FITC-albumin = Fluorescein + isothiocyanate tagged bovine serum albumin; HIST = Histamine; HRP = horse radish peroxidase; [125]I-BSA = [125]I tagged bovine serum albumin; KRBS = Krebs Ringer bicarbonate solution; KRBSG = KRBS containing 10 m*M* glucose; LIS = Lateral intercellular space; MAADV = Methoxysuccinyl-ala-ala-pro-val-chloromethyl; MC = Mast cell; MCM = Mast cell mediators; NADH = Nicotinamide-adenosine dinucleotide; NO = Nitric oxide; "Nonelectrolytes" = non electrolyte substances transported by carriers (sugars, amino acids, oligopeptides); PL = Platelet; PAF = Platelet aggregating factor; PE = Proteolytic enzymes; PEG-4000 = polyethylene glycol (4000); RL = Resident leukocyte; ROM = Reactive oxygen metabolites; SEM = Scanning electron microscopy; SOD = Superoxide dismutase; TEM = Transmission electron microscopy

## 10.1  INTRODUCTION

Small intestinal injury can occur as a result of acute administration of ethanol or as a consequence of prolonged intake by chronic alcoholics. While the mechanism of acute alcohol injury can be studied experimentally and considerable knowledge has been accumulated on the acute effects of ethanol, much less is known about the mechanism of the alcohol effect in chronic alcoholics. In humans, the intestinal alterations caused by chronic alcohol intake are modified by those caused by changes due to malnutrition, pancreatic maldigestion, abnormal bile secretion, and hematological changes. Experimental studies dealing with chronic alcohol administration are often difficult to compare as the length of administration and ethanol dosages vary among studies. Furthermore, publications by some investigators indicate careful adjustment for nutritional intake while in other studies caloric intake is not controlled. In some studies, the measurements were carried out in chronically treated animals without acute ethanol challenge, while other investigators administered alcohol before and during the experiments. These major variations in methods make comparison and interpretation of these studies difficult. Accordingly, the present treatise will not deal with changes caused by chronic alcohol intake and will concentrate on the mechanism of acute ethanol injury.

The effect of alcohol on any specific organ depends on its concentration, its duration of contact, and sensitivity of the tissue to its effect. For instance, 0.3 to 0.5% ethyl alcohol in the central nervous system induces coma and death[1] but a similar concentration of ethanol has no effect on small intestinal absorption.[2] Experiments with ethanol have been carried out with various concentrations, including the administration of 100% absolute ethanol into the stomach.[3-5] Results obtained with concentrations which do not occur in humans during moderate or heavy acute alcohol intake are of little value and are not helpful to assess the mechanism of the injury produced by acute alcohol ingestion. For this reason, this chapter will only review those studies which have been carried out with "relevant pharmacological" concentrations of ethanol.

The major primary functions of the small intestine are brush-border membrane (BBM) digestion, absorption, and secretion. Although these functions can be carried out by cell fractions, isolated BBMs, or basolateral membranes (BLM), under physiological conditions absorption and secretion are dependent on morphological integrity of the gut. The physiological efficacy of these primary functions is also dependent on a gradual passage of the chyme through the small intestine which relies on organized smooth muscle function. All of these elements need to be appropriately oxygenated and this is achieved by well-functioning microcirculation. The basic transport mechanisms are modified by neural and hormonal impulses and by substances released by cells of the immune system. All of these functions — BBM digestion,[6,7] transport,[8-12] contraction of the fibromyosites of the villus,[13] motility of the smooth muscle of the muscularis propria,[14] blood flow through the microcirculation,[15-17] and the release of neurotransmitters,[18] endocrine, paracrine, neurocrine, and immunological[19-21] substances — are affected by ethanol. Thus, the ethanol-induced injury is the result of a complex interaction of alcohol damage to multiple different functioning elements of the gut. Details of the effect of ethanol on permeability, absorption, motility, endocrine changes, free radicals, and immune defenses will be discussed in detail in other chapters of this book. Of the above aspects of alcohol actions, the present chapter will concentrate only on those which are directly implicated in ethanol injury of the small bowel. By correlating multiple ethanol effects on morphology, blood flow, and the agents involved in mediating these effects, the author hopes to provide an overall understanding of the mechanisms of acute ethanol injury to the small bowel.

## 10.2 METHODOLOGICAL PROBLEMS IN STUDIES WITH ACUTE ETHANOL CONSUMPTION

### 10.2.1 Ethanol Concentration in the Small Intestine After Moderate Drinking

#### 10.2.1.1 Intraluminal Ethanol Concentration

To assess alcohol injury at different depths of the small intestine, it is necessary to know the ethanol concentrations that occur in any specific region during moderate alcohol intake in humans. Intraluminal ethanol concentration after moderate drinking was first studied by Israel et al.,[22] who gave 40 g of ethanol in a 20% (w/v*) solution and found a maximum ethanol concentration in the jejunum of 2.5 to 3.0%. After ingesting 0.8 g ethanol/kg body weight, Halsted and co-workers[23] observed intraluminal ethanol peak concentrations of 1 to 5% in the duodenum and proximal jejunum during the first 45 min after ethanol ingestion. The intraluminal concentration in the ileum was only 0.2%. One hundred twenty minutes after administration, the ethanol concentration of the serum and the lumen of the entire gastrointestinal (GI) tract equalized and varied between 0.02 and 0.05%. Because ethanol diffuses through tissues as easily as water,[24] equalization of concentrations between blood and intraluminal fluid is the result of rapid diffusion of ethanol through the gut wall[15,25-28] into mesenteric veins,[29] rapid metabolism in liver,[30] redistribution of remaining ethanol to the peripheral blood, and extravascular fluid. From the latter, it enters intestinal secretions and achieves an equilibrium between blood and intraluminal fluid.

To assess the optimal concentrations to be used in our animal experiments, we studied the intraluminal ethanol concentrations in humans after moderate alcohol intake.[31] After intragastric administration of 45 to 60 g of ethanol (either in the form of alcohol or whisky, both diluted to a 20% w/v ethanol), the peak ethanol concentration in the intestinal lumen varied between 6.46 and 9.37% in the duodenum and 5.69 and 6.35% in the jejunum. With these intraluminal concentrations, the peak serum concentration was 100 to 150 times lower than that in the duodenal lumen and varied between 0.05 and 0.14%. Because few of the subjects had serum alcohol levels higher than 0.08% w/v, a concentration allowable for driving in Canada according to the Criminal Code of Canada, none of them was seriously inebriated. Taking the above studies into consideration, experiments on the effect of ethanol should be carried out with intraluminal small bowel concentration of 3 to 8% and a blood concentration not higher than 0.15%.

#### 10.2.1.2 Ethanol Concentration in Small Intestinal Tissues

While the alcohol concentration in the lumen of the gut has been well established, there is no knowledge regarding the concentration of ethanol in the subepithelial tissues. As different cells

---

* Unless otherwise stated, all ethanol concentrations are given as w/v.

(epithelial, immunocytes, nerves, smooth muscle, etc.) are located at different levels of the intestine, without information on the prevalent ethanol concentrations at different layers of the gut, meaningful concentrations cannot be established for *in vitro* experiments on various cell preparations. Because transepithelial absorption is isoosmotic[32,33] and because in isoosmotic transport the epithelial cell takes up the osmolality of the lumen,[34] the ethanol concentration for *in vitro* studies on epithelial cells or their cell fractions should be similar to that found in the intestinal lumen. To carry out meaningful *in vitro* studies on smooth muscle cells, fibrocytes, nerve cells, immunocytes, etc., further information needs to be experimentally obtained on the prevalent ethanol concentrations at the level of their normal habitat. Unfortunately, such data are not available in the literature and several attempts in our laboratory failed to accurately determine the ethanol concentrations at different levels of the villus core. However, in an attempt to obtain some data on which to base our *in vitro* experiments, we determined in dogs the ethanol concentration in the mesenteric veins closely adjacent to gut segments perfused with ethanol. We found that the vessel draining the 3 and 6% perfused segments had ethanol concentrations of 0.1 and 0.2%, respectively.[35] Because blood in the mesenteric veins was diluted by blood coming from areas of lower ethanol concentration (e.g., the muscularis and the serosa), the above data are only partially helpful to assess the tissue concentration in the villus core. Theoretically the subepithelial area of the villus should have a lower ethanol concentration than the lumen, and a considerably higher one than that measured in the mesenteric venules. Furthermore, the existence of a countercurrent multiplication system[36] would tend to concentrate the ethanol at the tip of the villus core. Taking all of this into consideration, it is not unreasonable to accept values between 0.5 and 6% as reasonable ethanol concentrations for tissues which are in close proximity to the subepithelial layer of the villus.

### 10.2.2    Osmolality of Intraluminal and Tissue Ethanol

Intraluminal concentrations of 1, 3, and 6% w/v ethanol have osmolalities of 215, 645, and 1290, respectively. It has been suggested by several investigators that a part, if not all, of the adverse effects of ethanol on intestinal function and morphology could be the result of the high osmolality of the intraluminal solution and have used urea,[37] mannitol,[38] or sodium chloride[39,40] as control solutions in their experiments with ethanol. Addition of ethanol to a solvent increases the "theoretical osmotic pressure" of the solution as measured by freezing point depression. This method measures the osmolality that ethanol would exert against a membrane which is permeable to the solvent (water) but not to the solute (ethanol). However, ethanol is a nonelectrolyte of small molecular weight with a molecular radius of only 2.6 Å even when it produces an azeotrope containing 4% water.[41] Its lipid/water partition coefficient is high (0.032).[26] Accordingly, it penetrates membranes rapidly and diffuses without resistance and can pass through the intestinal membrane as easily as the solvent. Therefore, the "effective osmotic pressure" produced by ethanol is less than the theoretical osmotic pressure measured by freezing point depression. The Staverman reflection coefficient measures the ratio of the effective to the theoretical osmotic pressure and is expressed as the reflection coefficient ($\sigma$) of a substance to a certain membrane.[26] The $\sigma$ may have a value between 1 and 0, where 1 indicates a completely semipermeable (impermeable to the solute) membrane where the effective osmotic pressure exerted by the solute is equal to the theoretical osmotic pressure determined by freezing point depression. A $\sigma$ of 0 indicates that the solute is so highly permeable that the membrane cannot discriminate between the solute and solvent. We measured the Staverman reflection coefficient of ethanol in the jejunum of the hamster[28] and the rabbit[15] and found it to be 0, indicating that ethanol in concentrations found in the intestinal lumen exerts no osmotic pressure on the mucosal membrane. The ideal osmotic control for any substance would be a solute which has similar physical character but has no specific pharmacological effect. Since water has a $\sigma$ of 0, it is the most suitable osmotic control for ethanol.

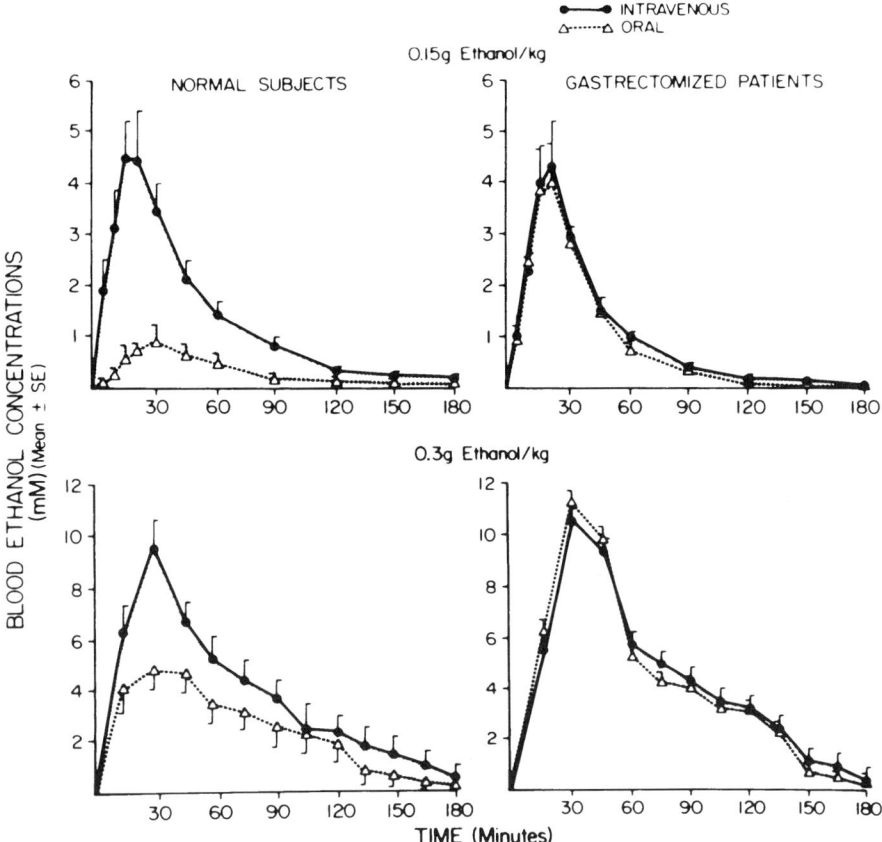

**FIGURE 10.1** Difference in blood ethanol levels between oral and intravenous administration of either 0.15 or 0.3 g/kg body weight of ethanol. Solid line = intravenous; broken line = oral. The difference between the two indicates first-pass metabolism. On the left: normal subjects; on the right: patients with Billroth II subtotal gastrectomy. Note the abolition of first-pass metabolism in gastrectomized patients. (Reprinted from Caballeria, J., Frezza, M., Hernandez-Munoz, R., Dipadova, C., Korsten, M. A., Baraona, E., and Lieber, C. S., *Gastroenterology,* 97, 1205, 1989. With permission.)

## 10.2.3 Ethanol Metabolism in the Small Intestine

It has been suggested that some of the actions of ethanol on the small intestine may be due to its metabolites, acetaldehyde and acetate.[42,43] However, experimental evidence indicates that very little if any of the ingested ethanol is metabolized in the small bowel. The intestinal alcohol dehydrogenase activity in the jejunum varies between species, but it is very low in all. In the hamster the activity of this enzyme is less than 0.1 U/ml protein.[44] Using gas chromatography we were unable to demonstrate the presence of acetaldehyde or acetate in the effluent of the intestinal perfusion solution which contained 3% or 6% ethanol (unpublished data), nor did we find acetaldehyde in villus scrapings or in BBM preparations incubated in ethanol.[6] Rats have a high alcohol dehydrogenase activity in their stomach, but none in their small intestine,[45,46] although the P450IIE1 enzyme is inducible by chronic alcohol intake.[47] Caballeria et al.[48] compared blood alcohol levels after administration of the same amount of ethanol intravenously and intragastrically to human volunteers and observed a considerably lower blood ethanol concentration after intragastric administration, indicating first-pass metabolism of ethanol in the stomach. They also found a high alcohol dehydrogenase activity in gastric biopsies.[49] In contrast, when ethanol was perfused into the jejunum of subjects with Billroth II gastrectomy, the blood alcohol concentration was similar to that obtained with intravenous administration, indicating that ethanol is not metabolized in the small intestine (Figure 10.1).[48] In view of this, experiments with ethanol on the small intestine do not need controls containing acetaldehyde or acetone and incorporation of these substances in studies on ethanol effect[50] may lead to erroneous conclusions.

## 10.3   EFFECT OF ETHANOL ON SMALL INTESTINAL MORPHOLOGY

### 10.3.1   Morphological Observations

The earlier literature on morphological lesions caused by ethanol is inconsistent, mainly because of differences in species, intraluminal ethanol concentrations, lengths of exposure, and timing of the histological examination after ethanol administration. Perfusion of the rat jejunum with 0.05% ethanol caused no structural changes,[51] while intragastric administration of 12 to 76% alcohol had no effect on the small intestine of well-nourished rats but caused hemorrhagic lesions in malnourished animals.[52] Concentration-dependent morphological changes were observed in the duodenum and the jejunum of rats following intragastric administration of ethanol in concentrations ranging from 5 to 49%. The most severe damage occurred at the epithelial layer with denudation of the epithelial cells.[37,39,53]

The first systematic investigation on the effect of ethanol on small intestinal morphology was undertaken in our laboratory. We studied the effect of pharmacologically relevant concentrations of ethanol on the jejunum of hamster,[54-57] rat,[56] rabbit,[15,58] dog,[16,59] and humans.[31]

In the *hamster*, perfusion with solutions of 4.8% ethanol caused separation of epithelium from the villus core, accumulation of proteinaceous subepithelial fluid, and the formation of subepithelial blisters[55,56] (Figure 10.2). There was a variable distribution of blebs. Normal areas without subepithelial blisters were interspersed with areas with blebs in clumps or with areas where there was a bleb on every villus. Over the blebs, the epithelial layer in the hamster was not disrupted and thus there was no denudation of the villus. Cells over blebs appeared to have normal brush border, but because of their distention the shape of the epithelial cells had become cuboidal with complete disappearance of the lateral intercellular spaces (LIS). The lamina propria of the villi with blebs were compacted and shortened, the capillaries were congested, and the lacteals appeared compressed. The subepithelial layer was filled with what appeared to be proteinaceous material. Transmission electron microscopy (TEM) revealed normal ultrastructure of those cells which were exposed to ethanol but which were not over blebs. Epithelial cells located over blebs exhibited diminished density and thickness of the glycocalyx. Because of this, the microvilli and the polygonal cell boundaries became clearly visible on scanning electron microscopy (SEM). On TEM, the epithelial cells were separated and shortened and as they detached from the basement membrane (BM), the lateral intercellular spaces disappeared and they became cuboidal in shape. In the detached cells, the granular endoplasmic reticulum was swollen, but except for this no other cellular abnormality was seen (Figure 10.3). There was, however, considerable vascular stasis in the capillaries and postcapillary venules of the lamina propria underlying blebs.

Observing the areas closely adjacent to blebs, it was possible to reconstruct the step-by-step development of the subepithelial blisters. As shown in Figure 10.4, the normal LIS is formed between the lateral portion of the BLM of the epithelial cells which are stretched by the attachment of the portion of the BLM to the basal lamina (basement membrane) of the villus core. Ethanol caused the LIS to widen. At this stage, the BLM of the cell remained attached only tenuously to the basement membrane of the villus core (Figure 10.4) indicating that blebs formed between the basal lamina of the villus core and the BLM of the epithelial cells.

Blebs started to appear within 5 min after the beginning of the ethanol administration and increased in number with the duration of the perfusion. The ratio of villi with blebs to normal villi was concentration dependent and a greater portion of villi developed blebs with increasing ethanol concentration.[55] The ethanol-induced changes were transient and, 45 min after discontinuation of ethanol perfusion, the separated epithelial layer reattached and villi regained normal appearance.[55]

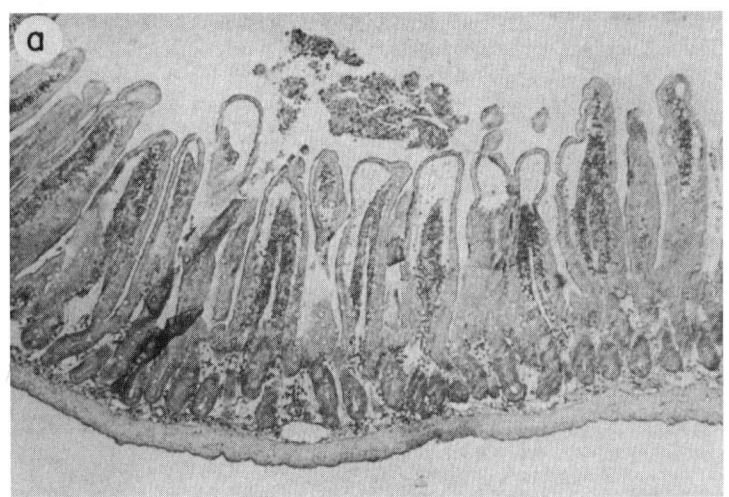

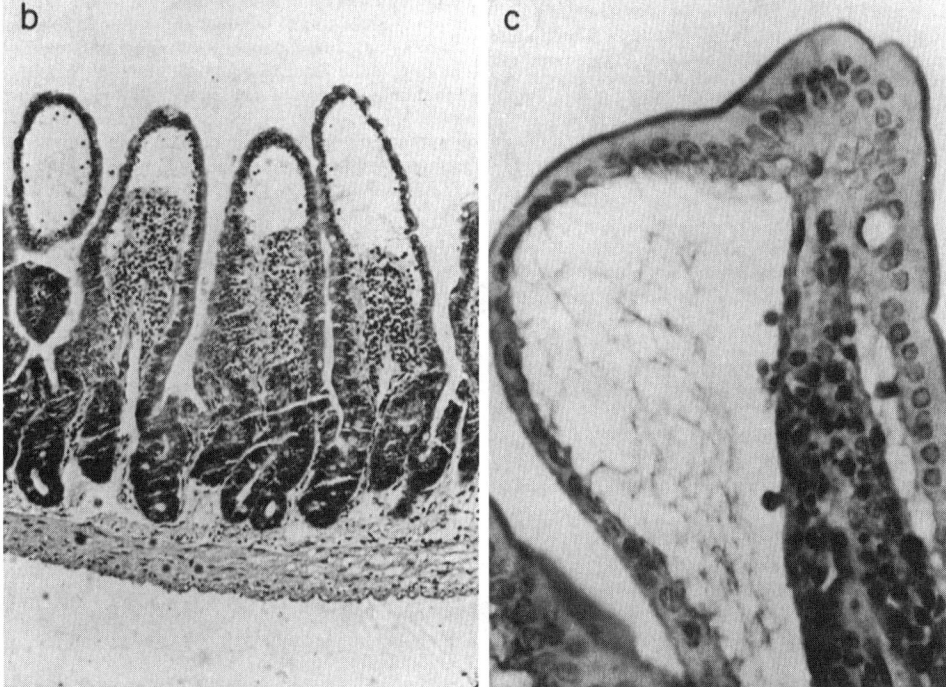

**FIGURE 10.2**    Photomicrograph of hamster jejunum perfused for 45 min with KRBSG containing 4.9% w/v ethanol. (a) Panoramic view with multiple subepithelial blebs. Blebs are unbroken. (Original magnification ×40.) (b) Higher magnification of some blebs. Note the underlying lamina propria is compact and the lacteals are closed. (Original magnification ×100.) (c) Stronger magnification of a villus seen in (a). The epithelial layer has been lifted away from the stroma, by what appears to be proteinaceous edema fluid. The epithelial cells have become cuboidal and no lateral intercellular spaces are visible. The brush-border membrane and the alignment of the nuclei over the blebs are normal. (Original magnification ×400.) (Reprinted from Fox, J. E., McElligott, T. F., and Beck, I. T., *Can. J. Physiol. Pharmacol.*, 56, 123, 1978. With permission.)

The morphological response of the rat jejunum is different from that of the hamster. Complete denudation of the villus tip was observed by some investigators.[37,39,53] To assess whether the differences in the findings in the rat, as compared to those in the hamster, were due to differences in species or to the higher ethanol concentrations used by the above investigators, we carried out

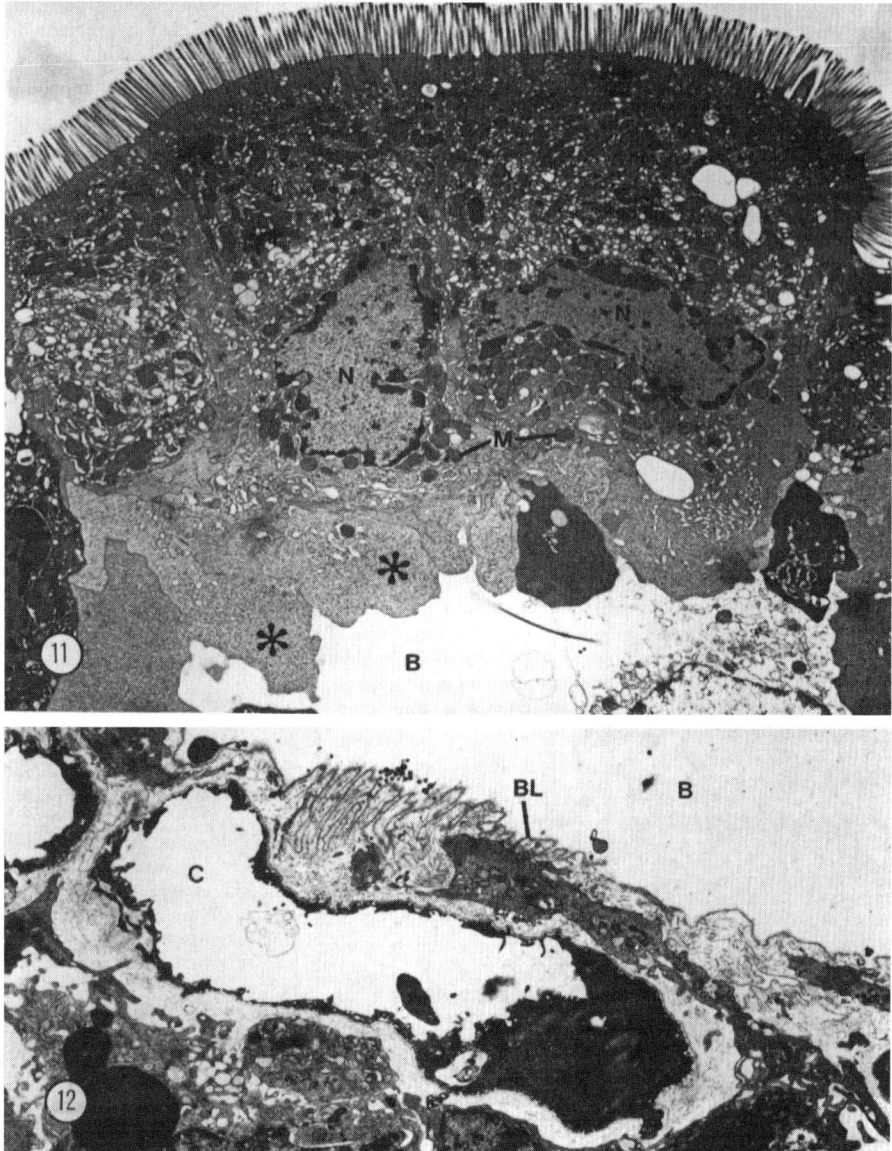

**FIGURE 10.3**    Transmission electron micrography of hamster jejunum perfused for 45 min with KRBSG containing 4.9% (w/v) ethanol. Top(11): Epithelium covering bleb (B). Note extensive swelling of endoplasmic reticulum and pseudopod-like extension of basal cytoplasm (indicated by asterisk). Also note absence of LIS between epithelial cells. Mitochondria (M) display normal morphology. N, nucleus. (Original magnification ×5200.) Bottom(12): Base of large bleb (B). The basal lamina (BL) remains adherent to the underlying propria. Note the vascular congestion in the capillary (C). (Original magnification ×6700.) (Reproduced from Fox, J. E., Morris, G. P., Beck, I. T., and McElligott, T. F., *Can. J. Physiol. Pharmacol.*, 57, 305, 1979. With permission.)

experiments on rats which reproduced identically the conditions used in the hamster experiments.[56] In agreement with others,[37,39,53] we also found denudation of the villus tip in the rat jejunum perfused with 4.9% ethanol. However, on careful assessment of our material, we were able to find many remnants of ruptured blebs and occasional unruptured ones (Figure 10.5). Thus, the denudation reported by others,[37,39,53] and observed by us, was likely the result of breakage of

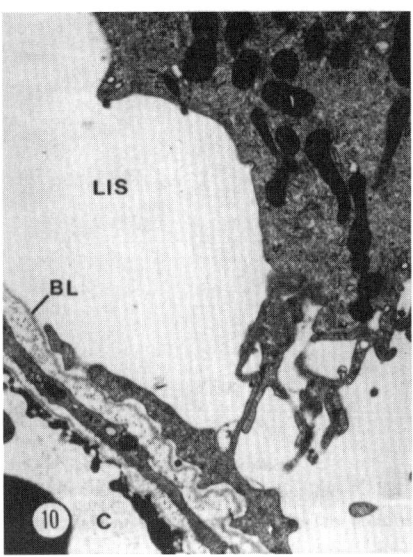

**FIGURE 10.4**   Transmission electronmicrography of the base of an epithelial cell near a bleb after 45-min perfusion with KRBSG containing 4.9% (w/v) ethanol. Note the swollen lateral intercellular space (LIS). Only tenuous connections remain between the base of the cell and the basal lamina (BL). C = capillary. (Original magnification ×11,000.) (Reproduced from Fox, J. E., Morris, G. P., Beck, I. T., and McElligott, T. F., *Can. J. Physiol. Pharmacol.*, 57, 305, 1979.)

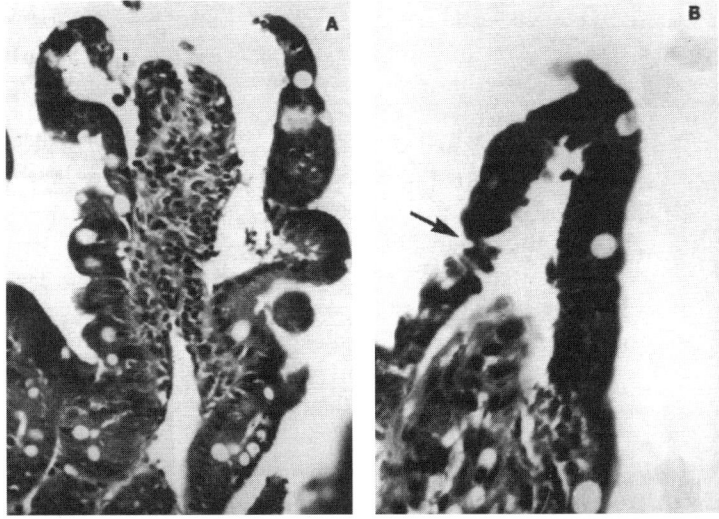

**FIGURE 10.5**   Photomicrograph of rat jejunum after perfusion for 45 min with KRBSG containing 4.9% (w/v) ethanol. (A) This villus shows typical extensive damage seen in the rat. The epithelial layer is broken and appears to be stripping away from the underlying stroma. Open lateral intercellular spaces are not obvious. There are necrotic cells at the edge of the break; (B) this shows an unbroken bleb with an epithelial layer which appears to be disintegrating (arrow). (Reprinted from Fox, J. E., McElligott, T. F., and Beck, I. T., *Am. J. Dig. Dis.*, 23, 201, 1978.)

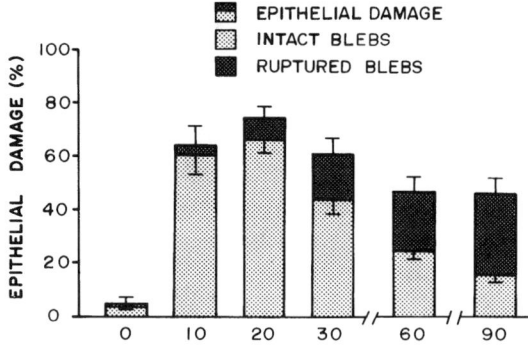

**FIGURE 10.6**    Time course of ethanol-induced epithelial damage in the dog. Ordinate = villi with epithelial damage as a percentage of the villi examined. Abscissa = duration in minutes of perfusion with KRBSG containing 6% w/v ethanol. The data for "0-min" ethanol perfusion represent those obtained from control segment (i.e., not perfused with ethanol). The full height of the bars represents total epithelial damage, i.e., percentage of villi with intact plus those with ruptured blebs. Note that the total damage decreases after a peak of 20 min but the percentage of broken blebs increases with time. Thus at 90 min, the total epithelial damage is less than at 20 min but the percentage of ruptured blebs is higher than at the peak. (Reproduced from Ray, M., Dinda, P. K., and Beck, I. T., *Gastroenterology*, 96, 345, 1989.)

the epithelium over the ethanol-induced blebs, possibly due to a relative weakness of the rat mucosa.[56] The fact that the mucosa of the rat jejunum is less resistant than that of the hamster has been observed by Levine et al.[60] and Faelli et al.,[61] who reported that in *in vitro* conditions, the rat jejunum disintegrates more rapidly than does the jejunum of the hamster.

In the rabbit,[15] 3% ethanol damaged only 20% of the villi and the majority of affected villi had intact blebs leaving very few broken ones. With 6% ethanol, however, 40% of the villi were damaged and the majority of the blebs had ruptured with very few intact ones, indicating that the breakage of the blebs is concentration dependent. Considering the proportion of breakage of blebs, the mucosa of the rabbit is less resistant than that of the hamster, but more resilient than that of the rat.

Morphological changes in the small intestine of the dog[16,17,59,62] were similar to those of other species. Perfusion with 3 to 6% ethanol for 90 min caused the development of subepithelial blebs at the tip of the villi. The blebs were either intact or broken. Intact blebs appeared to be filled with proteinaceous fluid. In some of the ruptured blebs there was exfoliation of most of the epithelial cells, while in others the broken epithelium remained attached to the stroma. The distribution of blebs and broken blebs was uneven with areas where epithelium remained entirely normal. The villus core appeared contracted, compressed, and this resulted in the compression of the central lymphatics of the villus.[59,62] The changes were more severe with 6% ethanol than with 3%.[16]

With continuous ethanol perfusion for 90 min, the peak damage occurred around 20 min after the beginning of the perfusion. After this, in spite of the continued intraluminal presence of ethanol, there was a diminution in the total number of damaged villi, probably because of the reattachment of unbroken blebs to the stroma. However, in spite of this overall improvement, the number of broken blebs increased (Figure 10.6).[59] The above findings suggest that there is a concentration-dependent increase in the ethanol-induced morphological damage, that there is rapid reattachment of unbroken blebs to the stroma and that prolonged exposure to ethanol increases the percentage of broken blebs. As will be discussed later, this biphasic morphological response to ethanol fits in timing with the biphasic reaction of the microvascular changes.[59,62]

The morphological changes in *humans* in response to the intragastric administration of 45 or 60 g of ethanol diluted to 20% (equivalent to 4.8 or 6.4 oz of 80 proof whisky) to normal

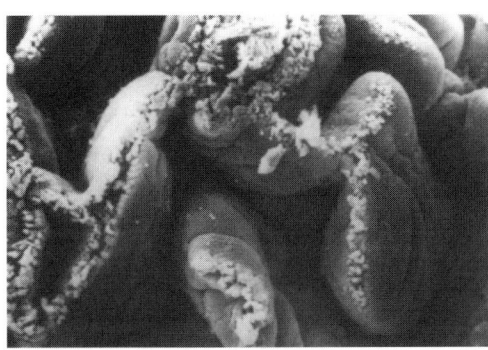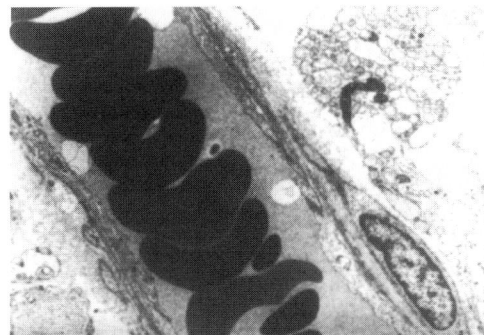

**FIGURE 10.7**    Ethanol effect on human duodenal mucosa. Left: Scanning electron microscopy 3 min after a spray
with 40% ethanol. Note that most of the villi are swollen and exhibit blebs. In the villi where the blebs
have broken and the superficial layer is lost, the villus core has retracted and cannot be seen. (Original
magnification ×150.) Right: Transmission electron microscopy: vascular engorgement 1 h after
superfusion with 40% ethanol. Note the stacking of red blood cells. (Original magnification ×2,600.)
(Reproduced from Foschi, D., Marazzi, M., Toti, G. L., Radaelli, E., Ferrante, F., Vaiani, G., Galeone,
M., and Trabucchi, E., *Am. J. Gastroenterol.*, 85, 1498, 1990. With permission.)

volunteers were similar to those observed in other species.[31] Hydraulic suction biopsies obtained
prior to ethanol administration yielded specimens with 18% damaged villi (7.5% with blebs and
10.3% with ruptured blebs). The damage in control biopsies may have been the result of
detachment of the epithelium and microvascular congestion caused by the hydraulic suction
biopsy equipment.[63] Biopsies taken 5 min after peak ethanol concentration (approximately 20
min after intragastric administration of alcohol) exhibited a significantly higher (45%) number
of damaged villi. Forty-five percent of villi were damaged, 26% with blebs, and 19% with broken
blebs. Approximately 90 to 120 min after peak ethanol concentration, the intraluminal ethanol
concentration returned to normal. At that time the mucosal biopsies appeared similar to those of
the controls, again demonstrating the rapidity by which the mucosa returns to normal after acute
exposure to ethanol.

Foschi et al.[64,65] sprayed 50 ml of 40% ethanol on duodenal mucosa of humans during
endoscopy and examined the area before alcohol administration and 3, 60, 180, and 300 min after
the challenge. This high concentration of ethanol caused severe damage in the duodenum with
extravasation of blood, and epithelial necrosis. The damage became progressively worse 3[64] to
5 h[65] after administration. Scanning and transmission electron microscopy showed a loss of
superficial epithelial cells. Their SEM pictures (Figure 10.7) indicate the presence of blebs, the
majority of which were ruptured. In those blebs where the epithelial layer has exfoliated the villus
core cannot be seen under the open end of the villus tip, probably because it had fully contracted
to the base of the villus. In addition to mucosal damage, there was severe microvascular
congestion (Figure 10.7).

In conclusion, in all species examined, the acute alcohol-induced morphological injury
consisted of villus core contraction and compaction, compression of lacteals, separation of the
epithelium from the normal appearing basal lamina of the villus core, congestion of villus
capillaries, and of postcapillary venules. Possibly, due to this vascular congestion, the subepithelial
blebs were filled with proteinaceous material. The extent of the loss of epithelial cells at the tip
of the villus appeared to depend on the concentration of ethanol, length of exposure to alcohol,
and species-dependent sensitivity of the mucosa to injury.

Recovery was rapid and occurred even during continuous exposure to ethanol. The probable
mechanism is reattachment of healthy epithelial cells to the normal basal lamina. In those villi
where epithelial cells were lost during rupture of the blebs, restitution must have occurred by
rapid migration of the still viable epithelial cells originating from cells adjacent to the exfoliated

ones. A similar mechanism of restitution has reportedly occurred in the stomach[66] and small intestines[67,68] during recovery from mucosal injury induced by various other agents.

### 10.3.2  Mechanism of Ethanol-Induced Morphological Changes

Morphological studies indicated that the mucosal and submucosal damage caused by ethanol was accompanied by severe vascular congestion of the villus.[15,16,31,55-57,64,65,69] This could suggest that alterations in the microvasculature play a considerable role in the development of epithelial injury. In contrast, the vascular and morphological changes could be independent from each other. To separate the mechanism(s) of the morphological alterations from that of ethanol's effect on the microcirculation, we have studied the ethanol-induced morphological changes in an *in vitro* preparation (i.e., in the absence of microcirculation), and compared the *in vitro* findings with those observed in *in vivo* (i.e., in the presence of microcirculation).[13] In an apparatus designed to study the behavior of the villus under *in vitro* conditions, we exposed excised hamster jejunum to a control solution [Krebs-Ringer bicarbonate solution (KRBS) containing 10 m$M$ glucose (KRBSG)] and to KRBSG solutions containing 0.8, 1.6, and 4.8% (w/v) ethanol. The morphological response of the mucosa was continuously examined for 20 min employing a videomicroscopic technique, and the changes were morphometrically evaluated. Ethanol caused a concentration-dependent increase in the number of villi with the accumulation of subepithelial clear fluid, resulting in blebs. This was accompanied by a decrease in the height of the villus core with contraction and compaction of the lamina propria. With 0.8 and 1.6% ethanol the contracted core remained partially attached to the epithelium and the total villus height (the sum of the height of the villus core plus epithelial layer) decreased. With 4.8% ethanol, the villus core contraction was so rapid (fully contracted in less than 1 min) that the stroma separated in its entire length from the epithelium (Figures 10.8 and 10.9). Thus among other factors, the rapidity of the villus core contractions appears to play a role in subepithelial bleb formation and the appearance of the blister. These *in vitro* experiments indicate that the effect of ethanol on morphology is independent from its action on the microcirculation.

Further studies in our laboratory seem to indicate that the development of subepithelial blebs does not depend solely on the rapidity and extent of villus core contraction but rather that the strength by which the epithelial cells adhere to the basement membrane and to each other plays a major role. For instance, under similar *in vitro* conditions, 1 m$M$ histamine (a pharmacological, rather than a physiological concentration*) causes rapid villus core contraction, but because the epithelium remains attached to the core, no blebs are formed (Table 10.1).[70] This would suggest that in addition to core contraction, the strength of the attachment of the epithelium to the subepithelial basal lamina also plays a role in bleb formation. Furthermore, when $H_1$ and $H_2$ receptors were blocked with promethazine and ranitidine, histamine did not cause villus core contraction, but in spite of the presence of $H_1$ and $H_2$ blockade, ethanol still exerted its usual effect on the villus core and blebs were formed. This suggests that the villus core contraction caused by ethanol is not mediated by histamine. Furthermore, these data also indicate that villus core contraction alone does not cause separation of the epithelium from the lamina propria. In order to form blebs, in addition to core contraction, ethanol may have some additional effect, possibly by loosening the adherence of the epithelium to the lamina propria (see Table 10.1). Further studies have demonstrated that calcium is necessary in the bathing solution for ethanol to produce subepithelial blebs and that calcium ionophores, even in the absence of ethanol, induce subepithelial blebs *in vitro*.[71] Ethanol has been shown to increase calcium entry into hepatocytes and gastric epithelial cells[72-74] and, if this is the case for small intestinal epithelium, it is possible that ethanol also affects enterocyte adhesion of the epithelium to the subjacent lamina propria by increasing calcium entry into the small intestinal epithelial cells.

---

* Smaller histamine concentrations had no effect on the villus morphology.

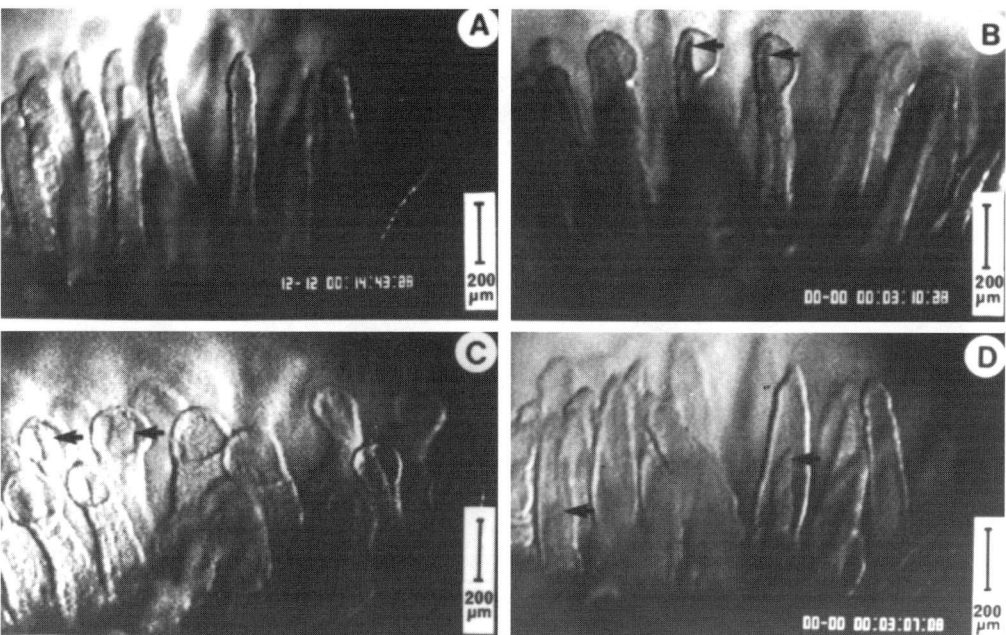

**FIGURE 10.8**    Villi after *in vitro* exposure of hamster jejunum for 3 min to different concentrations of ethanol in KRBSG. (A) Control solution; (B) a solution containing 0.8% (w/v) ethanol; (C) 1.6% (w/v) ethanol; and (D) 4.8% (w/v) ethanol. Note the ballooning of the epithelium with 0.8 and 1.6% ethanol and consequently a change in the shape of the villi. Villus cores are contracted, but in many instances they are still attached to the epithelium. With 4.8% ethanol the villus core was fully contracted, the bleb extended all along the villus and there was complete detachment of the epithelium from the stroma along the entire villus. Arrows indicate some of the denuded cores in (B) and (C) and the upper end of villus core in (D). (Reproduced from Dinda, P. K., Buell, M. G., Morris, G. P., and Beck, I. T., *Can. J. Physiol. Pharmacol.*, 72, 1186, 1994. With permission.)

## 10.4    EFFECT OF ETHANOL ON SMALL INTESTINAL MICROCIRCULATION

### 10.4.1    Mucosal Microcirculatory Changes

Bleb formation, followed in some cases by epithelial loss at the tip of the villi, has been observed in other conditions that interfere with villus drainage or cause vascular changes in the villus core. For instance, Lee[75] described subepithelial blisters in the dog when fluid drainage was inhibited by increasing pressure in the lymphatics of the villi. Similar morphological changes have been documented in portal hypertension in the dog[76] and in humans,[77] in diabetes,[78] in mucosal lesions adjacent to necrotic areas in patients with shock,[79] in small intestinal response to IgE,[80] and in microvascular injury caused by radiation.[81,82] The abundant vascular engorgement observed in the *in vivo* morphological studies suggest that ethanol has a considerable effect on the local microcirculation. Accepting that subepithelial blisters can be caused by ethanol *in vitro*, and therefore that the morphological changes cannot be primarily dependent on ethanol's effect on blood flow, there still may be an interaction between the alteration of blood flow in the microvasculature and the morphological injury. Accordingly a review of ethanol's effect on the vasculature, blood flow, and local microcirculation is necessary to fully understand the mechanisms of ethanol-induced small bowel injury. Depending on the route of administration, the dose, and the local concentration, acutely administered ethanol has variable quantitative and qualitative effects on blood flow. In the systemic circulation, blood ethanol concentrations are low and deep coma ensues at a concentration of 0.3%.[1] In spite of this upper limit for the pharmacologically relevant concentration, some investigators used up to 10% ethanol in *in vitro* vascular preparations.[83] Depending on whether low or well above toxic concentrations are used, ethanol can cause

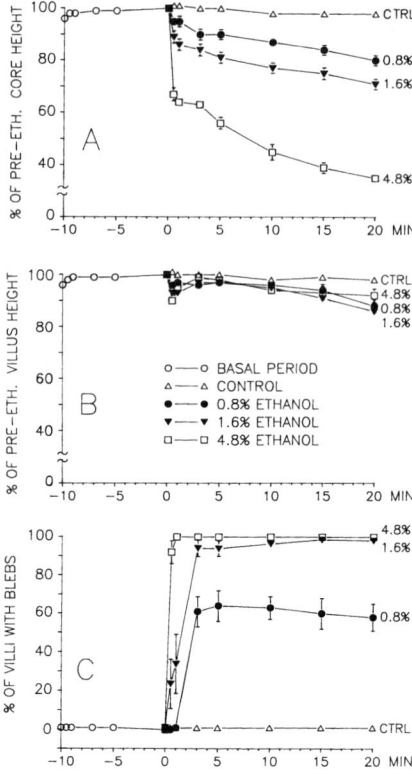

**FIGURE 10.9**    Morphometric assessment of the effect of exposure of hamster jejunum *in vitro* to control and 0.8, 1.6, and 4.8% (w/v) of ethanol in KRBSG before and after the experimental solution; (A) villus core height; (B) total villus height; (C) prevalence of villi with blebs. Abscissa time in minutes. Preexperimental measurements were done at –10, –9.5, –9, –7, –5, and 0 min, and after addition of experimental solutions at 0.5, 1, 3, 5, 10, 15, and 20 min, respectively. In (A) and (B), the ordinate represents percent change from the height as compared to the height at the end of the basal period. (At the basal period the villus core height of the four groups was $612 \pm 9$, $641 \pm 14$, $628 \pm 19$, and $633 \pm 15$ μm, respectively and for villus height it was $635 \pm 9$, $663 \pm 12$, $662 \pm 19$, and $660 \pm 15$ μm, respectively.) In (C), the ordinate shows the percentage of villi with blebs. Values are given as mean ± SE. ○—○ = combined basal values before the addition of the experimental solutions; △—△ = after addition of saline (control); ●—● = 0.8% (w/v) ethanol; ▼—▼ = 1.6% (w/v) ethanol; and □—□ = 4.8% (w/v) ethanol. (Reproduced from Dinda, P. K., Morris, G. P., Buell, M. G., and Beck, I. T., *Can. J. Physiol. Pharmacol.*, 72, 1186, 1994. With permission.)

vasoconstriction, vasodilation, or a biphasic response.[84] In the microcirculation of the canine small intestine, 4.5% intraluminal ethanol (a concentration observed in humans during moderate drinking) increased jejunal total gut wall blood flow, but decreased arteriovenous oxygen gradient.[85] Israel and co-workers[86] observed in the rat that total arterial inflow into the small intestine doubled after the administration of 4 g/kg of ethanol. In our laboratory 3 and 6% ethanol perfused intraluminally increased jejunal blood flow in the rabbit and the dog.[15,69] Using 15 μm microspheres, we could separately determine the blood flow of the mucosa and submucosa from that of the muscularis and serosa. In the rabbit, comparing blood flow in 3 loops perfused for 90 min with control KRBSG solution, KRBSG containing 3% ethanol, and KRBSG with 6% ethanol, we observed that ethanol increased arterial inflow into the mucosa and submucosa but did not affect the flow into the muscularis and serosa.[15] Thus ethanol exerts a local microvascular effect on the mucosa, but does not affect the microcirculation of the vessels of the deeper layers of the gut. Similar findings were obtained in the dog.[16]

The morphological studies suggested that ethanol caused mucosal vascular congestion and hemoconcentration. To confirm and quantitate this by physiological means, we determined

**TABLE 10.1    Effect of Ethanol, Histamine, and Histamine Antagonists on the Ethanol-Induced Bleb Formation in Hamster Jejunum *In Vitro***

|  | Control | 2% ETH | 1 mM HIST | HIST + P + R | ETH + P + R |
|---|---|---|---|---|---|
| Villus ht (μm) | 649 ± 15 | 629 ± 18 | 509 ± 20[a] | 627 ± 19 | 575 ± 17[a] |
| Villus core ht (μm) | 627 ± 15 | 488 ± 21[a] | 489 ± 21[a] | 615 ± 19 | 394 ± 15[a] |
| Villi with bleb (%) | — | 96 ± 2[a] | 3 ± 2 | 1 ± 1 | 94 ± 4[a] |

*Note:*  The agents were added into the incubation solution [Krebs-Ringer bicarbonate solution with 10 mM glucose (KRBSG)] in quantities to reach final concentrations as described below. $H_2$ antagonists were added 10 min before the addition of histamine or ethanol and the measurements in the table are those taken 10 min after the addition of histamine or ethanol. The difference between villus core height (ht) and villus height (ht) represents the thickness of the epithelial layer which in normal villi is 18 ± 8 μm. A greater difference indicates villus core contraction and a space (bleb) between the epithelial layer and the core. ETH = ethanol 2% (w/v); HIST = histamine (1 mM); P = promethazine (3 μM); R = ranitidine (3 mM).

[a]  Statistically ($p < 0.05$) different from appropriate control. Note that ethanol had only a minor effect on villus height but because of villus core contraction and consequent bleb formation the space between the two increased. In response to histamine an equal fall occurred in total villus height and the height of the villus core, indicating that in spite of villus core contraction the epithelium remained attached to the core and thus no blebs were formed. Antihistamines abolished the effect of histamine but not that of ethanol, indicating that the ethanol-induced morphological changes are not related to the effect of histamine, and that to produce blebs, ethanol, in addition to villus core contraction, loosens the attachment of the epithelial layer to the core.

Reproduced from Beck, I. T. and Dinda, P. K., *Gastroenterology*, 100, A561, 1991.

simultaneously the effect of ethanol on mucosal arterial blood flow, mucosal red blood cell volume, and mucosal plasma volume.[69] Three percent ethanol to some extent and 6% considerably increased mucosal arteriolar blood flow and mucosal red blood cell volume without an equivalent increase in the mucosal plasma volume, indicating that hemoconcentration occurred which was more severe with 6% alcohol than with 3% (Figure 10.10). The mucosal microvascular stasis was accompanied by an intraluminal loss of plasma protein (Table 10.2), which was barely significant with 3% ethanol but was disproportionally greater with 6%. A biphasic response of protein leakage was observed with a peak at 20 to 30 min, followed by a decline in spite of continued perfusion with ethanol for 90 min. Similar biphasic leakage of albumin into the gut lumen was observed during acute administration of ethanol in the rabbit,[19,20,58,62,87-90] but the peak of the curve occurred later and the protein loss was greater in this species (Figure 10.11). A similar biphasic curve was observed in humans by Lavo and co-workers.[91]

With the considerable loss of serum protein into the lumen, the question arises as to whether the protein loss was the result of increased *epithelial* or mainly of *microvascular* permeability. Protein could be lost simply because of alterations in Starling equilibrium due to an ethanol-induced increased blood flow, capillary pressure, capillary filtration coefficient, and thus an increase in oncotic pressure gradient. This would lead to leakage of serum protein through fenestrae of the endothelial cells into the interstitium and as a result of an increased mucosal permeability into the lumen.[17] A second possibility is that ethanol acts on the microvasculature in a similar manner as observed in response to injury caused by other agents (e.g., injection of turpentine, mustard oil, histamine or serotonin into the pleura, muscle, scrotum, etc.),[92-98] where endothelial cells retract, the intercellular junctions open and large quantities of macromolecules pass from capillaries and postcapillary venules into the interstitium. The large amount of protein lost into the lumen during 6% (w/v) ethanol perfusion made us consider that the second mechanism may play a more important role. To investigate whether this is the case, we used the colloidal carbon method of Majno and co-workers.[92,93] This technique is based on the observation that when endothelial cells temporarily retract a gap is created between the cells through which colloidal carbon particles can pass. Because the particles cannot traverse the BM, once the endothelial cells reexpand the carbon becomes trapped between the endothelial cells and the basal lamina of the microvessels. To assess whether ethanol causes a temporary retraction of endothelial cells, and thus intercellular exudation,

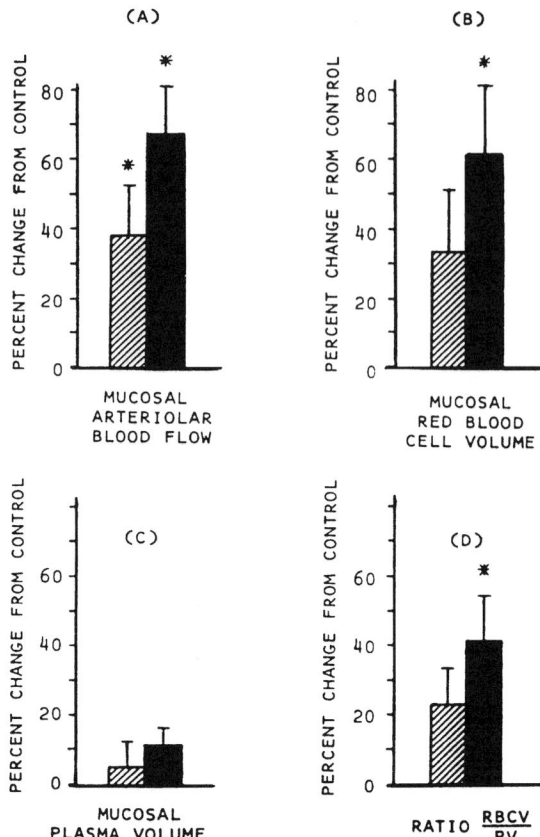

**FIGURE 10.10**    Effects of intraluminal perfusion with 3.0 and 6.0% (w/v) ethanol on canine jejunal mucosal arteriolar blood flow, red blood cell volume, and "plasma volume" (as reflected by mucosal total albumin volume). (A) Mucosal arteriolar blood flow (measured by 15 μm, $^{46}$Sc-labeled microspheres); (B) mucosal red blood cell volume (measured with $^{51}$Cr-labeled red blood cells); (C) mucosal "plasma volume" (measured with $^{125}$I-bovine serum albumin); (D) ratio of blood cell volume to plasma volume. (Reproduced from Buell, M. G. and Beck, I. T., *Gastroenterology,* 86, 413, 1984. With permission.)

we perfused three adjacent canine jejunal segments, one with control solutions (KRBSG), a second with KRBSG containing 3%, and the third with 6% ethanol in KRBSG. Subsequently, before sacrificing the animals we waited 1 h so that the circulating carbon could be cleared by the reticuloendothelial system so that in glycerin-cleared thick sections the vessels labeled in their walls would stand out and would not be confused with those in which the free carbon was still circulating. Six percent intraluminal ethanol caused accumulation of carbon particles in the microvessels of the villus tip.[99] Electron microscopy (Figure 10.12) showed that the carbon was

**TABLE 10.2    Effect of Ethanol on Vascular Permeability of the Dog Jejunum**

|  | Number of villi counted | Percentage of carbon-labeled villi | Significance of difference from control |
|---|---|---|---|
| Control | 1028 | $0.82 \pm 0.27$ | |
| 3% ethanol | 1125 | $9.62 \pm 4.13$ | $0.05 < p < 0.1$ |
| 6% ethanol | 1162 | $48.17 \pm 19.03$ | $p < 0.05$ |

*Note:*    Data present the percentage of villi with carbon labeling. The control segment was perfused with Krebs-Ringer bicarbonate solution containing 10 m*M* glucose (KRBSG); the other segments were perfused with KRBSG containing 3 and 6% (w/v) ethanol, respectively.

Reproduced from Beck, I. T., Morris, G. P., and Buell, M. G., *Gastroenterology,* 90, 1137, 1986. With permission.

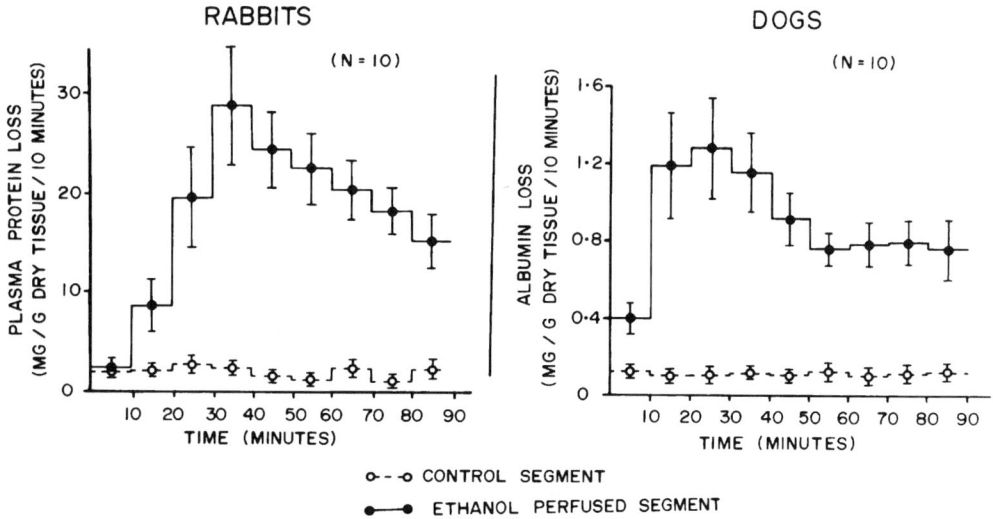

**FIGURE 10.11**   Comparison of time course of ethanol-induced intraluminal protein loss in rabbits (left) and in dogs (right). Broken lines depict control segments, solid line shows segments perfused with 6% ethanol in KRBSG. Ordinates on the left indicate plasma protein loss in rabbits in mg/g dry tissue/10 min and on the right albumin loss in dogs in mg/g dry tissue/10 min. Each square represents a 10-min collection. Note that in the rabbit the peak is achieved in 30 to 40 min while in the dog it is achieved between 20 and 30 min. In addition, protein loss in the rabbit is much greater than in the dog. (Reproduced from Beck, I. T., Dinda, P. K., Leddin, D. J., Ray, M., Prokopiw, I., and Boyd, A., Chemical mediators in ethanol-induced increased jejunal microvascular permeability, in *Microcirculation in Circulatory Disorders*, Manabe, H., Aweifach, B. W., and Messmer, K., Eds., Springer-Verlag, Tokyo, 1988, 171. With permission.)

localized between the endothelial cells and the basal lamina of the capillaries and postcapillary venules and was always adjacent to endothelial cell junctions. Thus, the escape of carbon particles (and of the much smaller albumin molecules) must have occurred through these intercellular gaps, suggesting that the protein loss observed during 6% ethanol perfusion was not only the result of the increased epithelial, but also of the enhanced microvascular permeability.

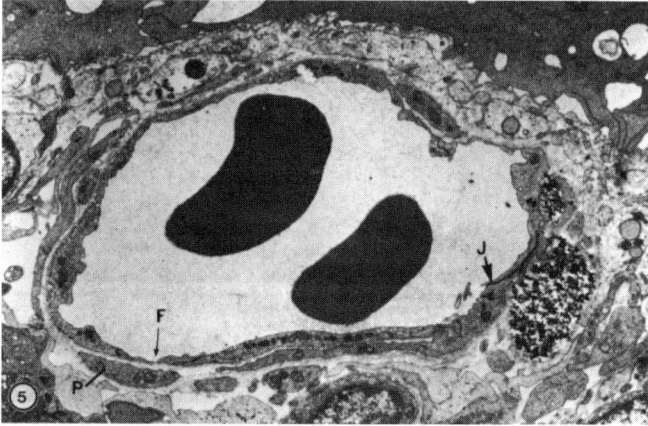

**FIGURE 10.12**   Venule from dog jejunal segment perfused with 6% w/v ethanol in KRBSG. Note that the carbon particles accumulate behind endothelial cell junctions (J). Carbon particles did not traverse the basement membrane. Carbon particles did not pass fenestrations (F). P = pericyte. (Original magnification ×7600.) (Reproduced from Beck, I. T., Morris, G. P., and Buell, M. G., *Gastroenterology*, 90, 1137, 1986. With permission.)

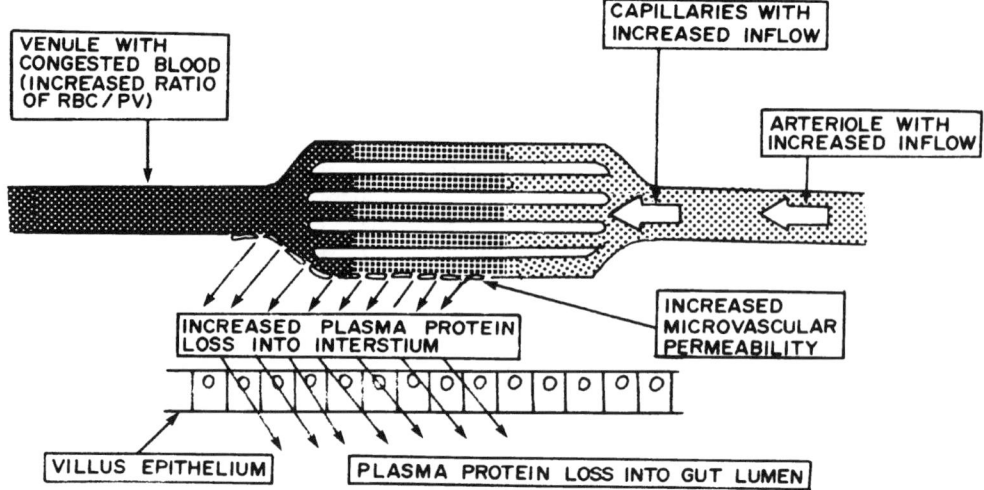

**FIGURE 10.13**   Schematic representation of ethanol-induced changes in the microcirculation. Note that there is an increased inflow of blood from the arterioles. The increased permeability of capillaries and postcapillary venules allows protein to leak into the interstitium. Due to leakage of protein from the capillaries, hemoconcentration occurs which causes vascular congestion. The protein that leaked into the interstitium passes through epithelial breakage into the intraluminal fluid.

Thirty minutes after the onset of the ethanol perfusion, some junctions were still open while the majority were already closed over the entrapped carbon. This indicates an ethanol-induced transient retraction followed by relaxation of endothelial cells. The early opening and subsequent closure of the interendothelial cell junctions in spite of ongoing ethanol perfusion may explain the biphasic curve of the intraluminal protein loss.

Entrapment of carbon was increased with 6% ethanol but not with the 3% solution (Table 10.2). This finding fits well with the high intraluminal loss of protein with 6% (w/v) ethanol and a relatively low protein loss with 3% w/v ethanol.[69] It also explains the observation of Kvietys et al.[17] that perfusion with lower concentrations [4% (w/v), 5% (v/v)] of ethanol did not increase capillary permeability. Thus protein loss with low intraluminal ethanol concentrations can be explained by alterations of the Starling equilibrium[17] but the more severe exudation of protein observed with 6% (w/v) ethanol is most likely due to microvascular damage.

To examine the time course of ethanol-induced microvascular permeability we studied the entrapment of monastral blue B dye into canine jejunal microvessels.[100] Monastral blue (particle diameter ≈ 500 Å) also passes through interendothelial gaps in injured blood vessels and becomes entrapped between the endothelial cells and the BM.[101] In this study on dogs, six jejunal segments were perfused, one loop with control solution, and five with 6% ethanol. Of the latter 5 segments, one was perfused for 10 min, the second for 20 min, the third, fourth, and fifth for 30, 40, and 50 min, respectively. The timing of the onset of the ethanol perfusion was such that all perfusions ended at the same time (i.e., at 50 min) and monastral blue was injected 5 min before the perfusion period ended. Protein loss was also measured and correlated with the timing of monastral blue entrapment. The highest proportion of monastral blue dyed vessels was observed 10 min after the onset of ethanol perfusion, indicating that the majority of endothelial cell junctions opened before the end of the 10-min perfusion period and were all closed by 20 min. Protein loss started to peak at 20 min and declined after 40 min, indicating that protein leakage was highest in the effluents collected immediately after the opening of endothelial cell junctions and fell soon after the closure of the gaps. Thus there is a close relationship between the opening and the closing of endothelial junctions and the biphasic curve of protein loss,[100] indicating that intraluminal protein loss is an accurate reflection of microvascular injury. The vascular mechanism involved in the first phase of protein loss is described in Figure 10.13. The possible mechanism(s) of the second part of the biphasic response are discussed in the section dealing with the role of inflammatory mediators.

## 10.4.2 Mechanism of Ethanol-Induced Microcirculatory Changes

The capillaries and postcapillary venules, as well as mast cells and other immunocytes, lay in close proximity to the epithelium. Ethanol, which traverses the epithelial layer rapidly, can reach these structures in relatively high concentration (see Section 10.2.1.2). Thus ethanol could act directly on the microvessels or through a cascade of inflammatory mediators. In a series of experiments, we investigated the role of these mediators on the ethanol-induced microvascular injury. The general approach of these experiments was to compare the ethanol-induced changes in the "untreated" (control) group to that of the "treated" (experimental) group. In the latter group(s), treatment consisted of the administration of mediators or their antagonists. In each animal of either group, one segment was perfused for 90 min with KRBSG (control segment), while the other with KRBSG containing 6% (w/v) ethanol (ethanol segment). In most experiments microvascular permeability (protein clearance into the lumen), epithelial permeability to small molecules ($^{51}$Cr-EDTA clearance*) and histamine and or other mediators in the tissues or effluents were measured. The effect of ethanol perfusion was assessed by comparing the results of the ethanol-perfused segment to those of the control segment. By comparing the results obtained in the ethanol segment of the treated group with those of the untreated group, it was possible to assess whether a specific treatment increased or decreased the ethanol-induced microvascular damage or influenced the release of mediators.

The ethanol-treated segment in all experiments demonstrated the typical biphasic response of protein loss and histamine release in spite of ongoing intraluminal ethanol perfusion. If mediators do play a role, this biphasic response could possibly be explained by the initial release of aggressive mediators followed by the adaptive release of protective substances. Studies on the aggressive mediators are available on the effect of ethanol on jejunal histamine release, and the interaction of histamine release and mast cell degranulation. The role of leukotrienes, reactive oxygen radicals, leukocyte adhesive factors, and leukocyte proteinases in the ethanol-induced changes of the microcirculation was also investigated. As regards the protective mediators, data are available only on the role of prostaglandins.

### 10.4.2.1 The Role of Aggressive Mediators

#### 10.4.2.1.1 Mast Cell Degranulation and Histamine Action

There are many reasons to suggest that histamine plays a major role in the ethanol-induced jejunal microvascular injury. The microcirculatory changes caused by ethanol resemble those reported for histamine. Similar to ethanol, intraarterial infusion of histamine into the canine small intestine increases blood flow and initiates protein loss and secretion.[102] Histamine in nonintestinal tissues causes gap formation between endothelial cells of postcapillary venules.[92,93,103,104] Like ethanol, histamine causes a large increase in microvascular permeability which lasts for only 15 to 30 min and then is followed by a rapid decline in microvascular transudation, in spite of ongoing administration of histamine.[105,106]

Several lines of evidence support the role of histamine in ethanol-induced jejunal microvascular injury. First, intraluminal ethanol releases histamine *in vivo* and *in vitro*. [19,58,88,90,107-111] Second, inhibition of histamine action with combined $H_1$ and $H_2$ receptor blockade partially abolishes the microvascular protein leakage in rabbits[19] and dogs.[107] Third, the time course of histamine release during a 90 min intraluminal ethanol perfusion parallels that of the protein loss, i.e., there is a progressive rise and fall of histamine content in the effluate of the perfusion solution

---

* The role of $^{51}$Cr-EDTA in determining epithelial permeability is discussed in Section 10.5.1. It probably measures not only permeability to small molecules, but also fluid movement due to secretory filtration.

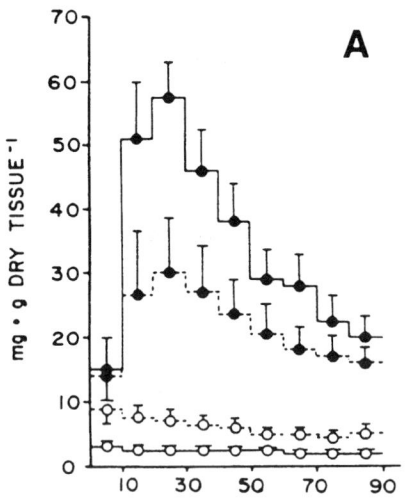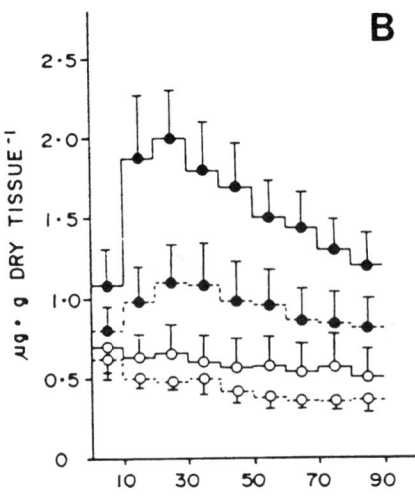

## PERFUSION TIME IN MINUTES

**FIGURE 10.14**    Time-course of action of 16, 16-dimethyl prostaglandin E$_2$ (dmPGE$_2$) on ethanol-induced interluminal plasma protein loss (A), and on histamine release into the luminal fluid (B) in the rabbit. Two groups of rabbits were studied: untreated and dmPGE$_2$-treated groups. In each animal of both groups, one jejunal segment was perfused with a control solution [control of untreated group (–○–) and control of dmPGE$_2$-treated (- -○- -)] and an adjacent segment with 6% (w/v) ethanol [ethanol segment of untreated group 6% (w/v) (–●–) and ethanol segment of dmPGE$_2$-treated group (- -●- -)]. The abscissa shows the 10-min effluent collection periods (which were 0 to 10 min, 10 to 20 min, 20 to 30 min, etc.) during the 90-min continuous intraluminal ethanol perfusion. The ordinates in (A) show plasma protein loss in mg/g dry tissue /10 min. In (B), histamine recovery is measured in the lumen/ 10 min in µg/g dry weight of the perfused jejunal segments. Data are given as mean ± SE. Note that dmPGE$_2$ decreased protein loss in the ethanol treated segment in parallel with the decrease in histamine release. (Reproduced from Dinda, P. K., Holitzner, C. A., Morris, G. P., and Beck, I. T., *Gastroenterology*, 104, 361, 1993. With permission.)

(Figure 10.14). Fourth, inhibition of protein loss with 16-16-dimethyl-prostaglandin[58] and several other protective agents decreases the ethanol-induced histamine release in parallel with a decrease in ethanol-induced protein exudation[88,90,108,110] indicating that a direct relationship exists between the histamine concentration of the effluate and the degree of microvascular damage.[58]

The main source of ethanol-induced histamine is the mast cell. The histamine release and concomitant protein loss caused by ethanol can be substantially decreased *in vivo* in the rabbit jejunum by the mast cell stabilizer ketotefin.[58] Furthermore, the mucosal mast cell stabilizer phloretin[112-114] decreases the ethanol-induced histamine release from the rabbit jejunum *in vitro*.[58]

Histamine, however, is not the only mediator of the microvascular injury. In the experiments with H$_1$ and H$_2$ receptor blockade, in spite of complete inhibition of both receptors, the decrease in protein loss was only 47% in the rabbit[19] and 49% in the dog.[107] Thus other inflammatory mediators (e.g., leukotrienes) may also be involved. However, because histamine release parallels fully the protein loss (i.e., the microvascular injury) and because it originates from mast cells, the assessment of its release provides an excellent measure of mast cell degranulation.

### 10.4.2.1.2    5-Lipoxygenase Products

Similar to histamine, the mediators derived from the action of 5-lipoxygenase on arachidonic acid, the leukotrienes (LT), specifically LTC$_4$, and LTD$_4$ increase the permeability of capillaries.[115,116] Ethanol stimulates leukotriene formation in the rat stomach[117] and in the rabbit[20] indicating that ethanol induces 5-lipoxygenase, and thus the enzymatic production of LTs. We studied the effect of 4-bromo-2,7-dimethoxy-3H-phenothiazine-3-1(L-651,392, Merck Frost, Canada), an inhibitor

**TABLE 10.3    Effect of Superoxide Dismutase and Catalase on Ethanol-Induced Microvascular and Epithelial Permeability and Histamine Release**

| | Untreated ($n = 8$) | | SOD + CAT Treated ($n = 9$) | |
| | Control segment | Ethanol segment | Control segment | Ethanol segment |
| --- | --- | --- | --- | --- |
| $^{15}$Cr-EDTA | $0.15 \pm 0.05$ | $2.7 \pm 0.3$[a] | $0.24 \pm 0.12$ | $1.3 \pm 0.1$[b] |
| $^{125}$I-BSA | $0.04 \pm 0.01$ | $2.1 \pm 0.3$[a] | $0.05 \pm 0.01$ | $1.0 \pm 0.2$[b] |
| HISTAMINE | $2.36 \pm 0.30$ | $5.8 \pm 0.9$[a] | $1.90 \pm 0.24$ | $2.9 \pm 0.7$[b] |

*Note:*  Superoxide dismutase (SOD) and catalase (CAT) were simultaneously infused intravenously at a dosage of 15,000 U/kg/h for each agent. The data represent $^{51}$Cr-labeled ethylene diamine tetra-acetic acid clearance (indicated by $^{51}$Cr-EDTA) and $^{125}$I-labeled bovine serum albumin clearance (indicated by $^{125}$I-BSA) and histamine release into intestinal lumen (indicated by HIST) during a 40-min perfusion period with control solution (KRBSG) or 6% w/v ethanol in KRBSG. Clearance data were calculated as µl plasma $^{51}$Cr-EDTA or µl of plasma $^{125}$I-BSA cleared into the jejunum per gram of dry tissue during the perfusion period. Histamine is expressed as µg/g dry tissue secreted into the lumen during the experimental perfusion period. Note that ethanol increased clearance of $^{51}$Cr-EDTA and $^{125}$I-BSA and increased histamine content in the ethanol segment of the untreated group. Combined treatment with CAT and SOD decreased these ethanol-induced increases in the treated group to below that of the ethanol segment of the untreated group.

[a]  Significantly ($p < 0.05$) different from control segments of untreated groups.

[b]  Significantly ($p < 0.05$) lower than the ethanol segment of the untreated group. The results are shown as mean ± SE.

From Dinda, P. K., Buell, M. G., and Beck, I. T., *Gastroenterology*, 102, A208, 1992.

of 5-lipoxygenase,[118] and found that it inhibited the LT formation in the rabbit jejunum and depressed the ethanol-induced intraluminal protein loss by 58%. Thus, leukotrienes, similar to histamine, have an important role in the production of ethanol-induced microvascular damage.

*10.4.2.1.3  Reactive Oxygen Metabolites (ROM) and Nitric Oxide*

Oxygen radicals are well-known causes of tissue injury,[119-121] and have been shown to play an important role in ischemia-reperfusion injury of the gut.[122,123] Thus, it was considered that they may have a role in the ethanol-induced microvascular damage. This chapter will not discuss in detail the complex biochemistry of their generation and the action of oxygen radicals on other tissues, as these will be reviewed in another chapter of this monograph. Briefly there are two main sources for the generation of active oxygen radicals. ROMs are either released from activated neutrophils or from the local tissue reaction of xanthine oxidase metabolism. When NADH dehydrogenase catalyzes the reaction of NADH with molecular oxygen ($O_2$) superoxide ($O_2^-$) is generated. Superoxide dismutase changes the highly toxic ($O_2^-$) to hydrogen peroxide ($H_2O_2$) which dissociates to $OH^-$. The hydroxy radical is more toxic than ($O_2^-$) or the $H_2O_2$. Another reaction catalyzed by neutrophil myeloperoxidase is the attachment of chloride ion leading to the highly toxic metabolite of $HOCl$ + N-chloramine.[120] Scavengers of oxygen radicals are superoxide-dismutase (SOD) and catalase.[124-126] The former converts ($O_2^-$) to $H_2O_2$ and the latter changes $H_2O_2$ to water. The second source of oxygen radicals in the intestine is the superoxide production during the enzymatic conversion of hypoxanthine to xanthine by xanthine oxidase.[121-123] This latter reaction can be arrested by allopurinol and oxypurinol.[121-123]

Recent studies in our laboratory have suggested that reactive oxygen radicals play an important role in the ethanol-induced microvascular injury. Pretreatment with a combination of SOD and catalase diminished the ethanol-induced release of histamine and the increased loss of protein and $^{51}$Cr-EDTA into the intestinal lumen (Table 10.3).[108] However, oxypurinol and allopurinol

**TABLE 10.4    Effect of Intraluminally Infused L-Arginine and D-Arginine on the Ethanol-Induced Microvascular and Epithelial Permeability**

|  | Control segment | 6% ETH segment | 6% ETH + L-A segment | 6% ETH + D-A segment |
|---|---|---|---|---|
| $^{51}$Cr-EDTA | $1.08 \pm 0.45$ | $3.56 \pm 0.88^a$ | $2.08 \pm 0.56^b$ | $3.31 \pm 0.84^a$ |
| $^{125}$I-BSA | $0.12 \pm 0.05$ | $1.18 \pm 0.58^a$ | $0.65 \pm 0.22^b$ | $1.61 \pm 0.51^a$ |

*Note:* In these experiments four segments were perfused: (1) control (KRBSG); (2) 6% w/v ethanol in KRBSG (6% ETH segment); (3) 6% ethanol plus 15 m*M* L-arginine in KRBSG (6% ETH + L-A segment); and (4) 6% ethanol plus 15 m*M* D-arginine in KRBSG (6% ETH + D-A segment) (*n* = 6). $^{51}$Cr-EDTA and $^{125}$I-BSA clearance were calculated as described for Table 10.3. Note that L-arginine and not D-arginine protected against ethanol-induced microvascular and epithelial permeability.

$^a$ Significantly ($p < 0.05$) different from control segment of untreated groups.

$^b$ Significantly ($p < 0.05$) lower than that of the ethanol segment of the untreated group. The results are shown as mean ±SE.

From Dinda, P. K., Kossev, P., Kosseva, V., and Beck, I. T., *Gastroenterology*, 104, A243, 1993.

diminished histamine release and protein and EDTA clearance only during the first 30 min of intraluminal ethanol perfusion and had no effect during the second part of the study.[88] Thus xanthine oxidase-derived ROMs (which do not originate from leukocytes) may initiate but do not sustain the ethanol-induced injury. Since the studies with SOD and catalase caused inhibition of ROM action throughout the perfusion period[88] the ongoing generation of ROMs must have derived from other sources probably from activated leukocytes,[88] similarly to what has been demonstrated in other types of intestinal injury.[124,126-128] Reactive oxygen metabolites cause inactivation of nitric oxide (NO), the endothelium derived relaxing factor.[121,129] Thus a ROM induced decrease in NO may be the cause of the endothelial cell contraction and increased microvascular permeability, and thus the intraluminal protein loss. It may also explain the ethanol-induced microvascular congestion. NO is synthetized from L-arginine by NO-synthase,* and its deficiency can be corrected by stimulating NO formation by L, but not D-arginine. Preliminary studies in our laboratory indicate that the ethanol-induced protein loss in the rabbit jejunum can be significantly diminished by adding L-(but not D-)arginine to the ethanol-containing perfusion solution (Table 10.4).[130] Thus the final step of the ethanol effect on endothelial cells could be a ROM-induced inactivation of NO.

### 10.4.2.1.4    *White Cell Adhesion Factors and Leukocyte Proteases*

It is today well accepted that the initiation of the inflammatory reaction is related to leukocyte adhesion and a release of leukocyte products.[120] This has been shown to be the case in many other types of intestinal injury[131,132] and their possible involvement in ethanol-induced injury has been suggested.[127] To assess whether the ethanol-induced microvascular permeability is also related to leukocyte adhesion and to the products released by activated leukocytes, we investigated whether inhibition of leukocyte adhesion could diminish the ethanol-induced histamine release and protein exudation. Using a monoclonal antibody against the CD-18 leukocyte adhesion molecule,[133-135] Dr. Dinda and co-workers found that its intravenous administration fully abolished histamine release and caused a 95% inhibition of protein and $^{51}$Cr-EDTA clearance.[110] A monoclonal antibody against the endothelial adhesive molecule ICAM-1 also depressed histamine release, protein loss, and $^{51}$Cr-EDTA clearance. However, the inhibition with anti-ICAM-1 antibody was less extensive than the complete abolition achieved with antibody to CD-18 (Table 10.5),[110] indicating that to achieve comparable inhibition, in addition to ICAM-1, to bind all activated leukocytes the endothelium must also express some additional ligands.[136]

---

* This chapter will not discuss details of NO synthesis by different enzymes.

**TABLE 10.5   The Effect of Anti-CD-18 and Anti-ICAM-1 Monoclonal Antibodies (Mab) on the Ethanol-Induced Microvascular and Epithelial Injury and Histamine Release in the Rabbit**

|  | Untreated | | Anti-CD-18 treated | | Anti-ICAM-1 treated | |
| --- | --- | --- | --- | --- | --- | --- |
|  | Control segment | Ethanol segment | Control segment | Ethanol segment | Control segment | Ethanol segment |
| $^{51}$Cr-EDTA | $0.20 \pm 0.05$ | $2.6 \pm 0.3^a$ | $0.2 \pm 0.04$ | $0.5 \pm 0.1^b$ | $0.2 \pm 0.0$ | $1.1 \pm 0.1^{a,b}$ |
| $^{125}$I-BSA | $0.05 \pm 0.01$ | $1.9 \pm 0.3^a$ | $0.0 \pm 0.00$ | $0.1 \pm 0.0^b$ | $0.0 \pm 0.0$ | $0.7 \pm 0.1^{a,b}$ |
| HISTAMINE | $2.00 \pm 0.56$ | $5.1 \pm 0.6^a$ | $0.8 \pm 0.30^a$ | $2.1 \pm 0.7^b$ | $1.2 \pm 0.4$ | $2.5 \pm 0.5^{a,b}$ |

*Note:* Three groups of rabbits were used ($n = 8$ in each). Rabbits were pretreated and treated with an i.v. infusion of saline (untreated group), 1 mg/kg CD-18 Mab (anti-CD-18 treated), or 1 mg/kg anti-ICAM-1 Mab (anti-ICAM-1 treated). Jejunal segments were perfused for 40 min. In each group the control segment (control) was perfused with KRBSG, and the ethanol segment (ethanol) with 6% (w/v) ethanol. Clearances and histamine release were calculated and expressed as described in Table 10.3. Note that anti-CD-18 Mab depressed all values in the ethanol perfused segments to that observed in the control segment of the untreated group. Anti-ICAM-1 Mab depressed the levels to below that of the ethanol perfused segment of the untreated group, but not to the level of the control segment of the untreated group.

[a] Significantly ($p < 0.05$) different from control segments of untreated groups.

[b] Significantly ($p < 0.05$) lower than that of the ethanol segment of the untreated group. The results are mean $\pm$ SE.

From Dinda, P. K., Kossev, P., and Beck, I. T., *Gastroenterology*, 106, A230, 1994.

The complete inhibition of histamine release and microvascular permeability by CD-18 monoclonal antibodies suggested that leukocyte-derived mediators play an important role in the ethanol-induced microvascular injury. We considered that as it occurs in other types of injury,[120] among other mediators, leukocyte proteases may be responsible for some of these effects. Further studies by Kosseva and Dinda et al. indicated that pretreatment with soybean trypsin inhibitor or the elastase inhibitor [methoxysuccinyl-ala-ala-pro-val-chloromethyl (MAAPV)] abolished the ethanol-induced histamine release and depressed by 80% the ethanol-induced increase in protein loss.[89,90] It appears therefore that the histamine release from mast cells (i.e., the degranulation of mast cells) and the resulting microvascular damage is caused by proteases released from circulating or possibly resident granulocytes.

### 10.4.2.1.5   Resident Leukocytes

The possibility that granulocyte proteases may be released from resident leukocytes was suggested by our previous observation that ethanol-induced mast cell degranulation and histamine release can occur in the jejunum *in vitro*, i.e., in the absence of circulating leukocytes.[19,58] The role of resident leukocytes was confirmed by our recent experiments which indicated that human granulocyte elastase caused histamine release (i.e., mast cell degranulation) *in vitro* and that the elastase inhibitor (MAAPV) counteracted the *in vitro* release of histamine.[111] Thus these enzymes can induce mast cell degranulation in the absence of circulating leukocytes. Furthermore, soybean trypsin inhibitor and the human elastase inhibitor (MAAPV) inhibited the ethanol-induced histamine release in everted rabbit jejunal sacs *in vitro*, suggesting that the ethanol-induced mast cell degranulation is mediated by leukocyte proteases originating from resident leukocytes.[111]

It is more difficult to explain the observation that the antibody to the leukocyte adhesive molecule (CD-18 antibody) also inhibited the *in vitro* release of histamine.[111] It is possible that in order to release their proteolytic enzymes resident leukocytes must adhere to some ligand in the tissue, which possibly may be located on the mast cell. Another, less likely possibility, is that mast cells may have CD-18 adhesion molecules and that the inhibition of these molecules leads to the degranulation of mast cells.

Further support for the role of resident leukocytes in causing the microvascular leakage has been obtained by our recent *in vivo* video microscopic findings.[137] These studies were carried out to correlate the time of onset of protein leakage with that of the adhesion of circulating leukocytes.

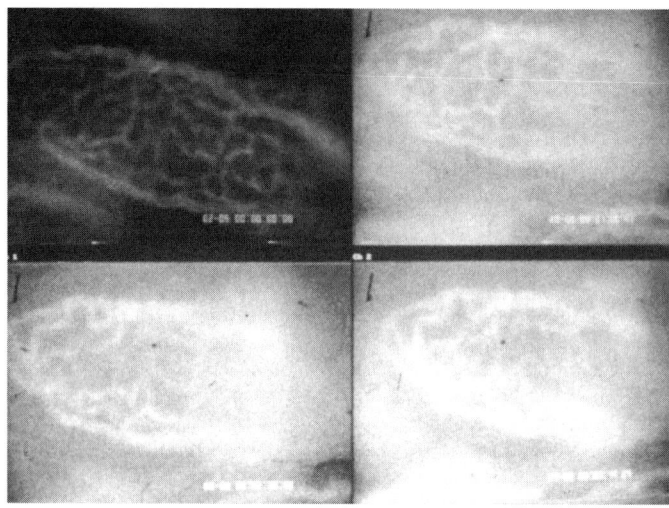

**FIGURE 10.15**  Effect of ethanol on early vascular permeability. Villus perfused with fluorescein-isothiocyanate labeled bovine serum albumin (FITC-albumin). Note on the upper left panel that, under control conditions (superfused with KRBSG), the vasculature is sharply outlined. All FITC-albumin is kept within the microvessels. On the upper right, 1 min after superfusion with 6% (w/v) ethanol in KRBSG the FITC tagged albumin has entered the interstitium of the villus. Vessel walls lack their sharpness and the background which was nonfluorescent during the control period became fluorescent (grayish-white). A somewhat greater leakage of FITC-albumin can be observed at 2 min (lower left) and 3 min (lower right) after ethanol superfusion. (Reproduced from Sukumar, P., Dinda, P. K., Buell, M. G., and Beck, I. T., *Gastroenterology*, 106, A1052, 1994.)

Vascularly well-perfused single hamster jejunal villi were examined *in situ* in a specially designed chamber, and the findings were recorded using a video microscopic set-up. Protein exudation from capillaries and postcapillary venules into villus interstitium was studied by observing the extravasation of fluorescein-isothiocyanate (FITC)-tagged bovine serum albumin (FITC-albumin); leukocyte adhesion was assessed by observing and measuring the passage of fluorescein labeled acridine-orange-tagged leukocytes through the microvessels. The villus was superfused with control solution and subsequently with 6% ethanol. Protein exudation started to occur immediately after ethanol superfusion and was severe within 1 min (Figure 10.15). The experiment had to be terminated at 3 min because by that time the villus was fully obscured by the extravasated fluorescent protein. In a separate set of experiments we observed that up to 3 min after superfusion with the same concentration of ethanol (6%) fluorescein-tagged leukocytes did not adhere to or traverse the villus capillaries or postcapillary venules. Thus the released substance that initiated the protein exudation did not originate from circulating leukocytes but possibly from resident leukocytes.[137]

### 10.4.2.1.6   Interaction of Aggressive Mediators

Considering the above described findings, ethanol does not appear to exhibit a direct effect on the endothelial cells because its action on vascular permeability can be counteracted by various substances that inhibit the cascade leading to endothelial cell contraction.[19,20,58,107,108,110] Mast cell degranulation must occur,[58,90,111] and histamine,[19,107] leukotriene,[20] and probably some other not as yet investigated inflammatory mediators need to be released from the mast cell to initiate the microvascular permeability.

These mediators may liberate ROMs from leukocytes and other tissues.[88,108] Possibly the inactivation of NO synthesis may be the final step which causes endothelial cell contraction,[130] exudation of protein, hemoconcentration, and stasis.[16,69] The cascade, however, does not start with the mast cell. Ethanol cannot release histamine from mast cells if the leukocyte adhesion molecule CD-18 is blocked by anti-CD-18 monoclonal antibody, suggesting that the primary target may be the leukocyte.[110,111] The active substances in resident and circulating white blood

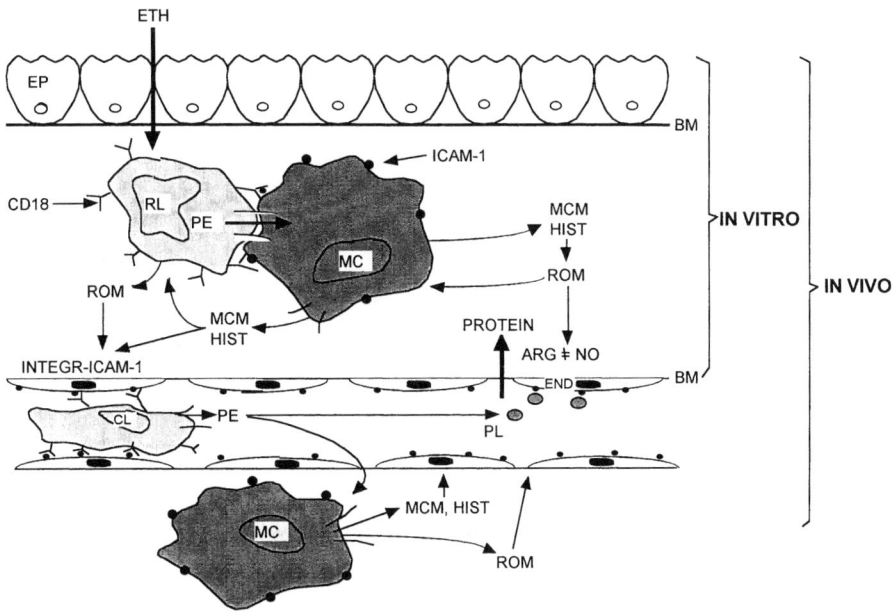

**FIGURE 10.16** Schematic representation of earliest stage of ethanol effects on immunocytes, mediators, and fluxes involved in the ethanol-induced microvascular alterations. ARG, L-arginine; BM, basement membrane; CL, circulating leukocyte with CD-18 receptors; END, endothelial cell with integrins; EP, epithelial cell; ETH, ethanol; HIST, histamine; MC, mast cell; MCM, mast cell mediators (leukotriene, PAF, etc.); MV, microvessel; NO, nitric oxide; PAF, platelet aggregating factor; PE, proteolytic enzymes; PL, platelets; RL, resident leukocyte with CD-18 receptors; ROM, reactive oxygen radicals. See text for details.

cells which lead to mast cell degranulation are the leukocyte proteases.[90,111] Because mast cell degranulation can be achieved *in vitro*[58] and because protein exudation precedes adhesion of circulating leukocytes,[58] the first effect of ethanol does not appear to be on the circulating leukocytes, but rather on the resident leukocytes. It is these cells which, by releasing proteases, initiate the entire process.[111] A major issue that has not been resolved is to identify the mechanism by which ethanol interacts with the CD-18 adhesion complex. The various possibilities are discussed in Section 10.4.2.1.5. It is likely that to become activated leukocytes need to adhere to cells and that several types of mucosal cells carry the ICAM-1 and other adhesion complexes. Once resident leukocytes have initiated mast cell degranulation, the released histamine, various other mast cell mediators, ROMs, etc., induce the formation of ICAM-1 and other selectins in the endothelial cells. This will result in the adhesion of activated circulating leukocytes.[90] Once this occurs, the proteases and mediators released from these adherent circulating white cells will participate in and aggravate the complex cascade described above for resident leukocyte-induced first phase of ethanol action. These possible interactions as developed by Dinda and the author are schematically presented in Figure 10.16.

## 10.4.2.2   The Role of Protective Mediators

### 10.4.2.2.1   Prostaglandins

Prostaglandins, especially the E types, have been shown to protect against the ethanol-induced gastric microvascular injury.[5,138] Similarly, 16,16-dimethyl-prostaglandin $E_2$ alleviated the jejunal microvascular effects of 6% (w/v) ethanol in the jejunum, as indicated by a 41% decrease of the ethanol-induced intraluminal albumin loss in the dog[21] and by a 31% decrease in the rabbit.[58] An important observation was that, like other observations in the stomach,[139] 16,16-dimethyl-prostaglandin decreased histamine release and improved the microvascular damage (see Figure

10.14), but it had no effect on ethanol-induced epithelial morphological injury, further supporting that the mechanism of the production of morphologic damage is unrelated to the mediators involved in causing microvascular injury.[58]

Foschi and co-workers[64,65] reported that 40% ethanol sprayed on the human duodenum caused severe vascular congestion and mucosal damage. They also observed that local administration of rosaprostol (9-hydroxy-19,20,bis-norprostanoic acid[64]) and the prostaglandin $E_1$ analog, misoprostol, protected against this ethanol-induced microvascular damage.[65] Lavo and co-workers [91] found that ethanol perfusion of the jejunum of human volunteers caused a tenfold increase in intraluminal albumin loss. The curve in the human was biphasic, similar to that observed in the dog and rabbit. Of interest is that, simultaneously with a decrease in albumin, there was a fourfold increase in intraluminal prostaglandin-$E_2$,[91] suggesting that the release of prostaglandin may have had a protective effect on the second (decreasing) phase of the microvascular leakage.

### 10.4.2.3    Evidence for Adaptive Protection

The concept of gastric "cytoprotection" was first conceived by Robert and co-workers in 1975[3] who found that one of the mediators involved in "cytoprotection" was the prostaglandins. They observed that intragastric administration of a mild irritant (ethanol 20%) 15 min before the administration of absolute alcohol attenuated the absolute alcohol-induced mucosal injury. This protection could be prevented by the administration of indomethacin, an inhibitor of prostaglandin production.[4,140] The word "cytoprotection" was unfortunately inappropriately chosen. Macroscopically, the protection of the rat mucosa by prostaglandin against absolute ethanol appeared dramatic, but histologic study by Lacy and Ito[139] demonstrated that prosta-glandins prevented injury to the microvessels and thus to deeper layers of the mucosa but did not protect the superficial gastric cells. Thus "cytoprotection" in the true sense did not occur. These findings are reminiscent of our observation that, in the small intestine, 16-16-dimethyl-prostaglandin protects against ethanol-induced microvascular damage, but not against mucosal injury.[58]

To examine whether similar "cytoprotection"* to that observed in the stomach also occurs in the small bowel, we investigated the effect of a 30 min preperfusion of rabbit jejunal segments with 1% ethanol on the microvascular changes caused by 6% ethanol. Indeed preperfusion partially protected against the 6% ethanol-induced histamine release and decreased the clearance of $^{51}$Cr-EDTA and plasma protein into the gut (Table 10.6).[109]

This adaptive vascular protection could be the underlying mechanism for the biphasic re-sponse of the microvasculature to ongoing ethanol perfusion. It is possible that after initial injury, the tissue responds with the generation of protective mediators. Mast cells which have already discharged some of their granules become stabilized, possibly due to the release of prostaglan-dins.[58] This should lead to decreased histamine release. The level of prostaglandin $E_2$ has been shown in humans to rise with ongoing ethanol perfusion.[91] However, the role of leukocytes, ROMs, NO, and many other agents in this recovery period remains to be investigated.

## 10.5    EFFECT OF ETHANOL ON INTESTINAL TRANSPORT

### 10.5.1    Effect on Permeability

The mucosa may be permeable in two directions: from the lumen toward the gut or from the tissues toward the lumen. Ethanol may alter both processes but changes affecting lumen to gut permeability have been studied in greater detail. The magnitude of permeability changes appears to be species and concentration dependent, and there is greater increase in permeability in those animals where ethanol causes breakage of the epithelium. For instance, in the hamster where

---

* In spite of the fact that cytoprotection against histologic injury does not occur, because of its general use in the literature, in this text it will occasionally be used to describe protection against microvascular injury.

**TABLE 10.6    Adaptive "Cytoprotection" Against Ethanol-Induced Injury by Low Concentrations of Ethanol**

|  | **Control SEG** | **Ethanol SEG** | **AD.CY. SEG** |
|---|---|---|---|
| $^{51}$Cr-EDTA | $0.78 \pm 0.19$ | $3.50 \pm 0.35^{a}$ | $1.45 \pm 0.21^{a,b}$ |
| $^{125}$I-BSA | $0.08 \pm 0.02$ | $2.10 \pm 0.26^{a}$ | $0.67 \pm 0.17^{a,b}$ |
| HISTAMINE | $2.09 \pm 0.58$ | $8.10 \pm 0.72^{a}$ | $4.51 \pm 0.81^{a,b}$ |

*Note:* Adaptive "cytoprotection" against ethanol-induced small bowel mucosal injury. Effect of preperfusion with 1% ethanol on the effect of 6% (w/v) ethanol perfusion was studied in three jejunal segments of the same rabbit (*n* = 6). Each segment was preperfused for 30 min as follows: The control (Control SEG) and the ethanol segments (Ethanol SEG) were preperfused with KRBSG. The adaptive "cytoprotected" segment (AD.CY.SEG) with 1% (w/v) ethanol in KRBSG. After this preperfusion, the segments were perfused for 90 min as follows: The control segment was continued to be perfused with KRBSG; the ethanol segment and the adaptive cytoprotective segment with 6% ethanol in KRBSG. Clearances and histamine release were calculated and expressed as in Table 10.3. Abbreviations and descriptions of statistical significance are the same as in Table 10.3. Note that preperfusion with 1% ethanol decreased histamine release and both clearances below that of the untreated ethanol segment, but did not return these values to those of the control segment.

From Dinda, P. K., Wassan, S., Kossev, P., and Beck, I. T., *Gastroenterology*, 104, A243, 1993.

blebs do not rupture, ethanol does not increase the mucosal permeability to polyethylene glycol (PEG)-MW-4000 and megluminediatrizoate (renographin) either *in vitro* or *in vivo*.[28] In the rat, however, which has mainly broken blebs, the ethanol-induced permeability to PEG-4000, horseradish peroxidase (HRP), bovine serum albumin,[141,142] and $^{51}$Cr-EDTA[143] is increased. In humans alcohol also increases the gut lumen to blood permeability for $^{51}$Cr-EDTA permeability.[144] Worthington and co-workers[145] were the first to demonstrate that in (chronic) alcoholic rats, macromolecules pass through the epithelium via the paracellular pathway. In acute experiments HRP penetrated the mucosa paracellularly in the rat[146] and in the presence of higher concentrations of ethanol (5 to 20%) both paracellularly and intracellularly via cytoplasmic vesicles in the guinea pig.[147] Although investigators find that the increased permeability is mainly through the paracellular route, it is likely that once the continuity of the epithelial layer has been broken due to rupture of blebs, the major route of unresisted transmucosal transport of macromolecules would occur through these openings of the mucosa.

Ethanol also increases gut wall to lumen permeability. For instance during acute ethanol perfusion in the dog, there is an increase in permeability to albumin[17,21,59,69,99,107] and lactoglobulin.[17] Similar loss of serum protein into the gut was observed in the rabbit[19,20,58] and humans.[91] Ethanol also increases gut wall to lumen permeability to EDTA.[58,88,89,90,130,148] This substance is a small molecule which traverses the vascular wall without difficulty and distributes rapidly into the extracellular fluid. It is easily measured as $^{51}$Cr-EDTA. If the permeability of the epithelium is normal, EDTA is cleared from the extracellular fluid into the gut lumen very slowly. However, once the epithelial resistance is broken, it passes this barrier easily and is rapidly lost into the lumen, probably at the rate of fluid secretion. Indeed in the case of ethanol-induced secretory filtration, EDTA passes the permeable epithelium rapidly and in experiments where the gut is exposed to a 90-min ethanol perfusion, the rise and fall of its excretion follows that of the biphasic curve of protein secretion. Furthermore, when the ethanol-induced protein exudation is diminished due to the administration of various agents which protect against *microvascular* leakage, EDTA excretion is decreased in parallel with that of serum protein. Thus it may be worth investigating whether EDTA clearance through broken epithelium is a measure for fluid secretion.

### 10.5.2 Effect on Absorption and Secretion

A considerable amount of work has been carried out to investigate the effect of ethanol on intestinal transport. Absorption of actively transported sugars, dipeptides, and amino acids is inhibited by ethanol in a concentration-dependent manner *in vivo* and *in vitro* and in preparation of BBM vesicles.[8,10-12,15,16,22,28,44,54,55,149-158] The effect of ethanol on lipid absorption and lipid metabolism is controversial. Several investigators have suggested an increase in lipid absorption,[159-162] while others have suggested diminished lipid transport.[163,164]

Acute intraluminal ethanol affects electrolyte and water transport. In the rabbit jejunal mucosa, translocation of $Na^+$ from mucosa (M) to serosa (S) is depressed in *in vitro* experiments.[38] Under similar conditions in the hamster jejunum, both M-S and S-M transport are inhibited.[54] Net sodium absorption was decreased by 52% in the dog[21] but in the human duodenum[165] and jejunum[166] net $Na^+$ transport was unaffected. The few data available in the literature indicate that net $K^+$[165] and $Cl^-$ absorption or secretion were unaffected by acute exposure to ethanol.[38,165] Under normal conditions water transport depends on $Na^+$ absorption and $Cl^-$ secretion, but in the presence of ethanol, the depression of water transport exceeds the inhibition of sodium absorption[21,54] and leads to fluid secretion in most *in vivo* studies.[15,16,21,56]

Alcohol affects the transport of many other substances.[167-172] Details of these actions of ethanol have recently been reviewed by Persson[173] and will be discussed in another chapter of this book. This chapter deals only with those aspects of ethanol-induced changes in transport in which specific steps of these alterations can be correlated with defined changes in small intestinal injury. The only transport system in which the effect of ethanol has been investigated sufficiently in detail to allow for such interpretation is the sodium-dependent glucose, $Na^+$, and water transport.

### 10.5.3 Mechanism of Ethanol-Induced Changes in Sodium-Dependent Glucose, Na⁺, and Water Transport

Ethanol affects glucose, sodium, and water transport through both the transcellular and extracellular pathway. The transcellular route passes through (1) the brush-border membrane, (2) the cytoplasm of epithelial cells (where it may undergo metabolism), and (3) the basolateral membrane. The extracellular route traverses (1) the unstirred water layer, (2) the extracellular shunt pathway between epithelial cells, (3) the lateral intercellular space, and (4) the connective tissue of the villus core.

#### 10.5.3.1   Transport Across the Cellular Route

The glucose and other "nonelectrolyte"* carriers of the BBM have high affinity to nonelectrolytes in the presence of high $Na^+$ and low $K^+$ concentration and low affinity (i.e., release glucose or other nonelectrolytes), when $K^+$ concentration is high and $Na^+$ concentration is low. The driving force of the transport of glucose and other nonelectrolytes by carrier systems across the BBM into the cell is the $Na^+$ and $K^+$ gradient between the high $Na^+$ and low $K^+$ concentration of the luminal fluid and the low $Na^+$ and high $K^+$ concentration inside the cell. This gradient is maintained by the $Na^+$, $K^+$ ATPase (the sodium pump) of the BLM which actively transports sodium out of the epithelial cell into the LIS and $K^+$ from LIS to the cell. Glucose traverses the intracellular space where it is partially utilized for epithelial cell metabolism. Glucose that has not been metabolized is extruded at the BLM by a nonsodium dependent carrier.[174]

#### 10.5.3.1.1   Effect on Brush-Border Membrane

Ethanol depresses the transport of glucose and other nonelectrolytes across purified BBM vesicles.[8-11] These vesicles are prepared in the absence of $Na^+$, so that the intravesicular space

---

*The definition "nonelectrolyte" will be used to denote only those nonelectrolyte substances which are transported by carriers (e.g., sugars, amino acids, oligopeptides).

does not contain any Na$^+$ and thus, with Na$^+$ present in the bathing solution, a Na$^+$ gradient is created. Two major mechanisms have been suggested to explain ethanol's inhibitory action on the glucose transport across the BBM and possibly both mechanisms may play a role. The first is that ethanol increases sodium permeability of the BBM.[9,157] This increased passive diffusion of sodium into the vesicles would lead to a faster collapse of the sodium gradient with a resulting diminished sodium-dependent glucose transport. The second mechanism is the distortion and thus inhibition of the carrier system. Considerable evidence supports this mechanism. BBM enzymes such as disaccharidases[6] and peptidases[7] are inhibited by ethanol in BBM vesicle preparations and these alterations in enzyme activity seem to be related to the distortion of the membrane.[6] A similar mechanism has been postulated for the glucose carrier by demonstrating that ethanol increases the fluidity of enterocyte membranes.[175] Bossmann and Hutter[176] observed that ethanol diminishes the cholesterol and phospholipid content of the BBM, changes its physical chemical properties, and causes distortion in its hydrophobic region. These alterations diminish the anchoring and the activity of the membrane bound enzymes.[176] It is likely that these changes would also alter carrier activity.

### 10.5.3.1.2 Effect on Intracellular Metabolism

Intracellular metabolism is depressed by ethanol. Tissue respiration is decreased[37,38] and protein synthesis per day and the amount of protein synthesized per unit RNA are depressed in the jejunal (but not duodenal) mucosa.[177] This may be the cause of the diminished jejunal mucosal ATP content[178,179] and decreased intracellular glucose utilization.[54]

### 10.5.3.1.3 Effect on Basolateral Membrane

The active transport of glucose, Na$^+$, and water depends on the Na$^+$, K$^+$ ATPase (the sodium pump) which maintains the intracellular low Na$^+$ and high K$^+$ concentration necessary for active BBM glucose transport. Water absorption is also linked to the Na$^+$ pump which is located at the lateral surface of the BLM. By pumping Na$^+$ into the narrow LIS, hyperosmolality is created in these spaces which then draw water through the cellular and the paracellular route into the LIS.[180] Indeed the morphological manifestation of water absorption is dilatation of the LIS.[181] An inhibition of glucose, sodium, and water transport could be explained by a diminished sodium pump activity. Several investigators have found that the activity of this enzyme is depressed[182-184] while others[179] have observed normal ATPase activity. Evidence on the activity of the sodium pump can also be obtained from the relative sensitivity of the mucosal and serosal surfaces to inhibitors of glucose and sodium transport. Phlorizin which acts on the glucose carrier depresses glucose transport *in vitro* only when placed on the mucosal surface but not when applied to the serosal side. In contrast ouabain which is an inhibitor of the sodium potassium ATPase acts on sodium (and glucose transport) only when applied to the serosal side but not when placed on the mucosa. Ethanol applied to the mucosal side of an *in vitro* jejunal preparation depresses glucose, sodium, and water transport but has no such effect when applied to the serosal side (i.e., the location of the sodium pump). This further supports that ethanol has no effect on the Na$^+$, K$^+$ATPase.[153,156]

Under normal conditions, 1 µmol of glucose is cotransported with 2 µmol Na$^+$ and 17.5 µl of water.[2] Ethanol disrupts this relationship. *In vitro* experiments have shown that the depression of the transfer of glucose is greater than that of the inhibition of Na$^+$ transport and that the depression of water absorption greatly exceeds that expected from the inhibition of glucose absorption and Na$^+$ movement.[54] Such a dissociation of transport could not be explained by a diminished Na$^+$ pump activity. However, a rise in intracellular Na$^+$ concentration could be achieved by the increased Na$^+$ permeation of the BBM, as demonstrated by Tillotson et al.[9] In the presence of normal Na$^+$, K$^+$ATPase activity this would decrease glucose absorption to a greater extent than Na$^+$ transport.

There are no data available on the effect of ethanol on the glucose carrier of the BLM. However, since application of alcohol to the serosal side of an *in vitro* preparation had no effect on glucose transport,[153] it is unlikely that the BLM glucose transport is affected by the ethanol.

### 10.5.3.2    Transport Across the Paracellular Route

The dissociation of water and Na$^+$ transport can be further explained by the ethanol-induced morphological alterations of the paracellular pathway. As blebs are formed, the LIS widens (Figure 10.4) and finally disappears (Figure 10.3). As a result, the narrow space necessary to create an intercellular hyperosmolar area is not present. Thus in spite of normal functioning of the Na$^+$, K$^+$ATPase water absorption is diminished to a greater extent than solute transport. In the presence of ethanol-induced microcirculatory changes due to protein exudation and resultant secretory filtration, water absorption is further depressed and fluid secretion occurs through the paracellular route.[15,28,55,69]

The possible alterations of the countercurrent multiplication system[36] caused by core contraction and compaction and by the changes in the microcirculation are unknown.

## 10.6    RELATIONSHIP BETWEEN THE ETHANOL-INDUCED MORPHOLOGICAL, MICROVASCULAR, AND ABSORPTIVE INJURY

Ethanol-induced morphological transport changes occur *in vitro* and thus are not primarily dependent on the microcirculation. However, under *in vivo* conditions, a close time relationship appears to exist between the morphologic alterations and microvascular injury[59,62] and the morphologic changes and fluid transport.[21,55,62] To investigate the role of morphology on absorption, we correlated in the hamster *in vivo* glucose absorption and fluid transport during ethanol perfusion and 45 min later when morphology returned to normal. We found that ethanol depressed glucose absorption and caused fluid secretion. Improvement in morphology reestablished normal fluid absorption without improving glucose absorption. The return to normal fluid absorption was correlated with reattachment of blebs and the reestablishment of normal LIS.[55] To study the relationship between morphological changes and microvascular effect of intraluminal ethanol, in a series of experiments we perfused jejunal segments of the dog with 6% ethanol for 10, 20, 30, 60, and 90 min and measured the time-dependent changes of the prevalence of epithelial damage, the height of the villus core, and the patency of lacteals. These data were correlated with time-dependent changes of intraluminal albumin loss and permeability of microvessels (as measured by the colloidal carbon vascular labeling). All events demonstrated a biphasic response in spite of the continuous presence of ethanol in the lumen. The first phase consisted of increasing impairment and the second of a phase of adaptive recovery.[59,62] These relationships are shown in Figure 10.17.[62] The epithelial damage and exudation of albumin increased for the first 20 min and then declined. Vascular permeability, as measured by the colloidal carbon method, also increased just prior to the increase in albumin loss.* In contrast, during the first phase, the height of the villus core decreased at 20 min and then spontaneously increased during the adaptation period. Villus core contraction resulted in compression of the lacteals and consequently the number of microscopically visible lymph vessels decreased at first and then returned toward normal with the expansion of the villus core. It appears that under *in vivo* conditions ethanol has three major effects and the relationship between these is schematically demonstrated in Figure 10.18 and described below. The *first* effect is on the epithelial cell causing depression of transport of nonelectrolytes (for references see Section 10.5.3). This effect is unrelated to the release of inflammatory mediators or villus core contraction since it occurs in BBM vesicles[8-11] and does not improve with normalization of the microvascular and morphological changes.[55] The *second* effect is on villus core contraction (for references see Sections 10.3.1 and 10.3.2). This action is unrelated to mast cell mediators since histamine in physiological

---

* A decrease in permeability using the colloidal carbon method could not be assessed because once the carbon was entrapped, it did not leave the microvessels.

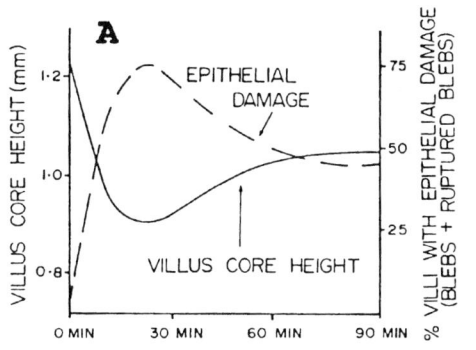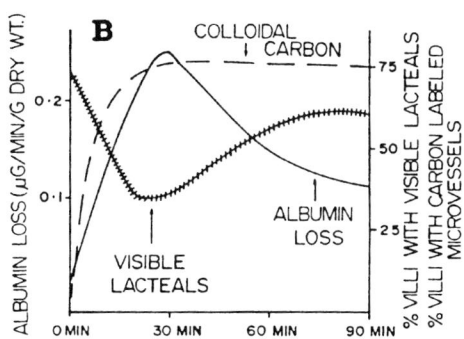

**FIGURE 10.17**  (A) Time course of the biphasic effect of ethanol on canine villus height and total damage. There is an inverse relationship between villus core contraction and epithelial damage. Epithelial damage consists of broken and unbroken blebs. Note that although the total damage decreases in the second phase, the percentage of broken blebs increases (see Figure 10.6); (B) demonstrates the biphasic fall and rise of visible lacteals, rise and fall of albumin loss, and the relation of albumin loss with increased microvascular permeability, as demonstrated by colloidal carbon entrapment. Note that once colloidal carbon is entrapped, it cannot leave the vessel, thus it does not decrease in the second phase. See text for details. (Reproduced from Beck, I. T., Leddin, D. J., Ray, M., and Dinda, P. K., *Proceedings of the Fourth World Congress of Microcirculation*, Tokyo, Japan, 2, 427, 1987. With permission.)

concentrations does not contract the villus core, and antihistamines do not inhibit ethanol-induced bleb formation.[70] The *third* effect is the release of aggressive mediators which precipitate the microvascular changes (for references see Sections 10.4.2.1 to 10.4.2.6).

There seems to be an interaction between the ethanol-induced microvascular and morphological alterations. The release of mediators results in opening of interendothelial junctions, leading to an increase in microvascular permeability. In the presence of increased arteriolar inflow and increased capillary pressure, plasma protein leaks into the interstitium.

Contraction of the villus core compresses the venules draining the villus, further increasing capillary pressure and thus contributing to the protein loss. Villus core contraction also results in bleb formation,[13] which may be facilitated by alcohol acting as a calcium donor.[13] Compression of lymphatics interferes with fluid drainage and causes the accumulation of the diminished but still ongoing absorption of fluid.[54,153] This subepithelially retained absorbed fluid further contributes to bleb formation. Epithelial cells in blebs become stretched and lose their LIS. This increases the paracellular permeability to small molecules (e.g., the permeability marker EDTA). Further interaction of morphological and microvascular changes occurs when the interstitially accumulated protein starts entering blebs. This increases the oncotic pressure in the blebs, and in time some of them will rupture, an event which further increases epithelial permeability. The plasma protein lost into the interstitium leaks through the damaged and thus easily permeable epithelium. The protein carries fluid which results in secretory filtration.[15,16,55] If small molecules are used as markers, these are carried out more rapidly by the increased fluid secretion, causing a parallel increase in EDTA and protein secretion.

Figure 10.19 demonstrates schematically the events in the second phase of ethanol action. The mechanisms involved in this phase have been less well investigated than those described above. It is likely that to achieve this adaptive response protective mediators are released. These may act on endothelial cells and thus close the endothelial junctions. This leads to a decrease in microvascular permeability and thus a diminished protein loss into the interstitium.[21,58,64,65,91] The oncotic pressure in the blebs decreases. Simultaneously, by mechanisms as yet unknown, the villus core expands.[59] The epithelium of unbroken blebs reattaches to the villus core and the number of unbroken blebs diminishes.[59,62] However, reepithelization of broken blebs will take somewhat

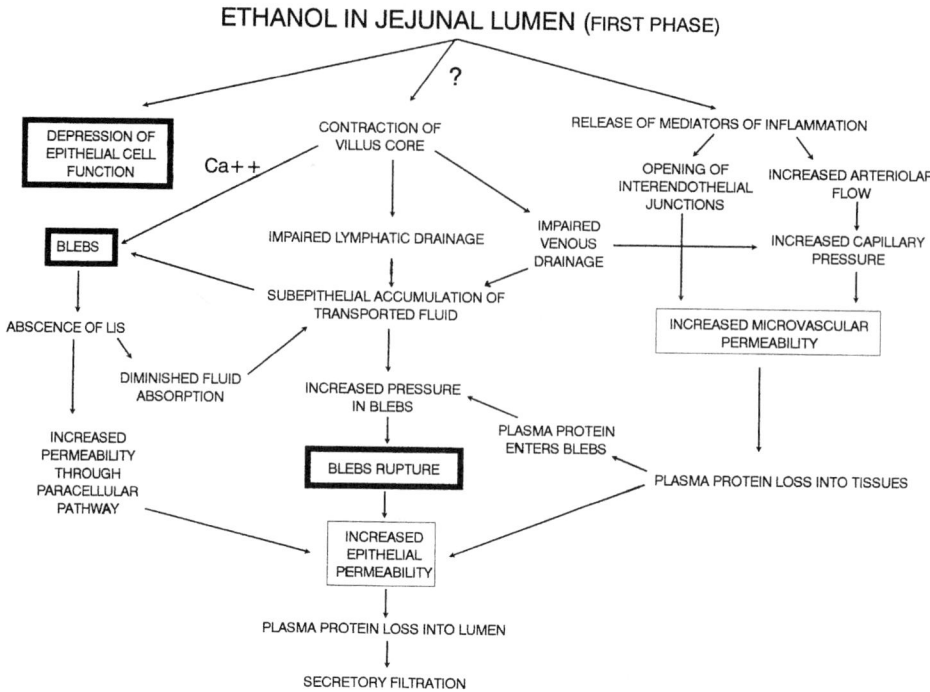

**FIGURE 10.18**   Schematic representation of the first phase of ethanol effect on the jejunum. See text for details.

longer,[59,67] and thus the permeability of the epithelium decreases but does not return immediately to normal. Once the villus core reexpands, better lymphatic and venous drainage ensues.[59,62] This should diminish capillary pressure and further reduce protein loss into the interstitium. Opening the lymphatics and better drainage of plasma protein, combined with decreased protein loss into the interstitium, leads to the diminished intraluminal protein loss.[59,62,87] Disappearance of the blebs diminishes the stretch of the epithelial cells and reestablishes the LIS, leading to a decrease in paracellular fluxes and a decrease in epithelial permeability. The reestablishment of LIS, combined with better drainage through the villus core, leads to improved fluid absorption.[55] The combination of decreased intraluminal protein loss and improved fluid absorption diminishes secretory filtration and decreases the intraluminal loss of small molecules (e.g., EDTA) used to detect epithelial permeability. In contrast, glucose and other nonelectrolyte transport remains depressed[55] because of the direct effect of ethanol on the BBM.[8-11] This longer lasting ethanol effect appears to be unrelated to any microscopically detectable morphological change (Figure 10.19).

## 10.7   UNRESOLVED PROBLEMS

There are numerous issues that still require elucidation. In the transport area, very little is known about the effect of ethanol on the BLM. As to secretion and absorption, there are no data available on the effect of ethanol on chloride secretion. Likewise, little is known about the role of the changes in the different mediators on nonelectrolyte, fat and fluid, and electrolyte transport. The exact role of secretory filtration in the fluxes of small molecules (e.g., EDTA) through membranes with increased permeability needs to be established by experimentation. The effect of ethanol on the enteric nervous system is unknown and whether it elicits local reflexes needs to be investigated. Since histamine does not affect villus core contraction, the mechanism by which ethanol causes this effect is unknown. The role of calcium on bleb formation needs to be further

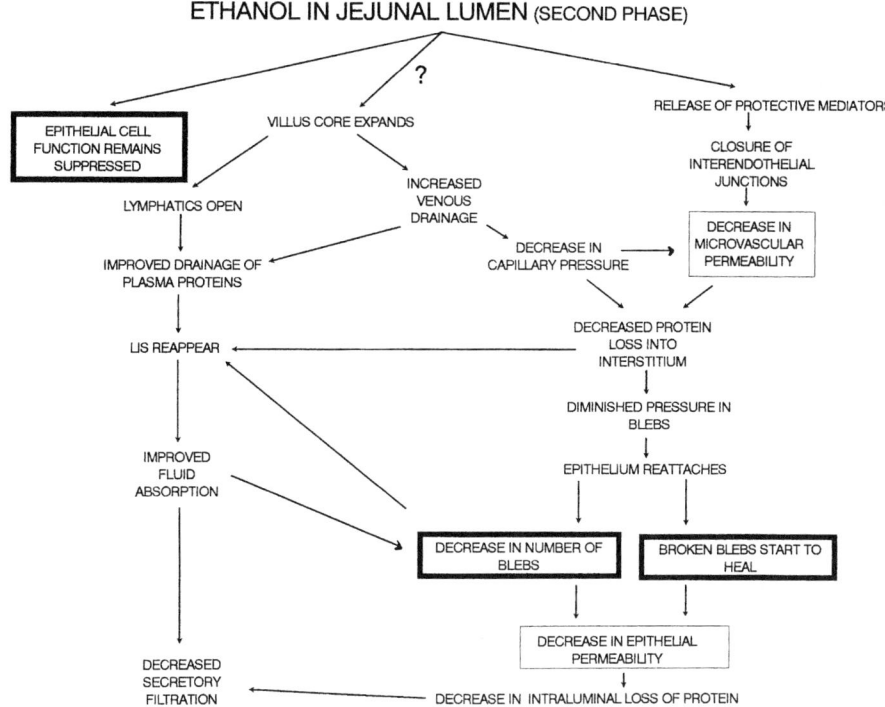

**FIGURE 10.19** Schematic representation of the adaptation of the small intestine to ongoing ethanol perfusion in the second phase of the ethanol effect on the jejunum. See text for details.

investigated. Although some evidence has been accumulated on the effect of ethanol on some mediators, as far as the small bowel is concerned there are no data on many of the other mediators such as serotonin, platelet aggregating factors, etc. Evidence seems to indicate that there is adaptation to ethanol but, except for some data on prostaglandin in the adaptation of the microcirculation, there is no knowledge on the overall mechanism.

In conclusion, ethanol affects intestinal transport, causes an acute inflammatory type reaction which alters the microcirculation and affects, by an as yet unknown mechanism, the morphology of the small bowel. In view of these multiple actions, the changes observed with acute ethanol toxicity provide an excellent prototype of acute small intestinal injury. By studying the mechanism(s) of these events, one may obtain in the future a better understanding of the interactions that occur in the course of acute damage to the small intestinal mucosa. The investigation of these interactions could be of major importance because their elucidation may help us better understand the mechanisms involved not only in small intestinal injury caused by ethanol, but possibly injury caused by other agents.

## 10.8 ACKNOWLEDGMENTS

The author would like to acknowledge the contribution of Dr. Paritosh K. Dinda, his co-worker of 20 years, without whose work and ideas the data presented in this review could not have been accumulated. The author would also like to thank Dr. Mikael Buell, his previous student, who recently returned to this unit, and who, in addition to his own research, continued to cooperate in some of the recent studies. Much of the morphological work could not have been carried out without the cooperation of Dr. Gerry P. Morris. The author would like to thank other co-workers and students mentioned in the bibliography, who have carried out many of the experiments.

The author also would like to acknowledge his wife, Marjorie Beck, who helped edit this chapter, and Wendy Gorski for typing the manuscript. The work carried out in our laboratory was supported by the Medical Research Council of Canada and the expenses of writing this chapter were supported by Janssen Pharmaceutica Inc., Canada.

## REFERENCES

1. **Kalant, H.,** Effects of ethanol on the nervous system, in *International Encyclopedia of Pharmacology and Therapeutics, Section 20,* Vol. 1, Tremolieres, J., Ed., Pergamon Press, Toronto, 1970, chapter 189.
2. **Dinda, P. K., Beck, M., and Beck, I. T.,** Isoosmotic transport of fluid across the hamster small intestine in the presence of phlorizin induced inhibition of sugar transport, *Can. J. Physiol. Pharmacol.,* 53, 375, 1975.
3. **Robert, A.,** Antisecretory, antiulcer, cytoprotective and diarrheogenic properties of prostaglandins, in *Advances in Prostaglandin and Thromboxane Research,* Raven Press, New York, 1975, 507.
4. **Robert, A., Nezamis, J. E., Lancaster, C., and Hanchar, A. J.,** Cytoprotection by prostaglandins in rats, prevention of gastric necrosis produced by alcohol, HCl, NaOH, hypertonic NaCl, and thermal injury, *Gastroenterology,* 77, 433, 1979.
5. **Leung, F. W., Robert, A., and Guth, P. H.,** Gastric mucosal blood flow in rats after administration of 16,16-dimethyl prostaglandin $E_2$ at a cytoprotective dose, *Gastroenterology,* 88, 1948, 1985.
6. **Dinda, P. K., Hurst, R. O., and Beck, I. T.,** Effect of ethanol on the disaccharidases of the hamster jejunal brush border membrane, *Am. J. Physiol.,* 237, E68, 1979.
7. **Dinda, P. K. and Beck, I. T.,** Effect of ethanol on peptidases of hamster jejunal brush-border membrane, *Am. J. Physiol.,* 242, 1982.
8. **Dinda, P. K. and Beck, I. T.,** Ethanol-induced inhibition of glucose transport across the isolated brush-border membrane of hamster jejunum, *Dig. Dis. Sci.,* 26, 23, 1981.
9. **Tillotson, L. G., Carter, E. A., Inui, K. I., and Isselbacher, K. J.,** Inhibition of $Na^+$-stimulated glucose transport function and perturbation of intestinal microvillus membrane vesicles by ethanol and acetaldehyde, *Arch. Biochem. Biophys.,* 207, 360, 1981.
10. **Beesley, R. C.,** Ethanol inhibits $Na^+$ — gradient-dependent uptake of L-amino acids into intestinal brush border membrane vesicles, *Dig. Dis. Sci.,* 31, 987, 1986.
11. **al-Balool, F. and Debnam E. S.,** The effects of acute and chronic exposure to ethanol on glucose uptake by rat jejunal brush border membrane vesicles, *Q. J. Exp. Phys.,* 74, 751, 1989.
12. **al-Balool, F., Debnam, E. S., and Mazzanti, R.,** Acute and chronic exposure to ethanol and the electrophysiology of the brush border membrane of rat small intestine, *Gut,* 30, 1698, 1989.
13. **Dinda, P. K., Buell, M. G., Morris, O., and Beck, I. T.,** Studies on the mechanism of the ethanol-induced subepithelial fluid accumulation and jejunal villus bleb formation. An *in vitro* video microscopic approach, *Can. J. Physiol. Pharmacol.,* 72, 1186, 1994.
14. **Robles, E. A., Mezey, E., Halsted, C. H., and Schuster, M. M.,** Effect of ethanol on motility of the small intestine, *Johns Hopkins Med. J.,* 135, 17, 1974.
15. **Buell, M. G. and Beck, I. T.,** Effect of ethanol on jejunal regional blood flow in the rabbit, *Gastroenterology,* 84, 81, 1983.
16. **Buell, M. G., Dinda, P. K., and Beck, I. T.,** Effect of ethanol on morphology and total, capillary, and shunted blood flow of different anatomical layers of the dog jejunum, *Dig. Dis. Sci.,* 28, 1005, 1983.
17. **Kvietys, P. R., Paterson, W. G., Russell, J. M., Barrowman, J. A., and Granger, D. N.,** Role of the microcirculation in ethanol-induced mucosal injury in the dog, *Gastroenterology,* 87, 562, 1984.
18. **Hallback, D. A., Eriksson, M., and Sjoqvist, A.,** Nerve-mediated effect of ethanol on sodium and fluid transport in the jejunum of the rat, *Scand. J. Gastroenterol.,* 25, 859, 1990.
19. **Dinda, P. K., Leddin, D. J., and Beck, I. T.,** Histamine is involved in ethanol-induced jejunal microvascular injury in rabbits, *Gastroenterology,* 95, 1227, 1988.
20. **Beck, I. T., Boyd, A., and Dinda, P. K.,** Evidence for the involvement of 5-lipoxygenase products in the ethanol-induced intestinal plasma protein loss, *Am. J. Physiol.,* 254, G483, 1988.
21. **Leddin, D. J., Ray, M., Dinda, P. K., Prokopiw, I., and Beck, I. T.,** 16,16-Dimethyl prostaglandin $E_2$ alleviates jejunal microvascular effects of ethanol but not the ethanol-induced inhibition of water, sodium, and glucose absorption, *Gastroenterology,* 94, 726, 1988.
22. **Israel, Y., Valenzuela, J. E., Salazar, I., and Ugarte, G.,** Alcohol and amino acid transport in the human small intestine, *J. Nutr.,* 98, 222, 1969.
23. **Halsted, C. H., Robles, E. A., and Mezey, E.,** Distribution of ethanol in the human gastrointestinal tract, *Am. J. Clin. Nutr.,* 26, 831, 1973.
24. **Pappenheimer, J. R. and Heisey, S. R.,** Exchange of material between cerebrospinal fluid and blood, in *Drugs and Membranes,* Vol. 4, Proc. 1st Int. Pharmacol. Meet., Hogben, C. A. M. and Lindgren, P., Eds., Pergamon Press, Oxford, 1963, 95.

25. **Falconer, B. and Gladnikoff, H.,** Ueber den Alkoholgehalt des Blutes verschiedener Gefasse beim Kaninchen nach Alkoholzufuhr, *Scand. Arch. Physiol.,* 68, 245, 1934.

26. **Wright, E. M. and Diamond, J. M.,** Patterns of non-electrolyte permeability, *Proc. R. Soc. London Biol.,* 172, 227, 1969.

27. **Beck, I. T.,** Effets de l'alcool sur l'intestin grele, *La vie medicale au Canada francais,* 6, 15, 1977.

28. **Fox, J. E., Bourdages, R., and Beck, I. T.,** Effect of ethanol on glucose and water absorption in hamster jejunum *in vivo,* methodological problems: anesthesia, non-absorbable markers and osmotic effect, *Am. J. Dig. Dis.,* 23, 193, 1978.

29. **Beck, I. T., Paloschi, G. B., Dinda, P. K., and Beck, M.,** Effect of intragastric administration of alcohol on the ethanol concentrations and osmolality of pancreatic juice, bile and portal and peripheral blood, *Gastroenterology,* 67, 484, 1974.

30. **Lieber, C. S.,** Interaction of alcohol with other drugs and nutrients. Implication for the therapy of alcoholic liver disease, *Drugs,* 40 (Suppl. 3), 23, 1990.

31. **Millan, M. S., Morris, G. P., Beck, I. T., and Henson, J. T.,** Villus damage induced by suction biopsy and by acute ethanol intake in normal human small intestine, *Dig. Dis. Sci.,* 25, 513, 1980.

32. **Lee, J. S.,** Isoosmotic absorption of fluid from rat jejunum *in vitro, Gastroenterology,* 54, 366, 1968.

33. **Dinda, P. K., Beck, M., and Beck, I. T.,** On the mechanism of isosmotic transport across the small intestine. The composition of the absorbate transported from a mucosal solution made hypertonic by the addition of mannitol, *Can. J. Physiol. Pharmacol.,* 51, 130, 1973.

34. **Dinda, P. K., Beck, M., and Beck, I. T.,** Effect of changes in the osmolality of the luminal fluid on intracellular concentration of solutes in the hamster jejunum, *Can. J. Physiol. Pharmacol.,* 50, 72, 1972.

35. **Coady, J. M.,** Isolation and purification of the basal lateral membrane of rat and enterocytes for investigation of intestinal transport, Ph.D. Thesis, Queen's University, Kingston, Ontario, Canada, (Thesis supervisor: Beck, I. T.) 1984.

36. **Haljamae, A. H., Jodal, M., and Lundgren, O.,** Countercurrent multiplication of sodium and intestinal villi during absorption of sodium chloride, *Acta Physiol. Scand.,* 89, 580, 1973.

37. **Baraona, E., Pirola, R. C., and Lieber C. S.,** Small intestinal damage and changes in cell population produced by ethanol ingestion in the rat, *Gastroenterology,* 66, 226, 1974.

38. **Kuo, Y. J. and Shanbour, L. L.,** Effects of ethanol on sodium, 3-0-methyl glucose, and l-alanine transport in the jejunum, *Am. J. Dig. Dis.,* 23, 51, 1978.

39. **Broitman, S. A., Gottlieb, L. S., and Vitale, J. J.,** Augmentation of ethanol absorption by mono- and disaccharides, *Gastroenterology,* 70, 1101, 1976.

40. **Pfeiffer, A., Schmidt, T., Vidon, N., and Kaess, H.,** Effect of ethanol on absorption of a nutrient solution in the upper human intestine, *Scand. J. Gastroenterol.,* 28, 515, 1985.

41. **Vyrodov, I. P., Bud'Ko, P. S., and Derkach, L. V.,** Use of kinetic concepts of the structure of a liquid to determine molecular dimensions, *Russ. J. Physiol. Chem.,* 38, 126, 1964.

42. **Gailis, L.,** Cardiovascular effects on acetaldehyde: evidence for the involvement of tissue SH groups, in *The Role of Acetaldehyde in the Actions of Ethanol,* Lindros, K. O. and Eriksson, C. J. P., Eds., Kartpakirjapaino, Helsinki, 1975, 135.

43. **Rix, K. J. B.,** *Alcohol and Alcoholism,* Eden, Montreal, 1977.

44. **Spencer, R. R., Brody, K. R., and Lutters, B. M.,** Some effects of ethanol on the gastrointestinal tract, *Am. J. Dig. Dis.,* 9, 599, 1964.

45. **Julkunen, R. J. K., DiPadova C., and Lieber, C. S.,** First pass metabolism of ethanol — a gastrointestinal barrier against the systemic toxicity of ethanol, *Life Sci.,* 37, 567, 1985.

46. **Julkunen, R. J., Tannenbaum, L., Baraona, E., and Lieber, C. S.,** First pass metabolism of ethanol: an important determinant of blood levels after alcohol consumption, *Alcohol,* 2, 437, 1985.

47. **Shimizu, M., Lasker, J., Tsutsumi, M., and Lieber, C.,** Immunohistochemical localization of ethanol-inducible P450IIE1 in the rat alimentary tract, *Gastroenterology,* 99, 1044, 1990.

48. **Caballeria, J., Frezza M., Hernandez-Munoz, R., Dipadova C., Korsten, M. A., Baraona, E., and Lieber, C. S.,** Gastric origin of the first-pass metabolism of ethanol in humans: effect of gastrectomy, *Gastroenterology,* 97, 1205, 1989.

49. **Frezza, M., di Padova, C., Pozzato, G., Terpin, M., Baraona, E., and Lieber, C. S.,** High blood alcohol levels in women: the role of decreased gastric alcohol dehydrogenase activity and first-pass metabolism, *N. Engl. J. Med.,* 322, 95, 1990 (published errata appear in *N. Engl. J. Med.,* 322, 1540, and 323, 553, 1990).

50. **Shinohara, T., Ijiri, I., Ameno, S., Fuke, C., and Ameno, K.,** A comparative study of ethanol absorption in the canine jejunum after pretreatment with cyanamide or pyrazole, *Alcohol Alcohol.,* 28, 423, 1993.

51. **Hayton, W. L.,** Effects of normal alcohols on intestinal absorption of salicylic acid, sulfapyridine, and prednisone in rats, *J. Pharmacol. Sci.,* 64, 1450, 1975.

52. **Gillespie, R. J. G. and Lucas, C. C.,** Effect of single intoxicating doses of ethanol on the gastric and intestinal mucosa of rats, *Can. J. Biochem. Physiol.,* 39, 237, 1961.

53. **Hoyumpa, A. M., Breen, K. J., Schenker, S., and Wilson, F. A.,** Thiamine transport across the rat intestine. II Effect of ethanol, *J. Lab. Clin. Med.,* 86, 803, 1975.

54. **Dinda, P. K., Beck, I. T., Beck, M., and McElligott, T. F.,** Effect of ethanol on sodium-dependent glucose transport in the small intestine of the hamster, *Gastroenterology,* 68, 1517, 1975.

55. **Fox, J. E., McElligott, T. F., and Beck, I. T.,** The correlation of ethanol-induced depression of glucose and water transport with morphological changes in the hamster jejunum *in vivo, Can. J. Physiol. Pharmacol.,* 56, 123, 1978.

56. **Fox, J. E., McElligott, T. F., and Beck, I. T.,** Effect of ethanol on the morphology of hamster jejunum, *Am. J. Dig. Dis.,* 23, 201, 1978.

57. **Fox, J. E., Morris, G. P., Beck, I. T., and McElligott, T. F.,** The ultrastructure of blebs induced in the hamster jejunum by ethanol, *Can. J. Physiol. Pharmacol.,* 57, 305, 1979.

58. **Dinda, P. K., Holitzner, C. A., Morris, G. P., and Beck, I. T.,** Ethanol-induced jejunal microvascular and morphological injury in relation to histamine release in rabbits, *Gastroenterology,* 104, 361, 1993.

59. **Ray, M., Dinda, P. K., and Beck, I. T.,** Mechanism of ethanol-induced jejunal microvascular and morphologic changes in the dog, *Gastroenterology,* 96, 345, 1989.

60. **Levine, R. R., McNary, W. F., Kornguth, P. J., and LeBlanc, R.,** Histological re-evaluation of everted gut technique for studying intestinal absorption, *Eur. J. Pharmacol.,* 9, 211, 1970.

61. **Faelli, A., Esposito, G., Burlini, N., Tosco, M., and Capraro, V.,** The rat and hamster jejunum during transintestinal transport *in vitro, Arch. Int. Physiol. Biochem.,* 87, 73, 1979.

62. **Beck, I. T., Leddin, D. J., Ray, M., and Dinda, P. K.,** Relationship between the ethanol (ETH) induced microvascular (MV) damage and absorption, in *Microcirculation, An Update, Proceedings of the Fourth World Congress for Microcirculation,* Tokyo, Japan, 2, 427, 1987.

63. **Loder, R., Mueller, V. C., Trier, J. S., Dobbins, W. O., Barrett, B., and Rubin, C. E.,** An improved design for a hydraulic biopsy tube, *Gastroenterology,* 46, 418, 1964.

64. **Foschi, D., Trabucchi, E., Galeone, M., Ferrante, F., Toti, G. L., Costoldi, L., Musazzi, M., Centemero, A., and Montorsi, W.,** Prostaglandin cytoprotection in humans: effectiveness of rosaprostol, *Int. J. Tissue React.,* 10, 53, 1988.

65. **Foschi, D., Marazzi, M., Toti, G. L., Radaelli, E., Ferrante, F., Vaiani, G., Galeone, M., and Trabucchi, E.,** Prostaglandin-stimulated recovery of the human duodenal epithelium: effects of misoprostol on ethanol damage, *Am. J. Gastroenterol.,* 85, 1498,1990.

66. **Fromm, D.,** Mechanisms involved in gastric mucosal resistance to injury, *Annu. Rev. Med.,* 38, 119, 1987.

67. **Moore, R., Carlson, S., and Madara, J. L.,** Rapid barrier restitution in an *in vitro* model of intestinal epithelial injury, *Lab. Invest.,* 60, 237, 1989.

68. **Kvietys, P. R., Specian, R. D., Grisham, M. B., and Tso, P.,** Jejunal mucosal injury and restitution: role of hydrolytic products of food digestion, *Am. J. Physiol.,* 261, G384, 1991.

69. **Buell, M. G. and Beck, I. T.,** Ethanol-induced mucosal microvascular stasis and enhanced plasma protein loss in the dog jejunum, *Gastroenterology,* 86, 413, 1984.

70. **Beck, I. T. and Dinda, P. K.,** The role of histamine (HIST) in the ethanol-induced morphological injury, *Gastroenterology,* 100, A561, 1991.

71. **Dinda, P. K., Morris, O., Buell, M. G., and Beck, I. T.,** Does Ca$^{++}$ play a role in the ethanol (ETH)-induced jejunal subepithelial bleb formation?, *Gastroenterology,* 106, A230, 1994.

72. **Rubin, R. and Hoek, J. B.,** Ethanol-induced stimulation of phosphoinositide turnover and calcium influx in isolated hepatocytes, *Biochem. Pharmacol.,* 37, 2461, 1988.

73. **Rutten, M. J. and Moore, C. D.,** Low doses of ethanol have Ca$^{2+}$ ionophore-like effects on apical membrane potential of *in vitro* Necturus antrum, *Am. J. Physiol.,* 261, G92, 1991.

74. **Konda, Y., Sakamoto, C., Nishisaki, H., Nakano, O., Matozaki, T., Nagao, M., Matsuda, K., Wada, K., and Baba, S.,** Ethanol stimulates pepsinogen release by opening a Ca$^{2+}$ channel of guinea pig gastric chief cells, *Gastroenterology,* 100, 17, 1991.

75. **Lee, J. S.,** Epithelial cell extrusion during fluid transport in canine small intestine, *Am. J. Physiol.,* 232, E408, 1977.

76. **Granger, D. N., Cook, B. H., and Taylor, A. E.,** Structural locus of transmucosal albumin efflux in canine ileum, a fluorescent study, *Gastroenterology,* 71, 1023, 1976.

77. **Astaldi, G. and Strosselli, E.,** Peroral biopsy of the intestinal mucosa in hepatic cirrhosis, *Am. J. Dig. Dis.,* 5, 603, 1960.

78. **Adrich, A., Boj, E., Kryszewski, A., and Rynkiewicz, H.,** Jejunal mucosa structure and small intestine function in diabetes, *Przegl. Lek.,* 32, 782, 1975.

79. **Haglund, U., Hulten, L., Ahren, C., and Lundgren, O.,** Mucosal lesions in the human small intestine in shock, *Gut,* 16, 979, 1975.

80. **Perdue, M., Roomi, N., Forstner, J., and Gall, D. G.,** Effect of IgE-mediated reactions on rat intestinal epithelium: goblet cell reaction and enterocyte damage, *Gastroenterology,* 86, 1209, 1984.

81. **Buell, M. G. and Harding, R. K.,** Proinflammatory effects of local abdominal irradiation of rat gastrointestinal tract, *Dig. Dis. Sci.,* 34, 390, 1989.

82. **MacNaughton, W. K., Leach, K. E., Purd'Homme-Lalonde, L., Ho, W., and Sharkey, K. A.,** Ionizing radiation reduces neurally evoked electrolyte transport in rat ileum through a mast cell-dependent mechanism, *Gastroenterology,* 106, 324, 1994.

83. **Altura, B. M., Ogunkoya, A., Gebrewold, A., and Altura, B. T.,** Effects of ethanol on terminal arterioles and muscular venules: direct observations on the microcirculation, *J. Cardiovasc. Pharmacol.*, 1, 97, 1979.

84. **Beck, I. T.,** The role of splanchnic circulatory and mucosal microvascular changes in the ethanol-induced acute small bowel injury, in *Pathophysiology of the Splanchnic Circulation,* Kvietys, P. R., Barrowman, J. A., and Granger, D. N., Eds., CRC Press, Boca Raton, FL, 1987, 1.

85. **Siregar, H. and Chou, C. C.,** Relative contribution of fat, protein, carbohydrate, and ethanol to intestinal hyperemia, *Am. J. Physiol.*, 242, G27, 1982.

86. **Israel, Y., MacDonald, A., and Orrego, H.,** Contribution of portal and arterial flow to the increase in liver blood flow induced by acute ethanol administration, *Gastroenterology*, 84, 1377, 1983.

87. **Beck, I. T., Dinda, P. K., Leddin, D. J., Ray, M., Prokopiw, I., and Boyd, A.,** Chemical mediators in ethanol-induced increased jejunal microvascular permeability, in *Microcirculation in Circulatory Disorders*, Manabe, H., Zweifach, B. W., and Messmer, K., Eds., Springer-Verlag, Tokyo, 1988, 171.

88. **Dinda, P. K., Kossev, P., Buell, M. G., and Beck, I. T.,** Ethanol-induced jejunal mucosal injury — role of xanthine oxidase (XO) and leukocytes, *Gastroenterology,* 104, A242, 1993.

89. **Kosseva, V., Dinda, P. K., and Beck, I. T.,** Ethanol-induced jejunal mucosal injury — role of elastase, *Gastroenterology*, 104, A1045, 1993.

90. **Kosseva, V., Kossev, P., Beck, I. T., and Dinda, P. K.,** Role of neutrophylic proteases in ethanol (ETH) induced increased jejunal mucosal permeability and degranulation of mast cells, *Gastroenterology*, 106, A1033, 1994.

91. **Lavo, B., Colombel, J. F., Knutsson, L., and Hallgren, R.,** Acute exposure of small intestine to ethanol induces mucosal leakage and prostaglandin E2 synthesis, *Gastroenterology,* 102, 468, 1992.

92. **Majno, G. and Palade, G. E.,** Studies in inflammation. 1. The effect of histamine and serotonin on vascular permeability: an electron microscopic study, *J. Biophys. Biochem. Cytol.,* 11, 571, 1961.

93. **Majno, G., Palade, G. E., and Schoefl, G. I.,** Studies in inflammation. II. The site of action of histamine and serotonin along the vascular tree: a topographic study, *J. Biophys. Biochem. Cytol.*, 11, 607, 1961.

94. **Cotran, R. S. and Majno, G.,** The delayed and prolonged vascular leakage in inflammation. I. Topography of the leaking vessels after thermal injury, *Am. J. Pathol.*, 45, 261, 1964.

95. **Ham, K. N. and Hurley, J. V.,** Acute inflammation. An electron-microscope study of turpentine-induced pleurisy in the rat, *J. Pathol. Bacteriol.*, 90, 365, 1965.

96. **Majno, G., Gilmore, V., and Leventhal, M.,** On the mechanism of vascular leakage caused by histamine-type mediators. A microscopic study *in vivo, Circ. Res.,* 21, 833, 1967.

97. **Hurley, J. V. and McQueen, A.,** The response of fenestrated vessels of the small intestine of rats to application of mustard oil, *J. Pathol.*, 105, 21, 1971.

98. **Wells, F. R.,** Standardization of biological ink for the study of vascular injury in inflammation, *Experientia,* 28, 371, 1972.

99. **Beck, I. T., Morris, G. P., and Buell, M. G.,** Ethanol-induced vascular permeability changes in the jejunal mucosa of the dog, *Gastroenterology*, 90, 1137, 1986.

100. **Holitzner, C. A., Dinda, P. K., Morris G. P., and Beck, I. T.,** Changes in microvascular permeability precede ethanol-induced plasma protein loss in the canine jejunum, *Gastroenterology,* 100, A217, l991.

101. **Joris, I., DeGirolami, U., and Wortham, K.,** Vascular labelling with monastral blue B, *Stain Technol.*, 57, 177, 1982.

102. **Lee, J. S. and Silverberg, J. W.,** Effect of histamine on intestinal fluid secretion in the dog, *Am. J. Physiol.*, 231, 793, 1976.

103. **Casley-Smith, J. R.,** Fine structural studies of passage across capillary walls, in *Progress in Microcirculation Research*, Garlick, D., Ed., University of South Wales, South Wales, 1981, 175.

104. **Svensjo, E., Adamski, S. W., Su, K., and Grega, G. J.,** Quantitative physiological and morphological aspects of microvascular permeability changes by histamine and inhibited by terbutaline, *Acta Physiol. Scand.,* 116, 265, 1982.

105. **Fox, J., Galey, F., and Wayland, H.,** Actions of histamine on the mesenteric microvasculature, *Microvasc. Res.,* 19, 102, 1980.

106. **Korthuis, R. J., Wang, C. Y., and Spielman, W. S.,** Transient effects of histamine on the capillary filtration coefficient, *Microvasc. Res.*, 28, 322, 1984.

107. **Leddin, D. J., Dinda, P. K., and Beck, I. T.,** The role of histamine$_1$ and histamine$_2$ receptors in the ethanol-induced jejunal plasma protein loss, *Agents Actions*, 35, 163, 1992.

108. **Dinda, P. K., Buell, M. G., and Beck, I. T.,** Role of oxygen derived free radicals in the ethanol-induced small intestinal mucosal injury, *Gastroenterology,* 102, A208, 1992.

109. **Dinda, P. K., Wasan, S., Kossev, P., and Beck, I. T.,** Adaptive cytoprotection against ethanol-induced small bowel mucosal injury, *Gastroenterology,* 104, A243, 1993.

110. **Dinda, P. K., Kossev, P., and Beck, I. T.,** Effect of anti-CD18 and Anti-ICAM-1 monoclonal antibodies (MAb) on ethanol (ETH)-induced jejunal mucosal injury, *Gastroenterology,* 106, A230, 1994.

111. **Kosseva, V., Kossev, P., Beck, I. T., and Dinda, P. K.,** Mechanism of ethanol (ETH)-induced degranulation of jejunal mast cells (MC), *Gastroenterology*, 106, A1033, 1994.

112. **Fewtrell, C. M. S. and Comperts, B. D.,** Quercetin: A novel inhibitor of $Ca^{2+}$ influx and exocytosis in rat peritoneal mast cells, *Biochim. Biophys. Acta,* 469, 52, 1977.

113. **Pearce, F. L., Befus, A. D., and Bienenstock, J.,** Mucosal mast cells. III. Effect of quercetin and other flavonoids on antigen-induced histamine secretion from rat intestinal mast cells, *J. Allergy Clin. Immunol.,* 73, 819, 1984.

114. **Grosman, N.,** Inhibitory effect of phloretin on histamine release from isolated rat mast cells, *Agents Action,* 25, 284, 1988.

115. **Williams, T. J. and Piper, P. J.,** The action of chemically pure SRS-A on the microcirculation *in vivo, Prostaglandins,* 19, 779, 1980.

116. **Vane, J. and Botting, R.,** Inflammation and the mechanism of action of anti-inflammatory drugs, *FASEB J.,* 1, 89, 1987.

117. **Peskar, B. M., Lange, K., Hoppe, U., and Peskar, B. A.,** Ethanol stimulates formation of leukotriene $C_4$ in rat gastric mucosa, *Prostaglandins,* 31, 283, 1986.

118. **Guidon, Y., Girard, A., Maycock, A., Ford-Hutchinson, A. W., Atkinson, P. C., Belanger, J. G., Dallob, A., DeSouse, D., Dougherty, H., Egan, R., Goldberg, M. M., Ham, E., Fortin, R., Hamel, P., Lau, C. K., Leblanc, Y., McFarlane, C. S., Piechuta, H., Therien, M., Yoakim, C., and Rokach, J.,** A novel, potent and selective 5-lipoxygenase inhibitor, in *Advances in Prostaglandin, Thromboxane, and Leukotriene Research,* Vol. 17, Samuelson, B., Paoletti, R., and Ramwell, P. W., Eds., Raven Press, New York, 1987, 554.

119. **Gutteridge, J. M. C.,** in *Oxygen Radicals and Tissue Injury, Proceedings of a Brook Lodge Symposium,* Halliwell, B., Ed., Upjohn Company, Bethesda, MD, 1988, 9.

120. **Weiss, S. J.,** Tissue destruction by neutrophils, *N. Engl. J. Med.,* 320, 365, 1989.

121. **Gutteridge, J. M. and Halliwell, B.,** Reoxygenation injury and antioxidant protection: a tale of two paradoxes, *Arch. Biochem. Biophys.,* 283, 223, 1990.

122. **Granger, D. N., McCord, J. M., Parks, D. A., and Hoellwarth, M. E.,** Xanthine oxidase inhibitors attenuate ischemia-induced vascular permeability changes in the cat intestine, *Gastroenterology,* 90, 80, 1986.

123. **Grisham, M. B., Hernandez, L. A., and Granger, D. N.,** Xanthine oxidase and neutrophil infiltration in intestinal ischemia, *Am. J. Physiol.,* 251, G567, 1986.

124. **Granger, D. N., Rutili, G., and McCord, J. M.,** Superoxide radicals in feline intestinal ischemia, *Gastroenterology,* 81, 22, 1981.

125. **Kvietys, P. R., Twohig, B., Danzell, J., and Specian, R. D.,** Ethanol-induced injury to rat gastric mucosa: role of neutrophils and xanthine oxidase-derived radicals, *Gastroenterology,* 98, 1, 1990.

126. **Miller, M. J. S., McNeill, H., Mullane, K. M., Caravella, S. J., and Clark, D.,** SOD prevents damage and attenuates eicosanoid release in a rabbit model of necrotising enterocolitis, *Am. J. Physiol.,* 255, G556, 1988.

127. **Kvietys, P. R., Perry, M. A., Gaginella, T. S., and Granger, D. N.,** Ethanol enhances leukocyte-endothelial cell interactions in mesenteric venules, *Am. J. Physiol.,* 259, G578, 1990.

128. **Zimmerman, B. J., Grisham, M. B., and Granger, D. N.,** Role of oxidants in ischemia/reperfusion-induced granulocyte infiltration, *Am. J. Physiol.,* 258, G185, 1990.

129. **Angus, J. A. and Cocks, T. M.,** Endothelium-derived relaxing factor, *Pharmacol. Ther.,* 41, 303, 1989.

130. **Dinda, P. K., Kossev, P., Kosseva, V., and Beck, I. T.,** L-arginine protects against ethanol(Eth)-induced jejunal mucosal injury, *Gastroenterology,* 104, A243, 1993.

131. **Kubes, P. and Gaboury, J. P.,** Mast cell degranulation causes granulocyte rolling and adhesion in venules, *Gastroenterology,* 106 (Abstract), 1027, 1994.

132. **Kubes, P., Hunter, J., and Granger, D. N.,** Ischemia/reperfusion-induced feline intestinal dysfunction: importance of granulocyte recruitment, *Gastroenterology,* 103, 807, 1992.

133. **Todd, R. F. and Arnaout, M. A.,** Monoclonal antibodies that identify Mo1 and LFA-1, two human leukocyte membrane glycoproteins: a review, in *Leukocyte Typing II,* Vol. 3, Reinherz, E. L., Haynes, B. F., Nadler, L. M., and Berstein, I. D., Eds., Springer-Verlag, New York, 1986, 95.

134. **Tuomanen, E. I., Saukkonen, K., Sande, S., Cloffe, C., and Wright, S. D.,** Reduction of inflammation, tissue damage, and mortality in bacterial meningitis in rabbits treated with monoclonal antibodies against adhesion-promoting receptors of leukocytes, *J. Exp. Med.,* 170, 959, 1989.

135. **Wallace, J. L., Arfors, K.-E., and McKnight, G. W.,** A monoclonal antibody against the CD18 leukocyte adhesion molecule prevents indomethacin-induced gastric damage in the rabbit, *Gastroenterology,* 100, 878, 1991.

136. **Lasky, L. A. and Rosen, S. D.,** The selectins: carbohydrate-binding adhesion molecules of the immune system, in *Inflammation: Basic Principles and Clinical Correlates,* 2nd ed., Gallin, J. I., Goldstein, I. M., and Snyderman, R., Eds., Raven Press, New York, 1992, 407.

137. **Sukumar, P., Dinda, P. K., Buell, M. G., and Beck, I. T.,** Ethanol induced microvascular and morphological injury precedes leukocyte adhesion to villus microvessels. A videomicroscopic study on hamster, *Gastroenterology,* 106, A1052, 1994.

138. **Pihan, G., Majzoubi, D., Haudenschild, C., Trier, J., and Szabo, S.,** Early microcirculatory stasis in acute gastric mucosal injury in the rat and prevention by 16,16-dimethyl prostaglandin $E_2$ or sodium thiosulfate, *Gastroenterology,* 91, 1415, 1986.

139. **Lacy, E. R. and Ito, S.,** Microscopic analysis of ethanol damage to rat gastric mucosa after treatment with a prostaglandin, *Gastroenterology*, 83, 619, 1982.

140. **Robert, A.,** Cytoprotection by prostaglandins, *Gastroenterology*, 77, 761, 1979.

141. **Stern, M., Carter, E. A., and Walker, W. A.,** Food proteins and gut mucosal barrier. IV. Effect of acute and chronic ethanol administration on handling and uptake of bovine serum albumin by rat small intestine, *Dig. Dis. Sci.*, 31, 1242, 1986.

142. **Carter, E. A., Harmatz, P. R., Udall, I. N., and Walker, W. A.,** Barrier defense function of the small intestine: effect of ethanol and acute burn trauma, *Adv. Exp. Med. Biol.*, 216A, 829, 1987.

143. **Bjarnason, I., Smethurst, P., Levi, A. J., and Peters, T. J.,** Intestinal permeability to $^{51}$Cr-EDTA in rats with experimentally induced enteropathy, *Gut*, 26, 579, 1985.

144. **Aabakken, L.,** Cr-ethylenediaminetetraacetic acid absorption test. Methodologic aspects, *Scand. J. Gastroenterol.*, 24, 351, 1989.

145. **Worthington, B. S., Meserole, L., and Syrotuck, J. A.,** Effect of daily ethanol ingestion on intestinal permeability to macromolecules, *Am. J. Dig. Dis.*, 23, 23, 1978.

146. **Draper, L. R., Gyure, L. A., Hall, J. G., and Roberston, D.,** Effect of alcohol on the integrity of the intestinal epithelium, *Gut*, 24, 399, 1983.

147. **Talbot, R. W., Foster, J. R., Hermon-Taylor, J., and Grant, D. A. W.,** Induced mucosal penetration and transfer to portal blood of luminal horseradish peroxidase after exposure of mucosa of guinea pig small intestine to ethanol and lysolecithin, *Dig. Dis. Sci.*, 29, 1015, 1984.

148. **Crissinger, K. D., Kvietys, P. R., and Granger, D. N.,** Pathophysiology of gastrointestinal mucosal permeability, *J. Intern. Med.*, 732 (Suppl.), 145, 1990.

149. **Chang, T., Lewis, J., and Glazko, A. J.,** Effect of ethanol and other alcohols on the transport of amino acids and glucose by everted sacs of rat small intestine, *Biochim. Biophys. Acta*, 135, 1000, 1967.

150. **Panowicz, H.,** Effect of ethyl alcohol on glucose absorption in the isolated segment of the small intestine of the rat, *Rocz. Pomor. Akad. Med. Swierczewski.*, 13, 385, 1967.

151. **Israel, Y., Salazar, I., and Rosenmann, E.,** Inhibitory effects of alcohol on intestinal amino acid transport *in vivo* and *in vitro*, *J. Nutr.*, 96, 499, 1968.

152. **Mezey, E.,** Intestinal function in chronic alcoholism, *Ann. N.Y. Acad. Sci.*, 252, 215, 1975.

153. **Dinda, P. K. and Beck, I. T.,** On the mechanism of the inhibitory effect of ethanol on intestinal glucose and water absorption, *Am. J. Dig. Dis.*, 22, 529, 1977.

154. **Fox, J. E., Dinda, P. K., and Beck, I. T.,** Is ethanol (ETH) toxicity in the jejunum due to osmotic damage?, *Gastroenterology*, 85, 1058, 1977.

155. **Jacobs, F. A., Crandall, J. C., and Fabel, C. B.,** An effect of ethanol in the bidirectional intestinal flux of amino acids, *Nutr. Rep. Int.*, 21, 397, 1980.

156. **Beck, I. T. and Dinda, P. K.,** Effect of ethanol on Na+K+-ATPase and active transport of sugars and amino acids, in *Alcohol and the Gastrointestinal Tract, INSERM*, 95, 423, 1980.

157. **O'Neill, B., Weber, F., Hornig, D., and Semenza, G.,** Ethanol selectively affects Na+-gradient dependent intestinal transport systems, *FEBS Lett.*, 194, 183, 1986.

158. **Money, S. R., Petroianu, A., Kimura, K., and Jaffe, B. M.,** The effects of short-term ethanol exposure on the canine jejunal handling of calcium and glucose, *Surgery*, 107, 167, 1990.

159. **Carter, E. A., Drummey, G. D., and Isselbacher, K. J.,** Ethanol stimulates triglyceride synthesis by the intestine, *Science*, 174, 1245, 1971.

160. **Mistillis, S. P. and Ockner, R. K.,** Effects of ethanol on endogenous lipid and lipoprotein metabolism in small intestine, *J. Lab. Clin. Med.*, 80, 34, 1972.

161. **Baraona, E. and Lieber, C. S.,** Intestinal lymph formation and fat absorption: stimulation by acute ethanol administration and inhibition by chronic ethanol feeding, *Gastroenterology*, 68, 495, 1975.

162. **Boquillon, M.,** Effect of acute ethanol ingestion on fat absorption, *Lipids*, 11, 848, 1976.

163. **Mansbach, C. M., II,** Effect of ethanol on intestinal lipid absorption in the rat, *J. Lipid Res.*, 24, 1310, 1983.

164. **Thomson, A. B.,** Effect of chronic ingestion of ethanol on *in vitro* uptake of lipids and glucose in the rabbit jejunum, *Am. J. Physiol.*, 246, G120, 1984.

165. **Himal, H. S. and Greenberg, L.,** The effect of ethanol and bile on electrolyte movement across canine proximal duodenal mucosa, *Am. J. Gastroenterol.*, 68, 45, 1977.

166. **Mekhjian, H. S. and May E. S.,** Acute and chronic effects of ethanol on fluid transport in the human small intestine, *Gastroenterology*, 72, 1280, 1977.

167. **Breen, K. J. Buttigieg, R., Iossifidis, S., Lourensz, C., and Wood, B.,** Jejunal uptake of thiamin hydrochloride in humans: influence of alcoholism and alcohol, *Am. J. Clin. Nutr.*, 42, 121, 1985.

168. **Said, H. M. and Strum, W. B.,** Effect of ethanol and other aliphatic alcohols on the intestinal transport of folates, *Digestion*, 35, 129, 1986.

169. **Krishnamra, N. and Boonpimol, P.,** Acute effect of ethanol on intestinal calcium transport, *J. Nutr. Sci. Vit.*, 32, 229, 1986.

170. **Krishnamra, N. and Limlomwongse, L.,** The *in vivo* effect of ethanol on gastrointestinal motility and gastrointestinal handling of calcium in rats, *J. Nut. Sci. Vit.*, 33, 89, 1987.

171. **Pinto, J., Huang, Y. P., and Rivlin, R. S.,** Mechanisms underlying the differential effects of ethanol on the bioavailability of riboflavin and flavin adenine dinucleotide, *J. Clin. Invest.,* 79, 1343, 1987.

172. **Barrio Lera, J. P., Alvarez, A. I., and Prieto, J. G.,** Effects of ethanol on the pharmacokinetics of cephalexin and cefadroxil in the rat, *J. Pharmacol. Sci.,* 80, 511, 1991.

173. **Persson, J.,** Alcohol and the small intestine, *Scand. J. Gastroenterol.,* 26, 3, 1991.

174. **Crane, R. K.,** Absorption of sugars, in *Handbook of Physiology: Section 6: Alimentary Canal,* Vol. 3, Code, C. F. and Heidel, W., Eds., Williams and Wilkins, Baltimore, 1968, 1323.

175. **Gray, J. P., Hoyumpa, A. M., Dunn, G. D., Henderson, G. I., Wilson, F. A., and Swift, L. L.,** Effect of ethanol (E) on fluidity of enterocyte membranes, *Clin. Res.,* 27, 683A, 1979.

176. **Bossmann, B. and Hutter, H. J.,** Beeinflussung membrangebundener Enzymaktivitaten durch Veranderung der Membranlipidzusammensetzung, *Eur. J. Clin. Chem. Clin. Biochem.,* 30, 381, 1992.

177. **Marway, J. S., Salisbury, J. R., and Preedy, V. R.,** Effects of acute ethanol toxicity on protein synthesis in three anatomically distinct regions of the rat gut, *Biochem. Soc. Trans.,* 19, 165S, 1991.

178. **Carter, E. A. and Isselbacher, K. J.,** Effect of ethanol on intestinal adenosine triphosphate (ATP) content, *Proc. Soc. Exp. Biol. Med.,* 142, 1171, 1973.

179. **Krasner, N., Carmichael, H. A., Russell, R. I., Thompson, G. G., and Cochran, K. M.,** Alcohol and absorption from the small intestine. 2. Effect of ethanol on ATP and ATPase activities in guinea-pig jejunum, *Gut,* 17, 249, 1976.

180. **Diamond, J. M. and Bossert, W. H.,** Standing-gradient osmotic flow. A mechanism for coupling of water and solute transport in epithelia, *J. Gen. Physiol.,* 50, 2061, 1967.

181. **Tomasini, J. T. and Dobbins, W. O.,** Intestinal mucosal morphology during water and electrolyte absorption. A light and electron microscopic study, *Am. J. Dig. Dis.,* 15, 226, 1970.

182. **Mitjavila, S., Lacombe, C., and Carrera, G.,** Changes in activity of rat brush border enzymes incubated with a homologous series of aliphatic alcohols, *Biochem. Pharmacol.,* 25, 625, 1976.

183. **Lacombe, C., Mitjavila, S., and Carrera, G.,** The action and interaction of three alimentary substances (ethanol, tannic acid, and sodium sulfite) on the activity of the ATPases in enterocyte brush borders, *Life Sci.,* 18, 1245, 1976.

184. **Hoyumpa, A. M., Jr., Nichols, S. G., Wilson, F. A., and Schenker, S.,** Effect of ethanol on intestinal (Na, K) ATPase and intestinal thiamine transport in rats, *J. Lab. Clin. Med.,* 90, 1086, 1977.

# 11

# Alcohol-Induced Malabsorption in the Gastrointestinal Tract

Allan D. Thomson, Laura C. Heap, and Roberta J. Ward

## CONTENTS

0-8493-2480-7/96/$0.00+$.50

## 11.1   INTRODUCTION

The principal role of the gastrointestinal tract is to deliver water, salts, and nutrients from the intestinal lumen to the bloodstream, and lymph and tissue fluids at a rate sufficient to maintain requirements for growth and reparative purposes. Malabsorption arises when such transport is impaired sufficiently to prevent optimum levels of nutrients to maintain functional processes. Ethanol causes malabsorption of certain nutrients, especially when taken in excessive amounts, although the precise mechanisms involved remain unclear.

The results in the literature pertaining to the adverse effects of ethanol administration on the absorption of a wide number of nutrients are conflicting and reflect the wide range of approaches used in the experimental design such as differences in the application of ethanol to the gut, either to the whole animal *in vivo,* or to isolated gut segments *in vitro*; acute vs. chronic ethanol administration; physiological or pharmacological doses of ethanol; the species of animal; and the nutritional status of the animal plus the diet in which the ethanol is administered. For example, feeding rats a diet enriched with saturated fatty acids prevents the inhibitory effects of chronic ethanol on the *in vitro* uptake of hexoses and lipids.[1] Such factors are further confounded by the extent to which it is possible to extrapolate the results from absorption studies in animals to humans. It would be presumptuous to assume that the mechanisms are identical. For example, low concentrations of thiamine are absorbed by an active, sodium-dependent mechanism in both animals and humans; however, at high thiamine concentrations the absorption of $B_1$ from the rat intestine occurs by diffusion, a mechanism which has not been demonstrated in humans *in vivo*. (See Reference 2 for further details.)

The effects of ethanol on absorptive processes of a variety of nutrients are highly complex and multifactorial. There are likely to be differences in the susceptibility of the rate of absorption for each nutrient to ethanol, which will depend on the precise mechanism of absorption, the nutritional status, the luminal content plus the tissue levels and stores of each nutrient, so that the optimum rate of absorption for each nutrient may decline at different rates. Furthermore, some functions of a particular nutrient may be more susceptible to a decrease such that maintenance of its optimal level is more critical. Despite the demonstration of $B_{12}$ malabsorption in alcoholics,[3] low serum $B_{12}$ levels are rarely encountered and tend to be normal or elevated in alcoholics with liver disease with or without cirrhosis.[4] In addition, $B_{12}$ may be high in patients with liver damage but it is in the bound form (having been released by the liver), and cannot be utilized. There are also many complex influential interactions between nutrients; for example, lack of niacin (a B group vitamin) is of little consequence provided that there is an adequate supply of the essential amino acid, tryptophan, which may be converted into niacin. Finally, questions such as how does the gut respond to changes in the absorption of nutrients, what signals are sent from the tissue as a result of decreased nutrient levels and to what extent is the gut capable of responding, particularly when there is continued presence of ethanol in the lumen often associated with malnutrition have not yet been answered.

This chapter addresses some of these questions by reviewing the various mechanisms involved in the transport of nutrients from the gastrointestinal tract into the blood stream and by discussing the effects of ethanol on these processes, highlighting common features, and illustrating general principles which may be applied to the effects of ethanol on absorption. Finally, the highly important evolutionary relationship between the interplay of ethanol and malnutrition will be discussed with reference to malabsorption in the gastrointestinal tract.

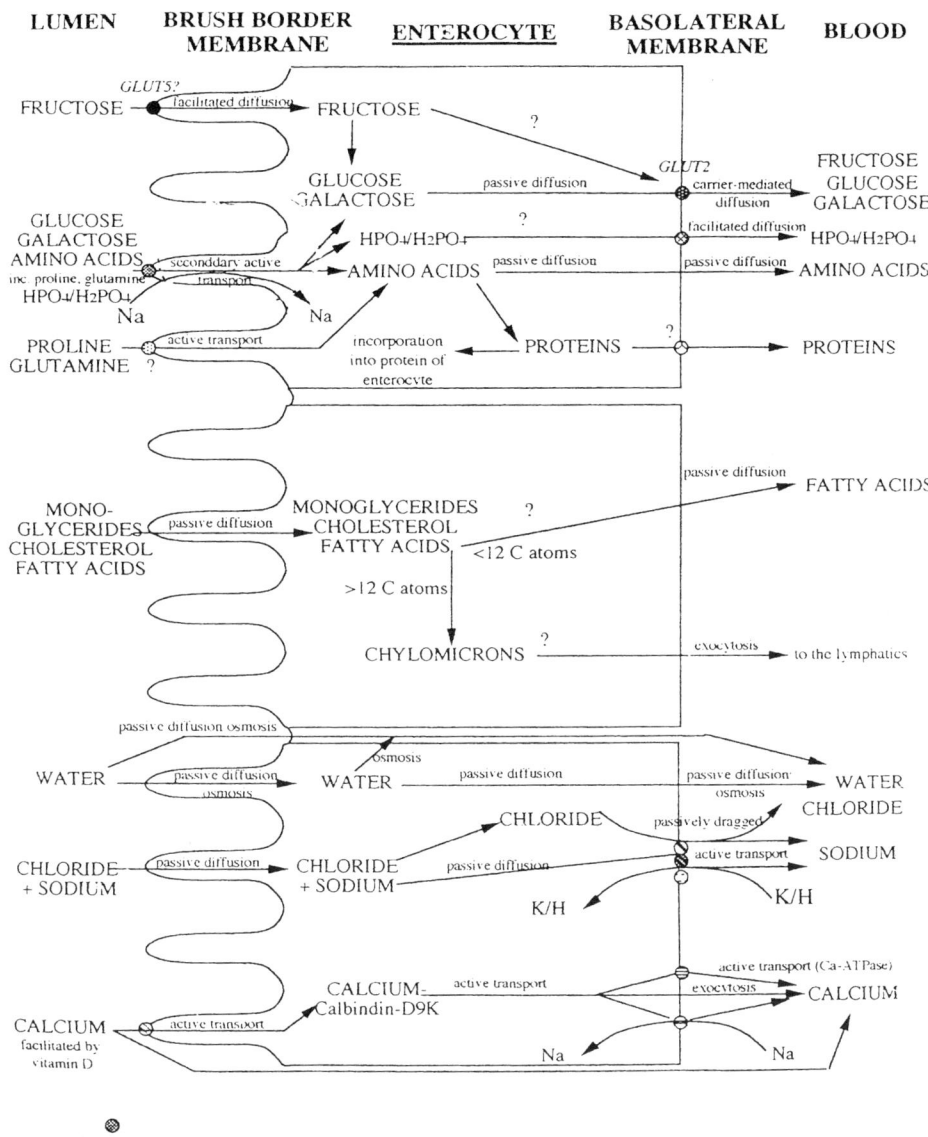

**FIGURE 11.1** Mechanism of nutrient transport across the gastrointestinal tract.

## 11.2   NUTRIENT ABSORPTION ACROSS THE ENTEROCYTE

There are three principal processes involved in the transfer of nutrients from the gastrointestinal tract to the bloodstream: (1) transport across the brush-border membrane, (2) its passage across the enterocyte, and (3) transport out of the enterocyte across the basolateral membrane. The precise mechanisms involved at each of these stages differs according to the particular nutrient, although general principles may be applied for several of the nutrients (Figure 11.1) and will subsequently be discussed together with some of the anomalies.

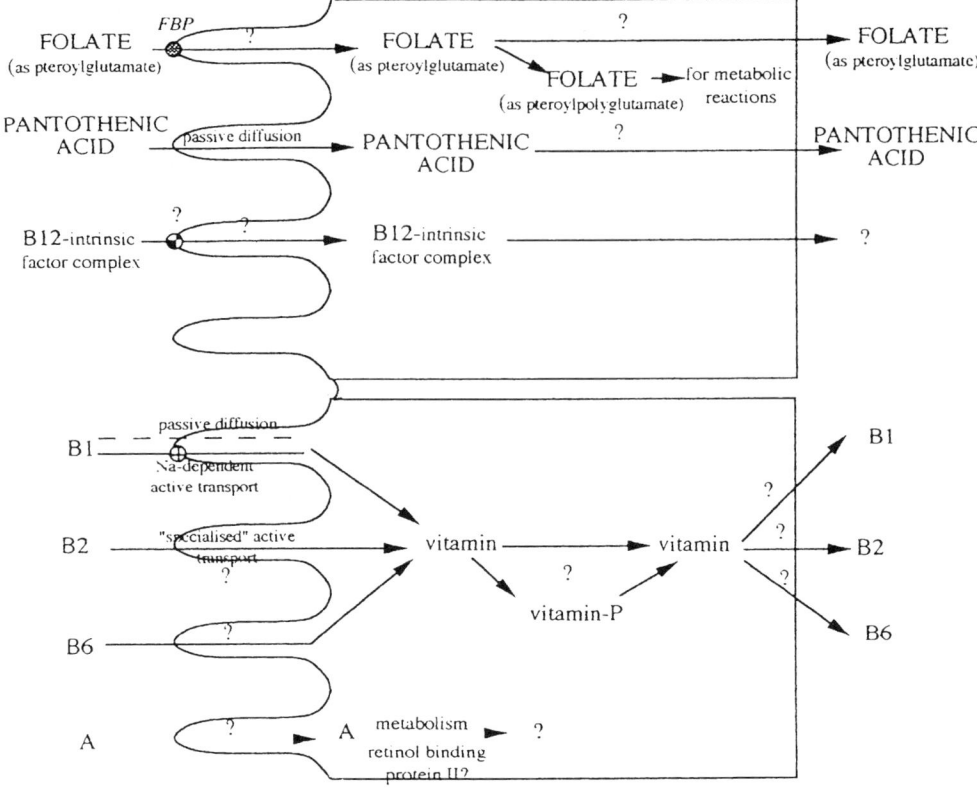

**FIGURE 11.1** *Continued.*

### 11.2.1   Interactions and Reactions Within the Lumen

The majority of nutrients are absorbed in the upper small intestine when they are first exposed to the absorbing surface. Prior to absorption, carbohydrates, fats, and proteins are generally digested to their primary constituents: monosaccharides, monoglycerides, cholesterol, fatty acids, and amino acids, respectively, by enzymes located either within the lumen or attached to the brush-border membrane. Specific sites for absorption of vitamin $B_{12}$ and bile salts are present in the distal ileum.

Many nutrients are dependent on the presence of various secretions, inorganic elements, or other factors for their adequate absorption. Interference with such parameters will have adverse effects on the absorption of the nutrient. The absorption of proteins, fats, and fat soluble vitamins (A, D, E, and K) is particularly dependent on adequate flow of bile and pancreatic secretions into the lumen.[5] High levels of sodium in the lumen are important for absorption of glucose and amino acids; conversely, glucose in the lumen facilitates reabsorption of sodium. Low dietary taurine intake appears to compromise vitamin D absorption, while the uptake of calcium is stimulated by vitamin D. Calcium absorption is also facilitated by the presence of lactose and protein in the lumen, while it is inhibited by phosphates and oxalates due to the formation of insoluble calcium salts. Such complex interactions highlight the possible effects which ethanol may have on the absorption of some nutrients by affecting the absorption of others.

The rate of absorption of some nutrients may be regulated by their level in the lumen. For example, in response to changes in carbohydrate content of the diet there is an increase in glucose transport across the enterocyte. Such a feedback mechanism is thought not to exist for proteins.

## 11.2.2    Transport Across the Brush-Border Membrane

Nutrient transport across the brush-border membrane may proceed by two principal mechanisms: diffusion or active transport. The brush border increases the surface of the epithelial cell by approximately 40 times, thus increasing the potential surface area over which both processes may occur.

### 11.2.2.1    Diffusion

Some nutrients diffuse across the brush-border membrane either (a) by passive diffusion, e.g., water (in response to osmotic gradients), sodium (and chloride which is passively "dragged" with sodium), D-amino acids, monoglycerides, cholesterol, and fatty acids or (b) by facilitated diffusion, e.g., fructose which binds to a carrier (possibly GLUT5) located on the brush-border membrane. These substances, with the exception of water, enter the enterocyte by diffusion, as there is a concentration gradient established across this membrane by the subsequent active transport of these substances across the basolateral membrane and out of the cell.

### 11.2.2.2    Active Transport

Some nutrients enter and traverse the brush-border membrane by active transport processes. Glucose, galactose, L-amino acids, phosphate, calcium, and the B vitamins thiamine and riboflavin enter the enterocyte by energy-dependent, active transport mechanisms after binding to highly specific protein "carriers" located on the brush-border membrane. Glucose and galactose bind to a protein known as SGLT1, while there are four separate carriers for the amino acids which are specific for basic, acidic, neutral amino acids and one that is specific for proline and hydroxyproline.

The transport of all these nutrients, with the exception of thiamine and calcium then proceeds by a "secondary active transport" mechanism. Such a process requires the cotransport of sodium which also binds to the relevant transporter protein, and the nutrients are then transported via the transmembrane electrochemical sodium gradient generated by the active transport of sodium out of the enterocyte at the basolateral membrane. In addition to this mechanism, proline may also be transported into the cell by a hydrogen-coupled, sodium-independent, active transport mechanism, while such a sodium-independent mechanism has also been proposed for glutamine. In contrast, calcium absorption may occur either by an active transport (ATP-dependent) pump or by sodium/calcium exchange.

The mechanism of absorption of some of the vitamins is unique. The absorption of thiamine occurs at low physiological concentrations (up to 2 m$M$) by a carrier-mediated, sodium-dependent, active transport mechanism. Riboflavin absorption occurs by a dual, sodium-independent mechanism, with a saturable component prevailing at low concentrations (< 2 $\mu M$) and a nonsaturable component prevailing at higher concentrations.[2] Vitamin $B_{12}$ binds to intrinsic factor, a protein secreted by the stomach and the complex is absorbed across the brush-border membrane. The mechanism of folic acid absorption is also unique to this vitamin. During intestinal absorption, dietary pteroylpolyglutamates (PteGlun) (a form in which dietary folates occur) are hydrolyzed to pteroylglutamate (PteGlu) by brush-border folate hydrolase and a zinc-dependent exopeptidase on the jejunal mucosal surface, followed by binding to folate-binding protein and transport into the enterocyte.

## 11.2.3    Intracellular Transport

Once inside the enterocyte, each nutrient must cross to the basolateral membrane prior to its transport into the bloodstream. Many nutrients traverse the enterocyte by diffusion down the concentration gradient, for example, glucose, galactose, sodium, chloride, fructose (although some fructose may be converted to glucose within the enterocyte), and amino acids, with some being incorporated into proteins within the enterocyte either for use within this cell or for their subsequent transport across the basolateral membrane.

Other nutrients undergo reactions/transformations within the enterocyte for utilization within the cell or prior to their exit. Some reactions may represent terminal stages of digestion, others are related to energy-yielding metabolism which provides power for pumping and synthetic reactions. For example, although fatty acids with less than 12 carbon atoms traverse the enterocyte to the basolateral membrane by diffusion, fatty acids with more than 12 carbon atoms and cholesterol are both reesterified to triglycerides in the cell. The triglyceride and cholesterol esters are then coated with a layer of lipoprotein, cholesterol, and phospholipid to form chylomicrons, which then cross the enterocyte by passive diffusion. Calcium is another such example because it binds to a specific protein within the enterocyte, Calbindin-D9K, and is then actively transported across the enterocyte. This process is rate limiting and is stimulated by vitamin D. Some B vitamins, such as $B_1$, $B_2$, and $B_6$, are phosphorylated within the enterocyte, only to be dephosphorylated again prior to their removal from the cell. The purpose of this process is not known.

Relatively little is known quantitatively of the efficiency of intestinal absorption of provitamin A carotenoids such as $\alpha$-, $\beta$- and $\gamma$-carotene and cryptoxanthin. Carotenoid absorption is by passive diffusion (in humans between 5 and 50% is absorbed); the absorption efficiency appears to depend on adequate amounts of dietary fat. The enzymatic mechanisms responsible for intestinal conversion of $\beta$-carotene to retinol are controversial. Recent work suggests that retinol binds to the intestinal cellular retinol-binding protein type II [cRBP(II)] and may be reduced by a membrane-bound microsomal enzyme.

Retinyl esters are hydrolyzed within the intestinal lumen. Several enzymes including pancreatic lipases, and one or more retinyl ester hydrolases are associated with BBM, and have been implicated in this hydrolysis. Retinol in physiological concentrations is absorbed by facilitated diffusion while at pharmacological levels it is by passive diffusion. Within the enterocytes, retinol is esterified to fatty acids before incorporation into chylomicrons. It is important that specific binding proteins carry retinol through the aqueous intracellular environment and deliver retinol to enzymes for esterification, thus limiting levels of the retinol in membranes. If free retinol is present it can disrupt normal membrane structure and function.

### 11.2.4   Transport Across the Basolateral Membrane

As with transport across the brush-border membrane, the mechanism differs with respect to individual nutrients in their ability to cross the basolateral membrane. Generally, substances may be actively transported into the enterocyte by a pump on the brush-border membrane and passively diffuse out (e.g., sugars or amino acids), or they may move passively into the cell and then be actively pumped out by a pump located on the basolateral membrane (e.g., salt transport). Examples of nutrients which utilize each method are discussed below.

Monosaccharides, amino acids, and phosphate (which enter the cell by active transport) traverse the basolateral membrane by diffusion, which may be passive (e.g., amino acids) or facilitated (e.g., monosaccharides). Such a facilitated process requires binding of the nutrient to a specific protein located on the membrane, as is the case for fructose, glucose, and galactose. The carrier is GLUT2, and this process is the rate-limiting step in glucose absorption.

In contrast, sodium (which enters the cell by passive diffusion) is transported out of the enterocyte by active transport processes, either with chloride, which is passively dragged with the sodium, or in exchange for potassium or hydrogen via specific membrane bound proteins. Similarly, the mechanism for calcium transport out of the enterocyte involves two active transport mechanisms, one which utilizes a Ca-ATPase (which is stimulated by 1,25-dihydroxycholecalciferol, the metabolite of vitamin D) and another which involves sodium exchange. In addition, calcium may also leave the cell by exocytosis, a mechanism also utilized by chylomicrons — the end products of fat absorption.

This principle is not maintained by thiamine which, in addition to entering the enterocyte by sodium-dependent active transport, also leaves the cell by a similar mechanism.

## 11.3 EFFECTS OF ETHANOL ON NUTRIENT ABSORPTION ACROSS THE GASTROINTESTINAL TRACT

Ethanol may potentially alter the net absorption of nutrients by affecting any one of the four processes discussed above. Few studies have precisely investigated which of the four processes are affected by ethanol; many studies merely report on the overall consequence of ethanol on the whole absorptive process. The following discussion will consider where ethanol may exert its deleterious effects on nutrient absorption with respect to each of the four processes and will attempt to highlight possible reasons why the absorption of some nutrients is adversely affected by ethanol while that of others remains unaltered.

### 11.3.1 Effects of Ethanol on Nutrient Absorption

#### 11.3.1.1 Passage of Ethanol Into and Across the Enterocytes Within the Jejunum

Most of ethanol (approximately 70%) will be absorbed directly from the stomach, passing via the portal vein to the liver (first-pass metabolism); the rate of absorption depending to a large extent on whether the ethanol is consumed with or without food. Although various isoenzymes of gastric alcohol dehydrogenase exist within the stomach it is unlikely that they play an important role in ethanol metabolism; perhaps 1%[7] such that acetaldehyde will not be formed to any large degree. The remainder of the ethanol (25%) passes into the duodenum and proximal jejunum, approximately 45 min after ethanol ingestion.[8] The concentration of ethanol within the jejunum lumen of humans during moderate drinking is thought to range from 200 to 2000 mmol/l (1 to 9% w/v).[9] Ethanol is transferred across the jejunum by simple diffusion, at least when its concentration is greater than 200 mmol/l and averages 65% irrespective of the intraluminal ethanol concentration in both humans[10] and rats.[11]

The possibility that the enterocytes will be able to metabolize ethanol by the presence of the microsomal P-450 enzymes has been investigated in two studies but with conflicting results. In one study, microsomes isolated from the small intestine of chronically alcohol treated rats showed enhanced ethanol metabolism;[12] in another study, a reduction in the isoenzymes of P-450 system, CYP1A and CYPSA was detected immunologically[13] in rats administered alcohol intragastrically. It therefore remains questionable as to whether acetaldehyde may be produced in the enterocytes by the oxidation of ethanol, either by cytosolic alcohol dehydrogenase, ADH, or by the microsomal P-450 system.

## 11.4 EFFECTS OF ETHANOL IN THE LUMEN

### 11.4.1 Luminal Contents

The presence of certain nutrients within the lumen may affect the absorption of other nutrients such that ethanol may affect the absorption of one nutrient indirectly by its effect on another. For example, feeding rats a diet enriched with saturated fatty acids prevents the inhibitory effects of chronic ethanol on the *in vitro* uptake of hexoses and lipids.[3] The intrinsic factor necessary for $B_{12}$ absorption is located within the gastric mucosa and may be reduced following chronic ethanol administration to rats,[21] although this could not be corrected by coadministration of intrinsic factor. However, impaired binding of the intrinsic factor-$B_{12}$ complex by intestinal homogenates was demonstrated. Similar findings were obtained in normal human volunteers chronically fed alcohol.[4] The most significant factor relating to luminal content that would affect nutrient absorption is the level of the nutrient itself.

### 11.4.2   Changes in Gut Motility

The synthesis rates of intestinal contractile proteins are reduced by acute ethanol dosage which may be responsible for, or reflect, alcohol-induced defects in intestinal motility. Oral or intravenous alcohol decreases Type I (impeding) wave motility in the jejunum, but has no effect on Type III (propulsive) wave motility, in either chronic alcoholics or in healthy volunteers.[14] The suppression of impeding waves in the jejunum and the stimulation of propulsive waves in the ileum may contribute to the increased sensitivity to osmotic loads, shortened transit time, and tendency to diarrhea frequently observed in alcoholics[15] which contributes to the nutrient malabsorption.

## 11.5   TRANSPORT OF NUTRIENTS ACROSS ENTEROCYTE AFTER ETHANOL EXPOSURE

### 11.5.1   Across the Brush-Border and Basolateral Membranes

Enterocytes are renewed approximately every 12 h. Therefore, the effects of ethanol on the structure/functioning of these cells is complex and depends on interactions with other factors, such as nutritional status. If the alcohol misuser is malnourished at the time of drinking, damaged enterocytes could potentially be replaced by "malfunctioning" enterocytes either due to the continued presence of ethanol in the intestinal lumen and/or as a result of inadequate nutritional status. For example, deficiency of folate (essential for DNA synthesis), which is frequently encountered in the alcohol misuser, results in enlarged, dysfunctional enterocytes and shortened villi in the jejunal mucosa.

### 11.5.2   Changes to Absorption Surface Area

The absorption of many nutrients depends on their initial diffusion across the brush-border membrane into the enterocyte. Therefore, the extensive morphological changes induced by ethanol in all areas of the gastrointestinal tract will have a devastating effect on their absorption; the enterocytes within the jejunum appear to be extremely sensitive to ethanol. The optimal rate of absorption may be decreased by a reduction in the absorbing surface area. Acute ethanol produces hemorrhagic erosions of the tips of jejunal villi of rats in a dose-dependent fashion,[16,17] in control humans[18] and in chronic alcoholics,[19] and will cause contraction of the villus core, accumulation of subepithelial fluid at the villus tip with the formation of blebs, and subepithelial blebs ultimately causing rupture of the epithelium.[20] Further changes in the structure of the brush-border membrane will then depend on the nutritional status of the ingested diet. Indeed, chronic administration of ethanol with an adequate diet to rats and humans does not necessarily produce the florid hemorrhagic changes seen with acute ingestion. It is suggested that the reduction in height of jejunal villi of chronic alcoholics is caused by an associated folate deficiency rather than by ethanol itself,[21,22] since severe folate deficiency is known to produce villus shortening, decreased mitosis in the crypts, and enlargement of epithelial cell nuclei.[23] In addition, a slight reduction in villus height in relation to crypt depth has been reported in alcoholics admitted for detoxification. On abstinence from ethanol ingestion the villi return to normal. There is evidence of small intestinal bacterial overgrowth in some patients with alcoholic liver disease which could contribute to the functional and/or morphological abnormalities of the small intestine commonly found in such patients. (For review see Reference 24.)

The jejunum will adapt to chronic ethanol ingestion by reducing the enterocyte turnover rate with the net result of enterocytes residing longer on the villus surface. This will produce an epithelium containing a greater proportion of mature cells.[25] Indeed, prolonged ethanol feeding has reportedly not caused a change in enterocyte number[25]; however, the efficiency of such enterocytes is unknown.

### 11.5.3    Changes in Intestinal Permeability and Fluidity

Chronic ethanol increases intestinal permeability to a number of substances, such as polyethyleneglycol (PEG) both in rats[26] and either chronic alcoholics or normal subjects following an acute oral administration of alcohol. Once ethanol was eliminated from the blood the intestinal permeability returned to normal in both groups.[27] Increased intestinal permeability may have serious implications because increased losses of nonprotein-bound substances from the blood to the gut lumen may occur. In the isolated rabbit mucosa, following ethanol (3 g/dl) administration, net transport of sodium, chloride, 3-*o*-methly-*D*-glucose, and L-alanine was inhibited mainly as a result of a back flux of these substances from the serosa to the mucosa.[28]

In addition to effects of ethanol on membrane permeability, the fluidity of the membrane may also be increased, resulting in changes in nutrient absorption. Maximal transport rates for proline by either the neutral brush-border membrane carriers or amino acid transport systems are reduced by ten times when the surrounding membrane environment is made of more fluid.[29] Biophysical studies have shown that ethanol, *in vitro*, dissociates the membrane and perturbs the fine structural arrangement of membrane lipids. In the chronic state, these membranes develop resistance to the disordering effects. However, measurement of membrane lipids, such as cholesterol content or fatty acid unsaturated phospholipid distribution, have not produced conclusive evidence that any of these parameters are directly involved in the action of ethanol It may be that small metabolically active pools located in certain subcellular fractions are more susceptible, e.g., $Na^+,K^+$ ATPase, lipid pool involved in the deacylation-reacylation mechanism. An increase in metabolic turnover of these phospholipid pools may have important implications for the membrane functional changes.

### 11.5.4    Indirect Damage

Chemical mediators of inflammation including free radicals,[30] histamine both *in vivo* and *in vitro*,[31,32] and leukotrienes[20] are released as a result of the enterocytes exposure to ethanol. The release of $PGE_2$ which occurs after these mediators of inflammation may play a protective role by limiting ethanol-induced effects on mucosal/microvascular permeability.[31,33] Nitric oxide production is known to be increased as a result of inflammation. However, there is no evidence, as yet, that nitric oxide is generated within the epithelial cell after acute or chronic ethanol ingestion. If an inhibitor of nitric oxide synthetase was administered, this could potentiate the adverse effects of ethanol by reducing the vascular tone of the gut thus allowing ethanol to accumulate in the gut rather than be washed away.

There does appear, however, to be a difference in the response of the enterocyte membrane to acute or chronic administration of ethanol. In one study where a defined jejunum segment was challenged with an acute dose of ethanol, (900 mmol/l) a tenfold increase in albumin and twofold increase in glycosaminoglycan hyaluronic acid were assayed in the perfusion fluid.[30] When a similar dose was administered over a longer period of time there was not such a dramatic effect on the enterocyte. Beck et al.[34] have suggested that ethanol increases microvascular permeability by causing the opening of the interendothelial junctions. Studying the intestine of dogs during perfusion with ethanol, Kvietys et al.[35] showed that ethanol decreased precapillary resistance, increased capillary pressure and capillary filtration coefficient, and increased intraluminal clearance of labeled albumin.

## 11.6    EFFECT OF ETHANOL ON NUTRIENT TRANSPORT

### 11.6.1    Changes to Active Transport Processes

The various discrepancies which are apparent between the different published studies for nutrient uptake and absorption are likely to be caused by such variables as the time scale of the ethanol ingestion and the alcohol and carbohydrate composition of the control and ethanol diets. A crucial factor of the dietary regime adopted is that the control diet should use fat as the calorie substitute for ethanol. Carbohydrate substitution should be avoided as variations in the dietary level of this nutrient have been shown to influence sugar uptake.[36] In addition rats should not be subjected to overnight starvation before experimentation as this procedure will cause profound changes in sugar absorption as well as changes in mucosal enzyme activity[37] and the electrophysiology of the brush-border membrane.[38] In addition, the maturity of the enterocytes present will also influence sugar transport.[39]

The transport rate will be affected by the composition of the diet, for example, diets with a high saturated fat content are associated with higher maximal transport rates. Low concentrations of ethanol ($< 200$ m$M$) do not significantly affect sodium coupled nutrient uptake,[40] while higher concentrations significantly inhibit such transport. The situation may be more complex, however. Although the mechanisms by which ethanol reduces intestinal glucose transport are not fully understood, it has been assumed to interfere with active transport across the brush-border membrane. Recently, studies have suggested that the inhibition of glucose transport is due to an effect of ethanol on passive diffusion, which results in a more prompt equilibration of the sodium gradient and a consequent reduction in the uptake velocities of sodium-dependent transport systems.[40]

Acute exposure of the intestinal mucosa to ethanol will adversely affect the nutrients which utilize the sodium-dependent gradient for their transport across the BBM, e.g., L-amino acids,[41] glucose,[42,43] and galactose.[44] On the other hand, acute/chronic ethanol has been shown to increase the polarization of the membrane thereby creating a higher electrical driving force for Na$^+$-coupled movement across the BBM.[45]

## 11.6.1.1 Sugars

Acute doses of ethanol will inhibit the sodium-dependent transport of galactose, glucose, and other hexoses across the jejunum both *in vivo* and *in vitro*.[46,47] Acute studies of gut sections from rats who had been administered chronic ethanol followed by a diet enriched with polyunsaturated fats were found to have significant reduced glucose uptake.[1] Another study in which no change in the active absorption of glucose was discernible might reflect the ability of the enterocyte to metabolize glucose.[48] Such inhibitory effects by acute ethanol doses on BBM sugar transport are not fully understood but could relate to a variety of factors including direct conformational effects on the hexose transporter, the increased fluidity of the BBM, or perhaps that there are different carriers for sugars. In one study where the *in vitro* effect of ethanol on D-glucose uptake was studied in isolated rabbit mucosa, it was the back flux from serosa to mucosa which particularly inhibited net transport.[26]

Chronic ethanol administration shows enhanced absorption of these nutrients which is likely to be caused by the increase in membrane permeability as a result of the increased presence of mature enterocytes,[49] a higher passive permeability to glucose, or to the presence of an increased maturity of the enterocyte population on the villus surface.[51] Galactose uptake is enhanced which is possibly due to the enhanced potential difference across the isolated BBM,[46] but not in another.[50] However, the composition of diet again may play a vital role in saccharide absorption, the jejunal uptake of glucose, and galactose being increased in ethanol fed rats who were given a diet supplemented with saturated fats.

## 11.6.1.2 Lipids

There is little evidence to indicate that acute ethanol inhibits the transport of lipids across the intestinal mucosa although changing the composition of the diet with regard to its polyunsaturated and saturated fat content may alter their transport especially in the case of rats fed ethanol supplemented with linoleic acid.[51]

There are conflicting reports regarding the transport of lipids after chronic ethanol ingestion, although most animal experiments indicate that, provided a nutritious diet particularly rich in protein is administered, no malabsorption of lipids occurs. Ethanol does alter lipid metabolism within the enterocyte, increasing the triglyceride content in the mucosa. Alterations in the uptake of most medium and long chain fatty acids and cholesterol could be detected when chronic ethanol feeding was combined with feeding a diet rich in polyunsaturated fat.

## 11.6.1.3   Amino Acids

It is important that the experimental conditions used in any of the studies of amino acids uptake and transfer by the gut reflect the true nutritional state often observed in chronic alcohol misusers, i.e., reduction in body wieght and a high calorific intake. In addition, ethanol ingestion enhances nitrogen loss in the urine of both rats[52] and humans[53] thereby increasing the protein requirement. It is also important that the morphological changes in the jejunum, described above, are present. If a good nutritional state exists, any inhibition of the active transport caused by ethanol will be compensated by the enhanced diffusion of amino acids across the intestine.

Acute ethanol administration either *in vivo* or *in vitro*, reversibly inhibits the active transport of amino acids in animals.[46,54,55] *In vivo* intestinal perfusion experiments in rats showed no inhibition of net amino acid transport unless alcohol was perfused at concentrations greater than 9.2 g/dl.[56] Efflux of a large number of amino acids was measured by adding ethanol at concentrations of 5 g/dl to the intestinal perfusate[57] which supported the *in vitro* finding that ethanol increased the serosal to mucosal back flux of L-alanine, which was responsible for the abolition of net transport of this amino acid by isolated rabbit mucosa preparations.[26]

Even though there are gross changes in the morphology of the jejunum after chronic ethanol consumption, the absorptive capacity of the membrane for amino acids appears to be maintained.[58] Chronic ethanol ingestion by rats caused a slight but not significant decrease in net leucine absorption at 5 m$M$ leucine concentrations. At higher concentrations (10 and 25 m$M$), minor increases were observed in the absorption values. Such results confirm that there is a diminution in the active mechanisms of leucine absorption but enhancement of diffusive processes. Since high alcohol concentrations increase membrane permeability, when luminal amino acid concentration is low, this will increase efflux of amino acids from the blood.[2]

## 11.6.1.4   Vitamins

### 11.6.1.4.1   Thiamine

The maximal rate of intestinal thiamine absorption is reduced in alcoholics and in healthy individuals following acute ethanol ingestion. In rats, using either intact intestinal loops or inverted jejunal segments, the active (low concentration) absorption of thiamine rather than passive (high concentration) absorption was susceptible to ethanol inhibition. Like the $Na^+, K^+$ ATPase inhibitor, ouabain blocked the exit of thiamine from the mucosal cell.[59] In agreement with this observation, the reduction of $Na^+, K^+$ ATPase activity at the basolateral enterocyte membrane produced by ethanol correlated with a reduction in serosal thiamine appearance.[60] It is suggested[61] that these animal experiments are not necessarily incompatible with clinical observations. However, since thiamine intake of alcoholics is extremely low, the critical process is the active absorption of the vitamin. This absorption process may be independently affected by ethanol and malnutrition in humans [62] and it has been suggested that the observed decrease in maximal thiamine absorption may be explained by damaged receptor sites by prolonged receipt of ethanol or nutritional deficiency, or by a combination of both factors.[63]

### 11.6.1.4.2   Riboflavin

Approximately 17% of chronic alcoholics may be riboflavin deficient. Neither animal nor clinical studies have indicated that the absorption of riboflavin is impaired after either acute or chronic administration of ethanol. Studies so far have indicated that a low dietary intake of the vitamin is the only mechanism suspected to cause deficiency.[64]

### 11.6.1.4.3   Pyridoxine

Chronic alcohol consumption has not been shown to influence the absorption of pyridoxine.

### 11.6.1.4.4   Biotin

Chronic ethanol feeding significantly decreases biotin transport in everted intestinal sac loops when given at physiological doses. There was little effect, however, on the absorption of biotin when given at pharmacological doses indicating selective inhibition of the carrier-mediated process for biotin by alcohol.[65]

### 11.6.1.4.5   Folate

Ethanol will inhibit the folate transport in proportion to the intestinal ethanol concentration.[66] Studies in humans have indicated that when the diet is adequate ethanol will not affect folate absorption. Intestinal perfusion through a triple-lumen tube has demonstrated a lower uptake of tritiated PteGlu into the enterocyte from the jejunum of malnourished or folate-deficient alcoholics by comparison to well-nourished alcoholics and controls.[67] Chronic ethanol studies using a minipig model, which were administered ethanol for 1 year, showed decreased hydrolysis of PteGlux but unchanged uptake of PteGlu.[68] *In vitro* isolated jejunum vesicles showed significantly lower activities of jejunum brush border folate hydrolase compared to controls but similar vesicle uptake of PteGlu.[69] By contrast, however, a decreased intestinal absorption of folate was identified in well-nourished monkeys after chronic ethanol feeding.[70]

### 11.6.1.4.6   Vitamin C

Absorption of ascorbic acid is reduced when ingested together with ethanol,[71] although inadequate intake is the more important cause. Since L-ascorbate is absorbed by the sodium gradient-dependent transport any change in its movement across the membrane will alter ascorbic acid status.

### 11.6.1.4.7   Fat-Soluble Vitamins

There is no evidence that alcohol consumption directly interferes with the absorption of fat soluble vitamins, which are generally absorbed by a saturable but not energy-dependent process. It is only when there is malabsorption of lipids secondary to chronic pancreatitis, cholestasis, cirrhosis, or bacterial overgrowth that malabsorption of these vitamins will occur.

### 11.6.1.5   Essential Elements

### 11.6.1.5.1   Calcium

Acute alcohol does not interfere with calcium transport[72,73] in nonalcoholic individuals and rats. Chronic alcohol ingestion inhibits duodenal absorption of calcium, independent of other factors.[74] Miller and Bronner[75] have described two types of calcium binding sites in rat duodenal BBMV when the uptake was prolonged until equilibrium. Acute doses of ethanol will adversely affect the carrier, inhibiting its transport at physiological concentration but having little effect at pharmacological concentrations. Exactly how this occurs is unknown but inhibition of energy metabolism and physiochemical alterations in enterocyte membrane has been implicated.

### 11.6.1.5.2   Magnesium

Absorption of magnesium has not been shown to be affected by alcohol ingestion.

### 11.6.1.5.3   Zinc

The intestinal absorption of zinc is a homeostatically regulated process located on the apical membrane of the enterocytes. Details of the membranous mechanisms involved in the transport of the metal from the intestinal lumen to the mucosal cell cytoplasm have not as yet been completely characterized. Zinc transport across the BBM is via a regulated saturable carrier-mediated process. A first step would involve nonspecific binding at the external surface of the membrane concomitant with the regulated and saturable passage of zinc across the BBM and a second step would consist of zinc binding to the internal surface and/or core components of the brush border leading to the formation of the intravesicular pools of zinc.[76] Although the importance of zinc has been recognized in chronic misusers of alcohol there are no published studies on the uptake and absorption of zinc by jejunum in the presence of ethanol.

### 11.6.1.5.4  Iron

Iron absorption can be divided into three distinct phases: luminal, mucosal, and systemic. The luminal stage concerns the delivery of iron to the BBM, and is determined by the type of food ingested and by its interaction with intestinal secretion. In chronic alcohol misusers there will be alterations in the acid content of the stomach as well as gastric juices, pancreatic, biliary, and other secretions which could influence the form of iron present as well as its uptake by the BBM. The mucosal phase involves the fate of iron that has been taken up by the mucosal epithelial cell, some of which will follow a direct pathway across the enterocyte to the BLM, some of which will be stored within the epithelial cell as ferritin and eventually be shed into the gastrointestinal tract at the end of the enterocyte's short lifespan. However, the mechanism of the uptake of iron across this mucosal membrane remains undefined. Clearly heme is able to rapidly traverse this membrane, while ferric iron will need to be reduced to ferrous, possibly by a ferri-reductase in the membrane and then transported across the membrane by a carrier-mediated and biologically regulated control mechansim. Exactly how ethanol influences this uptake and transfer of iron into the enterocyte is unclear. The effects of chronic alcohol consumption on iron absorption by the small intestine is, however, an unanswered question.

### 11.6.2  Summary

It is clear that both acute and chronic doses of ethanol will have an inhibitory effect on the uptake, transfer, and eventual utilization of many essential nutrients. The disadvantage of the numerous studies cited above will be that the majority have been undertaken in animals with adequate nutritional status where the morphological appearance of the gut will be essentially normal. It is an obvious prerequisite that the gut enterocytes, particularly the villi, should resemble that found in the chronic misuser of ethanol.

## 11.7  EVOLUTION OF ALCOHOL-INDUCED MALABSORPTION IN THE GASTROINTESTINAL TRACT

The effect of ethanol on gastrointestinal absorption may be considered as a progressive, evolutionary process. Beginning with a well-nourished individual who begins to drink heavily, the first disorder is likely to arise from the toxic effects of metabolizing large quantities of ethanol. It is likely that oxygen-derived cytotoxic free radicals will be generated, as a result of the inflammatory reponse by the enterocyte to ethanol, further damaging the capacity of the enterocyte to utilize nutrients within the intestinal mucosa and to transfer them across the cell to the basolateral membrane for absorption. In addition, ethanol-induced pancreatic malfunction will compromise digestion of fats and proteins while ethanol-induced liver damage will reduce storage of vitamins and other nutients. There will also be increased losses of nutients by renal excretion. Secondary nutritional losses will follow the development of gastritis causing vomiting or hematemesis. Similarly the development of diarrhea or steatorrhea will produce further depletion.

As the individual becomes more dependent on alcohol, malnutrition will increase, secondary to suppression of appetite and loss of social integration, and a preference to spend what little money is available on alcohol. The rate of evolution of this toxic alcohol malnutrition interaction will depend on a number of factors such as the individual susceptibility to damage to various organs. In addition, there will be a wide variation in alcohol intake, patterns of drinking, and the associated extent of poor nutrient intake in different patients. Some patients are thought to be particularly at risk of suffering brain damage due to thiamine deficiency and it is possible that extreme malabsorption in some drinking malnourished subjects may play a significant part in this deficiency. The consequence of such brain damage due to thiamine deficiency could be to interfere with further rehabilitation, to increase alcohol intake, and to cause the patient to deteriorate further. Reduced thiamine levels will increase alcohol intake directly and the development of folate deficiency will even more reduce the individual's ability to absorb thiamine.

The authors therefore see the evolution of the disease process where the interplay of ethanol toxicity will vary from time to time coupled with different degrees of nutrient depletion which, in turn, will impede enzyme function and retard reparative processes. Poor dietary intake in quantity and quality will potentiate the synergistic effects of alcohol and malnutrition. The onset of cirrhosis with portal hypertension or chronic brain damage such as Korsakoff psychosis with impaired memory will further compromise the patient.

Thus, the factors discussed in this chapter interact detrimentally to produce a progressively deteriorating condition unless alcohol intake can be kept below toxic levels and unless the patient is provided with the nutrients required in an environment where malabsorption can be reversed. The disease process usually occurs over many years with individual variations leading to diverse patterns of irreversible tissue and organ damage which are given a variety of diagnostic labels. Thus the primary disorder, excessive alcohol intake, evolves into a secondary stage of tissue damage (reversible in part) which interacts with chronic malnutrition to become episodically acute. From an early stage, varying degrees of damage to the gastrintestinal tract will be involved and in some patients the effects of malabsorption may ultimately become of decisive importance in limiting the ability of the patient to adapt because of the effects on the central nervous system.

## REFERENCES

1. **Thomson, A. B., Keelan, M., and Clandinin, M. T.,** Feeding rats a diet enriched with saturated fatty acids prevents the inhibitory effects of acute and chronic ethanol exposure on the *in vitro* uptake of hexoses and lipids, *Biochim. Biophys. Acta,* 1084, 122, 1991.
2. **World, M. J., Ryle, P. R., and Thomson, A. D.,** Alcoholic nutrition and the small intestine, *Alcohol Alcohol.,* 20, 89, 1985.
3. **Lindenbaum, J., Saha, J. R., Shea, N., and Lieber, C. S.,** Mechanism of alcohol induced malabsorption of vitamin $B_{12}$, *Gastroenterology,* 64, 762, 1973.
4. **Lindenbaum, J. and Lieber, C. S.,** Effects of chronic ethanol administration on intestinal absorption in man in the absence of nutritional deficiency, *Ann. N.Y. Acad. Sci.,* 252, 228, 1975.
5. **Watson, R. R. and Watzl, B., Eds.,** Interaction of nutrients and alcohol: absorption, transport, utilization and metabolism, in *Nutrition and Alcohol,* CRC Press, Boca Raton, FL, chap 18.
6. **Cheeseman, C. I.,** GLUT2 is the transporter for fructose across the rat intestinal basolateral membrane, *Gastroenterology,* 105, 1050, 1993.
7. **Seitz, H. K., Egerer, G., Simanowski, U. A., Waldherr, R., Eckey, R., Agarwal, D. P., Goedde, H. K., and von Wartburg, J.-P.,** Human gastric alcohol dehydrogenase activity: effect of age, sex and alcoholism, *Gut,* 34, 1433, 1993.
8. **Halsted, C. H., Robles, E. A., and Mezey, E.,** Distribution of ethanol in the human gastrointestinal tract, *Am. J. Clin. Nutr.,* 26, 831, 1973.
9. **Millan, M. S., Morris, G. P., Beck, I. P., and Henson, J. T.,** Villous damage induced by biopsy and by acute ethanol intake in normal human intestine, *Dig. Dis. Sci.,* 25, 513, 1980.
10. **Lavo, B., Colombel, J. F., Knutsson, L., and Hallgren, R.,** Acute exposure of small intestine to ethanol induces mucosal leakage and prostaglandin E2 synthesis, *Gastroenterology,* 102, 468, 1992.
11. **Leddin, D. J., Ray, M., Dinda, P.K., Prokopin, I., and Beck, I. T.,** Dimethyl prostaglandin E2 alleviates jejunal microvascular effects of ethanol but not the ethanol-induced inhibition of water sodium and glucose absorption, *Gastroenterology,* 94, 726, 1988.
12. **Seitz, H., Korsten, M., and Lieber, C.,** Ethanol oxidation by intestinal microsomes: increased activity after chronic ethanol administration, *Life Sci.,* 25, 1443, 1979.
13. **Hakkar, R., Ronis, M. J. J., and Badger, T. M.,** Effects of enteral nutrition and ethanol on cytochrome P450 distribution in small intestine, *Gastroenterology,* 104, 1611, 1993.

14. **Bode, J. C.,** Alcohol and the gastrointestinal tract, *Adv. Intern. Med. Pediatr.*, 45, 1, 1980.
15. **Keshavarzian, A., Iber, L., Dangleis, M. D., and Cornish, R.,** Intestinal transit and lactose intolerance in chronic alcoholics, *Am. J. Clin. Nutr.*, 44, 70, 1986.
16. **Baraona, E., Pirola, R. C., and Lieber, C. S.,** Small intestinal damage and changes in cell population produced by ethanol ingestion in the rat, *Gastroenterology*, 66, 226, 1974.
17. **Krawitt, E. L.,** Effect of acute ethanol administration on duodenal calcium transport, *Proc. Soc. Exp. Biol. Med.*, 146, 406, 1974.
18. **Millan, M. S., Morris, G. P., Beck, I. T., and Henson, J. T.,** Villous damage induced by suction biopsy and by acute ethanol intake in normal human small intestine, *Dig. Dis. Sci.*, 25, 513, 1980.
19. **Gottfried, E. B., Korsten, M. A., and Lieber, C. S.,** Gastrits and duodenitis induced by alcohol on endoscopic and histologic assessment, *Gastroenterology*, 70, 890, 1976.
20. **Ray, M., Dinda, P. K., and Beck, I. T.,** Mechanism of ethanol-induced jejunal microvascular and morphological changes in the dog, *Gastroenterology*, 96, 345, 1989.
21. **Langman, J. S. and Bell, G. D.,** Alcohol and the gastrointestinal tract, *Br. Med. Bull.*, 82, 71, 1982.
22. **Rubin, E., Rybak, B., Lindenbaum, J., Gezrson, C. D., Walker, G., and Lieber, C. S.,** Ultrastructural changes in the small intestine induced by ethanol, *Gastroenterology*, 63, 801, 1972.
23. **Hermos, J. A., Adams, W. H., et al.,** Mucosa of the small intestine in folate-deficient alcoholics, *Ann. Intern. Med.*, 76, 957, 1972.
24. **Persson, J.,** Alcohol and the small intestine, *Scand. J. Gastroenterol.*, 26, 3, 1991.
25. **Mazzanti, R. and Jenkins, W. J.,** Effect of chronic ethanol ingestion on enterocyte turnover in rat small intestine, *Gut*, 28, 52, 1987.
26. **Bode, C. H., Vollmer, E., Hug, J., and Bode, J. C.,** Increased permeability of the gut to polyethylene glycol and dextran in rats fed alcohol, *Ann. N.Y. Acad. Sci.*, 625, 837, 1991.
27. **Robison, G. M., Orrego, H., Israel, Y., Devenyi, P., and Kapur, B. M.,** Low molecular weight polyethylene glycol as a probe of gastrointestinal permeability after alcohol ingestion, *Dig. Dis. Sci.*, 26, 971, 1981.
28. **Kuo, Y. T. and Shanbour, L. L.,** Effect of ethanol on sodium, 3-O-methyl glucose and L-alanine transport in the jejunum, *Am. J. Dig. Dis.*, 23, 51, 1978.
29. **Thomson, A. D. and Majumdar, S. K.,** The influence of ethanol on intestinal absorption and utilization of nutrients, *Clin. Gastroenterol.*, 10, 263, 1981.
30. **Lavo, B., Colombel, J. F., Knutsson, L., and Hallgren, R.,** Acute exposure of small intestine to ethanol induces mucosal leakage and prostaglandin E2 synthesis, *Gastroenterology*, 102, 468, 1992.
31. **Beck, I. T., Leddin, D. J., and Beck, I. T.,** Histamine is involved in ethanol-induced jejunal microvascular injury in rabbits, *Gastroenterology*, 95, 1227, 1988.
32. **Beck, I. T., Dinda, P. K., Leddin, D. J., Ray, M., Prokopiw, I., and Boyd, A.,** Chemical mediators in the ethanol-induced increased jejunal microvascular permeability, in *Microcirculation in Circulatory Disorders*, Manabe, H., Zweifach, B. W., and Messmer, K., Eds., Springer-Verlag, Tokyo, 1988, 171.
33. **Beck, I. T., Boyd, A., and Dinda, P. K.,** Evidence for the involvement of 5-lipoxygenase products in the ethanol-induced intestinal plasma protein loss, *Am. J. Physiol.*, 254, G483, 1988.
34. **Beck, I. T., Morris, G. P., and Buell, M. G.,** Ethanol induced vascular permeability in the jejunal mucosa of the dog, *Gastroenterology*, 90, 1137, 1986.
35. **Kvietys, P. R., Patterson, W. G., Russell, J. M., Barrowwma, J. A., and Granger, D. N.,** Role of the microcirculation in ethanol induced mucosal injury in the dog, *Gastroenterology*, 87, 562, 1984.
36. **Diamond, J. M. and Karasov, W. H.,** Effect of dietary carbohydrate on monosaccharide uptake in mouse small intestine *in vitro*, *J. Physiol.*, 349, 419, 1984.
37. **Murrary, D. and Wild, G. E.,** Effect of fasting on Na-K-ATPase activity in rat small intestinal mucosa, *Can. J. Physiol. Pharmacol.*, 58, 643, 1980.
38. **Debham, E. S. and Thompson, C. S.,** Effect of fasting on the potential difference across the brush border membrane of enterocytes in rat small intestine, *J. Physiol.*, 355, 449, 1984.
39. **Mazzanti, R., Debham, E. S., and Jenkin, W. J.,** Effect of chronic ethanol intake on lactase activity and active galactose absorption in rat small intestine, *Gut*, 28, 56, 1987.
40. **O'Neill, B., Weber, F., Hornig, D., and Semenza, G.,** Ethanol selectively affects Na systems, $Na^+$-gradient dependent intestinal transport systems, *FEBS Lett.*, 194, 183, 1986.
41. **Beesley, R. C.,** Ethanol inhibits Na-gradient dependent uptake of L-amino acids into intestinal brush border membrane vesicles, *Dig. Dis. Sci.*, 31, 987, 1986.
42. **Tillotson, L. G., Carter, E. A., Inue, K.-I., and Isselbacher, K. J.,** Inhibition of Na-stimulated glucose transport function and perturbation of intestinal microvillous membrane vesicles by ethanol and acetaldehyde, *Arch. Biochem. Biophys.*, 207, 360, 1981.
43. **Chang, T., Lewis, J., and Glazko, A. J.,** Effect of ethanol and other alcohols on the transport of amino acids and glucose by everted sacs of rat small intestine, *Biochim. Biophys. Acta*, 135, 1000, 1967.
44. **Thomson, A. B. R.,** Acute exposure of rabbit jejunum to ethanol. *In vitro* uptake of hexoses, *Dig. Dis. Sci.*, 29, 267, 1984.

45. **Al-Balooi, F., Debham, E. S., and Mazzanti, R.,** Acute and chronic exposure to ethanol and the electrophysiology of the brush border membarne of rat small intestine, *Gut,* 30, 1698, 1989.

46. **Bode, J. C.,** Alcohol and the gastrointestinal tract, *Adv. Intern. Med. Pediatr.,* 45, 1, 1980.

47. **Lieber, C. S.,** Medical disorders of alcoholism: pathogenesis and treatment, in *Major Problems in Internal Medicine,* Vol. 22, Smith, L. D., Ed., W. B. Saunders, Philadelphia, 1982, 363.

48. **Debham, E. S.,** Effect of sodium concentration and plasma sugar concentration on hexose absorption by the rat jejunum *in vivo, Pflügers Arch.,* 393, 104, 1982.

49. **Mazzanti, R. and Jenkins, W. J.,** Effect of ethanol ingestion on enterocyte turnover in rar small intestine, *Gut,* 28, 52, 1984.

50. **Mazzanti, R., Debham, E. S., and Jenkins, W. J.,** Effect of ethanol intake on lactase activity and active galactose absorption in rat small intestine, *Gut,* 28, 52, 1987.

51. **Thomson, A. B. R., Keelan, M., and Clandinin, M. T.,** Feeding rats a diet enriched with saturated fatty acids prevents the inhibitory effects of acute and chronic ethanol exposure on the *in vitro* uptake of hexoses and lipids, *Biochim. Biophys. Acta,* 1084, 122, 1991.

52. **Rodrigo, C., Antezana, C., and Baraona, E.,** Fat and nitrogen balances in rats with alcohol-induced fatty liver, *J. Nutr.,* 101, 1307, 1971.

53. **McDonald, J. T. and Margen, S.,** Wine versus ethanol in human nutrition. I. Nitrogen and caloric balance, *Am. J. Clin. Nutr.,* 29, 1093, 1976.

54. **Bode, J. C.,** Alcohol and the gastrointestinal tract, in *Ergebnisse der Inneren Medizin und Klinderheilkunde,* Frick, P., von Harnack, G.-A., Martini, G. A., and Prader, B. A., Eds., Springer-Verlag, Berlin, 1980, 1.

55. **Israel, Y., Valenzuela, J. E., Salazar, J., and Ugarte, G.,** Alcohol and amino acid transport in the human intestine, *J. Nutr.,* 98, 222, 1969.

56. **Green, R. S., MacDermid, R. G., Scherg, R. L., and Hajjar, J. J.,** Effect of ethanol on amino acid transport across *in vivo* rat intestine, *Am. J. Physiol.,* 241, 9176, 1981.

57. **Jacobs, F. A., Crandall, J. C., and Fabel, C. B.,** An effect of ethanol on the bidirectional intestinal flux of amino acids, *Nutr. Reports Intern.,* 21, 398, 1980.

58. **Hajjar, J. J., Tomicic, T., and Scheig, R. L.,** Effect of chronic ethanol consumption on leucine absorption in rat small intestine, *Digestion,* 22, 170, 1981.

59. **Hoyumpa, A. M., Breen, K. J., and Schenker, S.,** Transport across the rat intestine; the effect of ethanol, *J. Lab. Clin. Med.,* 86, 803, 1975.

60. **Hoy, A. M., Nichols, S., Wilson, F. A., and Scherker, S.,** Effect of ethanol on intestinal (Na-K)-ATPase, *J. Lab. Clin. Med.,* 90, 1086, 1977.

61. **Thomson, A. D. and Pratt, O.,** Interaction of nutrients and alcohol: absorption, transport, utilization and metabolism, in *Nutrition and Alcohol,* Watson R. R. and Watzl, B., Eds., CRC Press, Boca Raton, FL, 1992, 75.

62. **Thomson, A. D.,** Vitamin deficiency and its role in alcoholic tissue damage, *J. Gastroenterol. Haematol.,* 2, 411 1990.

63. **Thomson, A. D. and Leevy, C. M.,** Observations on the mechanism of thiamine hydrochloride absorption in humans, *Clin. Sci.,* 43, 153, 1972.

64. **Bonjour, J. P.,** Vitamins and alcoholism: V. Riboflavin; VI. Niacin; VII. Pantothenic acid; VIII. Biotin, *Intern. J. Vit. Nutr. Res.,* 50, 425, 1980.

65. **Said, H. M., Shariform, A., Bagherzadeh, A., and Mock, D.,** Chronic ethanol feeding and acute ethanol exposure *in vitro*: effect on intestinal transport of biotin, *Am. J. Clin. Nutr.,* 52, 1083, 1990.

66. **Said, H. M. and Strum, W. B.,** Effect of ethanol and other aliphatic alcohols on the intestinal transport of folates, *Digestion,* 35, 129, 1986.

67. **Halsted, C. H., Robles, E. A., and Mezey, E.,** Decreased jejunal uptake of labelled folic acid ($^3$H-PGA) in alcoholic patients: roles of alcohol and malnutrition, *N. Engl. J. Med.,* 285, 701, 1971.

68. **Reisenauer, A. M., Buffington, C. A. T., Villanueva, J. A., and Halsted, C. H.,** Folate absorption in alcoholic pigs; *in vivo* intestinal perfusion studies, *Am. J. Clin. Nutr.,* 50, 1429, 1989.

69. **Naughton, C. A., Chandler, C. J., Duplantier, R. B., and Halsted, C. H.,** Folate absorption in alcoholic pigs: *in vitro* hydrolysis and transport at the brush border membrane, *Am. J. Clin. Nutr.,* 50, 1436, 1989.

70. **Halsted, C. H., Romero, J. J., Tamura,T., Ruebner, B., and French, S.,** Folate metabolism in the alcoholic monkey, *Gastroenterology,* 76, 1149, 1979.

71. **Lieber, C. S.,** The influence of alcohol on nutritional status, *Nutr. Rev.,* 46, 241, 1988.

72. **Verdy, M. and Caron, D.,** Ethanol et absorption du calcium chez l'human biol, *Gastroenterology,* 6, 157, 1973.

73. **Krawitt, E. L.,** Effect of acute ethanol administration on duodenal calcium transport, *Proc. Soc. Exp. Biol. Med.,* 146, 406, 1974.

74. **Krawitt, E. L., Sampson, W., and Katagiri, C. A.,** Effect of 1,25-dihydroxycholecalciferol on ethanol mediated suppression of calcium absorption, *Calcif. Tiss. Res.,* 18, 119, 1975.

75. **Miller, A. and Bronner, F.,** Calcium uptake in isolated brush-border vesicles from small rat intestine, *Biochem. J.,* 196, 391,1981.

76. **Tacnet, F., Watkins, D. W., and Ripoche, P.,** Zinc binding in intestinal brush-border membrane isolated from pig, *Biochim. Biophys. Acta,* 1063, 51, 1991.

# 12

## Alcohol and Small Intestinal Permeability

Ingvar Bjarnason and Andrew Macpherson

## CONTENTS

## 12.1 INTRODUCTION

There is considerable interest in the adverse effects of alcohol on the gastrointestinal tract. The previous chapters have covered the damage to the gastric mucosa and the association between alcohol ingestion and malabsorption. It is less well appreciated, however, that alcohol may disrupt the intestinal barrier function. This manifests as increased intestinal permeability across the epithelial cell layer and may have important practical and theoretical consequences for well being. Nevertheless, the findings of increased permeability in subjects misusing alcohol has not caused investigators dealing with these subjects to look closer at the mechanism of this effect or the possible consequences. One possible reason for the apparent lack of interest is that the techniques for noninvasive assessment of small intestinal function appear at first sight complex, and until recently, interpretation of results has lacked scientific justification.

This chapter will review briefly the history of development of noninvasive techniques for assessing intestinal permeability in humans, to outline the practical aspects of testing, and to draw attention to ways to localize the observed changes. The possible clinical consequences of increased intestinal permeability due to alcohol misuse will be examined in the context of what we have termed the Grand Unification Theory (GUT!) of the pathogenesis of small bowel disease.

## 12.2    ASSESSMENT OF INTESTINAL PERMEABILITY

With the introduction of nonmetabolized disaccharides as test substances it became practically possible[1] to assess intestinal permeability noninvasively in humans. The term permeability has become synonymous with assessing the intestinal barrier function. Acceptance of the technique was initially slow because of the confusion associated with the use of polyethylene glycol (PEG 400) as a permeability marker.[2,3] Increased specificity of permeability measurements was achieved in the early 1980s with the successful application of the principle of the differential urinary excretion of orally administered test probes. This resulted in wider acceptance of the tests for assessing intestinal permeability.

Practical and research applications of intestinal permeability tests are discussed in detail elsewhere[4] but relate in broad terms to diagnostic screening and confirmation of small intestinal disease, assessing responses to treatment, assessing intestinal toxicity of various drugs and evaluating the importance of the intestinal barrier function in the etiology, pathophysiology, and pathogenesis of intestinal and systemic disease. The latter has perhaps been the most exciting outcome of intestinal permeability testing and has resulted in the discovery of a number of low grade intestinal enteropathies. Collectively, the findings have led to the formulation of the GUT of the pathogenesis of small intestinal disease which will be discussed in some detail. First, how do we assess intestinal permeability reliably and noninvasively in humans?

### 12.2.1    Permeability Markers

The noninvasive testing of intestinal permeability involves an overnight fast with ingestion of a test solution at 8 am. This is followed by collection of timed urines, usually for 5 or 6 h, and the fraction of the probes excreted is measured. Although the principle is simple there are major constraints on the suitability of the test substances according to their physicochemical properties, and the method of analysis in urine also requires careful consideration.

The choice of probe (disaccharides, monosaccharides, PEG ranging in mean molecular weight from 400 to 4000 or $^{51}$Cr-EDTA) employed for assessing intestinal permeability can be viewed in a historical perspective. The tests were specifically designed by the desire to assess noninvasively the intestinal barrier function as opposed to its function as an absorptive organ. Initially a single probe such as lactulose or other nonmetabolized disaccharide (melibiose), trisaccharide (raffinose), or polysaccharide (dextrans), was used by itself.[1,5-7] The desired properties of the markers were found to include an appropriate molecular size (and perhaps shape), aqueous but no lipid solubility, resistance to metabolic degradation, lack of affinity for transport systems, no toxicity and a urinary excretion pattern resembling that of inulin following intravenous administration.[8-13] Even when the probes met the above criteria, however, it was clear that what appeared in urine following ingestion was influenced by a number of factors in addition to intestinal permeability, as explained in Table 12.1. This led to the formulation of the principle of differential urinary excretion of several simultaneously ingested test substances by Menzies, explained in Figure 12.1, which allows the specific assessment of intestinal integrity.[11] Two test substances are used together that only differ in the permeation pathways which they use during their passage across the intestinal epithelium. Monosaccharides (L-rhamnose or mannitol) and some disaccharides (lactulose and melibiose) are particularly well suited for simultaneous use and in these circumstances the differential urinary excretion of di-/monosaccharide provides a specific indication of the state of mucosal permeability. The ratio reflects the relative prevalence of large/small pores[14] in the intestine, an index which has become synonymous with intestinal permeability. The choice of test dose saccharides is based on their physicochemical properties as well as on practical issues. Lactulose is the most widely used disaccharide (obtained from a cheap syrup) in tests of intestinal permeability. It resists action of small intestinal disaccharidases and is not widely distributed in foods. Although commonly used as a laxative and in the treatment of hepatic encephalopathy

**TABLE 12.1  The Principle of the Differential Urinary Excretion of Orally Administered Test Substances**

| | Factors affecting the urinary excretion of orally administered test substances | Monosaccharide | Nonhydrolyzed disaccharide | Hydrolyzed disaccharide |
|---|---|---|---|---|
| Premucosal | Completeness of ingestion | = | = | = |
| | Gastric dilution | = | = | = |
| | Gastric emptying | = | = | = |
| | Intestinal dilution | = | = | = |
| | Intestinal transit | = | = | = |
| | Bacterial degradation | = | = | = |
| | Unstirred water layer | = | = | = |
| | Hydrolysis | 0 | 0 | + |
| Mucosal | Route of permeation | A | B | B |
| | Intestinal blood flow | = | = | = |
| Postmucosal | Metabolism | 0 | 0 | 0 |
| | Endogenous production[a] | 0 | 0 | 0 |
| | Tissue distribution | C | D | D |
| | Renal function | = | = | = |
| | Timing and completeness of urinary collection | ~ | ~ | ~ |
| | Bacterial degradation | = | = | = |
| | Analytical performance[b] | = | = | = |

*Note:*  When a nonhydrolyzed disaccharide (i.e., lactulose) and a monosaccharide (L-rhamnose or mannitol) are ingested together all the above factors will contribute to their (% of oral dose) excretion in urine. However, any change in the pre- and postmucosal factors will affect the two test substances equally so that the urinary excretion ratio (lactulose/L-rhamnose) will only be minimally or not at all affected. The two probes differ significantly in their routes of permeation across the intestine, with lactulose permeating between cells and monosaccharides through cells. The urinary excretion ratio of lactulose/L-rhamnose thereby becomes a specific index of intestinal permeability which is not affected to an appreciable extent by nonmucosal factors. The simultaneous administration of a nonhydrolyzed (lactulose) and a hydrolyzed disaccharide (lactose, sucrose, or palatinose), with subsequent analysis in urine, to assess the efficacy of intestinal disaccharidase activities (lactase, sucrase, and isomaltase, respectively) is an extension of the above principle. The disaccharides differ only in respect to the rate of hydrolyses in the intestine which in turn governs the amount of intact disaccharide available for transport across the mucosa. In normal subjects the urinary excretion (% dose) ratios of hydrolyzable to nonhydrolyzable disaccharides is less than 0.3 but with increasing severity of disaccharidase deficiency this ratio approaches 1.0 at which time there is no disaccharide hydrolyses. =, Identical or affects all the test substances equally; ~, Roughly equal; 0, Does not take place; +, Rate is determined mainly by intestinal disaccharidase activities; A and B, Indicates different routes of permeation. See text for detailed discussion; C and D, Mono- and disaccharides have a different volume of distribution following intravenous administration and hence there is a slight difference in the speed and completeness of their urinary excretions. This is not of major importance.

[a]  There may be some but minimal endogenous production of mannitol.

[b]  Excellent if thin layer chromatography is used.

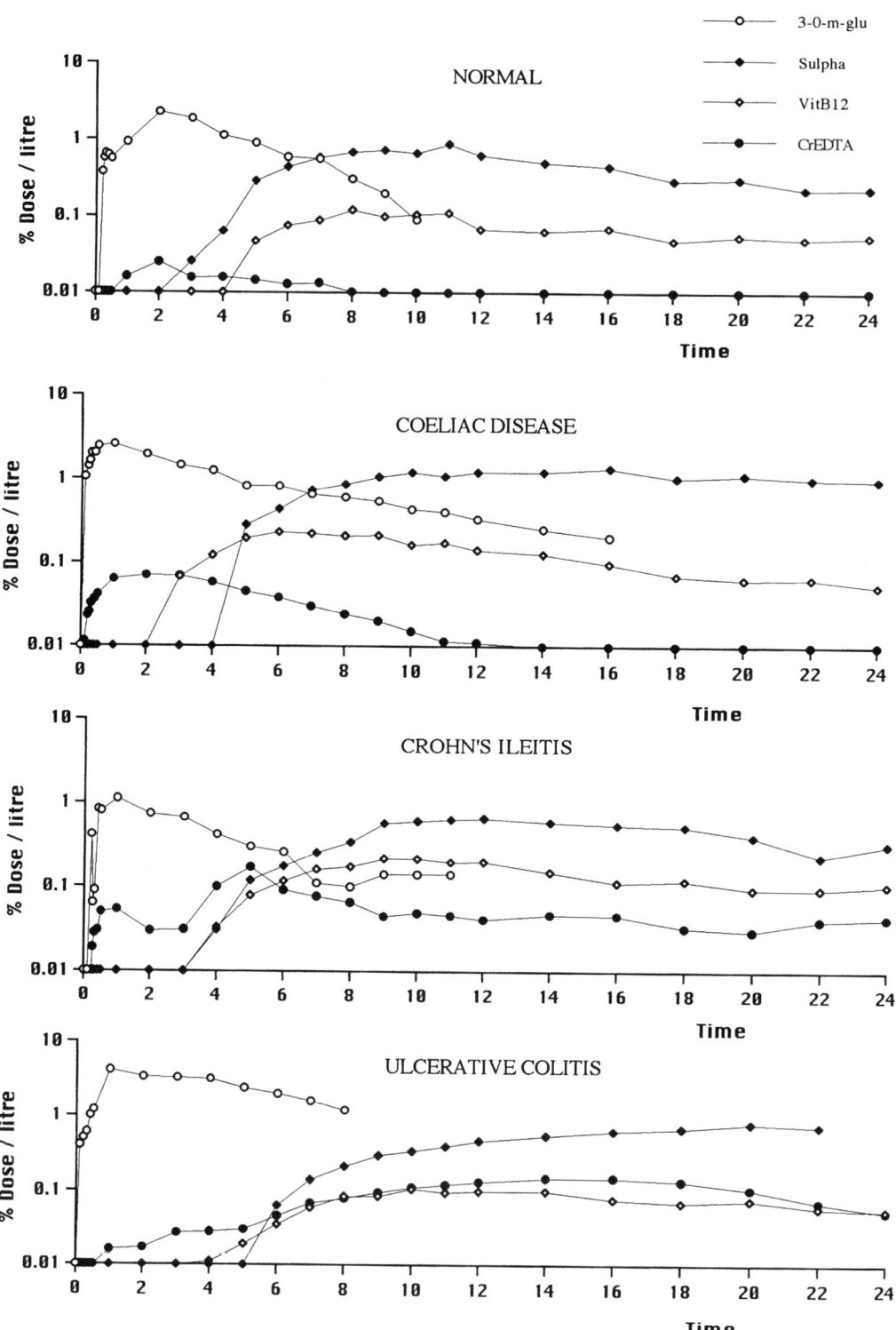

it can be substituted by melibiose in these circumstances. Raffinose, a trisaccharide, can equally be used but it is found in some foods especially in baked beans so that care needs to be taken with diet around the test. Of L-rhamnose or mannitol, the latter has theoretical advantages as its urinary excretion following intravenous administration simulates [51]Cr-EDTA and lactulose more closely than does L-rhamnose.[14-18]

The analyses of di- and monosaccharides are time consuming. The choice is between thin-layer chromatography, high pressure liquid chromatography, and enzyme assays.

[51]Cr-EDTA can be used alone, but adequate sensitivity necessitates a 24-h urinary collection which requires that a substantial amount of the probe pass across the colon as well as the small intestine. [51]Cr-EDTA can be substituted for lactulose as the two molecules have almost identical properties. However, because [51]Cr-EDTA is not degraded by intestinal bacteria it has been suggested that small intestinal bacterial overgrowth (causing degradation of L-rhamnose and mannitol) or a particularily rapid intestinal transit (reducing the effective mucosal contact time of L-rhamnose) may give rise to an increased [51]Cr-EDTA:monosaccharide urinary excretion ratio in the absence of a genuine alteration of permeability. In practice, however, this does not seem to be important.[19-26]

PEG 400 was popularized as a test substance by Chadwick et al. in 1977[2,3] and subsequently was used in several studies by a single Scandinavian group.[27-38] However, the use of PEG 400 has been controversial for a number of reasons. First, the PEG 400 polymers, despite physicochemical similarities with [51]Cr-EDTA and nonmetabolized di- and monosaccharides, permeate the small intestine 10 to 50 times more readily than other test substances. This is inconsistent with the desire to assess the intestinal barrier function. The precise reason for such atypical permeation is uncertain, but discussion has focused on the question of molecular shape or lipid solubility.[11,12,39-43] Second, recovery of PEG 400 in human urine following intravenous administration is incomplete and varies between 26 to 72% of the administered dose excreted within 5 h[14] depending on the polymer size. The low urinary recovery is surprising as PEG polymers are not metabolized. It has been suggested that the polymers must be retained in tissue following absorption. Third, PEG 400 is not appropriate for assessing the profile of intestinal permeability along the lines dictated by the differential urinary excretion principle of test substances, as the range of PEG 400 polymers all appear to use the same diffusion pathway. Lastly, altered permeation of PEG 400 recorded in various diseases does not correlate logically with other aspects of intestinal physiology. In particular, where increased intestinal permeability has been found with the differential urinary excretion of di-/monosaccharides (coeliac and small intestinal Crohn's disease, intestinal infections, etc.) or [51]Cr-EDTA, the permeation of PEG 400 is usually reduced. The implications are that while the permeation of [51]Cr-EDTA correlates significantly with macromolecular permeation,[44-46] the permeation of PEG 400 might relate inversely to macromolecular permeation. As a routine test to screen for small intestinal disease the PEG 400 test lacks sensitivity, and only a marginal improvement is achieved by mathematical manipulation (filter function or N1/2).[28,30,36,47]

### 12.2.2 Test Dose Composition

Test dose composition is determined by the purpose of the investigation, but there are also several practical issues involved in choosing the appropriate test for the problem at hand. Lactulose and

---

**FIGURE 12.1**  Sites of increased intestinal permeability. The permeation profile from a normal subject shows low serum levels of [51]Cr-EDTA following the appearance of 3-*o*-methyl-*D*-glucose, suggesting that [51]Cr-EDTA permeates across the small intestine somewhere distal to the duodenum. In the patient with untreated coeliac disease the [51]Cr-EDTA peaks earlier and serum levels are higher than in normal subjects suggesting that the diseased jejunum is the site of increased intestinal permeability. The patient with Crohn's ileitis shows an early rise of [51]Cr-EDTA and the second peak coincides with the appearance of the ileal and cecal markers. The permeation of [51]Cr-EDTA increases after the appearance of the ileal and cecal marker in the patient with panulcerative colitis.

monosaccharide probes should be administered at the lowest possible dose without compromising analytical performance. The reason for this is that the substances have limited intestinal permeation and therefore cause osmotic fluid retention within the bowel.[48] This reduces the contact time with the intestinal mucosa which affects the sensitivity of the procedure.[49] For routine assessment of small intestinal permeability and absorptive capacity in humans we use a 100-ml test solution which includes:

Lactulose 5 g
L-rhamnose (1.0 g) [or mannitol (no more than 2 g)]
3-O-methyl-D-glucose (0.2 g) which assesses an active carrier-mediated process in the enterocytes
D-xylose (0.5 g) which assesses a passive carrier-mediated transport system

A 5-h urine collection is made into a container with sufficient preservative (e.g., merthiolate 100 mg) to prevent bacterial degradation of sugars. A complete and accurate urine recovery is essential because an incomplete collection will give an erroneous underestimate of absorptive capacity and indeed the permeability ratio may alter slightly because the di- and monosaccharides have different rates of urinary excretion.

Apart from the osmotically active poorly absorbed disaccharide in intestinal permeability test solutions,[48] the tests may include "osmotic fillers" which are readily absorbed solutes used to increase the osmolarity of the test solutions up to 1500 mosm/l. The rationale for their use comes from the early years of permeability testing when lactulose was used by itself without a monosaccharide. The osmolarity of ingested test solutions was shown to be important in relation to urinary excretion of lactulose and other oligosaccharides.[1] Most readily absorbed compounds added to the test solution, apart from alcohol, increased intestinal permeation of the disaccharide[1,5-7,50] in normals, provided that the osmolarity was above 1500 mosm/l. However, patients with untreated coeliac disease were much more sensitive to this effect and solutions of less than 1500 mosm/l greatly increased the diagnostic discrimination of the test. These findings were then indiscriminately extrapolated to the use of the differential permeability test.[49] Several osmotic fillers were subsequently used by different workers including a mixture of sucrose, galactose and lactose, glycerol or glucose. However the results often failed to correspond because the osmotic fillers differ in their osmotic potency and because the osmolarity of test solutions employed by different workers varied.[26,51-58] Due to the lack of consensus regarding which osmotic filler should be used and the fact that they do not increase diagnostic discrimination of the procedure,[49] there has been a shift toward omitting them from the test solution altogether.

### 12.2.3 Assessment of Upper Gastrointestinal Permeability

It may be possible to assess the gastric side effects of alcohol selectively by using a sucrose permeation test[59] which has been validated in relation to the gastric toxicity of NSAIDs. A 100-g dose of sucrose was ingested before bedtime with subsequent analyses of morning urines. Patients with endoscopic gastric pathology due to NSAIDs had significant increases in urinary sucrose and it was suggested that it might be a useful screening test prior to deciding on endoscopy. The test has not yet been applied to subjects misusing alcohol.

### 12.2.4 Assessment of Colonic Permeability

One successful modification of the differential urinary excretion principle is to administer $^{51}$Cr-EDTA with lactulose and L-rhamnose followed by a 0 to 5 and a 5- to 24-h urine collection for marker analyses.[60,61] Lactulose and L-rhamnose are both rapidly degraded by colonic bacteria whereas $^{51}$Cr-EDTA is not. Any difference in the total 24-h urine excretion of $^{51}$Cr-EDTA and lactulose is thus due to colonic permeation because the two behave identically in all other respects. Recent studies have shown its application in patients undergoing radiation treatment for uterine malignancy demonstrating transient mild increases in small intestinal and substantial increases in colonic permeability.[62] Again, the test has not been applied to subjects misusing alcohol, but it is now possible to localize intestinal pathology noninvasively and accurately.

## 12.2.5 Localizing Intestinal Permeability Changes

Tne techniques described above localize intestinal disease and damage. Alternatively this may be achieved by a single combined investigation. The technique is, however, labor intensive, expensive, and requires an overnight stay in an investigational unit.[63] It was validated in patients with inflammatory bowel disease where the site of increased intestinal permeability was accurately located. The principle is that a mixture of test substances (whose absorptive site is localized to a particular region of the intestine) are given orally together with $^{51}$Cr-EDTA.[63] Serial serum samples are taken over 24 h and analyzed for appearance of the markers. The absorption profile of $^{51}$Cr-EDTA is then compared with the other markers allowing the site of increased intestinal permeability to be identified. The ingested test substances are:

a. 3-O-methyl-D-glucose; absorbed predominantly from the jejunum by the sodium coupled glucose carrier (active transport).
b. $^{57}$CoVitamin $B_{12}$ with intrinsic factor; absorbed from the terminal ileum by specific carriers.
c. Sulfasalazine, which passes unchanged into the cecum where it is cleaved into 5-aminosalicylic acid and sulfapyridine by azoreductase containing bacteria. Sulfapyridine is rapidly absorbed and its appearance in serum indicates when the test solution enters the cecum.

Figure 12.1 shows some representative results from patients with coeliac and inflammatory bowel disease. The absorption profile from a patient with untreated coeliac disease shows increased serum levels of $^{51}$Cr-EDTA which correspond to the 3-O-methyl-D-glucose absorption curve. Similarly the peak serum levels of $^{51}$Cr-EDTA in a patient with ileal Crohn's disease correspond to the appearance of the ileal and colonic markers whereas a patient with severe total colitis has increased serum levels of $^{51}$Cr-EDTA some time following the appearance of Vitamin $B_{12}$ or sulfapyridine.

## 12.2.6 Assessment of Intestinal Disaccharidase Activities

The principle of the differential urinary excretion of orally administered test substances has been used for noninvasive assessment and quantification of intestinal disaccharidase activities in humans.[64-66] As shown in Figure 12.1, simultaneous ingestion of lactulose and melibiose gives a urine excretion (% dose) ratio of melibiose/lactulose approaching 1.0 as these oligosaccharides are handled in an identical fashion. However, if a hydrolyzable disaccharide (say lactose) is substituted for melibiose all the variables in Figure 12.1 will affect the two test substances equally except the enzymatic degradation of the hydrolyzable disaccharide. The rate of hydrolysis therefore determines the amount of intact lactose available for permeation.

Based on the above findings, a test using sucrose, lactose, and palatinose (since they are substrates for sucrase, lactase and isomaltase), given with lactulose has been designed and validated.[64-66] Normal urinary excretion ratios of sucrose, lactose, and palatinose to that of lactulose in 10-h urines following their oral administration are in the range of 0.3 or below in subjects with active intestinal disaccharide hydrolysis. Ratios of 0.3 to 1.0 indicate increasing impairment of intestinal hydrolysis and clinically relevant impairments of lactase activity is associated with lactose/lactulose urinary excretion ratios of 0.45 or greater. The technique has been successfully used in Rotavirus enteritis in children[67] to demonstrate combined sucrase and palatinase deficiency in asucrasia[64,65,67] effectiveness of α-glucosidase inhibitors on sucrose hydrolysis, and to quantitate total small intestinal hydrolytic activity in patients with coeliac disease.[66] It could also be used to characterize the small intestinal damage in subjects misusing alcohol.

## 12.3   INTESTINAL PERMEABILITY IN INTESTINAL DISEASES

The preceding section has outlined some recent developments in intestinal function testing which represents an advance on preexisting tests in respect to sensitivity and specificity. As yet, however, there is limited data on the possible adverse effect of alcohol on the intestinal tract. One exception is that alcohol misuse is associated with increased intestinal permeability. By itself this appears no more than a curiosity. However, when viewed in the context of the possible role of increased intestinal permeability in the pathogenesis of small intestinal disease it may be that the consequences are more substantial. Before reviewing intestinal permeability changes induced by alcohol it is useful to review the studies that have led to the GUT of the pathogenesis of small intestinal disease and then to assess where alcohol may fit within this framework.

### 12.3.1   The GUT

Increased macromolecular permeation may play a pathogenic role in local as well as systemic disease.[68-70] The validity of this assumption depends on showing that increased intestinal permeability detected by low molecular weight markers is synonymous with macromolecular permeation. This has certainly been shown to be the case in respect to $^{51}$Cr-EDTA,[44-46] but the other permeability markers have not been studied. The GUT postulates that the intestinal barrier is a central pathophysiological mechanism for the development of a nonspecific enteropathy. It is suggested that the enteropathy is similar regardless of the initiating event causing the permeability changes[71-73] as the intestinal inflammatory response is nonspecifically directed at luminal aggressive factors which have gained access to the mucosa.

The initiation of the permeability changes can occur by three main mechanisms: (1) primary permeability breakers; (2) factors or diseases associated with enhanced luminal aggressiveness, and (3) diseases associated with diminished mucosal defense. The GUT emphasizes that there are different pathogenic stages of disease which start off as biochemical and ultrastructural damage but the common link is that the tissue reaction is driven by the permeability changes. Macroscopic damage only becomes evident if a number of additional factors are in play. It has been proposed that the tissue reaction (inflammation) is the common final pathway for the damage and that it is amenable to identical treatment. The following is a short summary of the studies which led to the GUT.

#### 12.3.1.1   Intestinal Permeability Breakers

NSAIDs are the prototype of the permeability breakers and are therefore discussed in some detail; however, a more complete assessment of NSAIDs on the entire intestine is found in Reference 73. NSAIDs increase intestinal permeability within 12 h of ingestion. The permeability changes occur in the period during drug absorption when the enterocytes are exposed to the highest concentration of the drugs.[21,24,61,74-85] The biochemical mechanism of damage is still unknown but the idea that it occurs simply as a result of inhibition of cyclooxygenase is no longer tenable.[86-90] The authors have suggested that the biochemical pathology of NSAIDs can be explained by their action on mitochondria.[73] It is suggested that NSAIDs uncouple oxidative phosphorylation or inhibit the electron transport chain, either of which would be followed by reduced ATP production and loss of control over the intercellular junctions. Increased intestinal permeability thus allows luminal aggressive factors access to the mucosa. In the small intestine the main luminal aggressive factors are bile, pancreatic secretions, bacteria, etc., all of which have been shown to be important in the pathogenesis of NSAID enteropathy in the rat.[91-99] The main neutrophil chemoattractant in humans appears to be metronidazole sensitive anaerobic bacteria.[100,101] Once the neutrophils are there (defining the presence of inflammation), they cause most of the tissue damage by oxygen radicals and lysosomal release of enzymes which occur following contact with the chemoattractant and internalization, respectively.

Although the permeability changes are immediate and seen in response to other drugs, the changes are more prolonged with NSAIDs because of their ability to prevent the generation of reparative prostaglandin in the intestinal mucosa.

The possibility that the permeability changes caused intestinal inflammation was studied with the technique of [111]indium-labeled leukocytes.[21,102] The results were clear: untreated patients had no evidence of intestinal inflammation while 65% of those receiving NSAIDs for more than 6 months had small intestinal inflammation. Two similar radioisotopic studies confirmed these findings.[103,104] Furthermore two morphological studies were also confirmatory. An enteroscopy study[105] showed small intestinal lesions in the mid-small intestine in about 50% of patients on NSAIDs, ranging from hemorrhagic blebs to frank ulceration, and a post-mortem study[106] showed frequent small intestinal ulcers at autopsy in patients receiving NSAIDs immediately before death. The latter estimated an incidence of 30% in these patients but fine detail was obscured by autolysis of the intestine. The enteropathy induced by NSAIDs is a low grade inflammatory process, with a fecal excretion of 1 to 6% (normal: less than 1%) and a mean of 3% which contrasts with classical inflammatory bowel disease (Crohn's disease and ulcerative colitis) where the excretion can go up to 50% in very active disease.

The clinical significance of NSAID enteropathy is clear. Patients bleed from the inflammatory site[73,101,107,108] and this contributes to the iron deficiency anemia which is common in these patients. Although the bleeding is usually mild (2 to 10 ml/day), it is no less than that found in patients with colonic malignancy who are also prone to an iron deficiency anemia. The other factors which contribute to iron deficiency in rheumatoid patients are their borderline adequate food intake and some have hypochlorhydria with a low baseline iron absorption. Most patients with NSAID enteropathy lose protein from the inflammatory site[107] which may play a significant role in hypoalbuminemia and the development of peripheral edema.

NSAIDs are also associated with specific if not pathognomic pathology in the small intestine[109,110] which fall into a range of pathology from single broad-based nonspecific strictures to that termed "diaphragm disease." These are multiple (numbering 3 to 70 in each patient) concentric, thin (2 to 4 mm), septate-like luminal projections, narrowing the lumen down to a few millimeters in most cases but at times causing complete obstruction. Most of the strictures have been localized to the mid-small intestine or the ileum; identical strictures in the cecum and the ascending colon have recently been described in patients on sustained release diclofenac sodium[111-115] (Voltaren). Prior to these findings there had been a number of case reports describing small intestinal ulcers and strictures in patients on NSAIDs but the connection between NSAIDs and the lesions were often not made.[116-121] In short, NSAIDs have a specific detrimental biochemical action on enterocytes which is not evident to the same extent in other tissues because of lower drug concentrations. The ultrastructural-biochemical alterations lead to increased intestinal permeability resulting in a low grade enteropathy. Collectively, the above represents the most compelling evidence that increased intestinal permeability leads to an intestinal inflammatory reaction.

Only a few studies have assessed intestinal permeability in alcoholic patients. One study looked at a group of middle class drinkers in Harrow, U.K. These were regular drinkers without significant liver disease but who, although clearly exceeding 70 g of ethanol per day, often held a job. When tested within 3 days of abstention they had increased intestinal permeability which was of comparable severity to that found in Crohn's and coeliac disease.[22] In most cases restoration of the permeability changes occurred within 2 weeks of cessation of alcohol. The precise cause of the permeability changes is unknown. It is not a reflection of associated liver disease as cirrhotic patients with portal hypertension have normal intestinal permeability.[122-125] Increased intestinal permeability is not seen when alcohol is included in the test solution,[1,126] even when the solution was made markedly hyperosmolar (3500 mosm/l). However, a modest dose of alcohol (0.5 g/kg) 15 h before the test caused a modest but significant increase in the permeation of [51]Cr-EDTA.[127] The permeation of PEG 400 on the other hand is increased only during intoxication.[128] Studies in animals show that chronic alcoholic consumption increases macromolecular permeation to horseradish peroxidase.[129,130] At the same time, there is damage to the intercellular junctions and increased permeability to $^{51}$Cr-EDTA.[131]

The possibility that the permeability changes lead to a low-grade enteropathy, similar to that seen with NSAIDs, has only been studied in a small number of patients. In a group of eight heavy drinkers, the authors found (unpublished) a low-grade enteropathy in five with fecal excretions ranging from 1.2 to 4.3%. The possibility that the inflammation is associated with intestinal blood and protein loss remains to be studied.

There are several other primary permeability breakers or situations where intestinal integrity is compromised.[62,132-142] Intestinal inflammation has been documented in the case of chronic renal failure and following abdominal radiation, but remains to be investigated in other situations.

### 12.3.1.2   Luminal Aggressive Factors

In the small intestine, the main luminal aggressors are bile, pancreas secretions, various hydrolytic and proteolytic enzymes, bacteria and their degradation products. There are not, however, many examples of human disease which are associated with increased luminal aggressiveness in the small intestine. One is the small intestinal bacterial overgrowth which occurs following intestinal bypass surgery for morbid obesity. The permeation of PEG 400 is reportedly increased in these patients[35] and there are certainly inflammatory changes present in the bypassed intestinal segment.

Intestinal infections increase intestinal permeability and quantitatively this is similar to that seen with the permeability breakers and in Crohn's and coeliac disease.[67] There is a moderately severe inflammatory response evident in these patients with $^{111}$indium leukocyte excretion levels between 1 and 9%[143] and a mean (6%) which is slightly higher than that found with the permeability breakers. The interrelationship between intestinal permeability and inflammation in specific intestinal infections is uncertain. Increased intestinal permeability could be a manifestation of the invasiveness of the microbe or a result of the inflammatory response. The slightly greater intensity of the inflammation, as assessed by the $^{111}$indium leukocyte technique, compared with the permeability breakers might be a reflection of greater antigen load. Patients with cystic fibrosis have striking increases in intestinal permeability[144-147] probably due to the viscous mucus providing a nidus for small intestinal microbial proliferation. The possibility that these patients develop an enteropathy remains to be examined, however.

### 12.3.1.3   Altered Mucosal Defense

Increased intestinal permeability is a universal feature in patients with hypogammaglobulinemia[148] and the fecal excretion of $^{111}$indium leukocytes in these patients ranges from 1.1 to 14.5% with a mean of 6.9%.[149]

Patients with acquired immune deficiency syndrome (AIDS) have increased intestinal permeability regardless of subgroup.[150,151] Those individuals recently infected and without an AIDS defining illness have normal intestinal permeability. $^{111}$Indium leukocytes in these patients show that those with increased intestinal permeability have a low-grade enteropathy, similar in severity to that found in NSAID enteropathy.[152]

When taken together, this suggests that there are a number of disease processes falling under the general description of permeability breakers, increased luminal aggressors, and reduced mucosal defense, which are characterized by increased intestinal permeability. The increased intestinal permeability then allows the luminal aggressors access to the intestinal mucosa where they initiate an inflammatory reaction. Certainly the intensity of the inflammatory response seems very similar in the various diseases where it has been studied. In the context of alcohol misuse, much work remains to be done on the early pathogenesis of the damage which leads to the permeability changes. Furthermore, by analogy with the findings in NSAID enteropathy, it seems possible that alcohol enteropathy in humans may be an important source of intestinal blood and protein loss.

## 12.4  CONCLUSION

This chapter reviewed the principles underlying the technique of the noninvasive assessment of small intestinal permeability. Some recent developments in the noninvasive assessment of small intestinal function have been described and how these may be used to characterize the possible damaging effects of alcohol on the small intestine. Most of the immediate consequences of increased intestinal permeability in relation to the etiology and pathogenesis of disease in humans have been formulated into the GUT. The GUT provides a logical framework for further investigation into the interaction between the intestinal barrier and intestinal luminal aggressors. The importance of the GUT is that it suggests that there is a number of small intestinal enteropathies still to be discovered — one of which probably relates to alcohol ingestion.

## REFERENCES

1.  **Menzies, I. S.,** Absorption of intact oligosaccharide in health and disease, *Biochem. Soc. Trans.,* 2, 1040, 1974.
2.  **Chadwick, V. S., Phillips, S. F., and Hofman, A. F.,** Measurements of intestinal permeability using low molecular weight polyethylene glycols (PEG 400). I. Chemical analysis and biological properties of PEG 400, *Gastroenterology,* 73, 241, 1977.
3.  **Chadwick, V. S., Phillips, S. F., and Hofman, A. F.,** Measurements of intestinal permeability using low molecular weight polyethylene glycols (PEG 400). II. Application to study of normal and abnormal permeability states in humans and animals, *Gastroenterology,* 73, 247, 1977.
4.  **Bjarnason, I., Macpherson, A. J. M., and Hollander, D.,** Intestinal permeability: an overview, *Gastroenterology,* 108, 1566, 1995.
5.  **Laker, M. F. and Menzies, I. S.,** Increase in human intestinal permeability following ingestion of hypertonic solutions, *J. Physiol. (Lond.),* 273, 881, 1977.
6.  **Laker, M. F.,** The effect of hypertonic solutions on intestinal permeability, MD Thesis, University of London, 1978.
7.  **Wheeler, P. G., Menzies, I. S., and Creamer, B.,** Effect of hyperosmolar stimuli and coeliac disease on the permeability of the human gastrointestinal tract, *Clin. Sci. Mol. Med.,* 54, 495, 1978.
8.  **Bjarnason, I., Peters, T. J., and Levi, A. J.,** Intestinal permeability: clinical correlates, *Dig. Dis. Sci.,* 4, 83, 1986.
9.  **Hamilton, I.,** Small intestinal permeability, in *Recent Advances in Gastroenterology,* Vol. 6, Pounder, R. E., Ed., Churchill Livingstone, Edinburgh, 1986, 73.
10.  **Cooper, B. T.,** The small intestinal permeability barrier, in *Gut Defenses in Clinical Practice*, Losowski, M. H. and Heatley, R. V., Eds., Churchill Livingstone, Edinburgh, 1986, 117.
11.  **Menzies, I. S.,** Transmucosal passage of inert molecules in health and disease, in *Intestinal Absorption and Secretion*, Skadhauge, E. and Heintze, K., Eds., Falk Symposium 36, MTP Press, 1984, 527.
12.  **Hollander, D.,** The intestinal permeability barrier. A hypothesis as to its regulation and involvement in Crohn's disease, *Scand. J. Gastroenterol.,* 27, 721, 1992.
13.  **Hollander, D.,** Permeability in Crohn's disease-altered barrier function in healthy relatives?, *Gastroenterology,* 104, 1848, 1993.
14.  **Maxton, D. G., Bjarnason, I., Reynolds, A. P., Catt, S. D., Peters, T. J., and Menzies, I. S.,** Lactulose, 51CrEDTA, L-rhamnose and polyethylene glycol 400 as probe markers for "*in vivo*" assessment of human intestinal permeability, *Clin. Sci.,* 71, 71, 1986.
15.  **Laker, M. F., Bull, H. J., and Menzies, I. S.,** Evaluation of mannitol for use as a probe marker of gastrointestinal permeability in humans, *Eur. J. Clin. Invest.,* 12, 485, 1982.
16.  **Cobden, I., Hamilton, I., Rothwell, J., and Axon, A. T. R.,** Cellobiose/mannitol test: physiological properties of probe molecules and influence of extraneous factors, *Clin. Chim. Acta,* 148, 53, 1985.
17.  **Dominguez, R., Corcoran, A. C., and Page, I. H.,** Mannitol: kinetics of distribution, excretion and utilization in human beings, *J. Lab. Clin. Med.,* 32, 192, 1947.
18.  **Newman, E. V., Bordlay, J., and Winternitz, J.,** The interrelationship of glomerular filtration rate (mannitol clearance), extracellular fluid volume, surface area of the body, and plasma concentration of mannitol, *Bull. Johns Hopkins Hosp.,* 75, 253, 1944.
19.  **Bjarnason, I., Peters, T. J., and Veall, N.,** A persistent defect of intestinal permeability in coeliac disease as demonstrated by a [51]Cr-labelled EDTA absorption test, *Lancet,* i, 323, 1983.

20. **Bjarnason, I., O'Morain, C., Levi, A. J., and Peters, T. J.,** The absorption of [51]Cr EDTA in inflammatory bowel disease, *Gastroenterology*, 85, 318, 1983.

21. **Bjarnason, I., Williams, P., So, A., Zanelli, G., Levi, A. J., Gumpel, M. J., Peters, T. J., and Ansell, B.,** Intestinal permeability and inflammation in rheumatoid arthritis; effects of non-steroidal anti-inflammatory drugs, *Lancet*, ii, 1171, 1984.

22. **Bjarnason, I., Ward, K., and Peters, T. J.,** The leaky gut of alcoholism: possible route of entry for toxic compounds, *Lancet*, i, 179, 1984.

23. **Bjarnason, I., Goolamali, S. K., Levi, A. J., and Peters, T. J.,** Intestinal permeability in patients with atopic eczema, *Br. J. Dermatol.*, 112, 291, 1985.

24. **Bjarnason, I. and Peters, T. J.,** Helping the mucosa make sense of macromolecules, *Gut*, 28, 1057, 1987.

25. **Hamilton, I., Fairris, G. M., Rothwell, J., Cunliffe, W. J., Dixon, M. F., and Axon, A. T. R.,** Small intestinal permeability in dermatological disease, *Q. J. Med.*, 56, 559, 1985.

26. **Judby, L. D., Rothwell, J., and Axon, A. T. R.,** Lactulose/mannitol test. An ideal screening test for coeliac disease, *Gastroenterology*, 96, 79, 1989.

27. **Magnusson, M., Magnusson, K. E., Sundqvist, T., and Dennebergz, T.,** Reduced intestinal permeability measured by differently sized polyethylene glycols in acute uremic rats, *Nephron*, 60, 193, 1992.

28. **Magnusson, K. E. and Sundquist, T.,** Mathematical modelling for determining intestinal permeability using polyethylene glycol, *Gut*, 25, 428, 1983.

29. **Magnusson, K. E., Sundquist, T., Sjodahl, R., and Tageson, C.,** Altered intestinal permeability to low-molecular-weight polyethylene glycols (PEG 400) in patients with Crohn's disease, *Acta Chir. Scand.*, 149, 323, 1983.

30. **Magnusson, K. E. and Sundqvist, T.,** Modelling of intestinal permeability in humans to polyethylene glycols (PEG 400 and PEG 1000), *Acta Physiol. Scand.*, 125, 289, 1985.

31. **Magnusson, M., Magnusson, K. E., Sundqvist, T., and Denneberg, T.,** Urinary excretion of differently sized polyethylene glycols after intravenous administration in uremic and control rats: effects of low- and high-protein diets, *Nephron*, 56, 312, 1990.

32. **Magnusson, M., Magnusson, K. E., Sundqvist, T., and Denneberg, T.,** Increased intestinal permeability to differently sized polyethylene glycols in uremic rats: effects of low- and high-protein diets, *Nephron*, 56, 306, 1990.

33. **Sundquist, T., Magnusson, K. E., Sjodahl, R., Stjernstrom, I., and Tageson, C.,** Passage of molecules through the wall of the gastrointestinal tract. II. Application of low-molecular weight polyethyleneglycol and a deterministic mathematical model for determining intestinal permeability in humans, *Gut*, 21, 208, 1980.

34. **Sundquist, T., Lindstrom, F., Magnusson, K. E., Skoldstram, L., Stjernstrom, I., and Tageson, C.,** Influence of fasting on intestinal permeability and disease activity in patients with rheumatoid arthritis, *Scand. J. Rheumatol.*, 11, 33, 1982.

35. **Sundquist, T., Magnusson, K. E., Larsson, L., Tageson, C., Backman, L., and Nordenvall, B.,** Reduced intestinal permeability to low-molecular-weight polyethylene glycols (PEG400) in patients with jejunoileal bypass, *Acta Chir. Scand.*, 150, 567, 1984.

36. **Sundquist, T., Tageson, C., and Magnusson, K. E.,** Simulation of a multicompartment model for the intestinal permeability to low-molecular-weight probes (polyethylene glycol 400), *Math. Biosci.*, 56, 287, 1981.

37. **Tageson, C., Anderson, P. A., Anderson, J., Bolin, T., Kallberg, M., and Sjodahl, R.,** Passage of molecules through the wall of the gastrointestinal tract. Measurement of intestinal permeability to polyethylene glycols in the range 634-1338 dalton range (PEG 1000), *Scand. J. Gastroenterol.*, 18, 481, 1983.

38. **Tageson, C. and Bengtsson, A.,** Intestinal permeability to different sized polyethylene glycols in patients with rheumatoid arthritis, *Scand. J. Rheumatol.*, 12, 124, 1983.

39. **Hollander, D., Rickets, D., and Boyd, C. A. R.,** Importance of "probe" molecular geometry in determining intestinal permeability, *Can. J. Gastroenterol.*, 2 (Suppl. A), 35A, 1988.

40. **Ma, T. Y., Hollander, D., Krugliak, P., and Katz, K.,** PEG 400, a hydrophyllic molecular probe for measuring intestinal permeability, *Gastroenterology*, 98, 39, 1990.

41. **Krugilak, P., Hollander, D., Ma, T. Y., Tran, D., Dadufalza, V. D., Katz, K. D., and Ce, K.,** Mechanism of polyethylene glycol 400 permeability of perfused rat intestine, *Gastroenterology*, 97, 1164, 1989.

42. **Krugliak, P., Hollander, D., Le, K., Ma, T., Dadufalza, V. D., and Katz, K. D.,** Regulation of polyethylene glycol 400 intestinal permeability by endogenous and exogenous prostanoids. Influence of non-steroidal anti-inflammatory drugs, *Gut*, 31, 417, 1990.

43. **Iqbal, T. H., Lewis, K. O., and Cooper, B. T.,** Diffusion of polyethylene glycol-400 across lipid barriers *in vitro*, *Clin. Sci.*, 85, 111, 1993.

44. **Davin, J. C., Forget, P., and Mahieu, P. R.,** Increased intestinal permeability to (51Cr)EDTA is correlated with IgA immune complex-plasma levels in children with IgA-associated nephropathies, *Acta Pediatr. Scand.*, 77, 118, 1988.

45. **Ferry, D. M., Butt, T. J., Broom, M. F., Hunter, J., and Chadwick, V. S.,** Bacterial chemotactic oligopeptides and the intestinal mucosal barrier, *Gastroenterology*, 97, 61, 1989.

46. **Ramage, J. K., Stanisz, A., Scicchitano, R., Hunt, R. H., and Perdue, M. H.,** Effects of immunologic reactions on rat intestinal epithelium. Correlation of increased intestinal permeability to chromium 51 labelled ethylenediaminetetraacetic acid and ovalbumin during acute inflammation and anaphylaxis, *Gastroenterology*, 94, 1368, 1988.

47. **Irving, C. S., Lifschitz, C. H., Marks, L. M., Nichols, B. C., and Klein, P. D.,** Polyethylene glycol polymers of low molecular weight as probes of intestinal permeability. I. Innovations in analyses and quantitation, *J. Lab. Clin. Med.*, 107, 290, 1986.

48. **Menzies, I. S., Jenkins, A. P., Heduan, E., Catt, S. D., Segal, M. B., and Creamer, B.,** The effect of poorly absorbed solute on intestinal absorption, *Scand. J. Gastroenterol.*, 25, 1257, 1990.

49. **Bjarnason, I., Maxton, D., Reynolds, A. P., Catt, S., Peters, T. J., and Menzies, I. S.,** A comparison of 4 markers of intestinal permeability in control subjects and patients with coeliac disease, *Scand. J. Gastroenterol.*, 26, 630, 1994.

50. **Menzies, I. S., Pounder, R., Heyer, S., Laker, M. F., Bull, J., Wheeler, P. G., and Creamer, B.,** Abnormal intestinal permeability to sugars in villus atrophy, *Lancet*, ii, 1107, 1979.

51. **Blomquist, L., Bark, T., Hedenborg, G., Svenberg, T., and Norman, A.,** A comparison between the lactulose/mannitol and $^{51}$CrEDTA/$^{14}$C-mannitol methods for intestinal permeability, *Scand. J. Gastroenterol.*, 28, 274, 1993.

52. **Elia, M., Beherens, R., Northrop, C., Wraight, P., and Neale, G.,** Evaluation of mannitol, lactulose and $^{51}$Cr labelled ethylenediaminetetraacetate as markers of intestinal permeability in humans, *Clin. Sci.*, 73, 197, 1987.

53. **Andre, F., Andre, C., and Emery, Y.,** Assessement of the lactulose-mannitol test in Crohn's disease, *Gut*, 29, 511, 1988.

54. **Kapembwa, M. S., Fleming, S. C., Sewankambo, N., Serwadda, D., Lucas, S., Moody, A., and Griffin, G. E.,** Altered small-intestinal permeability associated with diarrhoea in human-immunodeficiency-virus-infected Caucasian and African subjects, *Clin. Sci.*, 81, 327, 1991.

55. **Murphy, M. S., Eastham, E. J., Nelson, R., Pearson, A. D. J., and Laker, M. F.,** Intestinal permeability in Crohn's disease, *Arch. Dis. Child.*, 64, 321, 1989.

56. **Ukabam, S. O., Homeda, M. A., and Cooper, B. J.,** Small intestinal permeability in Sudanese subjects: evidence of tropical enteropathy, *Trans. R. Soc. Trop. Med. Hyg.*, 40, 204, 1986.

57. **van der Hulst, P. R. W. J., Kreel, B. K., Meyenfelt, M. F., Brummer, R.-J. M., Arends, J.-W., Deytz, N. E. P., and Soeters, P. B.,** Glutamine and the preservation of gut integrity, *Lancet*, 341, 1363, 1993.

58. **Wyatt, J., Vogelsang, H., Hubl, W., Waldhoer, T., and Lochs, H.,** Intestinal permeability and the predictor of relapse in Crohn's disease, *Lancet*, 341, 1437, 1993.

59. **Sutherland, L. R., Verhoef, M., Wallace, J. L., Rosendaahl, G. V., Crutcher, R., and Meddings, J. B.,** A simple, non-invasive marker of gastric damage: sucrose permeability, *Lancet*, 343, 998, 1994.

60. **Jenkins, A. P., Nukajam, W. S., Menzies, I. S., and Creamer, B.,** Simultaneous administration of lactulose and $^{51}$Cr-ethylenediaminetetraacetic acid. A test to distinguish colonic from small-intestinal permeability change, *Scand. J. Gastroenterol.*, 27, 769, 1992.

61. **Jenkins, A. P., Trew, D. R., Crump, B. J., Menzies, I. S., and Creamer, B.,** Do nonsteroidal anti-inflammatory drugs increase colonic permeability?, *Gut*, 32, 66, 1991.

62. **Qvist, H., Somasundaram, S., Macpherson, A., Menzies, I. S., Giercksky, K., and Bjarnason, I.,** The effect of pelvic radiation on small and large intestinal absorption and permeability in humans, *Gastroenterology*, 106, A430, 1994.

63. **Teahon, K., Smith, T., Smethurst, P., and Bjarnason, I.,** A technique for localizing alterations of intestinal permeability in man, *Gastroenterology*, 100, A251, 1991.

64. **Maxton, D. G., Catt, S. D., and Menzies, I. S.,** Intestinal disaccharidases assessed in congenital asucrasia by differential urinary disaccharide excretion, *Dig. Dis. Sci.*, 34, 129, 1989.

65. **Maxton, D. G., Catt, S. D., and Menzies, I. S.,** Combined assessment of intestinal disaccharidases in congenital asucrasia by differential urinary disaccharide excretion, *J. Clin. Pathol.*, 43, 406, 1990.

66. **Bjarnason, I., Smethurst, P., Batt, R., Catt, S., Maxton, D., and Menzies, I. S.,** Differential urine excretion of disaccharides for the non-invasive assessment of intestinal disaccharidase activities: effects of α-glucosidase inhibitors and primary hypolactasia, and the correlation between *in vivo* and *in vitro* measurements of sucrase, lactase and isomaltase activity in patients with coeliac disease, submitted, 1995.

67. **Ford, R. P. K., Menzies, I. S., Phillips, A. D., Walker-Smith, J. A., and Turner, M. W.,** Intestinal sugar permeability: relationship to diarrheal disease and small bowel morphology, *J. Pediatr. Gastroenterol. Nutr.*, 4, 568, 1985.

68. **Walker, A. W. and Isselbacher, K. J.,** Uptake and transport of macromolecules by the intestine. Possible role in clinical disorders, *Gastroenterology*, 67, 531, 1974.

69. **Walker, W. A.,** Mechanisms of antigen handling by the gut, *Clin. Immunol. Allergy*, 2, 15, 1982.

70. **Sanderson, I. R. and Walker, W. A.,** Uptake and transport of macromolecules by the intestine: possible role in clinical disorders (an update), *Gastroenterology*, 104, 622, 1993.

71. **Bjarnason, I., Macpherson, A., Somasundaram, S., and Teahon, K.,** Nonsteroidal anti-inflammatory drugs and inflammatory bowel disease, *Can. J. Gastroenterol.*, 7, 160, 1993.

72. **Bjarnason, I., Macpherson, A. J. S., Somasundaram, S., and Teahon, K.,** Non-steroidal anti-inflammatory drugs and Crohn's disease, in *Inflammatory Bowel Diseases: Pathophysiology as Basis of Treatment*, Scholmeric, J., Kruis, W., Goebbell, H., Hohenberger, W., and Gross, V., Eds., Falk Symposium No. 67, Kluwer Academic Publishers, Lancaster, 1993, 208.

73. **Bjarnason, I., Hayllar, J., Macpherson, A. J., and Russell, A. S.,** Side effects of nonsteroidal anti-inflammatory drugs on the small and large intestine, *Gastroenterology*, 104, 1832, 1993.

74. **Auer, I. O., Habscheid, W., Hiller, S., Gerhards, W., and Eilles, C.,** Nicht-steroidale antiphlogistika erhohen die darmpermeabilitat, *Dtsch. Med. Wochenschr.*, 112, 1032, 1987.

75. **Bjarnason, I., Williams, P., Smethurst, P., Peters, T. J., and Levi, A. J.,** The effect of NSAIDs and prostaglandins on the permeability of the human small intestine, *Gut*, 27, 1292, 1986.

76. **Bjarnason, I., Smethurst, P., Clarke, P., Menzies, I. S., Levi, A. J., and Peters, T. J.,** Effect of prostaglandins on indomethacin induced increased intestinal permeability in humans, *Scand. J. Gastroenterol.*, 29 (Suppl. 164), 97, 1989.

77. **Bjarnason, I., Fehilly, B., Smethurst, P., Menzies, I. S., and Levi, A. J.,** The importance of local versus systemic effects of non-steroidal anti-inflammatory drugs to increase intestinal permeability in humans, *Gut*, 32, 275, 1991.

78. **Bjarnason, I., Smethurst, P., Macpherson, A., Walker, F., McElnay, J. C., Passmore, A. P., and Menzies, I. S.,** Glucose and citrate reduce the permeability changes caused by indomethacin in humans, *Gastroenterology*, 102, 1546, 1992.

79. **Bjarnason, I., Smethurst, P., Fenn, G. C., Lee, C. F., Menzies, I. S., and Levi, A. J.,** Misoprostol reduces indomethacin induced changes in human small intestinal permeability, *Dig. Dis. Sci.*, 34, 407, 1989.

80. **Jenkins, R. T., Rooney, P. J., Jones, D. B., Bienenstock, J., and Goodacre, R. L.,** Increased intestinal permeability in patients with rheumatoid arthritis. A side effect of nonsteroidal antiinflammatory drug therapy, *Br. J. Rheumatol.*, 26, 103, 1987.

81. **Aabakken, L. and Osnes, M.,** $^{51}$Cr-ethylenediaminetetraacetic acid absorption test. Effects of naproxen, a non-steroidal, antiinflammatory drug, *Scand. J. Gastroenterol.*, 25, 917, 1990.

82. **Bjarnason, I., Smethurst, P., Menzies, I. S., and Peters, T. J.,** The effect of polyacrylic acid polymers (carbopol) on small intestinal function and permeability changes caused by indomethacin, *Scand. J. Gastroenterol.*, 26, 685, 1991.

83. **Davies, G. R. and Rampton, D. S.,** The pro-drug sulindac may reduce the risk of intestinal damage associated with the use of conventional non-steroidal anti-inflammatory drugs, *Aliment Pharmacol. Ther.*, 5, 593, 1991.

84. **Aabakken, L., Larsen, S., and Osnes, K.,** Sucralfate for prevention of naproxen-induced mucosal lesions, *Scand. J. Rheumatol.*, 18, 361, 1989.

85. **Aabakken, L., Larsen, S., and Osnes, M.,** Cimetidine tablets or suspension in the prevention of gastrointestinal mucosal lesions caused by nonsteroidal anti-inflammatory drugs, *Scand. J. Rheumatol.*, 18, 647, 1989.

86. **Levine, R. A., Petokas, S., Nandi, J., and Enthoven, D.,** Effects of nonsteroidal anti-inflammatory drugs on gastrointestinal injury and prostanoid generation in healthy volunteers, *Dig. Dis. Sci.*, 33, 660, 1988.

87. **Ligumski, M., Golanska, E. M., Hansen, D. G., and Kauffman, G. L.,** Aspirin can inhibit gastric mucosal cyclo-oxygenase without causing lesions in the rat, *Gastroenterology*, 84, 756, 1983.

88. **Rainsford, K. D.,** The biochemical pathology of aspirin induced gastric damage, *Agents Actions*, 5, 326, 1975.

89. **Redfern, J. S. and Feldman, M.,** Role of prostaglandins in preventing gastrointestinal ulceration: induction of ulcers by antibodies to prostaglandins, *Gastroenterology*, 96, 596, 1989.

90. **Whittle, B. J. R.,** Temporal relationship between cyclooxygenase inhibition, as measured by prostacyclin biosynthesis, and gastrointestinal damage induced by indomethacin in the rat, *Gastroenterology*, 80, 94, 1981.

91. **Brune, K., Dietzel, K., Nurnberg, B., and Schneider, H.-Th.,** Recent insight into the mechanism of gastrointestinal tract ulceration, *Scand. J. Rheumatol.*, 65 (Suppl.), 135, 1987.

92. **Del Soldato, P., Foschi, D., Benoni, G., and Velo, G. P.,** Early and late phases in the formation by anti-inflammatory drugs of intestinal lesions in the rat, in *Side Effects of Antiinflammatory Drugs*, Rainsford, K. D. and Velo, G. P., Eds., MTP Press, Lancaster, 1987, 67.

93. **Duggan, D. E., Hooke, K. F., Noll, R. M., and Kwan, C. K.,** Enterohepatic circulation of indomethacin and its role in intestinal irritation, *Biochem. Pharmacol.*, 25, 1749, 1975.

94. **Fang, W.-F., Broughton, A., and Jacobson, E. D.,** Indomethacin-induced intestinal inflammation, *Dig. Dis. Sci.*, 22, 187, 1977.

95. **Kent, T. H., Cardeli, R. M., and Stanler, F. U.,** Small intestinal ulcers and intestinal flora in rats given indomethacin, *Am. J. Pathol.*, 54, 237, 1969.

96. **Melrange, R., Moore, G., Blower, P. R., Coates, M. E., Ward, F. W., and Ronaasen, V.,** A comparison of indomethacin with ibuprufen on gastrointestinal mucosal integrity in conventional and germ free rats, *Aliment Pharmacol. Ther.*, 6, 67, 1992.

97. **Robert, A. and Asano, T.,** Resistance of germ free rats to indomethacin-induced intestinal lesions, *Prostaglandins*, 14, 331, 1977.

98. **Satoh, H., Guth, P. H., and Grossman, M. I.,** Role of bacteria in gastric ulceration produced by indomethacin in the rat: cytoprotective action of antibiotics, *Gastroenterology*, 84, 483, 1983.

99. **Rainsford, K. D.,** Mucosal lesions induced in the rat intestinal tract by the anti-inflammatory drug, Wy-41,770, a weak inhibitor of prostaglandin synthesis, contrasted with those from the potent prostaglandin inhibitor, indomethecin, *Toxicol. Pathol.*, 16, 366, 1988.

100. **Bjarnason, I., Hayllar, J., Smethurst, P., Price, A. B., Menzies, I. S., and Gumpel, M. J.,** Metronidazole reduces inflammation and blood loss in NSAID enteropathy, *Gut*, 33, 1204, 1992.

101. **Teahon, K. and Bjarnason, I.,** Comparison of leukocyte excretion and blood loss in inflammatory disease of the bowel, *Gut*, 34, 1535, 1993.

102. **Bjarnason, I., Zanelli, G., Smith, T., Prouse, P., Williams, P., DeLacey, G., Gumpel, M. J., and Levi, A. J.,** Nonsteroidal antiinflammatory drug induced intestinal inflammation in humans, *Gastroenterology*, 93, 480, 1987.

103. **Rooney, P. J., Jenkins, R. T., Smith, K. M., and Coates, G.,** 111-Indium-labelled polymorphonuclear scans in rheumatoid arthritis — an important clinical cause of positive results, *Br. J. Rheumatol.*, 15, 167, 1986.

104. **Segall, A. W., Isenberg, D. A., Hajirousow, V., Tolfree, S., Clark, J., and Snaith, M. L.,** Preliminary evidence for gut involvement in the pathogenesis of rheumatoid arthritis?, *Br. J. Rheumatol.*, 25, 162, 1986.

105. **Morris, A. J., Wasson, L. A., and Mackenzie, J. F.,** Small bowel enteroscopy in undiagnosed gastrointestinal blood loss, *Gut*, 33, 887, 1992.

106. **Allison, M. C., Howatson, A. G., Torrance, C. J., Lee, F. D., and Russell, R. I.,** Gastrointestinal damage associated with the use of nonsteroidal anti-inflammatory drugs, *N. Engl. J. Med.*, 327, 749, 1992.

107. **Bjarnason, I., Zanelli, G., Prouse, P., Smethurst, P., Levi, S., Gumpel, M. J., and Levi, A. J.,** Blood and protein loss via small intestinal inflammation induced by nonsteroidal anti-inflammatory drugs, *Lancet*, 2, 711, 1987.

108. **Hayllar, J., Price, A. B., Smith, T., Macpherson, A., Gumpel, M. J., and Bjarnason, I.,** Nonsteroidal antiinflammatory drug-induced small intestinal inflammation and blood loss: effect of sulphasalazine and other disease modifying drugs, *Arthritis Rheum.*, 37, 1146, 1994.

109. **Bjarnason, I., Zanelli, G., Smethurst, P., Burke, M., Gumpel, M. J., Price, A. B., and Levi, A. J.,** Clinico-pathological features of nonsteroidal antiinflammatory drug induced small intestinal strictures, *Gastroenterology*, 94, 1070, 1988.

110. **Lang, J., Price, A. B., Levi, A. J., Burk, M., Gumpel, J. M., and Bjarnason, I.,** Diaphragm disease: the pathology of non-steroidal anti-inflammatory drug induced small intestinal strictures, *J. Clin. Pathol.*, 41, 516, 1988.

111. **Halter, F., Weber, B., Huber, T., Eigenmann, F., Frey, M., and Rutchi, C.,** Diaphragm disease of the ascending colon associated with sustained release diclofenac, *J. Clin. Gastroenterol.*, 16, 74, 1993.

112. **Huber, T., Ruchti, C., and Halter, F.,** Nonsteroidal antiinflammatory drug-induced colonic strictures: a case report, *Gastroenterology*, 100, 1119, 1992.

113. **Sheers, R. and Williams, W. R.,** NSAIDs and gut damage, *Lancet*, ii, 1154, 1989.

114. **Fellows, I. W., Clarke, J. M., and Roberts, P. F.,** Non-steroidal anti-inflammatory drug-induced jejunal and colonic diaphragm disease: a report of two cases, *Gut*, 33, 1424, 1992.

115. **Monahan, W., Starnes, E. C., and Parker, A. L.,** Colonic strictures in a patient on long-term non-steroidal anti-inflammatory drugs, *Gastrointest. Endosc.*, 38, 385, 1992.

116. **Sturges, H. F. and Krone, C. L.,** Ulcers and strictures of the jejunum in a patient on long term indomethacin therapy, *Am. J. Gastroenterol.*, 59, 162, 1973.

117. **Neoptolemos, J. P. and Locke, T. J.,** Recurrent small bowel obstruction associated with phenylbutazone, *Br. J. Surg.*, 70, 244, 1983.

118. **Madhok, R., Mackenzie, J. A., Lee, F. D., Bruckner, F. E., Terry, T. R., and Sturrock, R. D.,** Small bowel ulceration in patients receiving NSAIDs for rheumatoid arthritis, *Q. J. Med.*, 58, 53, 1986.

119. **Saverymuttu, S. H., Thomas, A., Grundy, A., and Maxwell, J. D.,** Ileal stricturing after long term indomethacin treatment, *Postgrad. Med. J.*, 62, 267, 1986.

120. **Sukumar, L.,** Recurrent small bowel obstruction with piroxicam, *Br. J. Surg.*, 74, 186, 1987.

121. **Johnson, F.,** Recurrent small bowel obstruction with piroxicam, *Br. J. Surg.*, 74, 654, 1987.

122. **Budillon, G., Parrilli, G., Pacella, M., Cuomo, R., and Menzies, I. S.,** Investigation of intestine and liver function in cirrhosis using combined sugar oral loads, *J. Hepatol.*, 1, 513, 1985.

123. **Romiti, A., Merli, M., Martorano, M., Parilli, G., Martino, F., Riggio, O., Trucelli, A., Copocaccia L., and Budillion, G.,** Malabsorption and nutritional abnormalities in patients with liver cirrhosis, *Ital. J. Gastroenterol.*, 22, 118, 1990.

124. **Bac, D. J., Swart, R., van der Berg, J. W. O., and Wilson, J. H. P.,** Small bowel wall function in patients with advanced liver cirrhosis and portal hypertension: studies on permeability and luminal bacterial overgrowth, *Eur. J. Gastroenterol. Hepatol.*, 5, 383, 1993.

125. **Wicks, C., Somasundaram, S., Menzies, I. S., Bjarnason, I., and Williams, R.,** Intestinal function and postoperative enteral nutrition following liver transplants, *Gut*, 34 (Suppl. 1), S65, 1993.

126. **Smethurst, P., Menzies, I. S., Levi, A. J., and Bjarnason, I.,** Is alcohol directly toxic to the small bowel mucosa?, *Clin. Sci.*, 75, 50, 1988.

127. **Aabakken, L.,** $^{51}$Cr ethylenediaminetetraacetic acid absorption test. Methodological aspects, *Scand. J. Gastroenterol.*, 24, 351, 1989.

128. **Robinson, G. M., Orrego, H., Israel, Y., Deveny, P., and Kapur, B. M.,** Low-molecular weight polyethylene glycol as a probe of gastrointestinal permeability after alcohol ingestion, *Dig. Dis. Sci.*, 26, 23, 1981.

129. **Worthington, B. S., Meserole, L., and Syrotuck, J. A.,** Effect of daily ethanol ingestion on intestinal permeability to macromolecules, *Dig. Dis. Sci.*, 23, 23, 1978.

130. **Bode, C., Vollmer, E., Hug, J., and Bode, J. C.,** Increased permeability of the gut to polyethylene glycol and dextran in rats fed alcohol, *Ann. N.Y. Acad. Sci.*, 625, 837, 1991.

131. **Bjarnason, I., Smethurst, P., Levi, A. J., and Peters, T. J.,** Intestinal permeability to $^{51}$CrEDTA in rats with experimentally induced enteropathy, *Gut*, 26, 579, 1985.

132. **Parrilli, G., Iaffaioli, R. V., Martorano, M., Cuomo, R., Tafuto, S., Zampino, M. G., Budillon, G., and Bianco, A. R.,** Effects of anthracycline therapy on intestinal absorption in patients with advanced breast cancer, *Cancer Res.*, 49, 3689, 1989.

133. **Pledger, J. V., Pearson, A. D. J., Craft, A. W., Laker, M. F., and Eastham, E. J.,** Intestinal permeability during chemotherapy for childhood tumors, *Eur. J. Pediatr.*, 147, 123, 1988.

134. **Pearson, A. D. J., Craft, A. W., Pledger, J. V., Eastham, E. J., Laker, M. F., and Pearson, C. S.,** Small bowel function in acute lymphoblastic leukemia, *Arch. Dis. Child*, 59, 460, 1984.

135. **Selby, P. J., Lopes, N., Mundy, J., Crofts, M., Millar, J. L., and McElwain, T. J.,** Cyclophosphomide priming reduces intestinal damage in humans following high dose melphalan chemotherapy, *Br. J. Cancer*, 55, 531, 1987.

136. **Cooper, B. T., Ukabam, S. O., O'Brien, I. A. D., Hara, J. P. O., and Corrall, R. J. M.,** Intestinal permeability in diabetic diarrhoea, *Diabetic Med.*, 4, 49, 1987.

137. **Ohri, S. K., Somasundaram, S., Koak, Y., Macpherson, A., Keogh, B. E., Taylor, K. M., Menzies, I. S., and Bjarnason, I.,** The effect of intestinal hypoperfusion during cardiopulmonary bypass surgery on saccharide permeation and intestinal permeability in humans, *Gastroenterology*, 106, 318, 1994.

138. **Otamiri, T., Sjodahl, R., and Tagesson, C.,** An experimental model for studying reversible intestinal ischemia, *Acta Chir. Scand.*, 153, 51, 1987.

139. **Roumen, R. M., van der Vliet, J. A., Wevers, R. A., and Goris, R. J.,** Intestinal permeability is increased after major vascular surgery, *J. Vasc. Surg.*, 17, 734, 1993.

140. **Coltart, R. S., Howard, G. C., Wraight, E. P., and Bleehen, N. M.,** The effect of hyperthermia and radiation on small bowel permeability using $^{51}$Cr EDTA and $^{14}$C mannitol in humans, *Int. J. Hyperthermia*, 4, 467, 1988.

141. **Ruppin, H., Hotze, A., During, A., Reichert, M., Bauer, J., Stoll, R., Herbst, M., and Mahlstedt, J.,** Reversible funktionsstorungen des intestinaltraktes durch abdominelle strahlentherapy, *Z. Gastroenterol.*, 25, 261, 1987.

142. **Yeoh, E. K., Horowitz, M., Russo, A., Muecke, T., Robb, T., and Chatterton, B. E.,** Gastrointestinal function in chronic radiation enteritis — effects of loperamide-N-oxide, *Gut*, 34, 476, 1993.

143. **Kardossis, T., Joseph, A. E. A., Gane, J. N., and Bridges, C. E., Griffin, G. E.,** Fecal leucocytosis. Indium-111 labelled autologous polymorphonuclear leukocyte abdominal scanning, and quantitative fecal indium-111 excretion in acute gastroenteritis and enteropathogen carriage, *Dig. Dis. Sci.*, 33, 1383, 1988.

144. **Leclercq-Foucart, J., Forget, P., Sodoyez-Gouffaux, F., and Zappitelli, A.,** Intestinal permeability to $^{51}$CrEDTA in children with cystic fibrosis, *J. Pediatr. Gastroenterol. Nutr.*, 5, 384, 1986.

145. **Leclercq-Foucart, J., Forget, P., and Van Cutsem, J. L.,** Lactulose-rhamnose intestinal permeability in children with cystic fibrosis, *J. Pediatr. Gastroenterol. Nutr.*, 6, 66, 1987.

146. **Dalzell, A. M., Freestone, N. S., Billington, D., and Heaf, D. P.,** Small intestinal permeability and orocaecal transit time in cystic fibrosis, *Arch. Dis. Child*, 65, 585, 1990.

147. **Escobar, H., Perdomo, M., Vasconez, F., Camarero, C., del Olmo, M. T., and Suarez, L.,** Intestinal permeability to $^{51}$Cr-EDTA and orocecal transit time in cystic fibrosis, *J. Pediatr. Gastroenterol. Nutr.*, 14, 204, 1992.

148. **Pignata, C., Budillon, G., Monaco, G., Nani, E., Cuomo, R., Parrilli, G., and Ciccimarra, F.,** Jejunal bacterial overgrowth and intestinal permeability in children with immunodeficiency syndromes, *Gut*, 31, 879, 1990.

149. **Teahon, K., Webster, A. D., Price, A. B., and Bjarnason, I.,** Studies of gastrointestinal structure and function in patients with primary hypogammaglobulinaemia, *Gut*, 35, 1244, 1994.

150. **Keating, J., Bjarnason, I., Somasundaram, S., Macpherson, A., Francis, N., Price, A. B., Sharpstone, D., Smithson, J., Menzies, I. S., and Gazzard, I. S.,** Intestinal absorptive capacity, intestinal permeability and jejunal histology in HIV infected patients and their relation to diarrhea, *Gut,* in press, 1995.

151. **Lim, S. G., Menzies, I. S., Lee, C. A., Johnson, M. A., and Pounder, R. E.,** Intestinal permeability and function in patients infected with human immunodeficiency virus, *Scand. J. Gastroenterol.*, 28, 573, 1993.

152. **Bjarnason, I., Somasundaram, S., MacManus, T., and Macpherson, A.,** Small intestinal permeability and inflammation in HIV infected patients, *Gastroenterology*, 104, A670, 1993.

# 13

# Gastrointestinal Motility Disorders Induced by Ethanol

Ali Keshavarzian and Jeremy Z. Fields

## CONTENTS

## 13.1    INTRODUCTION

Both acute and chronic consumption of alcohol (ethanol) have been reported to cause significant gastrointestinal (GI) symptoms.[1-4] These symptoms include chest pain, heartburn, and other symptoms of gastroesophageal reflux, nausea, vomiting, postprandial fullness, and diarrhea.[4,5] Each of these symptoms could be a consequence of the effects of ethanol either on the GI mucosal lining and/or on GI motility. For example, the above mentioned symptoms are known to be associated not only with GI mucosal diseases such as ulceration and inflammation, but also have been noted in patients with GI dysmotility.[6,7] Indeed, these symptoms have been reported in alcoholic subjects that have intact gastroduodenal mucosal integrity.[8] Hence, GI dysmotility may be responsible, at least in part, for the various GI symptoms that have been reported after either acute or chronic alcohol ingestion.

Alcohol-induced GI dysmotility should not be a surprising finding since it is already known that ethanol can profoundly affect the function of both muscles and nerves in various organs.[9-14] Moreover, abnormalities in GI motor function and transit have been observed following either acute or chronic exposure to ethanol. It should be noted, however, that these motor abnormalities are not necessarily associated with symptoms.[1-3,15] Regardless, it appears that alcohol can affect motor functions of all segments of the GI tract. Additionally, the effects of acute and chronic ethanol on GI motility may profoundly differ.

The following sections will separately discuss the effects of ethanol on motor functions of esophagus, stomach, small and large intestine, and finally gallbladder and biliary tree. For each segment our discussions will include first the clinical picture, and then the *in vivo* and *in vitro* effects of both acute and chronic ethanol on motility of the organ.

## 13.2    ETHANOL-INDUCED ESOPHAGEAL DYSMOTILITY

### 13.2.1    Clinical Picture

#### 13.2.1.1    Acute Exposure to Ethanol

GI symptoms related to esophageal disorders such as postprandial chest pain and heartburn are believed to occur after an acute alcohol binge.[16] However, the authors found no reports of any systematic study evaluating the frequency and severity of these symptoms after an alcohol binge. On the other hand, it has been reported that acute exposure to alcohol can induce gastroesophageal reflux (GER) both postprandially[17] and nocturnally.[18]

Kaufman and co-workers[17] gave 180 ml of 100 proof vodka to 12 volunteers and then recorded GER of acid for 3 h after a meal. Blood alcohol levels (BAL) ranged from 63 to 129 mg/dl. Eleven of 12 of these subjects (92%) developed postprandial reflux after drinking alcohol while none of the 12 had GER when alcohol was not ingested. Vitale et al.[18] observed prolonged, nocturnal GER of acid in 7 of 17 volunteers (41%) who had consumed 120 ml of whisky 3 h after dinner. The maximum reflux occurred approximately 3 h after alcohol consumption. Impaired esophageal acid clearance at night was also noted after drinking alcohol.

These observations suggest that symptoms associated with acid reflux such as heartburn should be expected after alcohol consumption, and yet the majority of volunteers who developed GER did not complain of any heartburn.[17,18] Nonetheless, it is well accepted that patients with gastroesophageal reflux disease experience their symptoms more severely and more frequently after drinking alcohol.[19] The mechanism of ethanol-induced GER is not fully established. One possibility is ethanol-induced esophageal dysmotility which will be discussed in Section 13.2.2.

### 13.2.1.2   Chronic Exposure to Ethanol

Unlike acute exposure to ethanol, GI symptoms related to esophageal disorders are well documented following chronic exposure to ethanol.[4,5] Wegener et al.[5] reported chest pain in 17% of 46 alcoholics. Fields and co-workers[4] reported heartburn and chest pain in 33 and 14%, respectively, in 48 actively drinking alcoholics. These symptoms were reported significantly more often by alcoholics than by 48 control subjects (10% and 0%, respectively) and they resolved in the majority of alcoholics after a few weeks of sobriety. The underlying mechanism for these symptoms could be esophagitis, but only 1 of 18 actively drinking alcoholics had mild, microscopic esophagitis.[20] Another possibility is ethanol-induced esophageal dysmotility which will be discussed in Section 13.2.2.

The other major esophageal symptom that is sometimes experienced by alcoholics is difficulty in swallowing (dysphagia). Although dysphagia reportedly occurred more frequently in alcoholics than in controls (4% vs. 2%), this difference was not statistically significant.[4] Dysphagia in these alcoholics was transient and resolved completely after a short period of sobriety. Hence, the most likely explanation is esophageal dysmotility. However, none of the alcoholics with documented esophageal dysmotility complained of dysphagia.[20-23] Nonetheless, clinically significant dysphagia does sometime occur in alcoholics. Hodes and Korsten[24] reported a case of an alcoholic subject with dysphagia and "corkscrew esophagus." The manometric finding of this case can be labeled as "nutcracker esophagus." This manometric abnormality was subsequently reported in a group of asymptomatic alcoholics.[20,21] Additionally, transient pharyngeal dysphasia was reported by Weber et al.[25] in an alcoholic subject with myopathy who also appeared to have pharyngeal/upper esophageal sphincter dysfunction. Also, Howell[26] reported a fatal, progressive case of alcoholic myopathy who also had pharyngeal dysphasia. Hence, dysphagia, although it can occur in alcoholics, is rare and appears to be due to myopathy and pharyngeal/upper esophageal sphincter dysfunction rather than to esophageal dysmotility.

## 13.2.2   Esophageal Motility and Transit Studies

### 13.2.2.1   Acute Exposure to Ethanol

The clinical picture suggests, and reports confirm, that acute ethanol can induce esophageal dysmotility. For example, Mayer et al.[27] observed esophageal dysmotility in humans following acute exposure to ethanol. These abnormalities included a modest decrease in amplitude of esophageal contraction in both proximal and distal segments of the esophagus. Velocity and duration of esophageal contractions were not affected by ethanol. While ethanol did not affect resting lower esophageal sphincter (LES) pressure when studied 30 min after ethanol ingestion, it did blunt the rise in LES pressure in response to pentagastrin or to protein meals.[27] The effect of ethanol on esophageal motility occurred only when BAL levels were greater than 77 mg/dl. Also, the effect of ethanol appears to be systemic since p.o. and i.v. ethanol had similar effects. Additionally, there was no correlation between the magnitude of any of these effects and either BAL (range: 59 to 117 mg/dl) or administered dose of ethanol (range: 30 to 80 g). Hogan et al.[28] also evaluated the effect of acute ethanol on esophageal motility of both primary peristalsis and distension-induced secondary esophageal peristalsis. They, too, found a modest decrease in esophageal amplitude after ingestion of 300 ml of whisky over a 1-h period. They also noted that alcohol decreased the number of primary and distension-induced secondary esophageal peristaltic waves. In contrast to the report of Mayer et al.,[27] Hogan and co-workers[28] observed that basal LES pressure decreased from 17 to 9 mm Hg immediately after ethanol exposure. Again, no correlation was found between the magnitude of motility changes and BAL. This ethanol-induced esophageal dysmotility was reversible as no abnormality was noted 8 h after exposure to ethanol.

Recently, Keshavarzian et al.[21] evaluated the effect of acute ethanol on esophageal motility using a continuously perfused, low compliance motility apparatus with a manometric catheter equipped with a sleeve. This system can provide accurate and reproducible monitoring of LES pressure over several hours. They observed that intravenous ethanol transiently decreased LES pressure. LES pressure returned to normal after 30 min thus explaining the lack of inhibition of ethanol on LES pressure reported previously.[27] Again, a modest decrease in esophageal contraction amplitude was noted. All three studies demonstrate a deleterious effect of acute ethanol on esophageal motility, one which could increase the chance of GER and hamper the ability of the esophagus to cleanse refluxed acid, thereby explaining the observed GER induced by ethanol.[17,18]

The underlying mechanism of ethanol-induced esophageal dysmotility is not clear. In an attempt to better understand this mechanism, Keshavarzian et al.[29] evaluated the effect of acute intravenous ethanol (0.5 to 1.5 g/kg) on esophageal motility in cats. Feline esophageal abnormalities were similar to human ones. Acute ethanol decreased LES pressure and resulted in prolonged, low amplitude esophageal contractions.[29] Chronic ethanol appeared to result in tolerance to these acute effects of ethanol since acute ethanol had significantly less marked effects on esophageal contractions in cats previously exposed to daily alcohol for a minimum of 30 days.[29] The inhibitory effect of ethanol on LES pressure appeared to be predominantly due to its direct effect on muscle since tetrodotoxin, at a dose selective for neurotoxicity, did not prevent the inhibition. There was a weak and nonsignificant correlation ($r = 0.25$) between BAL and ethanol-induced dysmotility.

In contrast to the above effects of ethanol on LES and on distal esophagus areas containing smooth muscle, acute ethanol had no effect on amplitude of esophageal contractions of proximal esophagus, a segment of the esophagus that contains striated muscle.[29] However, ethanol did prolong and slow contraction of the proximal esophagus. Such an abnormality could disrupt normal transit of liquid or solid boluses in proximal esophagus. This abnormality in cats may, therefore, be analogous to the pharyngeal/upper esophageal functional abnormalities that were reported in two actively drinking alcoholics.[25,26] However, the effect of acute ethanol on the pharynx, upper esophageal sphincter and the striated portion of the upper esophagus in humans has not been reported.

*In vitro* studies are required to further evaluate the mechanism of esophageal dysmotility induced by acute ethanol. Fox and Daniel[30] observed inhibitory effects of ethanol on tension of LES muscle strips. Jacyno et al.[31] showed that ethanol at a concentration of 75 m$M$ significantly decreased resting LES tension in LES strips (–30%) in cats. Additionally, ethanol significantly increased the "on response relaxation" in these LES strips (–465 to –682 mg) that follows electrical field stimulation (EFS). Furthermore, ethanol inhibited the EFS-induced "off response contraction" of LES by 69%. Ethanol also dose dependently inhibited maximal carbachol-induced strip tension. This inhibition (–37%) was significant at 25 m$M$ ethanol and reached a maximum inhibition (–50%) at 75 m$M$ with, in fact, less inhibition (–36%) at 100 m$M$ ethanol. The magnitude of *in vitro* ethanol inhibition of LES muscle strips was similar to the magnitude of ethanol inhibition of LES pressure previously observed *in vivo*. Experiments on smooth muscle strips isolated from the distal esophagus also revealed an inhibition by ethanol. However, the inhibitory effects of ethanol were more substantial on the LES. A similar contrast was found during *in vivo* studies in that the magnitude of inhibition of LES pressure was more pronounced than the inhibition of the amplitude of distal esophageal contractions. For example, Mayer et al.[27] showed that the threshold for inhibition of LES pressure was a BAL of 70 mg/dl while the BAL level was 90 mg/dl for inhibition of contraction of the esophageal body. The ability of ethanol to inhibit contractility of isolated esophageal smooth muscle strips *in vitro* strongly suggests that the inhibitory effect of ethanol on esophageal motility is mediated through a direct effect of ethanol on the esophagus rather than through indirect mechanisms involving the CNS.

To determine whether these direct effects of ethanol on the esophagus are mediated by esophageal nerve or muscle, Fields et al.[32] evaluated the effect of ethanol on muscle tension in the presence of tetrodotoxin (1 μ$M$). Tetrodotoxin partially but significantly prevented ethanol's potentiation of the EFS-induced on response relaxation. However, it did not affect the ability of ethanol to inhibit the EFS-induced off response contraction. Similarly, ethanol inhibition of carbachol-induced LES tension was not affected by tetrodotoxin. These data indicate that some aspects of ethanol-induced inhibition of LES contractility are neurally mediated while other aspects appear to be due to direct effects of ethanol on esophageal muscle. The neurally mediated effects of ethanol could be through nitric oxide containing nerves since the nitric oxide synthase inhibitor L-NNA prevented the inhibition.[32] Recent studies by Muska et al.[33] support the idea that ethanol can have a direct inhibitory effect on esophageal smooth muscle since they demonstrated that acute ethanol inhibits carbachol-induced shortening of isolated muscle cells from both LES and esophageal body.

In summary, acute consumption of ethanol inhibits esophageal contractility. This effect is a result of interactions of ethanol with both esophageal muscles and their neural plexuses. This dysmotility could result in functional impairment of the esophagus that predisposes the esophagus to GER.

### 13.2.2.2 Chronic Exposure to Ethanol

Winship et al.[23] were the first to report esophageal dysmotility in chronic alcoholics. The abnormalities included nonperistaltic, low amplitude, distal esophageal contractions with normal LES pressure. This dysmotility, however, was observed only in alcoholics with peripheral neuropathy. The observed abnormality could therefore be secondary to peripheral neuropathy rather than to alcoholism. Indeed, Fischer et al.[34] reported similar findings in a group of patients with neuropathy, only some of whom had alcoholic neuropathy. It is important to note that Winship et al.[23] studied alcoholics 3 to 6 weeks after cessation of drinking. None of these patients had esophageal symptoms in spite of abnormal esophageal motility. Hodes and Korsten[24] reported a patient with dysphagia and persistent corkscrew esophagus who happened to be an actively drinking alcoholic. The manometric recording of the esophagus of this patient demonstrated high amplitude peristaltic contractions compatible with nutcracker esophagus.

Keshavarzian et al.[20] reported high amplitude peristaltic contractions in 9 of 18 actively drinking alcoholics 2 to 3 days after admission to the detoxification unit. LES pressure was also elevated in these patients. These abnormalities were transient and esophageal motility returned to normal after 3 to 4 weeks of sobriety. Esophageal dysmotility was noted in patients without neuropathy and was associated with delayed esophageal transit. Keshavarzian et al.[21] subsequently reported increased LES pressure and increased amplitude of esophageal contractions in an additional 13 actively drinking alcoholics. Again, the majority of alcoholics (77%) had esophageal dysmotility including 38% of patients with nutcracker esophagus. High amplitude esophageal contractions and elevated LES pressures appear to result from alcohol withdrawal since esophageal motility returned to normal immediately following i.v. administration of ethanol (0.8 g/kg). Similar findings were noted for secondary esophageal contractions.[35] In withdrawing alcoholics, acid-induced secondary esophageal contractions, similar to primary esophageal contractions, were prolonged and of high amplitude. Silver et al.[22] also noted high LES pressures in alcoholics which were reversible and which returned to normal values after a period of sobriety. They did not, however, observe nutcracker esophagus in their alcoholics. Instead, increased tertiary contractions were the common abnormality seen in their patients.

The mechanism of esophageal dysmotility in chronic alcoholics is not clear. One possibility is that the esophagus, similar to the CNS, undergoes a "withdrawal syndrome." That is, if acute ethanol causes inhibition of esophageal contractility (as discussed above), and if chronic ethanol results in tolerance, then withdrawal from ethanol might elicit a transient hyperexcitability associated with high amplitude esophageal contractions and increased LES pressures. To demonstrate this phenomenon one needs to evaluate inebriated subjects, a study which is not ethically possible since inebriated subjects cannot give informed consent. Hence, an animal model is needed. Keshavarzian et al.[36] studied esophageal motility in cats which were given daily intragastric doses of ethanol for at least 30 days. Motility studies were done initially when cats were still inebriated (BAL of $350 \pm 166$ mg/dl), and again during withdrawal. LES pressures and amplitudes of esophageal contractions in inebriated alcoholic cats were not significantly different from controls thus demonstrating the development of tolerance to the acute inhibitory effect of ethanol on these parameters. In contrast, during withdrawal, LES pressure and amplitude of esophageal contractions were significantly higher . This hyperexcitability reached statistical significance in male cats. Thus, esophageal dysmotility in withdrawing male cats mirrors abnormalities observed in withdrawing alcoholic men. That is, withdrawal is associated with prolonged, high amplitude, peristaltic, esophageal contractions. Since inebriated alcoholic cats did not demonstrate these changes, the authors conclude that the abnormality is more a result of withdrawal rather than of chronic ethanol exposure. It is interesting that these abnormalities were noted only in male and not in female alcoholic cats. To date the authors have not found any reports evaluating esophageal motility in alcoholic women. Hence, it is not known if this gender selectivity is unique to cats. Further studies are needed to elucidate the underlying mechanism of esophageal dysmotility in alcoholics.

These studies demonstrate that esophageal dysmotility is common in actively drinking alcoholics. These abnormalities are transient, however, and resolve after a short period of sobriety. They are rarely if ever symptomatic. The functional significance of these abnormalities remains to be seen. These abnormalities are associated with delayed esophageal transit which may disturb the ability of the esophagus to clear deleterious compounds such as refluxed gastric acid or carcinogens. If so, these abnormalities may contribute to the higher incidence of esophagitis[2,3,16,37,38] and esophageal cancer[3,16] that have been documented in alcoholics.

## 13.3   ETHANOL-INDUCED GASTRIC DYSMOTILITY

### 13.3.1   Clinical Picture

#### 13.3.1.1   Acute Exposure to Ethanol

Although there has been no systematic study of the ability of acute ethanol to elicit gastric-related symptoms, it is common knowledge that nausea and vomiting can occur after excessive alcohol consumption. These symptoms could be due to acute gastric mucosal injuries which are known to occur after alcohol ingestion[2,3] or to alcohol-induced gastroparesis/dysmotility. Ethanol-induced changes in gastric emptying not only can be responsible for these undesirable symptoms, but they also can be influential in the rate of delivery and absorption of medications. Additionally, various alcoholic beverages have been used as "apertifs" and/or "digestives" which may exert their alleged desired effects through their ability to alter gastric emptying. For example, digestives could increase gastric emptying. Reports on the effects of such beverages do not support this ancient notion, however.

#### 13.3.1.2   Chronic Exposure to Ethanol

Symptoms such as nausea, vomiting, epigastric pain, and postprandial fullness, which are typically related to gastric abnormalities, are common in alcoholics.[1-5] In one study, for example, 48% of 46 alcoholics had nausea and vomiting while 41% had postprandial fullness and 30% had epigastric pain.[5] In another study, these symptoms were reported significantly more often by alcoholics than by controls.[4] For instance, 27% of 48 inebriated alcoholics reported nausea compared to only 8% of controls. Nausea became less frequent after a short period of sobriety and was then reported by only 6% of abstinent alcoholics. Similarly, vomiting (29% vs. 0%) and abdominal pain (29% vs. 8%) were reported more commonly by inebriated alcoholics than by controls. Vomiting was transient being reported by only 5% and 0% of alcoholics after 3 and 14 days of sobriety, respectively. Abdominal pain was also transient, since it was reported by only 12% and 9% of alcoholics at 3 and 14 days, respectively. These symptoms could be due to either gastroduodenal inflammation/ulceration that is commonly reported in alcoholics,[1-3] or to gastroparesis. Since these symptoms are so transient, however, they are more likely to be due to functional problems (i.e., dysmotility) rather than to tissue injury since tissue injury typically takes longer to heal. Additionally, using a sucrose absorption test, Keshavarzian et al.[8] demonstrated that gastroduodenal mucosal integrity is intact in alcoholics even though they still had the symptom of nausea.

## 13.3.2   Gastric Motility and Emptying Studies

### 13.3.2.1   Acute Exposure to Ethanol

Although reported data on the effects of acute ethanol on gastric emptying are quite variable, it appears that ethanol *per se* delays gastric emptying. This effect depends, however, on the amount and type of alcoholic beverage, and on the manner in which ethanol is administered including parameters such as the speed of ingestion and the presence of food in the stomach. This is not surprising since the frequency and severity of nausea and vomiting also appear to be variable and to depend on these factors. Hence, any evaluation of studies on the effect of acute ethanol on gastric emptying should consider these variables.

In considering studies in which ethanol was given in the form of grain alcohol (pure ethyl alcohol) to either humans or animals, alcohol-induced delayed gastric emptying was reported[39] as early as 1936 and this was subsequently confirmed by others.[40,41] Recently, using far more accurate nuclear medicine techniques to quantify gastric emptying of radiolabeled meals, Jian et al.[42] showed that ethanol (1 g/kg) infused into the stomach delayed gastric emptying of solid meals and homogenized liquid meals. Using a similar technique, Willson et al.[43] demonstrated a similar delay in gastric emptying of high calorie liquid meals in cats by alcohol (1 g/kg) given 30 min before food. Peak BAL at 60 min after alcohol administration ranged from 105 to 260 mg/dl. Inhibition of gastric emptying did not correlate with BAL. Knight et al.[44] also demonstrated that ethanol dose dependently delays gastric emptying of solid food in dogs after either oral or i.v. ethanol administration that was given just before the meal. The effect of oral ethanol was more pronounced than i.v. ethanol. Delayed gastric emptying occurred only if the BAL was greater than 80 mg/dl.

When, instead of grain alcohol, different specific alcoholic beverages are used, reported data on the effect of alcohol on gastric emptying appear to be more variable. For instance, it was reported that wine[45] and beer[46] delayed gastric emptying in some studies while whisky or brandy did not influence gastric emptying.[46,47] However, Barboriak and Meade[48] observed delayed gastric emptying in 8 control subjects following ingestion of 120 ml of whisky immediately prior to consumption of a liquid meal. Mushambi et al.[49] also demonstrated that whisky taken over 20 min, 1 h before a low calorie liquid meal, can delay gastric emptying. This effect was dose dependent and occurred after 150 ml of whisky which resulted in a BAL of 86 mg/dl, while 75 ml of whisky, which elicited a BAL of 32 mg/dl, had no effect.

In contrast to whisky, and to the above mentioned report of Pihkanen,[46] in other studies wine did not have a significant effect on gastric emptying. Moore et al.[50] were not able to demonstrate a significant effect of red wine, given with meals, on emptying of either liquid or solid meals. But, the maximum BAL achieved was only 39 mg/dl. Pfeiffer et al.,[51] using white wine, also failed to show any effect of wine on gastric emptying of liquid meals. These investigators also did not observe any abnormalities when beer was used instead of wine. In contrast, when pure alcohol was used, gastric emptying of liquid meals was delayed.[51] Unfortunately, no BAL was reported. Hence it is not known whether a sufficiently high BAL was reached after wine or beer in their studies.

Although it may appear that the type of alcoholic beverage strongly influences whether alcohol will affect gastric emptying, it may be that BAL is an even more critical factor than the type of beverage. It seems that a minimum BAL ranging between 80 to 100 mg/dl is required to delay gastric emptying. Interestingly, BAL greater than 100 mg/dl does not appear to exert additional effects.[43] Nonetheless, the contribution of congeners in various alcoholic beverages to alcohol-induced gastroparesis requires further evaluation.

Various factors could be responsible for the effect of ethanol on gastric emptying. For example, the caloric content, osmolarity, and pH of the meal are known to affect gastric emptying,[6,52] and ethanol can clearly affect these factors. Hence, delayed gastric emptying by alcohol could be due to a low pH of the test meal.[53] This is unlikely, however, since the test meals containing wine or beer were more acidic than the test meals containing grain alcohol; yet, it was the grain alcohol that resulted in delayed gastric emptying.[51]

Alcohol-induced gastroparesis does not appear to be due to the fact that ethanol increases the caloric content of the test meal since delayed gastric emptying was noted even when control test meals were made isocaloric or when the ethanol was given a half hour before the test meal.[43] Similarly, ethanol-induced changes in osmolarity of the test meal do not appear to be responsible for delayed gastric emptying because test meals containing wine or beer had much higher osmolarities than meals containing pure alcohol; yet, it was only the grain alcohol that elicited delays in gastric emptying.[51] Furthermore, the delay in gastric emptying was observed even when alcohol was given intravenously[44] or even a half hour before meals.[43] In fact, it appears that either duodenal osmoreceptors are insensitive to ethanol-induced changes in osmolarity or ethanol cannot exert significant changes in the osmolarity of the gastrointestinal lumen. This conclusion is based on the fact that Kaufman and Kaye[54] demonstrated acceleration of gastric emptying of liquids by alcohol even when the osmolarity of the control test meals was adjusted by adding dextrose and sodium chloride. This observation is not surprising since ethanol is easily and rapidly absorbed across both stomach and intestine[55-57] and thus it may not have an opportunity to exert osmotic pressure in the lumen. In addition, the findings by Kaufman and Kaye[54] that alcohol accelerates gastric emptying can be explained since the control test meals were hyperosmolar and the food therein should be emptied from the stomach more slowly than the food in the less osmotic ethanol-containing test meals.

The mechanism for alcohol-induced gastroparesis appears to be due to the effect of ethanol on gastric contractility. Knight et al.[44] observed that oral alcohol abolished or decreased the amplitude of antral contractions in dog. The inhibitory effect of alcohol on muscle contractility was also confirmed by *in vitro* studies on gastric muscle strips.[58-61] Ethanol inhibited spontaneous and acetylcholine-induced contractility of antral muscle strips from dogs. This mechanical effect appears to be due to an effect of ethanol on electrical mechanisms.[58,61] At a concentration of 0.1 to 1.0%, ethanol reduced the force and frequency of phasic contractions of gastric muscle. It also hyperpolarized resting membrane potential and reduced the amplitude, duration, and frequency of slow waves.[61] Its inhibitory effect on contractility (−60%) was much greater than its inhibitory effect on electrical activity (−28%). But, due to a steep correlation between force and membrane potential, one can still conclude that the inhibitory effect of ethanol on muscle contractility is entirely due to the effect of ethanol on membrane conductance since a 10 to 20% change in membrane potential can completely abolish contractility.[61]

The inhibitory effect of ethanol on contractility of gastric muscle could be due to its direct effect on this muscle or on the myenteric plexus muscle, or to ethanol's ability to change the bioavailability of various hormones such as cholecystokinin and gastrin. In fact, both gastrin and cholecystokinin can result in delayed gastric emptying.[62,63] However, alcohol-induced delays in gastric emptying were reported without any change in either serum gastrin or cholecystokinin.[42,64] Additionally, it is well known that alcohol can directly inhibit contractility of other muscles[11,12] including other muscles of the GI tract.[13] Hence, acute alcohol, if given in high enough concentrations, can delay gastric emptying of both liquid and solid meals. This appears to be due to a direct effect of ethanol on gastric muscle contractility secondary to changes in membrane conductance.

## 13.3.2.2   Chronic Exposure to Ethanol

Unlike data on the effect of acute ethanol, studies on the effect of chronic alcohol on gastric motility and emptying are sparse. Keshavarzian et al.[65] were the first to study gastric emptying in alcoholics. Using a radionuclide technique, they showed that gastric emptying of $^{99m}$Tc-labeled sulfur colloid labeled egg was not significantly different in alcoholics compared to healthy volunteers 3 to 10 days after the alcoholics were admitted to the detoxification unit. Only 1 of 10 alcoholics (10%) had delayed gastric emptying. This is in spite of the fact that 5 of 10 patients reported nausea and postprandial fullness at the time of the study. Moreover, there was no correlation between the half time for gastric emptying and the presence or severity of symptoms. Similarly, Wegener et al.[5] failed to show any significant differences in gastric emptying of either solid or liquid meals comparing 30 controls to 46 sober alcoholics who had been admitted to the detoxification unit at least 7 days prior to the study. But, 24% of alcoholics had delayed gastric emptying. There was also a modest but significant correlation between gastric emptying and GI symptoms ($r = 0.48$). Also, daily ethanol ingestion significantly correlated with gastric emptying ($r = 0.42$).

Hence, it appears that unlike the effects of acute alcohol on gastric emptying, in which gastric emptying was clearly delayed, after chronic ethanol the inhibitory effect of ethanol is only modest and occurs only in a minority of subjects (10 to 24%). This suggests the development of tolerance to the effects of ethanol on gastric emptying. Both of these reports, however, studied alcoholics who had abstained from alcohol for several days and the effect of alcohol may have resolved by the time of each study.

Because studying inebriated alcoholics is not ethically feasible, Willson et al.[43] evaluated gastric emptying in inebriated cats chronically exposed to daily ethanol. Ethanol was given through an intragastric tube twice daily for a minimum of 30 days. Cats developed evidence of tolerance and dependence related to CNS behaviors. Using a radionuclide technique, gastric emptying of a liquid meal was evaluated in cats when the animals were still inebriated (BAL = $442 \pm 38$ mg/dl) and again 24 h after the last ethanol dose when the BAL was $58 \pm 40$ mg/dl. Inebriated alcoholic cats ($n = 9$) had significantly delayed gastric emptying ($t$ 1/2 = 90 min) compared to controls ($t$ 1/2 = 46 min; $n = 10$). The delays in gastric emptying diminished ($t$ 1/2 = 70 min) after 24 h of abstinence but still remained significantly abnormal. Hence, similar to acute alcohol, chronic ethanol also delays gastric emptying and does so to about the same extent. But this does not necessarily indicate a lack of development of tolerance since the BAL in the chronic alcoholic cats were two- to sixfold higher than BAL in acutely exposed cats. One can therefore infer from animal and human studies that both acute and chronic ethanol cause delays in gastric emptying. This effect is not universal and is transient, often resolving within 1 or 2 weeks of abstinence in most subjects.

## 13.4 ETHANOL-INDUCED INTESTINAL DYSMOTILITY

### 13.4.1 Clinical Picture

#### 13.4.1.1 Acute Exposure to Ethanol

It is widely believed that alcohol intake can either initiate or aggravate symptoms related to intestinal dysfunction such as diarrhea, cramps, or flatulence. For example, many patients with GI diseases such as irritable bowel syndrome or inflammatory bowel disease avoid alcohol because they believe that it aggravates their symptoms. However, the authors found no systematic studies evaluating the severity or frequency of these symptoms after acute exposure to ethanol. It appears, however, that acute alcohol causes diarrhea in some but not all individuals. For example, in one study 5 of 12 control subjects developed diarrhea within 8 h after i.v. administration of ethanol that resulted in BAL higher than 100 mg/dl.[66] In contrast, in studies of intestinal motility, diarrhea did not develop in any of 13 subjects given ethanol by Robels et al.[67] nor in 6 subjects given ethanol by Charles et al.[68] Hence, one can surmise that acute ingestion of ethanol should not cause significant diarrhea in most healthy subjects. But, ethanol still could be clinically important in susceptible individuals or in subjects with underlying GI disease. There are several possible mechanisms for alcohol-induced diarrhea including the effect of ethanol on intestinal absorption/secretion.[1-3] Another possibility is the effect of ethanol on small intestinal and colonic motility and transit which will be discussed in Section 13.4.2.

## 13.4.1.2   Chronic Exposure to Ethanol

Symptoms related to intestinal dysfunction such as diarrhea, cramps, and flatulence are common in alcoholics.[1-4] For example, 65% of 20 alcoholics in one study[69] and 26% of 46 alcoholics in another study[5] reported diarrhea for the period when they had been actively drinking. However, this does not necessarily mean that diarrhea is significantly more common in alcoholics since the frequency was not compared with appropriate control groups. However, Fields et al.[4] demonstrated that these intestinal symptoms are indeed significantly more common in inebriated alcoholics. For example, while 46% of 48 alcoholics reported diarrhea for the period when they were actively drinking, none of the 48 controls had this complaint. Diarrhea was mild, typically 3 to 5 bowel movements a day, and was transient in the majority of alcoholics since only 24% and 4% of subjects reported diarrhea 3 and 14 days, respectively, after abstinence. Similarly, a significantly greater fraction of alcoholics reported abdominal cramps (29% vs. 8%). Again, cramps were transient and reported in only 12% and 9% of alcoholics at 3 and 14 days, respectively. Flatulence was also reported significantly more often by alcoholics (50% vs. 21%). But, this complaint was not transient as it was reported by 47% and 49% of alcoholics on days 3 and 14, respectively.

The underlying mechanism for these intestinal symptoms in alcoholics is most likely multifactorial since several abnormalities of intestinal function have been reported in alcoholics.[1-3] These include mucosal injury, disaccharide malabsorption due to intestinal brush-border disaccharidase deficiency, abnormalities of intestinal absorption, and pancreatic insufficiency.[1-3] Another potentially important factor that could underlie or contribute to these symptoms is abnormal intestinal motility and transit. Intestinal dysmotility can result in diarrhea by either accelerated transit or delayed transit. Delayed intestinal transit can result in bacterial overgrowth and diarrhea. Indeed, 2 of 12 alcoholics with diarrhea had evidence of small intestinal bacterial overgrowth defined by hydrogen breath test.[5] Another clinical consequence of delayed intestinal transit, if it also involves the colon, is constipation. Six of 46 alcoholics (13%) reported less than 3 spontaneous bowel movements per week.[5] But, since the frequency of constipation in controls was not reported in this study, it is not clear whether constipation is more or even less common in alcoholics. Intestinal dysmotility in alcoholics, therefore, can have significant clinical impact, not only by causing symptoms, but also by contributing to malabsorption and malnutrition. Alcohol-induced intestinal dysmotility will be discussed in Section 13.4.2.

## 13.4.2   Intestinal Motility and Transit Studies

### 13.4.2.1   Small Intestinal Motility and Transit Studies

#### *13.4.2.1.1   Acute Exposure to Ethanol*

Although the effect of acute ethanol on motility of the small intestine was reported some time ago by Pirola and Davis[70] and again by Robels et al.,[67] the effect of ethanol on transit of the small intestine was only recently reported by Pfeiffer et al.[51] Pirola and Davis[70] studied the effect of i.v. ethanol (0.6 g/kg over 20 min) on duodenal motility using an open-tip, nonperfused catheter and cine radiography in eight controls. Manometrically, acute ethanol transiently increased the number of duodenal pressure waves and the average motility index. Radiographically, these pressure changes were associated with a burst of large contraction waves and marked narrowing of the second part of the duodenum. These authors concluded that ethanol increases intestinal transit and may result in diarrhea. No direct intestinal transit measurement was done, however. Similarly, Robels et al.[67] found that acute ethanol administration (0.8 g/kg, p.o. or i.v.) in 13 subjects (2 controls, 11 sober alcoholics) resulted in intestinal motility changes compatible with intestinal hurry. Using a balloon, they demonstrated decreases in Type 1 (impeding) and increases in Type 3 (propulsive) jejunal and ileal pressure waves. There was no difference between alcoholics and volunteers. The effect of alcohol appears to be systemic as there was no difference between oral and intravenous routes. Again, the authors concluded that their observations suggest that ethanol induces rapid intestinal transit which could account for alcohol-induced diarrhea; however, no direct measurement of transit was made.

Using a hydrogen breath test following ingestion of the nonabsorbable carbohydrate lactulose, Pfeiffer et al.[51] measured mouth to cecum transit time (MCT) following acute exposure to ethanol. While beer significantly shortened MCT (95 min vs. 158 min in controls), the effect of wine was less marked (130 min). It was surprising that equivalent doses of grain ethanol had no significant effect (150 min). The BAL was not provided in this report and it is possible that the higher doses of ethanol used in the studies by Robels et al.[67] and Pirola and Davis[70] still could have shortened intestinal transit times. However, Scroggs et al.[71] not only did not show rapid transit, but instead demonstrated inhibition of intestinal transit after 2 or 3 g of ethanol (s.c. or i.p.) in mice.[1-3]

Hence, it appears that acute alcohol has variable and sometimes subtle effects on small intestinal motility. This may not necessarily result in changes in transit time, however. For example, using micropressure transducers, Charles et al.[68] continuously monitored intestinal manometry for 24 h in 6 ambulatory control subjects. They observed only subtle postprandial changes after ingestion of wine (0.6 g/kg). That is, wine only increased the amplitude of small intestinal contractions at night and induced clustered contractions postprandially. Ethanol also abolished normal circadian variations of fasting, intestinal, migrating myoelectric complexes (MMC).

The effect of ethanol on intestinal electrical spikes and MMC in opossum have also been reported[72,73] with variable results. While Becker and Sharp[72] failed to demonstrate any effect of ethanol on duration or frequency of duodenal cyclical myoelectric spike activities, Coelho et al.[73] demonstrated that ethanol induces intense bursts of spike potentials similar to Type III MMC. This effect appears to be due to a combination of local and systemic factors. Although i.v. ethanol induced these spike potentials, they were more frequent (87% vs. 12% of experiments) and were seen in more animals when ethanol was given intraduodenally compared to intravenously. This effect of ethanol may be mediated through release of the intestinal peptide motilin since serum motilin was elevated in association with ethanol-induced spike potentials similar to spontaneous spike potentials.

It appears that both nerve and muscle tissues are involved in ethanol-induced intestinal dysmotility regardless of whether ethanol exerts its effects directly or through release of gut hormones. For instance, modification of the amplitude of contractions by ethanol reported by Charles et al.[68] suggests a direct effect of ethanol on intestinal smooth muscle cells. On the other hand, electromyographic data on the rabbit jejunum reported by Martin et al.[74] suggest an effect on nerves rather than on muscles because they demonstrated that low concentrations of intraluminally infused ethanol induce migrating action potential complexes and produce repetitive bursts of action potentials while having no effect on the slow wave frequency. As reported by Charles et al.,[68] the effect of ethanol on nerve appears not to be limited to the enteric system (ENS) since ethanol elicited alterations in the duration of the MMC cycle without changing the organization of the MMC or its propagation. This suggests that ethanol has effects on the extrinsic neural control of the gut.

### 13.4.2.1.2  Chronic Exposure to Ethanol

Studies on the effect of chronic ethanol on small intestinal motility are even more limited than studies on the acute effects of ethanol on this organ. Keshavarzian et al.[69] were the first to study small intestinal transit in chronic alcoholics. Using a hydrogen breath test following ingestion of lactulose, they observed that MCT was not significantly different in 20 alcoholics compared to healthy controls when this parameter was measured within 24 to 48 h following admission of the alcoholics to a detoxification program. But, alcoholics with diarrhea (MCT = 62 min) had significantly shorter transit times than controls (93 min) or alcoholics without diarrhea (98 min). The abnormally rapid intestinal transit in alcoholics with diarrhea was reversible since 8 to 10 days after abstinence, at a time when they no longer had diarrhea, their transit time returned to normal (101 min). In contrast, MCT in alcoholics without diarrhea did not change after 8 to 10 days of abstinence.

It also appears that withdrawing alcoholics have increased sensitivity to osmotic loads since 75% of alcoholics developed diarrhea when lactulose was given 24 to 48 h after admission compared to none of the controls. This hypersensitivity appears to be transient in most subjects since only 15% of alcoholics developed diarrhea after lactulose ingestion when retested 8 to 10 days later. Intestinal transit time could not predict diarrhea in each individual all of the time. Nonetheless, none of the subjects without diarrhea during the initial study had a transit time shorter than 90 min. Since gastric emptying in a similar, but not identical, group of alcoholics was normal,[65] the observed shortening of the MCT should be due to rapid small intestinal transit. Hence, a large percentage of actively drinking alcoholics have increased sensitivity to an osmotic load which is associated with shortened intestinal transit time and diarrhea.

Wegener et al.[5] also demonstrated shortened MCT in alcoholics with diarrhea; however, 14 of 37 alcoholics (38%) had delayed MCT. None of these alcoholics had diarrhea and four of them also had delayed gastric emptying. Hence, prolonged MCT in those four subjects could be secondary to delayed gastric emptying rather than to prolonged small intestinal transit. Thus, only 10 alcoholics (27%) clearly had prolonged small intestinal transit times. Ghimire et al.[75] in a preliminary study confirmed these findings. Using a hydrogen breath test following ingestion of beans, they demonstrated that MCT of solid food was also significantly shortened in alcoholics with diarrhea in whom gastric emptying was normal. Hence, chronic alcohol consumption can result in abnormal small intestinal transit. This effect is not seen in all subjects, appears to be transient, and exhibits a wide spectrum of abnormalities including both delayed and shortened transit. Interestingly, both abnormalities could contribute to diarrhea in alcoholics. Delayed transit can predispose alcoholics to small bowel bacterial overgrowth while shortened transit can compromise intestinal absorption. The mechanisms underlying these abnormalities are not known and require further investigation.

## 13.4.2.2   Colonic Motility and Transit Studies

### 13.4.2.2.1   *Acute Exposure to Ethanol*

To our knowledge, Elder et al.[76] and Berenson and Avner[66] were the only groups to evaluate the effect of acute ethanol on colonic motility. Using tandem balloons, Elder et al.[76] found that i.v. ethanol blunted saline-induced augmentation of colonic tone and motility of both right- and left-sided colon in four dogs. Intragastric ethanol (200 ml of 20% infused into the stomach) had a more profound effect and not only blunted the augmentation, but also inhibited colonic motility. These effects were not seen in all dogs and, in some experiments, ethanol had either no effect or even increased motility. In other experiments, when a balloon bolus technique was substituted for the fixed tandem balloon system, alcohol uniformly increased the rate of passage of the bolus. The contrasting results of the two types of balloon techniques suggests that while alcohol reduces the frequency of nonpropulsive types of motility, it initiates propulsive activity.

Elder et al.[76] also performed similar studies in two human subjects with colostomy, inserting the balloons through the colostomy into the splenic flexure. They found that 125 ml of 20% whisky given orally resulted in increased propulsive colonic motility. Subjects passed flatus and fecal material from the colostomy only after ingestion of whisky but not after drinking nonalcoholic beverages. Whisky also appeared to facilitate the gastrocolic reflex since subjects passed flatus and fecal material soon after ingesting the whisky when it was given after breakfast.

These limited animal and humans studies suggest that ethanol increases colonic motor activity which may result in more rapid colonic transit and emptying. The techniques used are less refined, however, thus limiting the accuracy of the data and also limiting the conclusions that can be drawn from such studies.

Using a more refined technique, i.e., a perfused water-filled motility catheter, Berenson and Avner[66] showed that i.v. ethanol reduces the rectosigmoid motility index. This inhibition was a result of a fall in both wave frequency and amplitude and was inversely correlated with BAL ($r = -0.84$). All subjects developed CNS-related evidence of alcohol intoxication with drowsiness; four developed nausea and vomiting, but none had diarrhea and BAL ranged from 112 to 155 mg/dl. The functional significance of these manometric changes remains to be determined. However, reduced segmental colonic motility has been associated with diarrhea.[77,78] Hence, the observed abnormality could contribute, at least in part, to alcohol-induced diarrhea. On the other hand it is possible that the rectosigmoid dysmotility is secondary to changes in chronic fluid flux induced by alcohol.

### 13.4.2.2.2  Chronic Exposure to Ethanol

Similar to data on acute effects of ethanol on colonic motility, data on the effects of chronic ethanol on colonic motility are sparse. Using a nonabsorbable marker, indigo carmine, Wegener et al.[5] demonstrated that whole gut transit which is predominantly influenced by colonic transit is normal in alcoholics that had just recovered from a withdrawal syndrome. But, whole gut transit was significantly more prolonged in alcoholics with constipation (21.9 h) compared to alcoholics without constipation (8.4 h) or normals (11.9 h). However, this abnormality could be more a result of constipation rather than of alcoholism.

Bouchoucha et al.,[79] on the other hand, observed more rapid rectosigmoid transit in alcoholics. Using radiopaque, nonabsorbable markers, Bouchoucha et al. estimated total and segmental colonic transit times in 20 alcoholics 4 days and again 10 days after admission to a detoxification unit. Total colonic transit time in withdrawing alcoholics (24.9 h) was similar to values for controls (27.7 h). Total colonic transit was significantly increased after 10 days of abstinence to 33.3 h. This change in total colonic transit can be explained by changes in rectosigmoid transit time. In fact, segmental colonic transit time was significantly decreased in the rectosigmoid area in withdrawing alcoholics (2.8 h) compared to controls (9.2 h); values returned to normal (9.9 h) after 10 days of sobriety. Segmental colonic transit time in the right or left colon were similar in alcoholics and controls. These data suggest that reversible, rapid rectosigmoid transit time in alcoholics could, at least in part, contribute to transient diarrhea in alcoholics. Whether this observed rapid rectosigmoid transit is secondary to inhibition of rectosigmoid motility reported by Berenson and Avner,[66] or to other colonic dysmotility, remains to be seen. The underlying mechanism of ethanol-induced colonic dysmotility requires further study.

## 13.5  ETHANOL-INDUCED GALLBLADDER AND BILIARY TREE DYSMOTILITY

### 13.5.1  Clinical Picture

#### 13.5.1.1  Acute Exposure to Ethanol

Acute ethanol ingestion is associated with pancreatitis. The mechanism underlying this association is not fully established. One possibility is an increase in intraductal pancreatic pressure. While various factors can affect intraductal pancreatic pressure, one of the most important of these factors is changes in contractility and tonicity of the sphincter of Oddi. Hence, changes in sphincter of Oddi motility and pressure induced by acute alcohol, outlined in Section 13.5.2, can contribute to alcohol-induced pancreatic injury. No biliary symptoms or syndromes have been firmly associated with acute ethanol exposure.

### 13.5.1.2   Chronic Exposure to Ethanol

Chronic ethanol ingestion appears to provide protection against development of cholesterol gallstones. This could be due to several factors including the effect of ethanol on water absorption by gallbladder mucosa and ethanol-induced changes in biliary lipids.[80,81] However, since changes in gallbladder emptying have been shown to be important in the genesis of gallstones, ethanol-induced changes in gallbladder motility can also contribute to the protective effect of ethanol against the development of gallstones. Although cholesterol gallstones are less frequent in alcoholics, pigment gallstones are more common in alcoholic cirrhosis.[82] This increased incidence of pigment gallstones can be explained by the established effect of ethanol on metabolism of biliary calcium and biliary pigments.[82]

## 13.5.2   Biliary Motility and Gallbladder Emptying Studies

### 13.5.2.1   Acute Exposure to Ethanol

#### 13.5.2.1.1   Effects of Acute Ethanol on Gallbladder Emptying

To our knowledge, only Modaine et al.[83] and Malmud et al.[84] have reported the effects of alcohol on gallbladder emptying. Using ultrasonography, Modaine et al.[83] evaluated the effect of 20 g of ethanol ingestion on gallbladder motility in response to a fatty liquid meal in 16 healthy males. Alcohol stimulated postprandial gallbladder emptying and accelerated gallbladder filling. The accelerated gallbladder filling suggests that alcohol may also increase sphincter of Oddi pressure since increased sphincter of Oddi pressure can result in accelerated gallbladder emptying. However, other possibilities for accelerated gallbladder filling exist and should be considered. This ethanol-induced stimulation of gallbladder emptying may, at least in part, be responsible for the protective effect of ethanol against the development of gallstones.

The above *in vivo* study[83] suggests that acute ethanol has a stimulatory effect on gallbladder and sphincter of Oddi muscle contractions. But, the *in vitro* studies by Masui et al.[85] do not support this notion. They demonstrated that *in vitro* alcohol attenuates contractility of muscle strips from guinea pig gallbladder. Ethanol, at concentrations greater than 50 m$M$, dose dependently attenuated the reactivity and sensitivity of contractile responses of muscle strips to various stimuli including potassium chloride, acetylcholine, and histamine. The mechanism of this inhibition appears to be calcium mediated. Ethanol appears to decrease the sensitivity of muscle to calcium as well as inhibiting calcium fluxes into the cells. This observed inhibition could, however, not be relevant to *in vivo* alcohol exposure since even the lowest concentration of ethanol (50 m$M$) is much greater than the typical BAL that is reached in the vast majority of moderate drinkers. Indeed, Masui et al.[85] did not find any change in muscle contractility of the strips obtained from guinea pigs receiving 3% ethanol *in vivo* for 4 weeks.

Malmud et al.[84] found a different result for the effect of ethanol on gallbladder emptying than Modaine et al.[83] Using a radionuclide technique, they observed that ethanol delays gallbladder emptying. However, this finding is reported in an abstract; thus, critical evaluation of the data is not possible. Further studies are needed to reconcile the discrepancy between human *in vivo* studies and also between *in vivo* findings and *in vitro* studies in animals. The underlying mechanism of ethanol-induced changes in gallbladder emptying is not known and requires additional studies.

#### 13.5.2.1.2   Effects of Acute Ethanol on Biliary Motility

Acute ethanol appears to affect both intrabile duct pressure and pancreatic duct pressure. For example, i.v. alcohol causes a rise in choledochotomy tube pressure in patients recovering from cholecystectomy.[86] This increased intraductal pressure could be a result of contraction of the sphincter of Oddi. Indeed, alcohol has been shown to induce duodenal contraction and to increase sphincter of Oddi pressure.[70] These changes were associated with decreased pancreatic outflow and hence may contribute to alcohol-induced pancreatitis.

The mechanism of ethanol-induced increases in sphincter of Oddi pressure have been studied in opossum.[72,73] Ethanol administration resulted in intense bursts of spike potentials in sphincter of Oddi[73] and increases in peak sphincter of Oddi spike burst frequency.[72] This ethanol-induced myoelectrical activity in sphincter of Oddi was independent of changes in activity of the duodenum or stomach[72] and did not correlate with BAL.[73] Hence, alcohol can induce myoelectrical activity in sphincter of Oddi that could increase sphincter pressure which in turn results in increases in intraductal pressure and a fall in the flow of pancreatic secretion. These ethanol-induced functional changes could either initiate or facilitate pancreatic injury.

### 13.5.2.2   Chronic Exposure to Ethanol

#### 13.5.2.2.1   Effects of Chronic Ethanol on Gallbladder Emptying

Gallbladder emptying has not been extensively studied in alcoholics. Using ultrasonography, Keshavarzian et al.[87] evaluated fasting gallbladder volume and postprandial gallbladder emptying rate in 10 patients with alcoholic cirrhosis and in 7 alcoholics without liver disease. Fasting gallbladder volume was not significantly changed in either alcoholic cirrhotics (43 ml) or in alcoholics (35 ml) compared to controls (34 ml). Similarly, gallbladder emptying was normal in alcoholics. Maximum gallbladder emptying occurred within 30 min of a meal and rates were similar in all 3 groups (54, 49, and 51%, respectively). There was no difference between alcoholics with and without gallstones. These data indicate that gallbladder emptying is normal in alcoholics regardless of whether they have liver disease or gallstones. Hence, gallbladder dysmotility does not appear to play a role in pigment stones commonly seen in alcoholic cirrhosis. Additionally, it appears that the effects of acute and chronic ethanol exposure on gallbladder emptying differs. The *in vitro* study in guinea pig muscle strips[85] is compatible with the above *in vivo* study[87] since contractility of muscle strips from chronically exposed animals was similar to values for control strips.[85]

#### 13.5.2.2.2   Effects of Chronic Ethanol on Biliary Motility

Pancreatic duct pressure and sphincter of Oddi have been studied in alcoholics with chronic pancreatitis[88,89] during endoscopic retrograde cholangiopancreatography. Pancreatic duct pressure was increased in 56 patients with alcoholic chronic pancreatitis, 34 patients with gallstone pancreatitis, and 45 patients with idiopathic pancreatitis. The frequency of sphincter of Oddi contractile waves was significantly higher in patients with pancreatitis but correlated with pancreatic duct pressure only in subjects with alcoholic pancreatitis. These changes could be secondary to pancreatitis rather than to alcoholism, but they appear to be more pronounced in alcoholic pancreatitis. Hence, both acute and chronic ethanol exposure can affect gallbladder and biliary motility. These effects can contribute to the pathogenesis of alcoholic pancreatitis but they do not appear to be important in pigment gallstones in alcoholic cirrhosis.

## 13.6   CONCLUSIONS

Both acute and chronic alcohol are capable of affecting the motility of the GI tract. The nature and magnitude of the changes induced by ethanol depend on the segment of the GI tract, the dose and duration of exposure to alcohol, and, in some cases, the type of alcoholic beverages or the presence of food. The effect of acute and chronic ethanol may differ as it does in ethanol's effect on the esophagus but it could also be similar to the effects of ethanol on the stomach. It seems that tolerance can occur to the effect of ethanol but the degree of tolerance does not appear to be profound and does not universally occur in all segments of the GI tract.

If the GI tract develops tolerance to the inhibitory effects of chronic ethanol, then, similar to findings in the CNS, a period of withdrawal-induced hyperexcitability could occur. Indeed, esophageal dysmotility observed in withdrawing alcoholics[20,21] could be secondary to esophageal hyperexcitability that is due to a state of "withdrawal" of the esophageal muscle.[90] This finding strongly suggests that a withdrawal syndrome is not limited to the CNS and all excitable tissues, including those of the GI tract, can develop such a state of hyperexcitability.

It also appears that there is a minimum BAL required for ethanol-induced dysmotility. This level is approximately 80 to 100 mg/dl. In most segments of the GI tract a higher BAL does not appear to elicit an effect of greater magnitude.

Interestingly, the overall effect of ethanol exposure on GI motility can vary from inhibition of function as in delayed esophageal and gastric emptying to pathologically accelerated function such as rapid intestinal transit. Ethanol-induced GI dysmotility can therefore hamper normal GI physiology and not only result in GI-related complaints but also contribute to ethanol-induced GI disorders such as malabsorption and pancreatitis that in turn cause malnutrition and impaired immunity which are commonly noted in alcoholics.

The mechanism of ethanol-induced dysmotility appears to be multifactorial. Ethanol can exert its effect either directly or through changes in secretion of gut hormones capable of modulating GI motility. Regardless, ethanol-induced dysmotility can be a result of ethanol's effects on muscle and/or nerve. Indeed, it is well established that ethanol can affect functioning of nerves[14] and muscles[9-12] in other tissues. Nonetheless, the cellular mechanisms of ethanol's effects on smooth muscles of the GI tract are not clear. However, primary effects of ethanol on neurohumoral receptors and on calcium kinetics in muscle and neural tissues[14,91-93] of other organs have been postulated and these putative mechanisms may also be operational in the GI tract. Indeed, the authors have recently shown that ethanol affects muscarinic receptor systems[94] and perturbs calcium homeostasis[95] of esophageal smooth muscle. Clearly, a better understanding of the mechanisms underlying ethanol-induced dysmotility could lead to more rational therapy of ethanol-induced GI disorders. This knowledge could also help us understand the mechanism of similar GI dysmotility disorders that are seen in nonalcoholic patients.

## 13.7   ACKNOWLEDGMENTS

This work was supported in part by a grant from NIAAA (Rol-AA07255). The authors are grateful to Mary McLernon and Ms. Heidi Heintz for preparing the manuscript.

## REFERENCES

1.  **Gazzard, B. G. and Clark, M. L.,** Alcohol and the alimentary system, *Clin. Endocrinol. Metab.,* 7, 429, 1978.
2.  **Nazer, H. and Wright, R. A.,** The effect of alcohol on the human alimentary tract: a review, *J. Clin. Gastroenterol.,* 5, 361, 1983.
3.  **Burbidge, E. J., Lewis, D. R., and Halsted, C. H.,** Alcohol and the gastrointestinal tract, *Med. Clin. North Am.,* 68, 77, 1984.
4.  **Fields, J. Z., Turk, A., Durkin, M., Ravi, N. V., and Keshavarzian, A.,** Increased gastrointestinal symptoms in chronic alcoholics, *Am. J. Gastroenterol.,* 89, 382, 1994.
5.  **Wegener, M., Schaffstein, J., Dilger, U., Coenen, C., Wedmann, B., and Schmidt, G.,** Gastrointestinal transit of solid-liquid meal in chronic alcoholics, *Dig. Dis. Sci.,* 36, 917, 1991.
6.  **Minami, H. and McCallum R. W.,** The physiology and pathophysiology of gastric emptying in humans, *Gastroenterology,* 86, 1592, 1984.
7.  **Malagelada, J. R., Rees, W. W., Mazzotta, L. J., and Go, V. L. W.,** Gastric motor abnormalities in diabetic and post-gastrectomy gastroparesis: effect of metaclopramide and bethanechol, *Gastroenterology,* 78, 286, 1980.
8.  **Keshavarzian, A., Fields, J. Z., Vaeth, J., and Holmes, E. W.,** The differing effects of acute and chronic alcohol on gastric and intestinal permeability, *Am. J. Gastroenterol.,* 89, 2205, 1994.
9.  **Urbano-Marquez, A., Estruch, R., Navarro-Lopez, F., Grau, J. M., Mont, L., and Rubin, E.,** The effects of alcoholism on skeletal and cardiac muscle, *N. Engl. J. Med.,* 320, 409, 1994.

10. **Inoue, F. and Frank, G. B.,** Effects of ethyl alcohol on excitability and on neuromuscular transmission in frog skeletal muscle, *Br. J. Pharmacol. Chemother.*, 30, 186, 1967.

11. **Altura, B. T., Pohorecky, L. A., and Altura, B. M.,** Demonstration of tolerance to ethanol in non-nervous tissue: effects on vascular smooth muscle, *Alcoholism: Clin. Exp. Res.*, 4, 462, 1990.

12. **DeTurck, K. H. and Pohorecky, L. A.,** Tolerance to ethanol in the rat vas deferens. Effect of a calcium channel antagonist, *Alcohol,* 4, 355, 1987.

13. **Sunano, S. and Miyazaki, E.,** Effects of ethanol and acetone on action potential and inhibitory potential of guinea pig taenia coli, *Nature,* 221, 380, 1969.

14. **Littleton, J.,** Basic science and alcoholism, *Br. J. Addict.*, 81, 450, 1986.

15. **Van Thiel, D. H., Lipsitz, H. D., Porter, L. E., Schade, R. R., Gottleib, G. P., and Graham, T. O.,** Gastrointestinal and hepatic manifestations of chronic alcoholism, *Gastroenterology,* 81, 594, 1981.

16. **Wienbeck, M. and Berges, W.,** Oesophageal lesions in the alcoholic, *Clin. Gastroenterol.*, 10, 375, 1981.

17. **Kaufman, S. E. and Kaye, M. D.,** Induction of gastro-oesophageal reflux by alcohol, *Gut,* 19, 336, 1978.

18. **Vitale, G. C., Cheadle, W. G., Patel, B., Sadek, S. A., Michel, M. E., and Cuschieri, A.,** The effect of alcohol on nocturnal gastroesophageal reflux, *JAMA,* 258, 2077, 1987.

19. **Kitchin, L. I. and Castell, D. O.,** Rationale and efficacy of conservative therapy for gastroesophageal reflux disease, *Arch. Intern. Med.*, 151, 448, 1991.

20. **Keshavarzian, A., Iber, F. L., and Ferguson, Y.,** Esophageal manometry and radionuclide emptying in chronic alcoholics, *Gastroenterology,* 92, 651, 1987.

21. **Keshavarzian, A., Polepalle, C., Iber, F. L., and Durkin, M.,** Esophageal motor disorder in alcoholics: result of alcoholism or withdrawal?, *Alcoholism,* 14, 561, 1990.

22. **Silver, L. S., Worner, T. M., and Korsten, M. A.,** Esophageal function in chronic alcoholics, *Am. J. Gastroenterol.*, 81, 423, 1986.

23. **Winship, D. H., Caflisch, C. R., Zboralske, F. F., and Hogan, W. J.,** Deterioration of esophageal peristalsis in patients with alcoholic neuropathy, *Gastroenterology,* 55, 173, 1968.

24. **Hodes, S. E. and Korsten, M. A.,** Fixed corkscrew pattern of the esophagus, *Am. J. Gastroenterol.*, 73, 249, 1980.

25. **Weber, L. D., Nashel, D. J., and Mellow, M. H.,** Pharyngeal dysphagia in alcoholic myopathy, *Ann. Intern. Med.*, 95, 189, 1981.

26. **Howell, L. P.,** An alcoholic woman who couldn't swallow, *Hosp. Pract.,* 21, 48A, 1986.

27. **Mayer, E. M., Grabowski, C. J., and Fisher, R. S.,** Effects of graded doses of alcohol upon esophageal motor function, *Gastroenterology,* 75, 1133, 1978.

28. **Hogan, W. J., Viegas de Andrade, S. R., and Winship, D. H.,** Ethanol-induced acute esophageal motor dysfunction, *J. Appl. Physiol.*, 32, 755, 1972.

29. **Keshavarzian, A., Urban, G., Sedghi, S., Willson, C., Sabella, L., Sweeny, C., and Anderson, K.,** Effect of acute ethanol on esophageal motility in cat, *Alcoholism: Clin. Exp. Res.,* 15, 116, 1991.

30. **Fox, J. E. T. and Daniel, E. E.,** Role of $Ca^{2+}$ in genesis of lower esophageal sphincter tone and other active contractions, *Am. J. Physiol.*, 237, E163, 1979.

31. **Jacyno, M., Keshavarzian, A., Urban, G., Wasyliw, R., Winship, D., and Fields, J.,** Ethanol dose dependently inhibits contractility of esophageal smooth muscle induced by carbachol or electrical stimulation, *Gastroenterology,* Suppl. 106, A516, 1994.

32. **Fields, J., Jacyno, M., Urban, G., Winship, D., and Keshavarzian, A.,** Role of myenteric nerves and nitric oxide (NO) on the inhibitory effects of ethanol (EtOH) on contractility of lower esophageal sphincter (LES) muscle, *Gastroenterology,* Suppl. 106, A498, 1994.

33. **Muska, B., Sundaresan, R., Fields, J. Z., Winship, D., and Keshavarzian, A.,** Ethanol dose-dependently inhibits carbachol-induced contraction of dispersed smooth muscle cells of cat esophagus, *Gastroenterology,* Suppl. 104, A556, 1993.

34. **Fischer, R. A., Ellison, C. W., Thayer, W. R., Spiro, H. M., and Glaser, G. H.,** Esophageal motility in neuromuscular disorders, *Ann. Intern. Med.,* 63, 229, 1965.

35. **Keshavarzian, A., Polepalle, C., Iber, F. L., and Durkin, M.,** Secondary esophageal contractions are abnormal in chronic alcoholics, *Dig. Dis. Sci.*, 37, 517, 1992.

36. **Keshavarzian, A., Rizk, R., Urban, G., and Willson, C.,** Ethanol-induced esophageal motor disorder: development of an animal model, *Alcoholism,* 14, 76, 1990.

37. **Banciu, T. and Sorian, E.,** Gastroesophageal reflux in chronic alcoholics. Endoesophageal pH determinations using Heidelberg telemetering capsule, *Med. Intern.,* 27, 279, 1989.

38. **Tonnesen, H., Andersen, J. R., Christofferson, P., and Kaas-Clasesson, N.,** Reflux esophagitis in heavy drinkers: effect of ranitidine and alginate/metaclopramide, *Digestion,* 38, 69, 1987.

39. **Barlow, O. W., Beams, A. J., and Goldblatt, H.,** Studies on the pharmacology of ethyl alcohol. A comparative study of pharmacologic effects of grain and synthetic alcohols, *J. Pharmacol. Exp. Ther.*, 56, 117, 1936.

40. **Tennent, D. M.,** The influence of alcohol on the emptying time of the stomach and the absorption of glucose, *Q. J. Stud. Alcohol,* 1, 271, 1941.

41. **Greenberg, L. A., Lolli, G., and Rubin, M.,** The influence of intravenously administered alcohol on the emptying time of the stomach. *Q. J. Stud. Alcohol,* 3, 370, 1942.

42. **Jian, R., Cortot, A., Ducrot, F., Jobin, G., Chayvialle, J. A., and Modigliani, R.,** Effect of ethanol ingestion on postprandial gastric emptying and secretion, bilio-pancreatic secretions, and duodenal absorption in man, *Dig. Dis. Sci.,* 31, 604, 1986.

43. **Willson, C. A., Bushnell, D., and Keshavarzian, A.,** The effect of acute and chronic ethanol administration on gastric emptying in cats, *Dig. Dis. Sci.,* 35, 444, 1990.

44. **Knight, L. C., Maurer, A. H., Wikander, R., Krevsky, B., Malmud, L. S., and Fisher, R. S.,** Effect of ethyl alcohol on motor function in canine stomach, *Am. J. Physiol.,* 262 (2 pt 1), G223, 1992.

45. **Franzen, G.,** Untersuchungen ueber alkohol. VII. Mitteilung alkoholwikungen auf die magenverdauung, *Arch. Exp. Pathol. Pharmakol.,* 134, 129, 1928.

46. **Pihkanen, T. A.,** Neurological and physiological studies on distilled and brewed beverages, *Ann. Med. Exp. Biol. Fenn.,* Suppl. 35, 9, 1957.

47. **Brewster, A. C., Lankford, H. G., Schwartz, M. G., and Sullivan, J. F.,** Ethanol and alimentary lipemia, *Am. J. Clin. Nutr.,* 19, 255, 1966.

48. **Barboriak, J. and Meade, R. C.,** Effect of alcohol on gastric emptying in man, *Am. J. Clin. Nutr.,* 23, 1151, 1970.

49. **Mushambi, M. C., Bailey, S. M., Trotter, T. N., Chadd, G. D., and Rowbotham, D. J.,** Effect of alcohol on gastric emptying in volunteers, *Br. J. Anaesth.,* 71, 674, 1993.

50. **Moore, J. G., Christian, P. E., and Datz, F. L.,** Effect of wine on gastric emptying in humans, *Gastroenterology,* 81, 1072, 1981.

51. **Pfeiffer, A., Hogl, B., and Kaess, H.,** Effect of ethanol and commonly ingested alcoholic beverages on gastric emptying and gastrointestinal transit, *Clin. Invest.,* 70, 487, 1992.

52. **Hunt, J. N. and Pathak, J. D.,** The osmotic effects of some simple molecules and ions on gastric emptying, *J. Physiol.,* 154, 254, 1960.

53. **Hunt, J. N. and Knox, M. T.,** The slowing of gastric emptying by four strong acids and three weak acids, *J. Physiol. (Lond.),* 227, 187, 1972.

54. **Kaufman, S. E. and Kaye, M. D.,** Effect of ethanol upon gastric emptying, *Gut,* 20, 688, 1979.

55. **Cortot, A., Jobin, G., Ducrot, F., Aymes, C., Giraudeaux, V., and Modigliani, R.,** Gastric emptying and gastrointestinal absorption of alcohol ingested with a meal, *Dig. Dis. Sci.,* 31, 343, 1986.

56. **Cooke, A. R. and Birchall, A.,** Absorption of ethanol from the stomach, *Gastroenterology,* 57, 269, 1969.

57. **Cooke, A. R.,** The simultaneous emptying and absorption of ethanol from the human stomach, *Am. J. Dig. Dis.,* 15, 449, 1970.

58. **Sanders, K. M. and Bauer, A. J.,** Ethyl alcohol interferes with excitation-contraction mechanisms of canine antral muscle, *Am. J. Physiol.,* 242, G222, 1982.

59. **Sanders, K. M. and Berry, R. G.,** Effects of ethyl alcohol on phasic and tonic contractions of the proximal stomach, *J. Pharmacol. Exp. Ther.,* 235, 858, 1985.

60. **Berry, R. G. and Sanders, K. M.,** Mechanical effects of ethyl alcohol on muscles of the proximal stomach, *Proc. West Pharmacol. Soc.,* 27, 115, 1984.

61. **Reed, J. B., Bauer, A. J., and Sanders, K. M.,** Electrical basis for the effects of ethyl alcohol on canine gastric corpus muscles, *Eur. J. Pharmacol.,* 119, 31, 1985.

62. **Hunt, J. N. and Ramsbottom, N.,** Effect of gastrin on gastric emptying and secretion during a test meal, *Br. Med. J.,* 4, 386, 1967.

63. **MacGregor, I. I., Zealous, D. W., and Martin, P. M.,** Effect of pentagastrin infusion on gastric emptying rate of solid food in man, *Am. J. Dig. Dis.,* 23, 72, 1978.

64. **Demol, P., Singer, M. V., Hotz, J., Eysselein, V., and Goebell, H.,** Different actions of intravenous ethanol on basal (= interdigestive) secretion of gastric acid, pancreatic enzymes and bile acids and gastrointestinal motility in man, *Alcohol Alcohol.,* 20, 195, 1985.

65. **Keshavarzian, A., Iber, F. L., Greer, P., and Wobbleton, J.,** Gastric emptying of solid meal in male chronic alcoholics, *Alcoholism: Clin. Exp. Res.,* 10, 432, 1986.

66. **Berenson, M. M. and Avner, D. L.,** Alcohol inhibition of rectosigmoid motility in humans, *Digestion,* 22, 210, 1981.

67. **Robels, E. A., Mezey, E., Halsted, C. H., and Schuster, M. M.,** Effect of ethanol on motility of the small intestine, *Johns Hopkins Med. J.,* 135, 7, 1974.

68. **Charles, F., Evans, D. F., Castillo, F. D., and Wingate, D. L.,** Daytime ingestion of alcohol alters nighttime jejunal motility, *Dig. Dis. Sci.,* 39, 51, 1994.

69. **Keshavarzian, A., Iber, F. L., Dangleis, M. D., and Cornish, R.,** Intestinal-transit and lactose intolerance in chronic alcoholics, *Am. J. Clin. Nutr.,* 44, 70, 1986.

70. **Pirola, R. C. and Davis, A. E.,** Effects of intravenous alcohol on motility of the duodenum and of the sphincter of Oddi, *Aust. Ann. Med.,* 19, 24, 1970.

71. **Scroggs, R., Abruzzo, M., and Advokat, C.,** Effects of ethanol on gastrointestinal transit in mice, *Alcoholism: Clin. Exp. Res.,* 10, 452, 1986.

72. **Becker, J. M. and Sharp, S. W.,** Effect of alcohol on cyclical myoelectric activity of the opossum sphincter of Oddi, *J. Surg. Res.*, 38, 343, 1985.

73. **Coelho, J. C., Gouma, D. J., and Moody, F. G.,** Sphincter of Oddi and gastrointestinal motility disturbance following alcohol administration in the opossum, *World J. Surg.*, 10, 990, 1986.

74. **Martin, J. R., Justus, P. G., and Mathias, J. R.,** Altered motility of the small intestine in response to ethanol: an explanation for the diarrhea associated with the consumption of alcohol, *Gastroenterology*, 78, 1218, 1980.

75. **Ghimire, M., Morris, A. L., Hill, D., Brownless, S. M., Stockdale, H. R., and Patten, M. D.,** A mechanism for diarrhea in alcoholics, *Gastroenterology*, 88, A1392, 1985.

76. **Elder, H. F., Beazell, J. M., Atkinson, A. J., and Ivy, A. C.,** The motor response of the colon to alcohol, *Q. J. Study Alcohol*, 10, 638, 1941.

77. **Connell, A. M.,** Significance of pressure waves in the sigmoid colon, *Am. J. Dig. Dis.*, 10, 455, 1965.

78. **Misiewicz, J. J.,** Colonic motility, *Gut*, 16, 311, 1975.

79. **Bouchoucha, M., Nalpas, B., Berger, M., Cugnenc, P. H., and Barbier, J. P.,** Recovery from disturbed colonic transit time after alcohol withdrawal, *Dis. Colon Rectum*, 34, 111, 1991.

80. **Kurtin, W. E., Schwesinger, W. H., and Stewart, R. M.,** Effect of dietary ethanol on gallbladder absorption and cholesterol gallstone formation in the prairie dog, *Am. J. Surg.*, 161, 470, 1991.

81. **Schwesinger, W. H., Kurtin, W. E., and Johnson, R.,** Alcohol protects against cholesterol gallstone formation, *Ann. Surg.*, 207, 641, 1988.

82. **Di Padova, C., Tritapepe, R., Rovagnati, P., Bessone, E., and Di Padova, F.,** Effect of ethanol on biliary unconjugated bilirubin and its implication in pigment gallstone pathogenesis in humans, *Digestion*, 24, 112, 1982.

83. **Modaine, P., Davion, T., Capron, D., and Capron, J. P.,** Ultrasound study of gallbladder motility in healthy subjects. Reproducibility of the method and effect of alcohol, *Gastroenterol. Clin. Biol.*, 17, 839, 1993.

84. **Malmud, L. S., Brody, S., Ryan, J., De Vegvar, M. L., and Fisher, R. S.,** Dual cholecystogastric scintigraphy: the mechanism of the effects of alcohol on the gallbladder, *J. Nucl. Med.*, 23 (Abstr.), 84, 1982.

85. **Masui, H., Wakabayashi, I., Hatake, K., Yoshimoto, S., and Sakamoto, K.,** Effects of ethanol on contractile response of gallbladder isolated from guinea pig, *Eur. J. Pharmacol.*, 248, 103, 1993.

86. **Pirola, R.C. and Davis, A.E.,** Effects of ethyl alcohol on sphincteric resistance at the choledochoduodenal junction in man, *Gut*, 9, 557, 1968.

87. **Keshavarzian, A., Medhat, A., Dunne, M., and Iber, F.,** The role of gallbladder emptying in gallstone formation in alcoholic cirrhosis, *Gastroenterology*, 92, A1743, 1987.

88. **Okazaki, K., Yamamoto, Y., Nishimori, I., Nishioka, T., Kagiyama, S., Tamura, S., Sakamoto, Y., Nakazawa, Y., Morita, M., and Yamamoto, Y.,** Motility of the sphincter of Oddi and pancreatic main ductal pressure in patients with alcoholic, gallstone-associated, and idiopathic chronic pancreatitis, *Am. J. Gastroenterol.*, 83, 820, 1988.

89. **Okazaki, K., Yamamoto, Y., Kagiyama, S., Tamura, S., Sakamoto, Y., Moriata, M., and Yamamoto, Y.,** Pressure of papillary sphincter zone and pancreatic main duct in patients with alcoholic and idiopathic chronic pancreatitis, *Int. J. Pancreatol.*, 3, 457, 1988.

90. **Keshavarzian, A., Willson, C., Urban, G., Sweeney, C., and Fields, J. Z.,** Muscle contraction as a peripheral correlate of the central nervous system withdrawal syndrome following chronic alcohol, *Res. Commun. Sub. Abuse*, 12, 81, 1991.

91. **Thomas, A. P., Sass, E. J., Tun-Kirchmann, T. T., and Rubin, E.,** Ethanol inhibits electrically-induced calcium transients in isolated rat cardiac myocytes, *J. Mol. Cell. Cardiol.*, 21, 555, 1989.

92. **Danell, L. C., Brass, E. P., and Harris, R. A.,** Effect of ethanol on intracellular ionized calcium concentrations in synaptosomes and hepatocytes, *Mol. Pharmacol.*, 32, 831, 1987.

93. **Lynch, M. A. and Littleton, J. M.,** Possible association of alcohol tolerance with increased synaptic $Ca^{2+}$ sensitivity, *Nature*, 303, 175, 1983.

94. **Keshavarzian, A., Gordon, J. H., Willson, C., Urban, G., and Fields, J. Z.,** Chronic ethanol feeding produces a muscarinic receptor upregulation, but not a muscarinic supersensitivity in lower esophageal sphincter muscle, *J. Pharmacol. Exp. Ther.*, 260, 601, 1992.

95. **Keshavarzian, A., Zorub, O., Sayeed, M., Sweeney, M., Urban, G., Winship, D., and Fields, J. Z.,** Acute ethanol inhibits calcium influxes into esophageal smooth but not striated muscle: a possible mechanism for ethanol-induced inhibition of esophageal contractility, *J. Pharmacol. Exp. Ther.*, 270, 1057, 1994.

# 14

# Protein Synthesis in the Gastrointestinal Tract and Its Modification by Ethanol

Jaspaul S. Marway, Adrian Bonner, Timothy J. Peters, and Victor R. Preedy

## CONTENTS

## 14.1 INTRODUCTION

Ethanol (ethyl alcohol) is also commonly known as alcohol and throughout this chapter, these terms will be used interchangeably. The orogastrointestinal tract is the first organ that comes into contact with ethanol. Tissues such as the mouth, esophagus, and stomach are therefore exposed to the highest concentrations of ethanol. Taken orally alcohol is partially absorbed slowly into the bloodstream through the stomach and more rapidly through the small intestine.[1] The rate of absorption varies greatly and depends on such factors as the time since the last intake of food, the fat and carbohydrate content of the stomach, and the nature of the beverage itself.[2,3] Any factor that delays or enhances gastric emptying will influence the rate of absorption of alcohol.

As ethanol is a small molecule and slightly polar, it is both water and fat soluble. Therefore, ethanol is easily absorbed and can traverse cell membranes by simple diffusion, without any expenditure of energy.[4,5] Thus, ethanol is swiftly distributed throughout the body and its organs in proportion to their water content.

As a consequence of ethanol consumption, numerous pathological changes arise in most mammalian organs, including the gastrointestinal tract. The variety of ethanol-induced abnormalities in the small intestine (see References 2, 6–9 for review) include partial villus atrophy, smooth muscle damage, and various defects in nutrient absorption[5,10-12] and disturbances in intestinal motility.[13-15] Extensive investigations have been made into the pathogenic mechanisms of the deleterious effects of ethanol on the alimentary tract, particularly by examining the mucosal regions of the stomach or small intestine.[8,10,12,16-19] These pathological changes may possibly be explained by changes in protein metabolism and especially protein synthesis. This chapter briefly reviews the effects of ethanol on the gastrointestinal tract, details the effects of ethanol on gastrointestinal protein synthesis, and attempts to provide possible mechanisms for the ethanol-induced inhibition of protein synthesis.

### 14.1.1 Effect on Smooth Muscle and Seromuscular Layer: A Defect in Protein Synthesis

The functions of the small intestine involve the digestion and absorption of various nutrients that pass from the stomach. The movement of material along the alimentary canal is primarily due to the peristaltic movement of the smooth muscle layers (longitudinal and circular muscles) of the gut. This motility is carefully controlled so that nutrients are exposed to the largest possible surface area for efficient absorption. Intestinal motility is also responsible for the passage or transmission of nondigestible products into the large intestine. The physiological and biochemical control of intestinal motility is complex (see References 20 and 21 for review). Contraction of the smooth muscle is involuntary and under the control of the sympathetic nervous system via the myenteric (Auerbach's) plexus which is located between the circular and longitudinal muscle layers.

Comparatively, very little work has been done on the effects of ethanol on gastrointestinal smooth muscle. One can speculate that because contractile proteins represent the major "business parts" of the muscle, any derangement in its molecular structure, biochemistry, or physiology will have important implications for gut motility. Diarrhea and malabsorption are commonly encountered in alcoholics which may partly be a consequence of changes in gut motility due to changes in contractile biochemistry, etc.[22] Keshavarzian et al.[14] have assessed intestinal mouth to cecum transit time of lactulose and malabsorption of lactose in male chronic alcoholics. They reported that 65% of the subjects investigated complained of diarrhea; small intestinal transit was also shorter in alcoholics with diarrhea than normal subjects. After lactulose, 75% of alcoholics developed diarrhea after 1 to 2 days compared to only 15%, 8 to 10 days after drinking stopped. Acute ethanol dosage (2 or 3 g of ethanol/kg i.p.) has been shown to have a dose-dependent inhibitory effect on gastrointestinal transit in mice. The small intestine was found to be more sensitive than the stomach to alcohol-induced inhibition of transit.[23] The study by Scroggs et al.[23] showed that i.p. injections of moderate doses of ethanol did not alter gastric emptying. However, in a recent study, Krishnamra and Limlomwongse[15] showed that acute intragastric ethanol administration delays gastric emptying in rats. From the polyethylene glycol (PEG) profile distribution, administration of ethanol directly into the duodenum was found to enhance intestinal motility. Delays in gastric emptying have also been demonstrated in cats during both acute and chronic exposure to ethanol.[24] In chronic alcoholics the small intestine and the stomach appear to be the most likely to be affected by transit disorders[25] although esophageal motility disorders in both acute and chronic exposure to ethanol have also been reported.[26-28] These transit abnormalities as a result of acute and chronic ethanol dosage are potentially related to toxic damage of gastrointestinal smooth muscle. However, there is no study that has looked at the relationship between protein synthesis and ethanol-induced motility disorders. One can speculate that motility disorders so commonly encountered in alcohol misusers may be due to or reflect perturbations in contractile protein synthesis.

### 14.1.2 Experimental Alcohol Toxicity Studies for Protein Synthesis

There are several ways to administer ethanol for investigative studies in laboratory animals. They are: (a) acute and (b) chronic treatment regimens. For acute studies, ethanol is usually given as a single bolus, either intraperitoneally (i.p.) or intragastrically (i.g.). The i.p. method where 75 mmol/kg body weight is injected as described by Tiernan and Ward[29] is particularly favored because it achieves high plasma ethanol levels that are sustained for up to 4 h. In addition, this route of administration also ensures more complete bioavailability of ethanol and in acute periods (i.e., 2.5 h) does not appear to cause overt morphological tissue damage as shown by histological analysis at the light microscopy level.[30] The i.g. administration of ethanol is another way to introduce ethanol but with this method lower plasma ethanol levels are attained for some doses when compared with i.p. dosing. The method is also prone to producing cytotoxic damage on contact with tissues of the gastrointestinal tract. For chronic studies, it is essential to consider the nutritional implications of ethanol administration, as over a prolonged period ethanol induces anorexia. To resolve these problems ethanol is mixed with a nutritionally complete liquid diet so that it is the animal's only source of water, ethanol, macro-, and micronutrients.[31,32] Using this technique animals can be made to consume as much as 40% of their calories as ethanol; this is similar to the proportion of ethanol-derived calories consumed by alcoholics. Control animals are fed the same diet in which ethanol is substituted by isocaloric glucose, i.e., pair feeding. In relation to intestinal protein turnover, this is an important point because nutritional status is a potent modulator of mammalian tissue protein synthesis.[33] Liquid dietary regimes in alcohol toxicity studies are reviewed in further detail by Lieber and DeCarli.[31,32] Likewise, the application of the liquid diet regimen to protein turnover studies have been reviewed by Preedy et al.[34]

## 14.2 PROTEIN TURNOVER IN THE SMALL INTESTINE

### 14.2.1 Basic Concepts

Protein turnover is a dynamic process whereby tissue proteins are continuously being synthesized and broken down. In the steady-state situation, tissue protein content is maintained. This is achieved by the fact that the fractional rates of protein synthesis and degradation are equal. Perturbations in one or both of these processes will lead to an alteration in tissue protein content (Figure 14.1). Reductions in protein content need not necessarily arise solely as a consequence of a decrease in the fractional rates of synthesis. In catabolic states, such as occur in alcoholism (or during injury, trauma or infection), degradation rates are greater than rates of protein synthesis. However, both degradation and synthesis may increase or decrease simultaneously: whether protein content is reduced or maintained depends on the magnitude of their relative changes. Only if degradation exceeds synthesis will protein content be reduced, as shown by Figure 14.1. Thus, protein content can be reduced if (a) synthesis falls and protein degradation increases, (b) degradation increases, (c) synthesis decreases, (d) degradation increases and exceeds an increase in synthesis, and (e) synthesis falls and the change exceeds a fall in degradation (Figure 14.1). Thus, experimental observations should be interpreted in the context of both synthesis and degradation as both these processes are intimately related.

### 14.2.2 The Measurement of Protein Synthesis

There are various reliable methods for measuring tissue protein synthesis *in vivo*. However, there are no direct methods for reliably measuring degradation *in vivo* (reviewed in References 35 and 36). Therefore we have concentrated mainly on protein synthetic pathways and processes.

Most methods for assessing the rate of protein synthesis involve the measurement of the incorporation of radiolabeled amino acids into protein. Theoretically, the most precise and desirable method for measuring protein synthesis is by accurately defining the specific radioactivity of the precursor amino acid at the site of protein synthesis, i.e., the aminoacyl-tRNA ($S_{ERNA}$), and the product, i.e., the labeled protein. Although there is little difficulty in measuring the latter, measuring the former presents immeasurable practical difficulties. The measurement of aminoacyl-tRNA specific radioactivies is technically difficult because they are exceedingly labile, occur in small quantities, and may be compartmentalized.

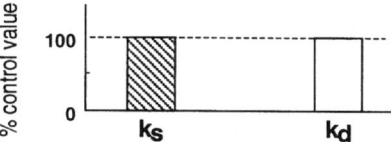

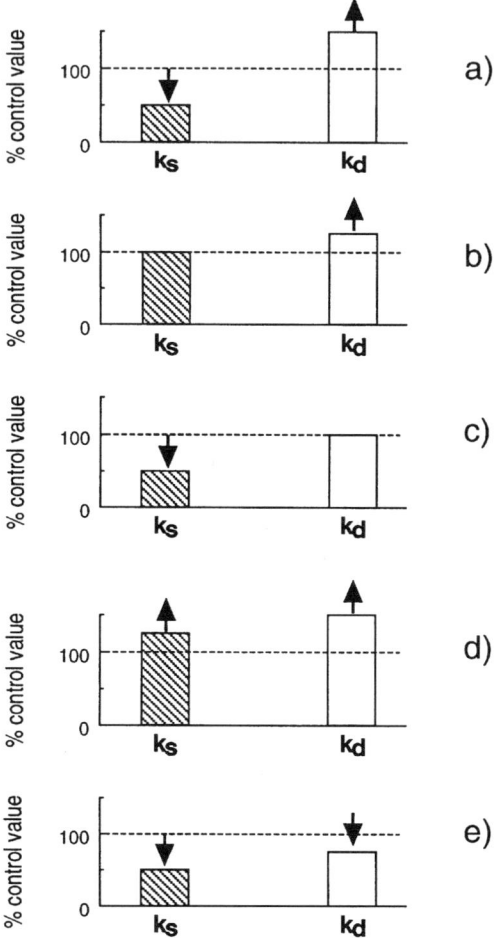

**FIGURE 14.1**   Relationship between protein synthesis, protein degradation, and protein content. Traditionally, schools of thought have considered that a fall in protein synthesis and an increase in protein breakdown are responsible for reductions in tissue protein content. However, the histograms demonstrate various other situations whereby tissue protein is also reduced. (Adapted from Marway, J. S., PhD thesis, University of London, 1993.)

To resolve this problem the specific radioactivity of the free amino acid in the intracellular ($S_i$) or extracellular ($S_p$) pools are usually measured with the assumption that they reflect $S_{tRNA}$. Acid supernatants of tissue homogenates and plasma are usually taken to represent $S_i$ and $S_p$, respectively. However, measurement of synthesis rates may become inaccurate if it is not known whether $S_{tRNA}$ is best represented by $S_i$ or $S_p$. This is especially compounded when there are large differences between $S_i$ and $S_p$. The specific radioactivity of the amino acid in the tissue protein also needs to be isolated and assayed.

There are three main methods for administering the radiolabeled amino acid: (a) single pulse injection of a tracer amount of labeled amino acid; (b) constant infusion of a tracer amount of labeled amino acid; and (c) single injection of a large "flooding" dose of labeled amino acid (all these methods are reviewed in References 33 and 36 to 40).

There are various disadvantages of using tracer methods. These include the release of protein-bound label back into the various free amino acid pools, which will underestimate the fractional rate of protein synthesis (denoted by the symbol $k_s$, i.e., %/day). Also, these methods are not amenable for acute measurements and as much as 6 h of labeling is required to measure $k_s$ with the constant infusion technique.[39,40] Large differences between $S_i$ and $S_p$ can also arise which will lead to uncertainty as to the true synthesis rates of the tissue. The changes in $S_i$ and $S_p$ may also be relatively complex. Using a single pulse injection of a tracer amount of labeled amino acid, a large number of measurements (and thereby many animals) need to be made during the course of the labeling period to accurately define the $S_i$ and $S_p$ curves.[33] Constant infusion methods can overcome this latter criticism, but rats require cannulation and immobilization to facilitate the infusion of the labeled amino acid. This procedure *per se* may on occasion alter tissue protein synthesis.[41] There are also specific problems pertaining to the measurement of protein synthesis which are unique to the gut, namely that precursor amino acids cannot only be derived from the plasma or tissue, but also from the intestinal lumen.[42,44] Nevertheless, the attributes of the constant infusion method has been detailed by Rennie et al.[40] In the laboratory rat, the gold standard method is probably the flooding dose technique, which is described in detail below, and also has the advantages of being able to simultaneously measure protein synthesis in virtually every mammalian organ.[39]

### 14.2.3 The Flooding Dose Technique

The flooding dose technique for reliably measuring $k_s$ entails the intravenous administration of a large concentration (usually 150 µmol/100 g rat) of labeled amino acid (usually leucine or phenylalanine) and killing rats at two time points, usually 2 and 10 min.[37,38,45,46] The flooding dose effectively saturates all free amino acids pools so that all endogenous free amino acids attain similar or identical specific radioactivities.[37,45-49] As a consequence, differences between $S_i$ and $S_p$ are minimal and approximate $S_{tRNA}$.[37,39,45] Synthesis rates can also be measured over a relatively shorter period of time, i.e., 10 min. The shorter incorporation periods diminish any probability of recycling of labeled amino acid and the shorter incorporation periods also have the added advantage that the effects of dietary influences on protein synthesis are avoided. In tissues with low turnover rates (such as skeletal muscle and cardiac muscle), there are very little differences between $S_i$ and $S_p$ after a short period of labeling. In the gut, and in other tissues with high rates of protein synthesis, there can be a 30% difference between $S_i$ and $S_p$.[50] This can further add to the difficulty in precisely assuming the value of the specific radioactivity in the precursor pool, especially as physiological perturbations cause only relatively small changes in protein synthesis. Nevertheless, the flooding dose technique reduces the requirement for a large number of measurements and synthesis rates can be determined in single animals. The radiolabel can either be administered intravenously or intraperitonally.[51,52] However, despite being technically difficult, the intravenous route of administration of radioisotope is preferred as ethanol inhibits the transfer of [$^3$H]phenylalanine from the extracellular to the intracellular compartments of the intestine.[53]

Originally leucine was used as the labeled amino acid in the flooding dose technique.[45] This amino acid has reportedly played a role in the regulation of tissue protein synthesis.[54,55] However, the part played by leucine in protein synthesis remains controversial as McNurlan et al.[56] have shown that leucine does not itself affect protein synthesis in *in vivo* studies on the small intestine.

Currently, the most commonly used amino acid to measure protein synthesis by the flooding dose technique is phenylalanine. Phenylalanine also has the further advantage of being more soluble than leucine. Garlick et al.[37] have suggested that a flooding dose of phenylalanine does not affect protein synthesis as measured with lysine or threonine tracers.

The fractional rates of protein synthesis ($k_s$) are calculated from a basic equation in which the specific radioactivity of the protein was divided by the product of the free specific radioactivity and radiolabeling period, i.e.,

$$k_S = \frac{S_B \times 100}{S_i \,(or\, S_p) \times t} \,(\% / day) \tag{1}$$

where $S_B$ is the specific radioactivity of phenylalanine in protein, $S_i$ is the specific radioactivity of phenylalanine in the tissue-free amino acid pool, $S_p$ is the specific radioactivity of phenylalanine in the plasma-free amino acid pool, and t is the actual time of radioisotope incorporation (in days).

There are, however, certain methodological limitations associated with measuring protein synthesis in the gastrointestinal tract with the flooding dose technique. In particular, the specific radioactivity of free amino acid falls significantly between 2 and 10 min. This fall in $S_i$ is due to the high turnover rate of proteins in the gastrointestinal tract. For example, in the jejunal mucosa a drop of 25% in the value of $S_i$ occurs over the 2- to 10-min period, whereas only a 2% decrease occurs in skeletal muscles.[57] As the fall in intestinal $S_i$ is linear with time, this problem is overcome by sacrificing animals at two time points (i.e., usually 2 and 10 min) and using the mean specific radioactivity of the free labeled amino acid during this period. For the accurate determination of $k_s$ it is assumed that there is no delay in the charging of the amino acyl-tRNA with labeled amino acid. However, although we have shown this to be true for various regions of the gastrointestinal tract (Figure 14.2), Samarel[58] has suggested there may be a brief delay in cardiac aminoacyl-tRNA charging. This will lead to a lag in the appearance of the protein bound isotope, and as a consequence underestimated $k_s$. The data in Figure 14.2 appear to refute this suggested limitation of the flooding dose method.

In the study by McNurlan et al.,[45] jejunal mucosa synthesis rates in young male rats were determined with a flooding dose of [$^{14}$C]leucine and were found to be 104%/day or 136%/day when calculated using plasma or tissue precursor specific radioactivities, respectively. This contrasts with a rate of 10 to 15%/day in skeletal muscles of similar sized rats.[37] Subsequent studies by McNurlan and Garlick[59] showed that the fractional rates of protein synthesis of liver, stomach, small intestine, and large intestine were very high, i.e., 105, 74, 103, and 62%/day, respectively, while whole body synthesis rates were found to be 33%/day. The studies by McNurlan and Garlick[59] also established for the first time the fact that the gastrointestinal tract is a very important contributor to whole body protein metabolism. For example, absolute rates of protein synthesis in the combined stomach and small and large intestines contributed to 19% of the whole body value.[59]

McNurlan and Garlick[59] and Goldspink et al.[42] also showed that the synthesis rates of the large intestine were approximately 40% lower than the small intestine. Heterogeneity in the small intestine could reflect the different biochemical roles of each anatomically distinct region. The gastrointestinal tract can also be further divided into other physiological compartments as described below.

## 14.2.4   Heterogeneity of Protein Synthesis in the Gastrointestinal Tract

Using the flooding dose method to measure $k_s$, fractional synthetic rates of proteins in the mucosal layer of the gastrointestinal tract have been shown to be two to three times higher than

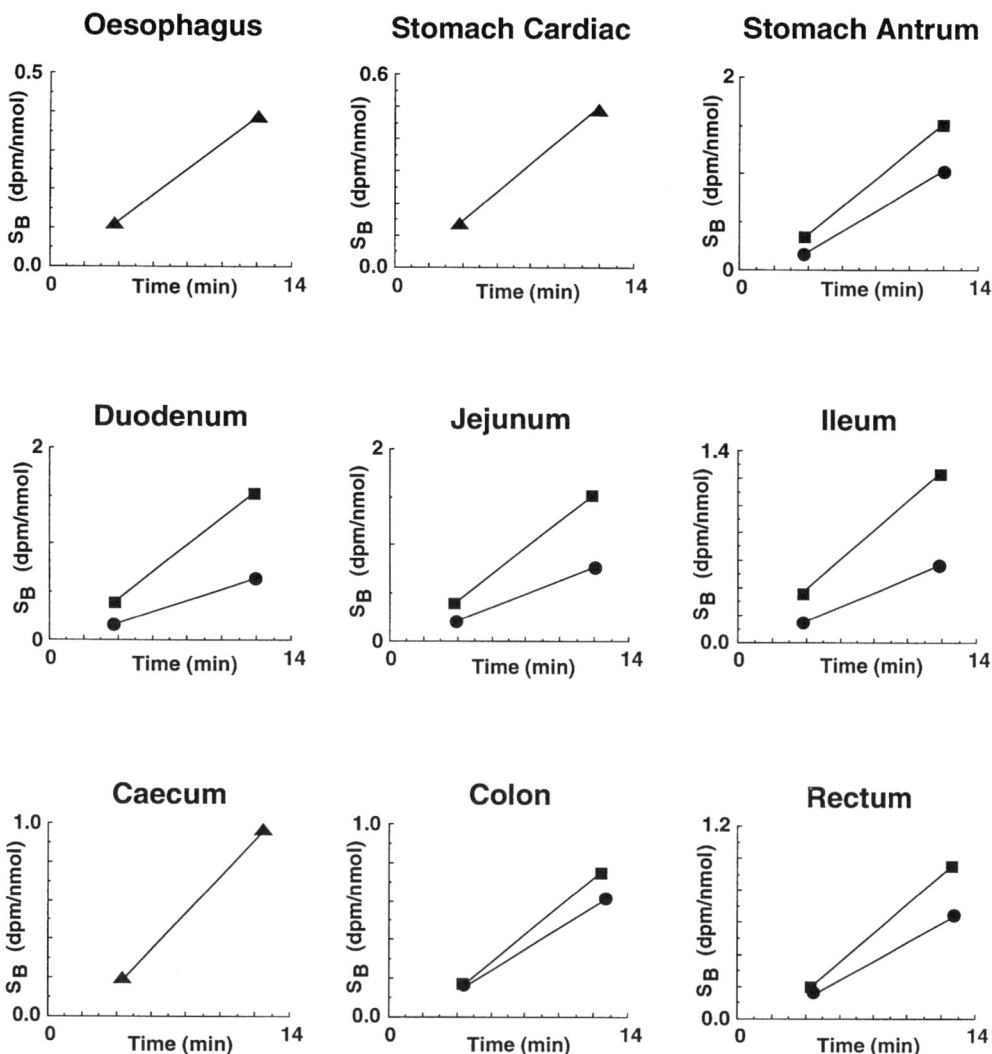

**FIGURE 14.2** Protein-bound phenylalanine specific radioactivities. Various tissues of the rat gastrointestinal tract were removed after the injection of a large flooding dose of L-[4-$^3$H] phenylalanine (at time 0 min) and analyzed for protein-bound phenylalanine specific radioactivities ($S_B$). All data are the means ± S.E.M. of 4 to 8 observations in each group (S.E.M. are very small and are contained within the symbols). ■, mucosa; ●, seromuscular layers; ▲, mixed. (From Marway, J. S., PhD thesis, University of London, 1993.)

proteins in the seromuscular layer.[30,57,60] This might have been expected as luminal mucosal cells are continually being shed and replaced via the process of cell turnover. Lewis et al.[61] also determined $k_s$ values in smooth muscle regions of the rat esophagus (i.e., 42%/day), which were considerably lower than rates in either the jejunum seromuscular or mucosal layers of the stomach. Protein metabolism has also been investigated by Schaefer and Krishnamurti[62] in different regions of the gastrointestinal tract in the developing ovine fetus. Synthesis rates in the recticulorumen, omasum, abomasum, proximal duodenum, and distal colon were found to be 49, 10, 14, 93, and 15% per day, respectively.[62] Thus synthesis in the small intestine were relatively higher than any other region and particularly the large intestines, essentially confirming the results of Goldspink et al.[42] Attaix and Arnal[63] examined fractional synthesis rates along the gastrointestinal tract of preruminant lambs. Fractional synthesis rates increased from the esophagus (27%/day), reticulorumen (30%/day), omasum (41%/day), abomasum (56%/day) to the small intestine (88%/day) and then declined significantly toward the cecum (45%/day) and the colon (38%/day). There were no significant differences between fractional synthesis rates in the duodenum, jejunum, or ileum. Thus there is considerable variability in synthesis rates between different regions of the gastrointestinal tract. In addition, Attaix and Arnal[63] reported that the relative contribution of the esophagus, stomachs, small intestine, and large intestine to gastrointestinal protein synthesis was 1, 13, 76, and 10%, respectively. The gastrointestinal tract accounted for approximately 12% of whole body protein synthesis. However, in the studies by Goldspink et al.,[42] McNurlan and Garlick,[59] Lewis et al.,[61] and Attaix and Arnal[63] there was a paucity of information on mucosa and values were not determined in pathophysiological states but in normal growth. Rates of protein synthesis in different protein fractions are also heterogeneous. Preedy et al.[64] determined rates of protein synthesis in subcellular fractions of the entire small intestine and showed that in young rats $k_s$ in the cytoplasmic and myofibrillar fraction were 129 and 99%/day, respectively.

## 14.2.5    Effects of Ethanol on Protein Synthesis in the Small Intestine

Chronic ethanol feeding has a major effect on protein metabolism in the small intestine. Studies by Preedy and Peters[50] showed that rats fed on ethanol as 36% of total calories in a nutritionally complete liquid diet for 6 weeks produced a 21% reduction in the absolute wet weight of the whole small intestine compared with pair fed controls. The total amounts of protein, RNA, and DNA were also significantly reduced as a result of ethanol feeding by 23, 16, and 28%, respectively. However, there was a 15% increase in the RNA/DNA ratio.[50] Also, fractional rates of mixed protein synthesis were measured using the flooding dose of L-[4-³H]phenylalanine and were found to be only slightly reduced, suggesting that protein breakdown may have been elevated.

In a similar chronic ethanol feeding study, Preedy et al.[65] showed that the wet weight of the stomach decreased by 17% ($p < 0.025$), while the large intestine wet weight decreased by only 6% ($p > 0.05$) after 6 weeks of alcohol ingestion. Thus it can be seen that ethanol may selectively affect different parts of the gastrointestinal tract considering that the large intestine was relatively unaffected. The mechanism for this differential sensitivity is unknown.

The study by Preedy et al.[65] also showed that the ethanol-induced changes in the small intestine occurred in the absence of changes in blood supply. This is an important point as alterations in the blood supply could conceivably affect the availability of precursor amino acids for protein synthesis.[44]

In most studies of the chronic effects of ethanol feeding on the gastrointestinal tract, the effects on the seromuscular layer have been relatively ignored. In a recent study, however, seromuscular layers of various regions of the gastrointestinal tract were examined in rats fed a nutritionally adequate liquid diet containing 35% of total calories as ethanol. After 6 weeks of chronic ethanol feeding, the wet weights of the antrum and whole jejunum were reduced by 31% and the wet weights of the duodenum, jejunum and distal ileum seromuscular layers decreased by 19 to 25%. However, the wet weight of the large intestine seromuscular layer was unaltered.[66] The total amounts of contractile and noncontractile protein in the small intestinal seromuscular layers were reduced by 16 to 52% (Figure 14.3). In the jejunal seromuscular layer, the total RNA contents were reduced by 29%, but total RNA contents in seromuscular layers of the ileum and duodenum were not significantly altered. The purpose of measuring total RNA is to assess the contribution of the ribosomes. Ribosomal RNA comprises a major proportion (approx. 80%) of total RNA[67] and is a predictor of protein synthesis.[30] Chronic ethanol feeding had no apparent effect on either contractile or noncontractile total protein, total RNA, or DNA contents in colonic and rectal

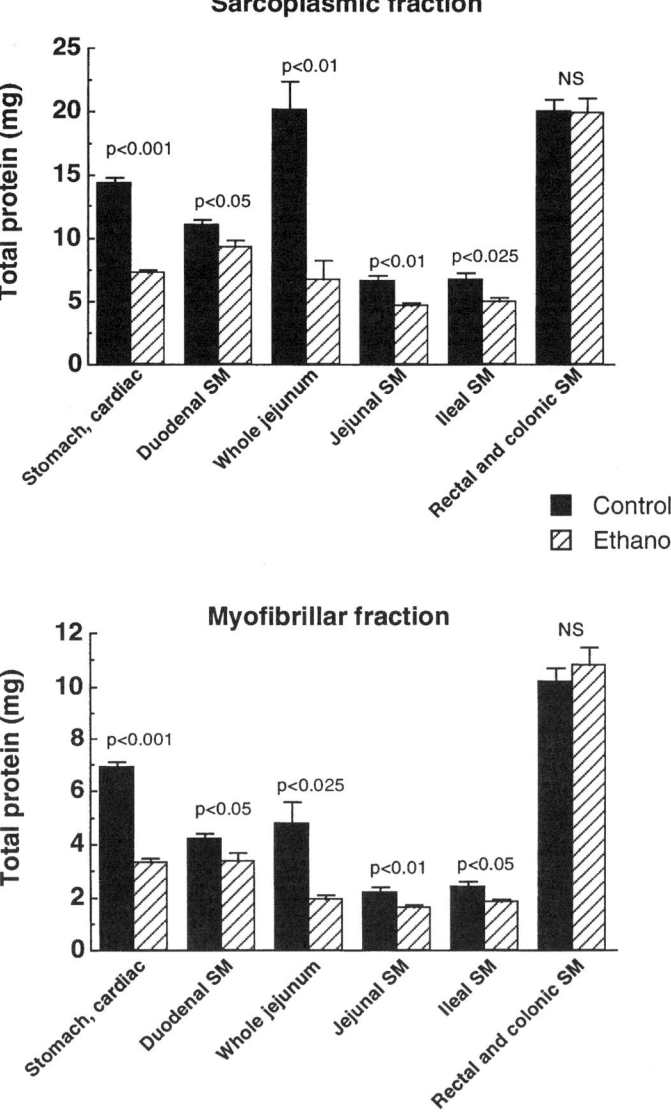

**FIGURE 14.3** The effect of chronic ethanol ingestion for 6 weeks on subcellular protein composition in various regions of the gastrointestinal tract. Protein composition was determined in subcellular protein fractions of various regions of the gastrointestinal tract. SM, seromuscular layer. All data are presented as means ± S.E.M. of 5 to 9 pairs of observations. Differences between means were assessed by Student's *t* test for paired samples as differences were normally distributed. NS, *p* >0.05, not significant. (From Marway, J. S. and Preedy, V. R., *Alcohol Alcohol.*, 26, 549, 1991.)

seromuscular layer.[66] The results reaffirmed that the small intestine and antral region of the stomach are generally sensitive to chronic ethanol toxicity. The authors have also shown that protein synthesis in different regions of the gastrointestinal tract show varying sensitivities to chronic ethanol ingestion. Chronic ethanol ingestion for 3 weeks led to significant decreases in $k_s$ in mixed protein fractions of the jejunal seromuscular layer and the esophagus, whereas mixed $k_s$ in the cardiac region of the stomach and seromuscular layers of the colon and rectum were unaffected.[68] The targeting of the seromuscular layer *per se*, and in particular the contractile

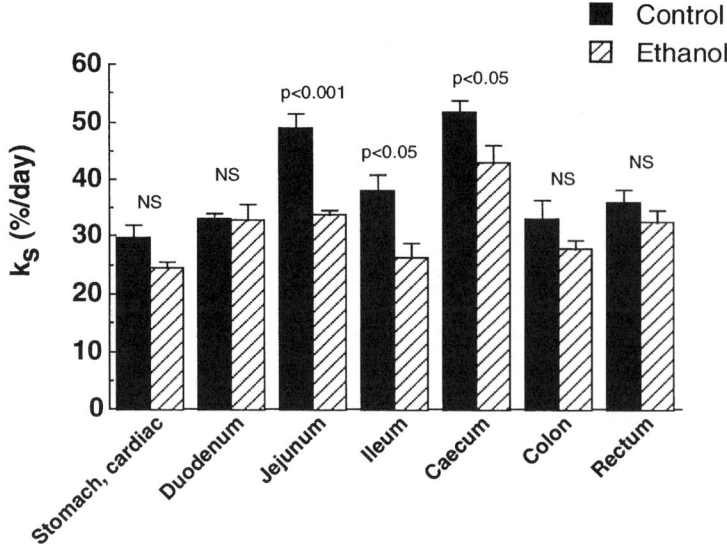

**FIGURE 14.4**  Contractile protein synthesis in gastrointestinal tissues and their response to acute ethanol toxicity. Young male Wistar rats (approx. 100 g body weight) were either injected (i.p.) with ethanol at a dosage of 75 mmol/kg body weight or an equal volume of 0.15 mol/l NaCl (controls). Fractional rates of myofibrillary (contractile) protein synthesis ($k_s$) were measured after 2.5 h with a flooding dose of L-[4-³H]phenylalanine. Contractile proteins were isolated from the seromuscular layers by combined differential solubility and high-speed centrifugation procedures. All data are means ± S.E.M. ($n$ = 6 to 9). NS, not significant, $p$ >0.05. (From Marway, J. S., et al., *Biochem. Soc. Trans.*, 22, 194S, 1994.)

proteins contained therein, may have important implications as loss of contractile proteins may contribute to the development of gastrointestinal motility-related disturbances so commonly found in chronic alcohol misusers.[12,25]

Using an acute (2.5 h) dose of ethanol (75 mmol/kg body weight) to investigate protein synthesis on the myofibrillar fraction of the small intestine, Preedy et al.[64] showed that ethanol reduced the rates of protein synthesis of contractile proteins by 40 to 50%. This study was the first to investigate how different protein fractions of the small intestine responded to acute ethanol dosage. Rates of mixed protein synthesis fell by approximately 20%, from 120%/day to 100%/day as a result of ethanol administration. The decrease in sarcoplasmic protein synthesis rates showed a similar response, but the fall in myofibrillar $k_s$ was greater (i.e., 40 to 50%; Preedy et al.[64]). It was suggested that perhaps there may be a very important relationship between loss of contractile protein (implicated by a fall in synthesis rates) and motility disorders seen in alcohol abusers.[64] The original studies by Preedy et al.[64] have now been extended to include all the regions of the rat gastrointestinal tract and data show that there is selective sensitivity between different regions in that myofibrillar rates of protein synthesis are decreased in the seromuscular layers of the stomach (cardiac region), jejunum, and ileum but protein synthesis in the seromuscular layers of the duodenum, colon, and rectum are not affected (Figure 14.4; Marway et al.[69]). Similarly, seromuscular layer mixed protein synthesis in various regions of the gastrointestinal tract also shows selective sensitivity to acute ethanol dosage, as shown in Figure 14.5.[30] Furthermore the study by Marway et al.[30] showed that with acute ethanol dosage mucosal protein synthesis in the colon and rectum was unaltered though mucosal protein synthesis in other regions, such as the stomach, duodenum, and jejunum were reduced.

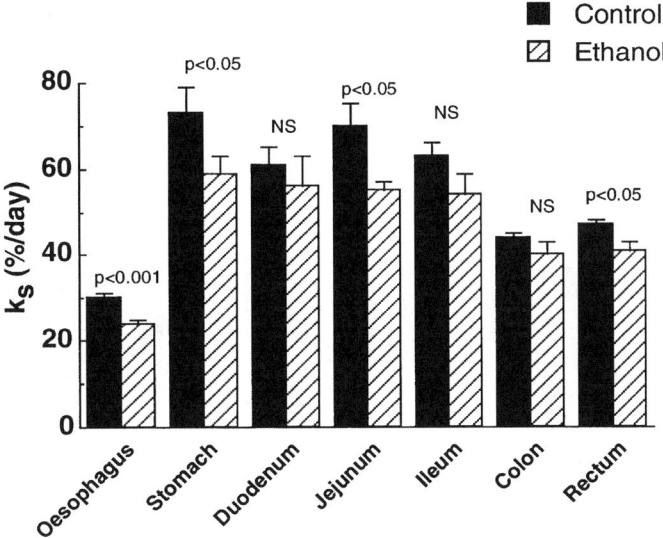

**FIGURE 14.5** The effects of acute ethanol dosage on protein synthesis in the seromuscular layers of the rat gastrointestinal tract. Young male Wistar rats (approx. 100 g body weight) were either injected (i.p.) with ethanol at a dosage of 75 mmol/kg body weight or an equal volume of 0.15 mol/l NaCl (controls). Fractional rates of protein synthesis ($k_s$) were measured after 2.5 h with a flooding dose of L-[4-$^3$H]phenylalanine. All data are means ± S.E.M. ($n$ = 6 to 9). Esophagus pertains to the mixed seromuscular layer plus mucosa, while the remaining regions of the gastrointestinal tract pertain to the isolated seromuscular layers. (From Marway, J. S., et al., *Eur. J. Gastroenterol. Hepatol.*, 5, 27, 1993.)

## 14.3 MECHANISMS FOR THE ETHANOL-INDUCED INHIBITION IN PROTEIN SYNTHESIS

Investigations into the acute and chronic effects of ethanol toxicity[50,53,64,65,70] have enhanced our understanding of protein synthesis in the small intestine. However, the exact mechanisms for the ethanol-induced inhibition of gastrointestinal protein synthesis are not yet known, although there are a number of possibilities. Some of the effects of ethanol dosage may be mediated by the highly reactive intermediate metabolite, acetaldehyde, as well as ethanol *per se*. By the concomitant administration of ethanol and inhibitors of ethanol metabolism, namely 4-methylpyrazole [which inhibits alcohol dehydrogenase (ADH)] and cyanamide [which inhibits aldehyde dehydrogenase (ALDH)] we have shown that even when acetaldehyde formation is inhibited, protein synthesis declines, indicating a direct effect of ethanol itself. However, profound inhibition of protein synthesis occurs when endogenous acetaldehyde is raised with cyanamide treatment (Figure 14.6; Marway and Preedy[71]). This is similar to the effects in heart and skeletal muscle.[72,73]

Endocrine function, i.e., adrenal and thyroid hormones, are also important regulators of intestinal function. Studies have shown that glucocorticoids are essential for intestinal maturation[74-77] and gastrointestinal motility,[78] as are thyroid hormones.[79,80] Ethanol has been found to have a variety of effects on the endocrine system,[81-84] more specifically, acute ethanol has been shown to increase plasma corticosterone in a dose–response manner.[85] In humans, both acute and chronic ethanol consumption occasionally results in hypercortisolemia[86,87] and can lead to pseudo-Cushing's syndrome.[88,89] Thyroid hormones have also been shown to be influenced by ethanol dosage.[90] Triiodothyronine decreases hepatic ADH and ALDH activity by 36 to 45%[91] whereas thyroidectomy causes an increase in rat liver ADH activity.[92] There is the possibility that the synthesis rates of small intestinal proteins are modulated by ethanol-induced endocrine

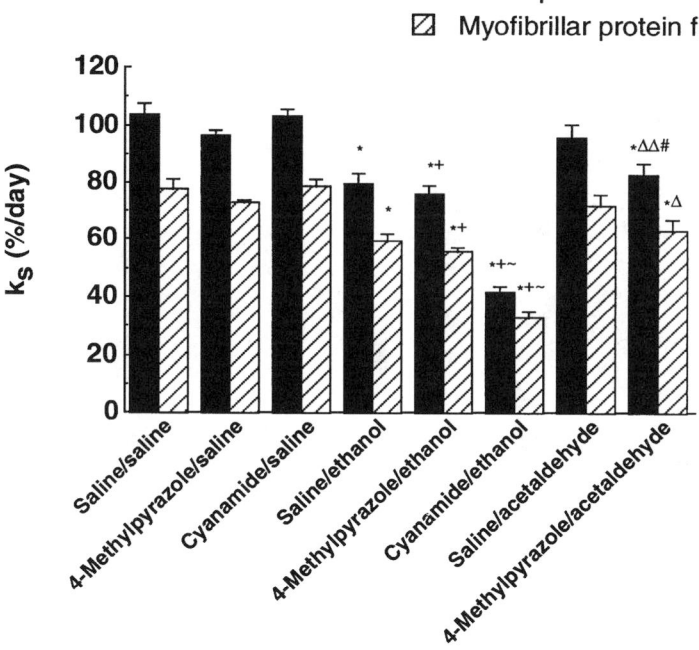

**PRETREATMENT / TREATMENT**

**FIGURE 14.6**  Effects of ethanol with or without enzyme inhibitors on fractional rates of protein synthesis in mixed and myofibrillar protein fractions of whole jejunum. Fractional rates of protein synthesis ($k_s$) were determined in mixed and contractile proteins of whole jejunum. All data are the means ± S.E.M. of 6 to 13 observations. Differences between means were assessed by Student's *t* test using the pooled estimate of variance. Saline plus saline versus all other groups: *$p$ <0.001. 4-Methylpyrazole plus saline vs. 4-methylpyrazole plus ethanol or cyanamide plus saline vs. cyanamide plus ethanol: +$p$ <0.001. Saline plus ethanol vs. 4-methylpyrazole plus ethanol or cyanamide plus ethanol: ~$p$ <0.001. 4-Methylpyrazole plus saline versus 4-methylpyrazole plus acetaldehyde: $^{\triangle}p$ <0.025; $^{\triangle\triangle}p$ <0.01. Saline plus acetaldehyde vs. 4-methylpyrazole plus acetaldehyde: #$p$ <0.05. (From Marway, J. S. and Preedy, V. R., *Alcohol Alcohol.*, 30, 211, 1995.)

dysfunction. Recently, the authors have shown that acute ethanol dosage significantly (*p* <0.025) reduced protein synthesis in all subcellular protein fractions of the whole jejunum and jejunal seromuscular layer in sham-thyroidectomized, thyroidectomized, sham-adrenalectomized, and adrenalectomized rats (Tables 14.1 and 14.2). In most protein fractions, however, the inhibition of protein synthesis was greater in thyroidectomized rats than in sham-thyroidectomized rats, whereas the reverse was true in adrenalectomized rats. Neither treatment abolished the ethanol-induced inhibition in protein synthesis. It is thus conceivable that motility disturbances or biochemical adjustments in response to alcohol toxicity may be modulated by endocrine status.

In eukarocytes, nucleotide concentrations regulate protein synthesis[93,94] and acute ethanol has been shown to reduce jejunal ATP.[95,96] Recently, the authors have showed that acute ethanol dosage reduced ATP and GTP levels whereas ADP and GDP concentrations were increased in conditions that reduce protein synthesis in the jejunum (Figure 14.7; Marway et al.[97]). Thus the energy status of cells could possibly offer some explanation as to why protein synthesis is inhibited. However, interpretation of data requires caution as ethanol may cause the shifting of nucleotides between different pools.[98] Nevertheless, the changes in nucleotide content may occur

**TABLE 14.1  The Effects of Ethanol and Thyroidectomy on Whole Jejunal and Jejunal Seromuscular Layer Protein Synthesis**

| | Control | Ethanol | Difference (% of control) | $p$ |
|---|---|---|---|---|
| Whole jejunum | | | | |
| $k_s$ (%/day) | | | | |
| Mixed | | | | |
| Sham-Tx | 116 ± 4 | 90 ± 3 | −22 | <0.001 |
| Tx | 93 ± 6 | 57 ± 4 | −39[b] | <0.001 |
| Sarcoplasmic | | | | |
| Sham-Tx | 135 ± 5 | 112 ± 6 | −17 | <0.025 |
| Tx | 107 ± 8 | 73 ± 5 | −32[b] | <0.001 |
| Myofibrillar | | | | |
| Sham-Tx | 110 ± 5 | 71 ± 4 | −35 | <0.001 |
| Tx | 81 ± 5 | 49 ± 3 | −40[b] | <0.001 |
| Jejunal seromuscular layer | | | | |
| $k_s$ (%/day) | | | | |
| Mixed | | | | |
| Sham-Tx | 78 ± 5 | 53 ± 3 | −32 | <0.001 |
| Tx | 70 ± 4 | 35 ± 2 | −50[a] | <0.001 |
| Sarcoplasmic | | | | |
| Sham-Tx | 107 ± 7 | 77 ± 5 | −28 | <0.001 |
| Tx | 94 ± 5 | 48 ± 3 | −49[b] | <0.001 |
| Myofibrillar | | | | |
| Sham-Tx | 42 ± 4 | 29 ± 2 | −31 | <0.01 |
| Tx | 42 ± 3 | 19 ± 1 | −55[c] | <0.001 |

*Note:* Sham-thyroidectomized (sham-Tx) or thyroidectomized (Tx) male Wistar rats were fed on solid laboratory diet and water. The quantity of food presented to the Tx group of rats was *ad libitum* whereas for the sham-Tx group, food was restricted (based on the quantity of food consumed by the Tx group of rats). On the day of measurement of protein synthesis, rats were injected (i.p.) with saline or ethanol (75 mmol/kg body weight). After 140 min rats were injected (i.v.) with a flooding dose of L-[4-³H]phenylalanine and 10 min later killed and the intestine rapidly dissected out and cooled in ice-cold saline. Whole jejunal sections and jejunal seromuscular layer (20 cm) of tissue were prepared, frozen in liquid nitrogen, and stored at −70°C until analysis. Fractional rates of protein synthesis ($k_s$) were determined in protein fractions. All data are presented as means ± S.E.M. of 5 to 8 observations. Differences between means were assessed by Student's *t* test. The superscript notation in the column headed "Difference (% of control)" pertains to two-way analysis of variance to test for any statistically significant differences as a result of acute ethanol dosage between sham-Tx and Tx groups.

[a] $p < 0.01$.

[b] $p < 0.001$.

[c] $p > 0.05$ (i.e., not significant).

due to decreased activity of nonmitochondrial enzymes, mitochondrial abnormalities, or via the formation of acetaldehyde-protein adducts.

Consideration must also be given to the involvement of free radicals in the ethanol-induced reductions in protein synthesis. Free radicals are an important component of gastrointestinal tract injury in ischemia,[99,100] inflammatory bowel disease,[101] and gastric ulceration.[102] Free radicals have also been implicated in ethanol-induced cellular damage in various tissues including the gastrointestinal tract.[103] Oxidative stress has also been proposed as altering intestinal motility; however, studies by Van der Vliet et al.[104] have indicated that smooth muscle dysfunction can occur in the absence of free radical-mediated damage. However, at present, there are no studies that have attempted to address the question of whether a relationship exists between free radicals

**TABLE 14.2    The Effects of Ethanol and Adrenalectomy on Whole Jejunal and Jejunal Seromuscular Layer Protein Synthesis**

| | Control | Ethanol | Difference (% of control) | $p$ |
|---|---|---|---|---|
| Whole jejunum | | | | |
| $k_s$ (%/day) | | | | |
| Mixed | | | | |
| Sham-Adx | $120 \pm 5$ | $71 \pm 6$ | –41 | <0.001 |
| Adx | $100 \pm 4$ | $68 \pm 5$ | –32[b] | <0.001 |
| Sarcoplasmic | | | | |
| Sham-Adx | $136 \pm 5$ | $82 \pm 6$ | –40 | <0.001 |
| Adx | $116 \pm 7$ | $81 \pm 7$ | –30[a] | <0.001 |
| Myofibrillar | | | | |
| Sham-Adx | $102 \pm 3$ | $56 \pm 5$ | –45 | <0.001 |
| Adx | $87 \pm 5$ | $57 \pm 4$ | –34[c] | <0.001 |
| Jejunal seromuscular layer | | | | |
| $k_s$ (%/day) | | | | |
| Mixed | | | | |
| Sham-Adx | $71 \pm 6$ | $42 \pm 6$ | –41 | <0.001 |
| Adx | $90 \pm 5$ | $45 \pm 5$ | –50[c] | <0.001 |
| Sarcoplasmic | | | | |
| Sham-Adx | $92 \pm 7$ | $72 \pm 5$ | –22 | <0.05 |
| Adx | $114 \pm 9$ | $63 \pm 5$ | –45[c] | <0.001 |
| Myofibrillar | | | | |
| Sham-Adx | $42 \pm 3$ | $26 \pm 2$ | –38 | <0.001 |
| Adx | $50 \pm 4$ | $28 \pm 3$ | –44[c] | <0.001 |

*Note:* Sham-adrenalectomized (sham-Adx) or adrenalectomized (Adx) male Wistar rats were fed on solid laboratory diet and water. The quantity of food presented to both groups of rats was restricted (based on the quantity of food consumed by the Tx group of rats). On the day of measurement of protein synthesis, rats were injected (i.p.) with saline or ethanol (75 mmol/kg body weight). After 140 min rats were injected (i.v.) with a flooding dose of L-[4-³H]phenylalanine and 10 min later killed and the intestine rapidly dissected out and cooled in ice-cold saline. Whole jejunal sections and jejunal seromuscular layers (20 cm) of tissue were prepared, frozen in liquid nitrogen, and stored at –70°C until analysis. Fractional rates of protein synthesis ($k_s$) were determined in protein fractions. All data are presented as means ± S.E.M. of 5 to 8 observations. Differences between means were assessed by Student's *t* test. The superscript notation in the column headed "Difference (% of control)" pertains to two-way analysis of variance to test for any statistically significant differences as a result of acute ethanol dosage between sham-Adx and Adx groups.

[a]  $p$ <0.05.

[b]  $p$ <0.01.

[c]  $p$ >0.05 (i.e., not significant).

and ethanol-induced inhibition of gastrointestinal tissue protein synthesis. In a preliminary study the authors have shown that although acute ethanol dosage does not affect the antioxidant enzyme, superoxide dismutase (SOD), in seromuscular layers of the jejunum, colon, and rectum, the distribution of SOD varies between tissues. In our preliminary study we found that SOD activities in seromuscular layers of the colon were significantly ($p$ <0.001) higher than in either the jejunum or the rectum.[105] Obviously there is still a considerable amount of work to be carried out in this area.

## 14.4   CONCLUSION

This chapter has reviewed the effects of ethanol on protein synthesis in the gastrointestinal tract and identified a few ways in which the mechanisms responsible for ethanol-induced perturbations

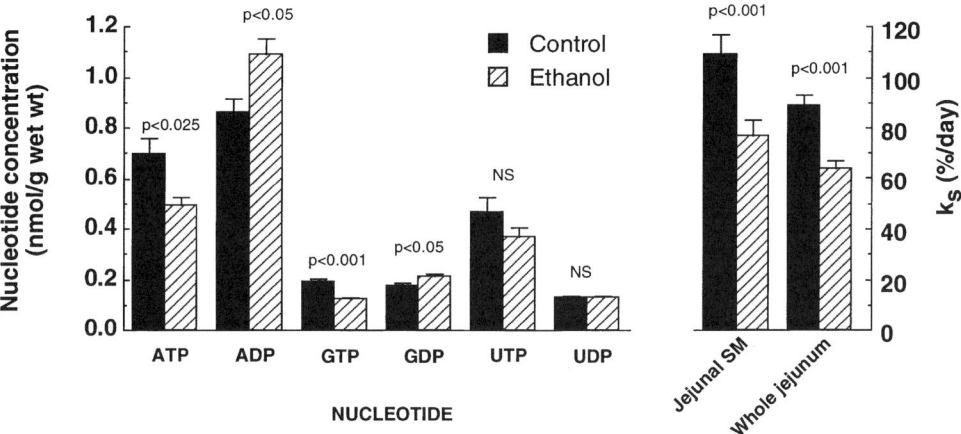

**FIGURE 14.7** Effect of acute ethanol dosage on jejunal nucleotides and protein synthesis. Male Wistar rats (approx. 100 g body weight) were injected (i.p.) with either saline (controls) or ethanol (75 mmol/kg body weight). After 2.5 h rats were killed and the proximal jejunum (20 cm) rapidly dissected and freeze clamped. Tissues were subsequently pulverized under liquid nitrogen and nucleotides extracted into perchloric acid followed by neutralization with potassium hydroxide. Nucleotides were measured in neutralized supernatants by high-performance liquid chromatography. All data are presented as means ± S.E.M. of 4 to 6 observations in each group. Differences between means were assessed by Student's *t* test, where data are normally distributed. NS, *p >0.05, not significant*; ATP, adenosine triphosphate; ADP, adenosine diphosphate; GTP, guanine triphosphate; GDP, guanine diphosphate; UTP, uridine triphosphates; UDP, uridine diphosphate; SM, seromuscular layer; $k_s$, fractional rate of protein synthesis. (From Marway, J. S., et al., *Alcohol Alcohol.*, 28, 521, 1993.)

may occur. There are, of course, numerous other areas that can be investigated. It is important to point out that compared to the liver, skeletal muscle, and the heart, the factors that regulate intestinal protein synthesis are not well understood.

## REFERENCES

1. **Halsted, C. H., Robles, E. A., and Mezey, E.,** Distribution of ethanol in the human gastrointestinal tract, *Am. J. Clin. Nutr.*, 26, 831, 1973.
2. **Lake-Bakaar, G.,** Gastrointestinal complications of alcoholism, in *Clinical Biochemistry of Alcoholism*, Rosalki, S. B., Ed., Churchill Livingstone, London, 1984, 227.
3. **Pikaar, N. A., Wedel, M., and Hermus, R. J. J.,** Influence of several factors on blood alcohol concentrations after drinking alcohol, *Alcohol Alcohol.*, 23, 289, 1988.
4. **Wallgren, H.,** Absorption, diffusion, distribution and elimination of ethanol, Effect on biological membranes, in *International Encyclopedia of Pharmacology and Therapeutics*, Bovet, D., Burgen, A. S. V., Cheymol, J., and Heymans, C., Eds., Pergemon Press, Oxford, 1972, 161.
5. **Geokas, M. C.,** Ethanol, the liver, and the gastrointestinal tract, *Ann. Intern. Med.*, 95, 198, 1981.
6. **Langman, M. J. S. and Bell, G. D.,** Alcohol and the gastrointestinal tract, *Br. Med. Bull.*, 38, 71, 1982.
7. **Nazer, H. and Wright, R. A.,** The effect of alcohol on the human alimentary tract: a review, *J. Clin. Gastroenterol.*, 5, 361, 1983.
8. **Mezey, E.,** Effect of ethanol on intestinal morphology, metabolism, and function, in *Alcohol Related Diseases in Gastroenterology*, Seitz, H. K. and Kommerell, B., Eds., Springer-Verlag, Berlin, 1985, 342.
9. **Persson, J.,** Alcohol and the small intestine, *Scand. J. Gastroenterol.*, 26, 3, 1991.
10. **Hajjar, J. J., Tomicic, T., and Scheig, R. L.,** Effect of chronic ethanol consumption on leucine absorption in the rat small intestine, *Digestion*, 22, 170, 1981.
11. **Bikle, D. D., Gee, E. A., and Munson, S. J.,** Effect of ethanol on intestinal calcium transport in chicks, *Gastroenterology*, 91, 870, 1986.
12. **Mazzanti, R., Debnam, E. S., and Jenkins, W. J.,** Effect of chronic ethanol intake on lactase activity and active galactose absorption in rat small intestine, *Gut*, 28, 56, 1987.
13. **Berenson, M. M. and Avner, D. L.,** Alcohol inhibition of rectosigmoid motility in humans, *Digestion*, 22, 210, 1981.

14. **Keshavarzian, A., Iber, F. L., Dangleis, M. D., and Cornish, R.,** Intestinal-transit and lactose intolerance in chronic alcoholics, *Am. J. Clin. Nutr.*, 44, 70, 1986.

15. **Krishnamra, N. and Limlomwongse, L.,** The *in vivo* effect of ethanol on gastrointestinal motility and gastrointestinal handling of calcium in rats, *J. Nutr. Sci. Vitaminol.*, 33, 89, 1987.

16. **Baraona, E., Pirola, R. C., and Lieber, C. S.,** Small intestinal damage and changes in cell population produced by ethanol ingestion in the rat, *Gastroenterology*, 66, 226, 1974.

17. **Guslandi, M.,** Effects of ethanol on the gastric mucosa, *Dig. Dis.*, 5, 21, 1987.

18. **Mazzanti, R., and Jenkins, W. J.,** Effect of chronic ethanol on enterocyte turnover in rat small intestine, *Gut*, 28, 52, 1987.

19. **Sellers, L. A., Allen, A., and Bennett, M. K.,** Formation of a fibrin based gelatinous coat over repairing rat gastric epithelium after acute ethanol damage: interaction with adherent mucus, *Gut*, 28, 835, 1987.

20. **Scratcherd, T. and Grundy, D.,** The physiology of intestinal motility and secretion, *Br. J. Anaesth.*, 56, 3, 1984.

21. **Surprenant, A.,** Control of the gastrointestinal tract by enteric neurons, *Annu. Rev. Physiol.*, 56, 117, 1994.

22. **Robles, E. A., Mezey, E., Halsted, C. H., and Schuster, M. M.,** Effect of ethanol on motility of the small intestine, *Johns Hopkins Med. J.*, 135, 17, 1974.

23. **Scroggs, R., Abruzzo, M., and Advokatt, C.,** Effects of ethanol on gastrointestinal transit in mice, *Alcoholism: Clin. Exp. Res.*, 10, 452, 1986.

24. **Willson, C. A., Bushnell, D., and Keshavarzian, A.,** The effect of acute and chronic ethanol administration on gastric emptying in cats, *Dig. Dis. Sci.*, 35, 444, 1990.

25. **Wegener, M., Schaffstein, J., Dilger, U., Coenen, C., Wedmann, B., and Schmidt, G.,** Gastrointestinal transit of solid-liquid meal in chronic alcoholics, *Dig. Dis. Sci.*, 36, 917, 1991.

26. **Mayer, E. M., Grabowski, C. J., and Fisher, R. S.,** Effect of graded doses of alcohol upon esophageal motor function, *Gastroenterology*, 76, 1133, 1978.

27. **Keshavarzian, A., Iber, F. L., and Ferguson, Y.,** Esophageal manometry and radionuclide emptying in chronic alcoholics, *Gastroenterology,* 92, 651, 1987.

28. **Keshaverzion, A., Polepalle, C., Iber, F. L., and Durkin, M.,** Secondary esophageal contractions are abnormal in chronic alcoholics, *Dig. Dis. Sci.*, 37, 517, 1992.

29. **Tiernan, J. M. and Ward, L. C.,** Acute effects of ethanol on protein synthesis in the rat, *Alcohol Alcohol.*, 21, 171, 1986.

30. **Marway, J. S., Keating, J. W., Reeves, J., Salisbury, J. R., and Preedy, V. R.,** Seromuscular and mucosal protein synthesis in various anatomical regions of the rat gastrointestinal tract and their response to acute ethanol toxicity, *Eur. J. Gastroenterol. Hepatol.*, 5, 27, 1993.

31. **Lieber, C. S. and DeCarli, L. M.,** The feeding of ethanol in liquid diets, *Alcoholism: Clin. Exp. Res.*, 10, 550, 1986.

32. **Lieber, C. S. and DeCarli, L. M.,** Liquid diet technique of ethanol administration: 1989 update, *Alcohol Alcohol.*, 24, 197, 1989.

33. **Waterlow, J. C., Garlick, P. J., and Millward, D. J.,** *Protein Turnover in Mammalian Tissues and The Whole Body*, North-Holland, Amsterdam, 1978.

34. **Preedy, V. R., Duane, P., and Peters, T. J.,** Biological effects of chronic ethanol consumption: a reappraisal of the Lieber-DeCarli liquid-diet model with reference to skeletal muscle, *Alcohol Alcohol.*, 23, 151, 1988.

35. **Hasselgren, P.-O., Pedersen, P., Sax, H. C., Warner, B. W., and Fischer, J. E.,** Methods for studying protein synthesis and degradation in liver and skeletal muscle, *J. Surg. Res.*, 45, 389, 1988.

36. **Preedy, V. R., Siddiq, T., Cook, E., Black, D., Palmer, T. N., and Peters, T. J.,** Alcohol and protein turnover, in *Alcoholism: A Molecular Perspective*, Palmer T. N., Ed., Plenum Press, New York, 1991, 253.

37. **Garlick, P. J., McNurlan, M. A., and Preedy, V. R.,** A rapid and convenient technique for measuring the rate of protein synthesis in tissues by injection of [$^3$H]phenylalanine, *Biochem. J.*, 192, 719, 1980.

38. **Preedy, V. R., Siddiq, T., Why, H. J. F., and Richardson, P. J.,** Ethanol toxicity and cardiac protein synthesis *in vivo*, *Am. Heart J.*, 127, 1432, 1994.

39. **Garlick, P. J., McNurlan, M. A., Essén, P., and Wernerman, J.,** Measurement of tissue protein synthesis rates *in vivo*: a critical analysis of contrasting methods, *Am. J. Physiol.*, 266, E287, 1994.

40. **Rennie, M. J., Smith, K., and Watt, P. W.,** Measurement of human tissue protein synthesis: an optimal approach, *Am. J. Physiol.*, 266, E298, 1994.

41. **Preedy, V. R. and Garlick, P. J.,** The influence of restraint and infusion on rates of muscle protein synthesis in the rat, *Biochem. J.*, 251, 577, 1988.

42. **Goldspink, D. F., Lewis, S. E. M., and Kelly, F. J.,** Protein synthesis during the developmental growth of the small and large intestine of the rat, *Biochem. J.*, 217, 527, 1984.

43. **Egan, C. J. and Rennie, M. J.,** Relative importance of luminal and vascular amino acids for protein synthesis in rat jejunum, *J. Physiol.*, 378, P49, 1986.

44. **Egan, C. J.,** Changes in structure and function of rat jejunum, PhD thesis, University of Dundee, 1988.

45. **McNurlan, M. A., Tomkins, A. M., and Garlick, P. J.,** The effect of starvation on the rate of protein synthesis in rat liver and small intestine, *Biochem. J.*, 178, 373, 1979.

46. **McNurlan, M. A.,** Protein synthesis in the liver and small intestine of the rat, PhD thesis, University of London, 1980.

47. **Khairallah, E. A. and Mortimore, G. E.,** Assessment of protein turnover in perfused rat liver: evidence for amino acid compartmentation from differential labelling of free and t-RNA-bound valine, *J. Biol. Chem.*, 251, 1375, 1976.

48. **McKee, E. E., Cheung, J. Y., Rannels, D. E., and Morgan, H. E.,** Measurement of the rate of protein synthesis and compartmentation of heart phenylalanine, *J. Biol. Chem.*, 253, 1030, 1978.

49. **Watkins, C. A. and Rannels, D. E.,** Measurement of protein synthesis in rat lungs perfused *in situ*, *Biochem. J.*, 188, 269, 1980.

50. **Preedy, V. R. and Peters, T. J.,** Protein metabolism in the small intestine of the ethanol-fed rat, *Cell Biochem. Funct.*, 7, 235, 1989.

51. **Jepson, M. M., Pell, J. M., Bates, P. C., and Millward, D. J.,** The effects of endotoxaemia on protein metabolism in skeletal muscle and liver of fed and fasted rats, *Biochem. J.*, 235, 329, 1986.

52. **Martinez, J. A.,** Validation of a fast, simple and reliable method to assess protein synthesis in individual tissues by intraperitoneal injection of a flooding dose of [³H]phenylalanine, *J. Biochemical. Biophys. Methods*, 14, 349, 1987.

53. **Preedy, V. R. and Peters, T. J.,** Protein synthesis of muscle fractions from the small intestine in alcohol fed rats, *Gut*, 31, 305, 1990.

54. **Buse, M. and Reid, S. S.,** Leucine: a possible regulator of protein turnover in muscle, *J. Clin. Invest.*, 58, 1250, 1975.

55. **Fulks, R. M., Li, J. B., and Goldberg, A. L.,** Effects of insulin, glucose and amino acids on protein turnover in rat diaphragm, *J. Biol. Chem.*, 250, 290, 1975.

56. **McNurlan, M. A., Fern, E. B., and Garlick, P. J.,** Failure of leucine to stimulate protein synthesis *in vivo*, *Biochem. J.*, 204, 831, 1982.

57. **Fern, E. B., McNurlan, M. A., and Garlick, P. J.,** Effect of malaria on rate of protein synthesis in individual tissues of rats, *Am. J. Physiol.*, 249, E485, 1985.

58. **Samarel, A. M.,** *In vivo* measurements of protein turnover during muscle growth and atrophy, *FASEB J.*, 5, 2020, 1991.

59. **McNurlan, M. A. and Garlick, P. J.,** Contribution of the rat liver and gastrointestinal tract to whole body protein synthesis in the rat, *Biochem. J.*, 186, 381, 1980.

60. **McNurlan, M. A. and Garlick, P. J.,** Protein synthesis in liver and small intestine in protein deprivation and diabetes, *Am. J. Physiol.*, 241, E238, 1981.

61. **Lewis, S. E. M., Kelly, F. J., and Goldspink, D. F.,** Pre- and post-natal growth and protein turnover in smooth muscle, heart and slow-and fast-twitch skeletal muscles of the rat, *Biochem. J.*, 217, 517, 1984.

62. **Schaefer, A. L. and Krishnamurti, C. R.,** Protein synthesis in the gastrointestinal tissues of the ovine fetus, *Growth*, 48, 309, 1984.

63. **Attaix, D. and Arnal, M.,** Protein synthesis and growth in the gastrointestinal tract of the young preruminant lamb, *Br. J. Nutr.*, 58, 159, 1987.

64. **Preedy, V. R., Duane, P., and Peters, T. J.,** Acute ethanol dosage reduces the synthesis of smooth muscle contractile proteins in the small intestine of the rat, *Gut*, 29, 1244, 1988.

65. **Preedy, V. R., Venkatesan, S., Peters, T. J., Nott, D. M., Yates, J., and Jenkins, S. A.,** The effect of chronic ethanol ingestion on tissue RNA in skeletal muscle with comparative reference to blood flow in bone and tissues of the gastrointestinal tract of the rat, *Clin. Sci.*, 76, 243, 1989.

66. **Marway, J. S. and Preedy, V. R.,** Contractile and non-contractile proteins and nucleic acids in the stomach, whole-jejunum and seromuscular layers of the duodenum, ileum and large intestine in response to chronic ethanol feeding, *Alcohol Alcohol.*, 26, 549, 1991.

67. **Gunning, P. W., Shooter, E. M., Austin, L., and Jeffrey, P. L.,** Differential and coordinate regulation of the eukaryotic small molecular weight RNAs, *J. Biol. Chem.*, 255, 6663, 1981.

68. **Marway, J. S., Bonner, A. B., and Preedy, V. R.,** Variable responses of chronic ethanol feeding on protein metabolism in different regions of the gastrointestinal tract, *Biochem. Soc. Trans.*, 22, 350S, 1994.

69. **Marway, J. S., Siddiq, T., Gibbs, P., Edwards, P., and Preedy, V. R.,** Contractile and non-contractile protein synthesis in the small and large intestine and their response to acute ethanol dosage, *Biochem. Soc. Trans.*, 22, 194S, 1994.

70. **Preedy, V. R. and Peters, T. J.,** Acute effects of ethanol on protein synthesis in different muscles and muscle protein fractions of the rat, *Clin. Sci.*, 74, 461, 1988.

71. **Marway, J. S. and Preedy, V. R.,** The acute effects of ethanol and acetaldehyde on the synthesis of mixed and contractile proteins of the jejunum, *Alcohol Alcohol.*, 30, 211, 1995.

72. **Siddiq, T., Richardson, P. J., Mitchell, W. D., Teare, J., and Preedy, V. R.,** Ethanol-induced inhibition of ventricular protein synthesis *in vivo* and the possible role of acetaldehyde, *Cell Biochem. Func.*, 11, 45, 1993.

73. **Preedy, V. R., Keating, J. W., and Peters, V. R.,** The acute effects of ethanol and acetaldehyde on rates of protein synthesis in Type I and Type II fibre-rich skeletal muscles of the rat, *Alcohol Alcohol.*, 27, 241, 1992.

74. **Henning, S. J.,** Postnatal development: coordination of feeding digestion and metabolism, *Am. J. Physiol.*, 241, G199, 1981.

75. **Trahair, J. F., Perry, R. A., Silver, M., and Robinson, P. M.,** Studies on the maturation of the small intestine of the fetal sheep. I. The effects of bilateral adrenalectomy, *Q. J. Exp. Physiol.*, 72, 61, 1987.

76. **Black, H. E.,** The effects of steroids upon the gastrointestinal tract, *Toxicol. Pathol.*, 16, 213, 1988.
77. **Lee, S., Szlachetka, M., and Christakos, S.,** Effect of glucocorticoids and 1,25-dihydroxvitamin $D_3$ on the developmental expression of the rat intestinal vitamin D receptor gene, *Endocrinology*, 129, 396, 1991.
78. **Valenzuela, G. A., Smalley, W. E., Schain, D. C., Vance, M. L., and McCallum, R. W.,** Reversibility of gastric dysmotility in cortisol deficiency, *Am. J. Gastroenterol.*, 82, 1066, 1987.
79. **Brown, T. R.,** The effect of hypothyroidism on gastric and intestinal function, *JAMA*, 97, 511, 1931.
80. **Kowalewski, K. and Kolodej, A.,** Myoelectrical and mechanical activity of stomach and intestine in hypothyroid dogs, *Dig. Dis. Sci.*, 22, 235, 1977.
81. **Morgan, M. Y.,** Alcohol and the endocrine system, *Br. Med. Bull.*, 38, 35, 1982.
82. **Noth, R. H. and Walter, R. M.,** The effects of alcohol on the endocrine system, *Med. Clin. North Am.*, 68, 133, 1984.
83. **Van Thiel, D. H. and Gavaler, J. S.,** Ethanol and the endocrine system, in *Alcohol Related Diseases in Gastroenterology*, Seitz, H. K. and Kommerell, B., Eds., Springer-Verlag, Berlin, 1985, 324.
84. **Van Thiel, D. H. and Gavaler, J. S.,** Endocrine consequences of alcohol abuse, *Alcohol Alcohol.*, 25, 341, 1990.
85. **Ellis, F. W.,** Effect of ethanol on plasma corticosterone levels, *J. Pharmacol. Exp.*, 153, 121, 1966.
86. **Jenkins, J. S. and Connolly, J.,** Adrenocortical response to ethanol in man, *Br. Med. J.*, 2, 804, 1968.
87. **Wright, J.,** Endocrine effects of alcohol, *Clin. Endocronol. Metab.*, 7, 351, 1978.
88. **Rees, L. H., Besser, G. M., Jeffcoate, W. J., Goldie, D. J., and Marks, V.,** Alcohol-induced pseudo-Cushing's syndrome, *Lancet* i, 726, 1977.
89. **Lamberts, S. W. J., Klijn, J. G. M., de Jong, F. H., and Birkenhager, J. C.,** Hormone secretion in alcohol-induced pseudo-Cushing's syndrome, differential diagnosis with Cushing's disease, *JAMA*, 242, 1640, 1979.
90. **Loosen, P. T.,** Thyroid function in affective disorders and alcoholism, *Endocrinol. Neuropsychiatric Disord.*, 17, 55, 1988.
91. **Smith, M. M. and Dawson, A. G.,** Effect of triiodothyronine on alcohol dehydrogenase and aldehyde dehydrogenase activities in rat liver: implications for the control of ethanol metabolism, *Biochem. Pharmacol.*, 34, 2291, 1985.
92. **Mezey, E. and Potter, J. J.,** Effects of thyroidectomy and triiodothyronine administration on rat liver alcohol dehydrogenase, *Gastroenterology*, 80, 566, 1981.
93. **Freudenberg, H. and Mager, J.,** Studies on the mechanism of the inhibition of protein synthesis induced by intracellular ATP depletion, *Biochim. Biophys. Acta, 232,* 537, 1971.
94. **Van Venrooij, W. J. W., Henshaw, E. C., and Hirsch, C. A.,** Effects of deprival of glucose or individual amino acids on polyribosome distribution and rate of protein synthesis in cultured mammalian cell, *Biochim. Biophys. Acta, 259,* 127, 1972.
95. **Krasner, N., Carmichael, H. A., Russel, R. I., Thompson, G. G., and Cochran, K. M.,** Alcohol and absorption from the small intestine. 2. Effect of ethanol on ATP and ATPase in guinea-pig jejunum, *Gut*, 17, 249, 1976.
96. **Carter, E. A. and Isselbacher, K. J.,** Effect of ethanol on intestinal adenosine triphosphate (ATP) content, *Proc. Soc. Exp. Biol. Med.*, 142, 1171, 1973.
97. **Marway, J. S., Rodrigues, L. M., Griffiths, J. R., and Preedy, V. R.,** Effect of acute ethanol dosage on nucleotide levels in the rat jejunum: relationship to protein synthesis, *Alcohol Alcohol.*, 28, 521, 1993.
98. **Hardman, J. G.,** Cyclic nucleotides and hormone action, in *Textbook of Endocrinology*, Williams, R. H., Ed., W. B. Saunders, Philadelphia, 1974, 869.
99. **Granger, D. N., Hollwarth, M. E., and Parks, D. A.,** Ischemia-reperfusion injury: role of oxygen-derived free radicals, *Acta Physiol. Scand.*, Suppl. 548, 47, 1986.
100. **Perry, M. A., Wadhwa, S., Parks, D. A., Pickard, W., and Granger, D. N.,** Role of oxygen radicals in ischemia-induced lesions in the cat stomach, *Gastroenterology*, 90, 362, 1986.
101. **Craven, P. A., Pfanstiel, J., and DeRubertis, F. R.,** Role of reactive oxygen in bile salt stimulation of colonic epithelial proliferation, *J. Clin. Invest.*, 77, 850, 1986.
102. **Korthuis, R. J. and Granger, D. N.,** Ischemia, reperfusion injury: role of oxygen derived free radicals, in *Physiology of Oxygen Radicals*, Taylor, A. E., Malaton, S., and Ward, P., Eds., American Physiological Society, Bethesda, MD, 1986, 217.
103. **Szelenyi, I. and Brune, K.,** Possible role of oxygen free radicals in ethanol-induced gastric mucosal damage in rats, *Dig. Dis. Sci.*, 33, 865, 1988.
104. **Van der Vliet, A., Van der Poel, K. I., and Bast, A.,** Intestinal smooth muscle dysfunction after intraperitoneal injection of zymosan in the rat: are oxygen radicals involved?, *Gut*, 33, 336, 1992.
105. **Marway, J. S., Heap, L., Bonner, A., and Preedy, V. R.,** Regional variations in superoxide dismutase activities in seromuscular layers from the small and large intestine, *Clin. Sci.*, submitted.
106. **Marway, J. S.,** The effects of ethanol on protein synthesis in the gastrointestinal tract, PhD thesis, University of London, 1993.

# 15

## Cell Turnover in the Gastrointestinal Tract and the Effect of Ethanol

Helmut K. Seitz and Ulrich A. Simanowski

## CONTENTS

## 15.1 INTRODUCTION

Cell proliferation is an important measure and characteristic of tissues. Its evaluation must relate quantitative as well as morphological proliferative activity to morphological structure. Cell proliferation is dynamic and therefore measurement of it should include time; moreover, it could even change with time. Therefore single time point measurements are always equivocal, and even observations over time may neglect acceleration or slowing of proliferative activity, unless experiments are tremendously laborious with multiple time point observations. It is not surprising that there are only sporadic and often indirect observations of cell proliferation in the gastrointestinal tract relating to ethanol treatment.

In general, there are two different entities of changes in mucosal cell proliferation. One is related to tissue damage and indicates reparative growth, i.e., healing, and the other is concerned with the acute and chronic proliferative changes during cancer development. This chapter discusses gastrointestinal cell proliferation in association with carcinogenesis. Changes of cell turnover are especially described in the colon where an enormous body of literature has been recently accumulated linking proliferation with molecular biology. The major emphasis, however, will be on the effect of ethanol ingestion on mucosal cell regeneration, its possible mechanisms, and its consequences.

## 15.2   NORMAL GASTROINTESTINAL CELL PROLIFERATION AND DIFFERENTIATION

The epithelium of the gastrointestinal tract is one of the great renewal systems of the mammalian body. The basic organization of crypt systems in the intestine is similar, and largely independent of site.[1] Cell production occurs in tubular crypts, themselves housed in the lamina propria, a supporting matrix of connective tissue. The esophagus and the oropharynx exhibit a squamous epithelium with a basal layer of cuboid replicating cells resting on the basement membrane.[2] Because of these differences in the mucosal architecture of the upper and lower alimentary tract the process of proliferation and differentiation in these two parts of the gastrointestinal tract should be briefly discussed.

### 15.2.1   Esophagus

In the esophagus, cell replication occurs only in the basal cells of the esophageal epithelium. In the rat, the majority of basal cells divide every 3 days, with mitosis occurring 12 h after DNA synthesis.[3,4] Replication is not focal but has a random distribution along the epithelium. The newly replicated cells migrate into the spinous layer and various factors such as the state of the microenvironment (cell pressure, supply of nutrients) control the speed of migration. The turnover time from basal cell replication to their final shedding into the lumen is 4 to 5 days in the rat[3,4] and in mice and hamsters.[5] In the normal esophagus, during migration, differentiation is triggered.

The rate of replication in the basal cells must be adjusted to the rate of loss into the lumen, as the thickness of the epithelium normally remains unchanged. The maintenance of this steady state is affected by the process of food consumption.[6] Thus, in mice, cell replication increases during and after food intake.[7] Food consumption also influences cell turnover during the recovery period following irradiation.[8]

### 15.2.2   Colorectum

In common with gastrointestinal tissues, the colonic crypt is divided into proliferative and functional compartment; cells being born in the proliferative compartment and migrating into the functional compartment. Between the two compartments cells lose their proliferative capability and acquire the characteristics of mature functional cells.

Colonic crypts are regulated open systems where the origin of the cell flux is at the base of the crypt. A stem cell compartment exists at this location. All cell lineages are considered to originate in this zone, coming from a multipotential stem cell.[9-11] In the rat, colonocytic cells appear to divide about every 50 h, depending on site, and DNA synthesis takes about 9 h. The proliferative compartment occupies some 30% of the crypt, and about 7% of the crypt population is labeled by a single injection of tritiated thymidine.[2] In humans, indirect calculations indicate that colonocytes divide once every 70 to 90 h and DNA synthesis lasts between 10 to 15 h; about 15% of the crypt population is labeled with a flash exposure to tritiated thymidine.[2]

Although many experiments have been performed in which colonic cell production was modulated by manipulations or exogenous agents, it is still unclear what controls colonic cell proliferation in physiological conditions. Although there is strong evidence for a negative feedback mechanism involving a tissue specific chalone which selectively represses cell production in the small intestine,[12] data for the colon are lacking.[1] There is general agreement that the presence of luminal content is essential for maintenance of mucosal mass. Starvation or bypass of the colon reduces colonic cell proliferation and mucosal epithelial cells which is reversed by refeeding or reversal of the bypass operation. There are two possible mechanisms which could account for such an observation:

a. The presence of luminal contents could stimulate cell production via the putative mechanisms of luminal nutrition and/or mucosal workload. It has been shown that products of fermentation can be utilized by the gut epithelial cells as nutrients[13] and that hindgut fermentation occurs both in animals and in humans. A major component of the fermentation process is the short-chain fatty acids such as butyrate. There is now strong evidence that short-chain fatty acids, produced by hindgut fermentation, stimulate colonic cell proliferation.[14]

b. The second way in which food in the lumen could stimulate cell proliferation is by the production of local or systemic hormones which stimulate cell proliferation. For example, there is a close correlation between crypt cell production rates in the small intestine and blood levels of enteroglucagon in a variety of adaptive situations.[15] However, recent investigations have indicated that colonic regeneration is not associated with increases in blood enterglucagon levels.[16] In addition, epidermal growth factor (EGF) can stimulate crypt cell production rates in the rat colon,[17] and high doses can produce a hyperplastic response in the colonic epithelium.

Cyclic nucleotides and polyamines are undoubtedly involved in the mediation of adaptive responses in the colon. EGF stimulates ornithine decarboxylase (ODC) and polyamine production in the intestine, an effect abolished by difluoromethylornithine (DFMO), a competitive inhibitor of ODC.[2] Sudies on inositol lipids and diacylglycerol in intestinal responses have not been conclusive, but early evidence indicates that calcium, which is closely concerned with the transfer of intracellular information, can modify cell proliferation rates in the colon.[18]

## 15.3 MUCOSAL CELL REGENERATION IN CARCINOGENESIS WITH SPECIAL EMPHASIS ON THE COLON

Abnormal cellular proliferation is a hallmark of neoplasia. Actively proliferating cells are more susceptible to initiators of carcinogenesis and genetic alterations. A substantial body of literature indicates that in the colon, the sequence of events after crypt cell production during migration and differentiation is disordered in carcinogenesis.[19] Thus, an increased proliferative activity has been found in the colon of patients with familial polyposis, Gardner's syndrome, and nonfamilial colorectal neoplasia,[20,21] while populations with low risk for colorectal cancer such as Seventh Day Adventists have reduced colonic cell proliferation.[22] Ornithine decarboxylase, an enzyme marker of rapid cellular proliferation, is elevated in the mucosa of family members with familial polyposis kindreds.[23] Likewise, it increases in the colonic mucosa during chemically induced colonic carcinogenesis in the rat.[24] Experimental evidence also suggests that protein C kinase may be involved in the stimulation of colonic epithelial cell proliferation by tumor promoters.[25]

Recently, it has been shown that various molecular events leading to quantitative or qualitative alterations in gene expression do occur during carcinogenesis.[26] In particular, alterations in protooncogene expression and deletion of so-called tumor suppressor genes have been studied intensively. As an early event in carcinogenesis during hyperproliferation and before adenoma development DNA hypomethylation and the loss of one of the alleles at the 5q location, which encodes a putative tumor suppressor gene, have to be considered. Later, but still early, ras point mutation (oncogene activation) occurs and later in the sequence inactivations of tumor suppressor oncogene on chromosome 17 (p53 gene) and 18 (DCC gene) take place. For more detailed information, the reader is referred to References 19, 26, and 27.

### 15.3.1 Acute and Late Effects of Carcinogen Treatment

The initial reaction of the gut mucosa to carcinogen treatment is to inhibit DNA synthesis, which is paralleled by crypt cell necrosis.[28,29] It has been suggested that the severity and distribution of acute mucosal changes parallels the distribution pattern of neoplasms which arise if treatment with the carcinogen is continued.[30] In human colonic mucosa, maintained in cell culture, several carcinogens inhibit or stimulate DNA synthesis, but in the doses used do not induce toxic changes either in tissues taken from cancerous or noncancerous colons.[31,32] Immediately 1 to 2 days after acute carcinogen application a compensatory proliferative response occurs, resulting in crypt cell hyperplasia at about 4 days after treatment.[33,34] This early response, however, cannot be observed longer than 1 week. At that time both morphology and kinetic state apears normal again.

Chronic treatment with carcinogens results in a variety of hyperplastic changes in colonic as well as other gastrointestinal epithelia.[35] Although there are some controversial results in rodents, most studies concur that the chronic dimethylhydrazine (DMH) model, in both rats and mice, is associated with a diffuse crypt hyperplasia in both small and large intestine. The expanded hyperplastic crypts are hyperproliferative with increasing labeling indices[28] and this is generally associated with an expansion of the proliferative compartment. The net effect of several kinetic changes is an increase in the cell production rate.[34] Analysis of cell cycle times during carcinogenesis depend on the animal species studied; it shows a decrease in cell cycle time only in the rat during chronic DMH administration.[34] A great amount of experimental literature suggests that chronic carcinogen treatment causes a large increase in population size. It occurs at some time after the initial proliferative response to acute cell death initiated by the first carcinogen application and is continuous right up to and indeed past the appearance of the first neoplasma. Hyperplasia and kinetic changes are persistent even 4 months after cessation of carcinogen treatment, indicating a mutation based alteration of the mucosa.[36] The best available data indicate a sustained hyperplasia during carcinogenesis, with a progressive reduction of cell cycle time. For more detailed information dealing with the complexity of cell kinetics during colonic carcinogenesis, the reader is referred to References 2 and 28.

## 15.3.2 Effects of Mucosal Proliferative Status on Carcinogenesis

If hyperplasia is to be considered important, then what are the effects of hyperplasia itself on carcinogenesis? Stimulation of cell regeneration generally enhances carcinogenesis. This was found to be true after ligature insertion in the rat cecum,[37] after large bowel transection and reanastomosis,[38] in *Citrobacter freundii*-infected mice[39] and after cholic acid feeding.[40] The work of Williamson[41] and Williamson and Malt[42] has approached the concept of hyperplasia and carcinogenesis in the rat dimethylhydrazine/azoxymethane (AOM) model on a systemic basis. It appeared that the compensatory response to maneuvers such as small bowel resection were led to hyperplastic changes in the colon. This seems to be a general principle of intestinal carcinogenesis in experimental models as well as in the human intestine. Hyperproliferation linked with an increased cancer risk is found in the human small bowel in coeliac disease,[43,44] and in the human colon in a variety of conditions including ulcerative colitis,[45,46] familial polyposis syndromes, Peutz-Jeghers syndrome, juvenile polyposis, and familial colon cancer without polyposis.[20,21] Lipkin[47] reported an extended proliferative compartment (PC) in those conditions, with labeled cells displaced toward the colonic lumen. This feature was utilized to identify high risk populations. Subsequently, this proliferative pattern was found to be present in animals particularly susceptible to chemical carcinogens.[48,49]

The cause of the association of hyperproliferation with tumorigenesis is naturally interesting: If the carcinogenic event is a somatic mutation which is arguably proliferation dependent, then increasing the proliferative rate will increase the chances of a mutation. Pozharisski[37] speculated that induced hyperplasia could act by "an increased entry of stem cells into the cell cycle." Although Pozharisski evidently assumed that all proliferating enterocytes were stem cells and did not demonstrate that there was an enhanced proliferative rate in the presumptive stem cell zone (i.e., the crypt base), this hypothesis would be consistent with the concept that functional stem cells need periods of Go (a well-characterized phase of the cell cycle) to affect genetic housekeeping, without which irreparable damage to stem cell DNA (which may possess an immortal DNA strand) may occur.[50,51]

There are other instances where this association between stimulated mucosal proliferation and enhanced carcinogenesis holds as well: after colostomy closure in the distal colon,[52] following jejunoileal bypass surgery,[53] in the vicinity of colonic suture lines,[54,55] after bile acid application,[40,56] in increased fecal bulk due to dietary fibers,[57-59] and after abdominal irradiation.[60,61] These instances represent mucosal states where proliferation is increased because of functional demand and/or compensatory due to injury-related cell death. This must be distinguished from increased mucosal proliferation due to changes in cell cycle regulation either in normal tissue or as part of malignant transformation. At this point it becomes crucial, although extremely difficult, to decide what the causes of the stimulation of cell proliferation are and what is merely expression of the subsequent, regulatory mechanisms. Epidermal growth factor (EGF) may be involved in either event,[62-64] as well as oncogenes,[65] growth hormone and/or somatomedins,[66] and other so-called growth factors.[28]

Perhaps supporting the hypothesis that induced hyperproliferation leads to increased carcinogenesis are the observations that reductions in the proliferative rate leads to decreased incidences of tumors in most sites. In several studies animals with defunctioned bowel segments have been treated with colonic carcinogens.[67-70] Most of these studies have concluded that the reduced incidence was due to the lack of the carcinogen or promoter in the fecal stream, but since defunctioning does lead to hypoplasia and atrophy, an alternative explanation could be the reduced proliferative state, a view which is substantiated by observations following total parenteral nutrition and DMH treatment.[71] Inhibition of proliferation may therefore be one important principle of tumor protection. Candidates for this approach are retinoids,[72] calcium,[18,73] guar gum,[74] selenium,[75] ODC inhibitors,[76-78] plant sterols,[79,80] and antioxidants.[81]

On the other hand, reduced cellular proliferation may, however, reflect different underlying mechanisms. Bile acids, generally implicated in tumor promotion, have not invariably been demonstrated to increase proliferation. There have also been reports of unchanged or decreased proliferative activity following administration of cocarcinogenic bile acids.[82,83] Because of possible interaction of the tumor promoter with nucleic acids and consequent hinderance of the normal cell cycle, reduced proliferation may in these instances indicate tumor promotion instead of protection.[84,85] Thus, one cannot just measure changes in cell proliferation, but instead must search for the underlying mechanisms.

## 15.4 EFFECTS OF ACUTE AND CHRONIC ETHANOL CONSUMPTION ON GASTROINTESTINAL CELL PROLIFERATION

Acute alcohol ingestion, depending on the concentrations, may result in moderate to severe mucosal injury of the upper gastrointestinal tract.[86] In addition, chronic ethanol consumption is a risk factor for cancer of the oropharnyx, larynx, esophagus, and rectum in humans.[87,88] Because of these facts and in the context of the discussed topic, it is very important to collect data on the effect of ethanol consumption on mucosal cell regeneration in the gastrointestinal tract.

### 15.4.1 Oropharynx

Chronic alcohol consumption is a major risk factor for oropharyngeal cancer.[87,88] Many early epidemiologic studies have described alcohol as a risk enhancer among smokers, but not as an independent risk factor. Recent studies, however, have provided evidence that chronic consumption of alcohol, independently from the exposure to tobacco smoke, increases the risk of head and neck cancer.[89] The cocarcinogenic action of ethanol in the upper alimentary tract such as the oral cavity, the oropharynx and the esophagus, has been related to a variety of mechanisms, including cytotoxic and mitogenic effects of ethanol, increased procarcinogen activation, generation of free radicals and acetaldehyde.[90-92] Alcohol may also affect cell membrane permeability and act as a solvent for certain carcinogens, thus increasing their cellular uptake.[90-92] Chronic ethanol consumption also causes a lipomathic atrophy of the salivary glands with a consecutive decrease of saliva secretion.[93] This may result in a reduced clearance of the mucosal surface and subsequently lead to higher local concentrations of procarcinogens or carcinogens. Finally, chronic alcohol consumption is often associated with malnutrition and a depletion of certain vitamins and trace elements with known cancer protective potential.[94]

The mucosa of the upper aerodigestive tract is directly exposed to high ethanol concentrations, which could damage epithelial cells.[95] Cellular injury may also be caused by acetaldehyde, a highly toxic metabolite of ethanol, which can be produced by oropharyngeal bacteria[96] and by mucosal alcohol dehydrogenase.[97,98] As mentioned, cellular injury is often answered by hyperregeneration.

The authors have investigated the effect of chronic ethanol consumption given as liquid diets over 6 months on cell regeneration in male Wistar rats.[99] Morphometric analysis showed that in the ethanol rats the size of the nuclei of the basal cells of the oral mucosa from the floor of the mouth, the edge of the tongue, and the base of the tongue were significantly enlarged when compared to controls. The size of the basal cell layer in these rats was also increased and the stratification of the cells was altered. The percentage of cells in the S-phase of the cell cycle was significantly higher in ethanol-fed rats as compared to controls. Mean epithelial thickness of the mucosa from the floor of the mouth was significantly reduced after chronic alcohol ingestion. This indicates an atrophy of the mucosa and it is remarkable that this finding was most pronounced for a location within the oral cavity which is believed to have most intensive contact with alcoholic beverages. A reduction of epithelial thickness increases the vulnerability of epithelium toward chemical and physical noxae. It is noteworthy that patients suffering from Plummer-Vinson Syndrome, a disease associated with an atrophy of the mucosa, have an increased risk of head and neck cancer.[100] These findings in the animal experiment are in agreement with the data of the post-mortem study performed by Valentine et al.[101] When ethanol diets were supplemented with vitamin A (10,000 U retinol palmetate per kg body weight) mucosal atrophy was only slightly affected by vitamin A, while parameters of mucosal hyperregeneration were significantly influenced by vitamin A supplementation. Vitamin A suppressed the ethanol-induced mucosal hyperregeneration in almost every location of the oropharynx.[102] In this context, chronic ethanol consumption resulted in increased rather than decreased vitamin A concentrations in the esophagus of experimental animals.[103,104] Also in humans, alcoholics with oropharyngeal carcinoma exhibited a similar or increased concentrations of a great variety of carotinoids.[105] Thus, the protective role of vitamin A or carotenoid supplementation in alcohol-associated oropharyngeal cancer is still questionable.

## 15.4.2 Esophagus

Long-term drinking of alcohol is also a major risk for esophageal cancer in humans.[87,88,106] Pathogenic factors seem to be similar as those already discussed for the oropharynx. Under normal conditions, the passage of liquids through the esophagus is rapid, and the duration of contact with the surface is very brief. However, it has been shown in humans that ethanol given orally or intravenously decreases the frequency of peristalsis.[107] This would delay clearance of the esophagus, and prolong the time of contact of the contents with the lumen surface. It also has been found that moderate alcohol intake in humans increases the frequency of gastric reflux into the esophagus.[108] The acidic gastric content damages the esophageal mucosa. When isolated rabbit esophagus was perfused for 3.5 h, a solution containing 20% ethanol was relatively harmless, whereas 40% ethanol caused edema and erythema.[109] In these experiments no effect was seen on cell replication. Using 20-min perfusion period, rat esophagus was perfused with either 2 ml apple brandy or 2 ml ethanol of the equivalent concentration through a catheter sewn into position *in situ*.[110] Animals were then killed at intervals, 1 h after receiving an injection of radiolabeled thymidine. In both groups of animals the labeling index began to increase after 6 to 12 h and the mitotic index after 12 to 18 h. As there was no histological evidence for superficial desquamation, the proliferative response did not appear to be a reaction secondary to cellular shedding.

Chronic ethanol consumption also enhances cell replication in the rat esophagus. Thus, 8 weeks of feeding an ethanol containing Lieber-DeCarli diet doubled the labeling index in the esophagus.[111] The thickness of the epithelium was increased, but no overt changes in morphology were detected. Recent studies by Simanowski et al.[112] confirmed these data. It was shown that long-term ethanol consumption of 6 months resulted in a significant increase of cell proliferation in the middle part of the esophagus of male F344 rats. This enhancement of cell proliferation was particularly obvious in young and middle aged animals. Age alone did not significantly affect cell regeneration. When the effect of ethanol was investigated in Wistar rats with and without sialoadenectomy, using a PCNA method, proliferative index values were significantly increased in the intact alcohol consuming animal, whereas this effect of alcohol was completely abolished in sialoadenectomized animals. No detectable mucosal damage was observed by light micros-copy. In our study the stimulating effect of alcohol on cell proliferation was especially pro-nounced in youg rats. This observation is interesting because epidemiologic data indicate that occurrence of esophageal cancer in humans at a relatively young age is more frequently associ-ated with heavy alcohol abuse than in occurrence of other types of gastrointestinal cancer. In the U.S., cancer-related mortality resulting from cancer of the esophagus among African Americans aged 35 to 54 years was second only to that from lung cancer in 1980.[113] The reason for the suppressing effect of sialoadenectomy remains speculative, but EGF could be involved, since saliva is relatively rich in epidermal growth factor. In addition, mucosal cells may contain EGF receptors, and it has been shown that the amount of these receptors could be correlated with carcinogenesis.[114,115] Alcohol is known to change receptor density and also the affinity of various cell receptors, including those for insulin, low density lipoproteins, and EGFs on hepato-cytes.[116,117] It is also known that chronic ethanol consumption increases mucosal EGF, and EGF receptors in the stomach.[118]

In an attempt to mimic more closely the situation as it occurs in humans, alcoholic solutions were administered to rats using an intubation tube long enough to prevent the solution from passing into the lungs, but as short as possible to allow maximum flow through the esopha-gus.[119,120] One day after treatment the animals were given a 1-h pulse of bromodeoxyuridine and were killed, and cell replication was measured. It was found that the intubation of 64% ethanol had no detectable effect on basal cell replication, but when 2-methylbutanol was dissolved in the ethanol the mixture produced a dramatic increase in replication. This effect could well explain the dependence of the degree of risk on the type of beverage consumed.

It is probable that the increase in cell replication seen after alcohol treatment is not only due to ethanol itself, but also to acetaldehyde — the first and most toxic intermediate of ethanol metabolism. It has been shown that the stomach and the esophagus contain sigma alcohol dehydrogenase (ADH), a class IV ADH with a much higher $K_m$ compared to Class I ADH.[97,98,121,122] The activity of this ADH isozyme is extremely high in the esophagus compared to all other locations in the gastrointestinal tract.[98] Therefore sufficient acetaldehyde can be produced by this ADH isozyme in the esophagus. Normally, as in the liver, acetaldehyde is rapidly removed by the action of acetaldehyde dehydrogenase. In the esophagus, however, the oxidative capacity for acetaldehyde is much lower.[106,119] Therefore, acetaldehyde and other aldehydes formed in the esophagus may persist *in situ* and react with cellular macromolecules, in some way triggering cell replication as already demonstrated for the rectum.[123] Formaldehyde has been shown to stimulate cell replication in the rat stomach[124] and benzaldehyde in rat lung.[125]

### 15.4.3 Stomach and Small Intestine

Acute and chronic ethanol consumption can severely damage the gastric mucosa. However, chronic ethanol consumption does not seem to lead to an increased risk of gastric cancer.[87,88,126]

Although a few reports have found a correlation between ethanol ingestion and cancer of the cardia, some of those cases probably reflect distal esophageal cancer.[127]

There is histological damage of the gastric mucosa in the rat after acute exposure to as little as 10% ethanol concentrations.[128] In humans, endoscopically diagnosed erosions and hemorrhages in the stomach and duodenum have been described after alcohol ingestion[129] as well as histological disturbancies of duodenal structure[130] and shortage of villi.[131] This seems to be associated with initial depression and subsequent increase of DNA synthesis as indicated in *in vitro* labeling and incorporation studies with tritiated thymidine.[132,133] This sequence is thought to represent initial toxic epithelial damage, followed by secondary reparative growth. In the rat intragastric ethanol administration produced hemorrhagic erosions in stomach, duodenum, and proximal jejunum,[134] whereas chronic alcohol treatment induced no changes in crypt cell production rates in the rat stomach or duodenum.[135] Adaptation of gastric mucosa to chronic ethanol administration is associated with increased cell proliferation and increased expression of mucosal EGF, transforming growth factor α and EGF receptor.[118] Together with carcinogen treatment, ethanol may not influence labeling indices in the rat stomach, depending on the time of observation and part of the stomach.[136]

There are numerous and sometimes conflicting reports concerning alcohol-induced changes in the jejunum and ileum, covering morphology and proliferative indices like mitotic and labeling index. Most data arrived from animal studies. After chronic ethanol feeding, Baraona et al.[134] demonstrated shortage of jejunal villi, jejunal and ileal crypt hyperplasia, and increased mitotic indices only in the ileum of rats but not in the jejunum. In this study small intestinal villus cells of chronically alcohol fed rats exhibited enzyme characteristics for immature cells, which may also indicate sustained mucosal injury due to ethanol. Although they did not observe small intestinal damage in light microscopy, Rubin et al.[137] demonstrated ultrastructural alterations in electron microscopy in similarly treated animals. Others also demonstrated smaller intestinal villi and smaller crypts after chronic ethanol feeding. In addition, they observed decreased mitotic indices in the jejunum and ileum.[138] Results from thymidine incorporation studies on isolated small intestinal cells would support the presence of increased epithelial proliferation after chronic ethanol feeding,[139] whereas more reliable evaluation of small intestinal cell proliferation by the dynamic metaphase arrest method showed decreased crypt cell production rates following chronic ethanol ingestion in the jejunum as well as in the ileum.[140] However, with a similar investigation we could not detect any changes of ileal morphology and cell proliferation in chronically ethanol fed rats.[135] In contrast to chronic ethanol ingestion, exposure of intestinal epithelial cells to 1 to 3% of ethanol in cell culture for 24 to 72 h significantly decreased cell growth.[141]

### 15.4.4   Colorectum

It has long been suspected that ethanol is cocarcinogenic for the rectum. This suspicion is strongly supported by a great variety of retrospective, case-control, and prospective studies.[142-144] Considering an adenoma carcinoma sequence in colorectal tumor development, it is of special interest that there seems to be also an association between alcohol consumption and the prevalence of colonic adenomas.[145] Similarily, in the rat model ethanol seems to be cocarcinogenic for the rectum.[146,147]

To study the effect of chronic ethanol consumption on colorectal cell turnover, the authors used the metaphase arrest technique in the rat. After 4 weeks of feeding liquid diets, cell production rates were unchanged in the proximal colon, but were markedly elevated in the distal colon of ethanol-fed animals.[123,135,147] This was accompanied by an extension of the proliferative compartment and reduced lifespan of functional epithelial cells.[135] Because age by itself increases intestinal cell proliferation, and because large bowel cancer is predominantly a disease of advanced age, the authors studied large intestinal cell proliferation after chronic ethanol ingestion in various age groups. In the proximal colon, cell turnover was unaffected by age and ethanol.

Crypt cell production rates in the rectum were increased after chronic ethanol treatment (134% of controls in young rats, 182% in middle-aged rats, and 239% in old rats). Therefore, the ethanol-related stimulation of rectal cell proliferation seems to be especially effective in old age. A hint that this may also be true in humans can derive from data showing a strong association of beer drinking and colonic adenomas in older subjects.[145]

Our studies have now been extended to humans. Rectal bioposies were taken from chronic alcoholics and from age- and sex-matched controls with no history of alcohol abuse. PCNA labeling techniques were used to measure cell regeneration. It could be shown that the proliferative index was significantly increased in all three crypt compartments which are located toward the base of the rectal crypt.[148] In other words, there was an increased proliferative index in the middle part of the crypt, where regenerativity is usually not observed and where differentiation starts. This observation may represent an underlying pathogenic mechanism for the increased rectal cancer risk in chronic alcoholics.

In an attempt to elucidate the mechanism of this ethanol-related rectal hyperregeneration the authors focused on acetaldehyde. With its known toxicity, acetaldehyde seems to be a good candidate for the transmission of ethanol-related tissue damage. After ethanol infusion, the authors recorded surprisingly high acetaldehyde concentrations in the rectum, even exceeding those measured in the liver when calculated per gram of tissue.[149] From studies with germfree and conventional animals it was concluded that some of the acetaldehyde (probably most of it) may be produced by fecal bacteria.[147] Recently, Jokelainen et al.[150] found that indeed a great variety of fecal microorganisms are capable of producing huge amounts of acetaldehyde from ethanol *in vitro*. In the rat, bacterial flora between proximal colon and rectum is strikingly different with more aerobes in the rectum leading to a significant enhanced acetaldehyde accumulation in the rectal mucosa.[147] These mucosal acetaldehyde concentrations show a highly significant positive correlation with crypt cell production rates in the large intestine demonstrating that acetaldehyde, at least in part, is responsible for the mucosal hyperregeneration. However, this hyperregeneration is not accompanied by hyperplasia. Thus, acetaldehyde likely injures the rectal mucosa and this tissue damage is answered by secondary compensatory hyperregeneration. This is supported by the fact that some alcoholics reveal severe morphological alterations in their rectal mucosa which completely return to normal following a few weeks of abstinence.[151] Also the fact that the functional compartment of the rectal crypt is reduced after alcohol ingestion underlines the toxic theory of acetaldehyde to the rectal mucosa. It has to be pointed out, however, that the mucosal hyperregeneration observed after chronic ethanol ingestion is paralleled by a significant increase of rectal mucosal ODC activity, a marker for high risk with respect to colorectal cancer.[147]

It is also interesting that chronic ethanol consumption in the rat leads to a significant increase of enteroglucagon and this increase is even more pronounced when an acute dose of ethanol is given in addition to chronic treatment.[152] Enteroglucagon has been reported to be associated with increased gastrointestinal cellular regeneration.[153] Although this increase in enteroglucagon after alcohol consumption could contribute to the hyperregeneration, it is noteworthy that high serum concentrations of enteroglucagon after intestinal resection correlate with an increased tumor development in the duodenum but not in the large intestine.[154]

In summary, chronic alcohol consumption results in mucosal hyperregeneration in the rectum of experimental animals and in humans. This hyperregeneration is associated with an expansion of the proliferative compartment of the rectal crypt and with an increase in ODC activity — both indicators of high risk for cancer development. Experimental data has shown that it is likely that acetaldehyde produced by fecal bacteria injures the rectal mucosa and may therefore initiate hyperregeneration. How acetaldehyde exerts its action, e.g., by binding to DNA or by other mechanisms, is still unknown. Although no local folate deficiency was found in the rat rectum after chronic ethanol feeding,[155] it is not known whether acetaldehyde, a substance which is capable of destroying folate *in vitro*,[156] may lead to a local folate deficiency in humans, since there is indirect evidence that folate deficiency may be involved in the local occurrence of colorectal tumors.

## 15.5  SUMMARY AND CONCLUSION

Acute and chronic ethanol ingestion has deleterious effects on the gastrointestinal mucosa. While acute alcohol intake (depending on the concentration) leads mainly to cell damage of the mucosa of the upper gastrointestinal tract including inflammation, erosions, and hemorrhages, chronic ethanol consumption results in changes of the mucosal cell populations and possibly to acetaldehyde-induced morphological alterations. In both situations the mucosa respond with hyperregeneration. This ethanol-associated mucosal hyperregeneration is particularly relevant in the oropharynx, esophagus, and rectum and is closely related to carcinogenesis since chronic ethanol ingestion leads to an increased risk of cancer in these gastrointestinal sites.

## REFERENCES

1. **Wright, N. A. and Alison, M. R.,** *The Biology of Epithelial Cell Population*, Vol. 2, Clarendon Press, 1984, 540.
2. **Wright, N. A.,** The control of cell proliferation in colonic epithelium, in *Colorectal Cancer: From Pathogenesis to Prevention*, Seitz, H. K., Simanowski, U. A., and Wright, N. A., Eds., Springer-Verlag, Berlin, Heidelberg, New York, 1989, 237.
3. **Leblond, C. P., Greulich, R. C., and Pereira, J. P. M.,** Relationship of cell formation and cell renewal of stratified squalous epithelia, in *Advances in Biology of Skin*, Vol. 5, *Wound Healing*, Montagna, W. and Billingham, R. E., Eds., Pergamon Press, Oxford, 1964, 39.
4. **Leblond, C. P., Clermont, Y., and Nadler, N. J.,** The pattern of stem cell renewal in three epithelia, esophagus, intestine and testis, in *Proc. 7th Canadian Cancer Conference*, Vol. 7, Morgan, J. F., Noble, R. L., Rossiter, R. J., Taylor, R. M., Wallace, A. C., and Whitelaw, D. M., Eds., Pergamon Press, Oxford, 1966, 3.
5. **Blenkinsopp, W. K.,** Absence of effect of multiple intraperitoneal injections on cell cycle time in epithelium of esophagus and forestomach in mice, hamsters and rats, *Cell. Tissue Kinet.*, 3, 83, 1970.
6. **Craddock, V. M.,** Biology of the esophagus, in *Cancer of the Esophagus*, Craddock, V. M., Ed., Cambridge University Press, New York, 1993, 4.
7. **Burholt, D. R., Etzel, S. L., Schenken, L. L., and Kovacs, C. J.,** Digestive tract cell proliferation and food consumption pattern of Ha/ICR mice, *Cell. Tissue Kinet.*, 18, 369, 1985.
8. **Burholt, D. R.,** Esophageal epithelial cell proliferation and food consumption patterns following irradiation, *Br. J. Cancer*, 53 (Suppl. VII), 7, 1986.
9. **Chang, W. W. L. and Leblond, C. P.,** A unitarian theory of the origin of the three populations of epithelial cells in the mouse large intestine, *Anat. Rec.*, 169, 293, 1971.
10. **Ponder, B. A. J., Schmidt, G. H., Wilkinson, M. A., Wood, M. J., Monk, M., and Reid, A.,** Derivation of mouse intestinal crypts from single progenitor cell, *Nature*, 313, 689, 1985.
11. **Williams, G. T. and Williams, E. D.,** Evidence that colonic crypts are maintained by a single stem cell, *Nature*, 334, 87, 1988.
12. **Wright, N. A. and Al-Nafussi, A.,** Kinetics of villous cell populations in the mouse small intestine. II. Negative feedback after death of proliferative cells, *Cell. Tissue Kinet.*, 15, 618, 1982.
13. **Sakata, T., Hitosaka, K., Shiomara, Y., and Tawate, H.,** The stimulatory effect of butyrate on epithelial cell proliferation in the lumen of the sheep, and its mediation by insulin: differences between *in vivo* and *in vitro* studies, in *Cell Proliferation in the Gastrointestinal Tract*, Appleton, D. R., Sunter, J. P., and Watson, A. J., Eds., Piman Medical, London, 1980, 123.
14. **Goodlad, R. A., Lenton, W., Ghatei, M. A., Adrian, T. E., Bloom, S. R., and Wright, N. A.,** Proliferative effects of fibre on the intestinal epithelium; relationship to plasma gastrin, enteroglucagon and PYY levels, *Gut*, 28, 221, 1987.
15. **Al-Mukhtar, M. Y. T., Sagor, G. R., Ghatei, M. A., Polak, J. M., Koopmans, H. S., Bloom, S. R., and Wright, N. A.,** The relationship between gastrointestinal hormones and cell proliferation in models of intestinal adaptation, in *Mechanisms of Intestinal Adaptation*, Robinson, J. W. L., Dowling, H. R., and Riecken, E. O., Eds., MTP Press, Lancaster, 1982, 243.
16. **Bristol, J. B., Ghatei, M. A., Smith, J. A., Bloom, S. R., and Williamson, R. C. N.,** Elevated plasma enteroglucagon alone fails to alter distal colonic carcinogenesis in rats, *Gastroenterology*, 92, 617, 1987.
17. **Goodlad, R. A., Wilson, T. G., Lenton, W., Wright, N. A., Gregory, H., and McCullagh, K. C.,** The proliferative effects of urogastrone (epidermal and growth factor) on the intestinal epithelium, *Gut*, 28, 37, 1987.
18. **Lipkin, M. and Newmark, H.,** Effects of added dietary calcium on colonic epithelial cell proliferation in subjects at high risk for familial colonic cancer, *N. Engl. J. Med.*, 313, 1381, 1985.
19. **Bresalier, R. S. and Kim, Y. S.,** Malignant neoplasms of the large intestine, in *Gastrointestinal Disease*, 5th ed., Sleisenger, M. H. and Fordtran, J. S., Eds, W. B. Saunders, Philadelphia, 1993, 1449.

20. **Lipkin, M., Blattner, W. E., Fraumeni, J. F., Jr., Lynch, H. T., Deschner, E., and Winaver, S.,** Tritiated thymidine labeling distribution as a marker for hereditary predisposition to colon cancer, *Cancer Res.*, 43, 1899, 1984.

21. **Lipkin, M., Blattner, W. A., Gardner, E. J., Burt, E. W., Lynch, H., Deschner, E., Winawer, S., and Fraumeni, J. F., Jr.,** Classification and risk assessment of individuals with familial polyposis. Gardner's Syndrome, and familial nonpolyposis colon cancer from [3]H-thymidine labeling patterns in colonic epithelial cells, *Cancer Res.*, 44, 4102, 1984.

22. **Lipkin, M., Uehara, K., Winaver, S., Sanchez, A., Burt, R. W., Lynch, H., Blattner, W. A., and Fraumeni, J. F., Jr.,** Seventh Day Adventist vegetarians have a quiescent proliferative activity in colonic mucosa, *Cancer Lett.*, 26, 139-143, 1985.

23. **Luk, G. D. and Baylin, S. B.,** Ornithine decarboxylase as a biological marker in familial colonic polyposis, *N. Engl. J. Med.*, 311, 80, 1984.

24. **Luk, G. D., Hamilton, S. R., Yang, P., Smith, P. A., O'Ceallaigh, D., McAvinchey, D., and Hyland, J.,** Kinetic changes in mucosal ornithine decarboxylase activity during azoxymethane-induced colonic carcinogenesis in the rat, *Cancer Res.*, 46, 4449, 1986.

25. **Craven, P. A., Pfanstiel, J., and DeRubertis, F. R.,** Role of activation of protein kinase C in the stimulation of colonic epithelial proliferation and reactive oxygen formation by bile acids, *J. Clin. Invest.*, 79, 532, 1987.

26. **Vogelstein, B., Fearon, E. R., Hamilton, S. R., Kern, S. E., Preisinger, A. C., Leppert, M., Nakamura, Y., White, R., Smits, A. M. M., and Bos, J. L.,** Genetic alterations during colorectal tumor development, *N. Engl. J. Med.*, 319, 525, 1988.

27. **Fearon, E. R. and Vogelstein, B.,** A genetic model for colorectal tumorigenesis, *Cell*, 61, 759, 1990.

28. **Simanowski, U. A., Wright, N. A., and Seitz, H. K.,** Mucosal cellular regeneration and colorectal carcinogenesis, in *Colorectal Cancer from Pathogenesis to Prevention*, Springer-Verlag, Berlin, Heidelberg, New York, 1989, 225.

29. **Zedeck, M. S., Sternberg, S. S., Poynter, R. W., and McGowan, J.,** Biochemical and pathological effects of methylazoxymethanol acetate, a potent carcinogen, *Cancer Res.*, 30, 801, 1970.

30. **Zedeck, M. S., Grab, D. J., and Sternberg, S. S.,** Differences in the acute response of the various segments in the rat intestine to treatment with the intestinal carcinogen methylazoxymethanol, *Cancer Res.*, 37, 32, 1977.

31. **Mak, K. M., Slater, G. I., and Hoff, M. B.,** Inhibition of DNA synthesis by carcinogens in human colon mucosa in organ culture, *J. Natl. Cancer Instit.*, 63, 1305, 1979.

32. **Mikol, Y. B. and Lipkin, M.,** Effects of carcinogens on indices of cell proliferation in human colonic epithelial cells, *Proc. Ann. Meet. Am. Assoc. Cancer Res.*, 25, 78, 1984.

33. **Deschner, E. E.,** Early proliferative effects induced by six weekly injections of 1,2-dimethylhydrazine in epithelial cells of mouse distal colon, *Z. Krebsforsch.*, 91, 205, 1978.

34. **Sunter, J. P.,** Cell proliferation studies on normal, carcinogen damaged and neoplastic intestinal epithelia, M.D. thesis, University of Newcastle at Tyne, U.K.

35. **Altmann, G. G. and Snow, A. D.,** Effects of 1,2-dimethylhydrazine on the number of epithelial cells present in the villi, crypts, and mitotic pool along the rat small intestine, *Cancer Res.*, 44, 5522, 1984.

36. **Barthold, S. W.,** Relationship of colonic mucosal background to neoplastic proliferative activity in dimethylhydrazine treated mice, *Cancer Res.*, 41, 2616, 1981.

37. **Pozharisski, K. M.,** Morphology and morphogenesis of experimental epithelial tumors of the intestine, *J. Natl. Cancer Instit.*, 54, 1115, 1975.

38. **Roe, R., Fermor, B., and Williamsson, R. C. N.,** Proliferative instability and experimental carcinogenesis at colonic anastomoses, *Gut*, 28, 808, 1987.

39. **Barthold, S. W. and Jonas, A. M.,** Morphogenesis of early 1,2-dimethylhydrazine-induced lesions and latent period of colonic carcinogenesis in mice by a variant of *Citrobacter freundi*, *Cancer Res.*, 37, 4352, 1977.

40. **Cohen, B. I., Raicht, R. F., Deschner, E. E., Takahashi, M., Sarwal, A. N., and Fazzini, E.,** Effects of cholic acid feeding on N-methyl-N-nitrosourea-induced colon tumors and cell kinetics in rats, *J. Natl. Cancer Instit.*, 64, 573, 1980.

41. **Williamson, R. C. N.,** Hyperplasia and neoplasia of the intestinal tract, *Ann. R. Coll. Surg. Engl.*, 61, 341, 1979.

42. **Williamson, R. C. N. and Malt, R. A.,** Promotion of intestinal carcinogenesis by adaptive mucosal hyperplasia, in *Cell Proliferation in the Gastrointestinal Tract*, Appleton, D. R., Sunter, J. P., and Watson, A. J., Eds., Pitman, London, 1980, 303.

43. **Wright, N. A., Watson, M., Morley, A., Appleton, D., and Marks, J.,** Cell kinetics in flat avillous mucosa of the human small intestine, *Gut*, 14, 701, 1973.

44. **Swinson, C. M, Slavin, G., Coles, E. C., and Booth, C. C.,** Coeliac disease and malignancy, *Lancet*, i, 111, 1983.

45. **Bleiberg, H., Mainguet, P., Galant, P., Chretien, J., and Dupont-Marisse, N.,** Cell renewal in the human rectum; *in vitro* autographic study on active ulcerative colitis, *Gastroenterology*, 58, 851, 1970.

46. **Collins, R. H., Feldman, M., and Fordtran, J. S.,** Colon cancer, dysplasia, and surveillance in patients with ulcerative colitis: a critical review, *N. Engl. J. Med.*, 316, 1654, 1987.

47. **Lipkin, M.,** Method for binary classification and risk assessment of individuals with familial polyposis based on [3]H-TdR labeling of epithelial cells in colonic crypts, *Cell Kinet.*, 17, 209, 1984.

48. **Deschner, E. E., Long, F. C., Hakissian, M., and Herrmann, S. L.,** Differential susceptibility of AKR, C57BL/ 6J, and CF1 mice to 1, 2-diemthylhydrazine-induced colonic tumor formation predicted by proliferative characteristics of colonic epithelial cells, *J. Natl. Cancer Instit.*, 70, 279, 1983.

49. **Deschner, E. E., Long, F. C., Hakissian, M., and Cupo, S. H.,** Differential susceptibility of inbred mouse strains forecast by acute colonic proliferative response to methylazoxymethanol, *J. Natl. Cancer Instit.*, 72, 195, 1984.

50. **Cairns, J.,** Mutation selection and the natural history of cancer, *Nature*, 225, 197, 1975.

51. **Potten, C. S., Hume, W. J., Reid, P., and Cairns, J.,** The segregation of DNA in epithelial stem cells, *Cell*, 15, 899, 1978.

52. **Terpstra, O. T., Peterson Dahl, P., Williamson, R. C. N., Ross, J. S., and Malt, R. A.,** Colostomy closure promotes cell proliferation and dimethylhydrazine-induced carcinogenesis in the rat distal colon, *Gastroenterology*, 81, 475, 1981.

53. **Bristol, J., Wells, M., and Williamson, R. C. N.,** Jejunoileal bypass stimulates cell proliferation and enhances experimental carcinogenesis in rat large bowel, *Proc. Am. Assoc. Cancer Res.*, 23, 233, 1982.

54. **Williamson, R. C. N., Davies, P. W., Bristol, J. B., and Wells, M.,** Intestinal adaptation and experimental carcinogenesis after partial colectomy; increased tumor yields are confined to the anastomosis, *Gut*, 23, 316, 1982.

55. **Barkla, D. H. and Tutton, P. M.,** The influence of surgical transection and anastomosis on the rate of cell proliferation in the colonic epithelium of normal and DMH treated rats, *Carcinogenesis*, 4, 1323, 1983.

56. **Deschner, E. E., Cohen, B. I., and Raicht, R. F.,** Acute and chronic effects of dietary cholic acid on colonic epithelial cell proliferation, *Digestion*, 21, 290, 1981.

57. **Jacobs, L. R.,** Enhancement of rat colon carcinogenesis by wheat bran consumption during the stage of 1,2-dimethylhydrazine administration, *Cancer Res.*, 43, 4057, 1983.

58. **Jacobs, L. R. and Lupton, J. R.,** Relationship between colonic luminal pH, cell proliferation, and colon carcinogenesis in 1,2- diemthylhydrazine treated rats fed high fibre diets, *Cancer Res.*, 46, 1727, 1986.

59. **Goodlad, R. A., Lenton, W., Ghatei, M. A., Adrian, T. E., Bloom, S. R., and Wright, N. A.,** Proliferative effect "fibre" on the intestinal epithelium: relationship to gastrin, enteroglucagon and PYY, *Gut*, 28, 221, 1987.

60. **Sharp, J. G., Crouse, D. A., Jackson, J. D., Mann, S. L., and Murphy, B. O.,** Abdominal irradiation is a potent promoter of diemthylhydrazine induced colon tumors in rats, *Proc. Am. Assoc. Cancer Res.*, 26, 144, 1985.

61. **Sandler, R. S. and Sandler, D. P.,** Radiation induced cancers of the colon and rectum: assessing the risk, *Gastroenterology*, 84, 51, 1983.

62. **Malt, R. A., Chester, J. F., Gaissert, H. A., and Ross, J. S.,** Augmentation of chemically induced pancreatic and bronchial cancers by epidermal growth factor, *Gut*, 28, 249, 1987.

63. **Kingsnorth, A. N., Abu-Khalaf, M., Ross, J. S., and Malt, R. A.,** Potentiation of 1,2-dimethylhydrazine induced anal carcinoma by epidermal growth factor in mice, *Surgery*, 97, 696, 1985.

64. **Ulsen, M. H., Lyn-Cook, L. E., and Raasch, R. H.,** Effects of intraluminal epidermal growth factor on mucosal proliferation in the small intestine of adult rats, *Gastroenterology*, 91, 1134, 1986.

65. **Weinberg, R. A.,** The action of oncogenes in the cytoplasm and nucleus, *Science*, 230, 770, 1985.

66. **Ituarte, E. A., Petrini, J., and Hershman, J. M.,** Acromegaly and colon cancer, *Ann. Intern. Med.*, 101, 627, 1984.

67. **Rubio, C. A.,** Experimental colon cancer in the absence of intestinal contents in Sprague Dawley rats, *J. Natl. Cancer Instit.*, 64, 569, 1980.

68. **Cleveland, J. C., Litvak, S. F., and Cole, J. W.,** Identification of the route of action of the carcinogen 3,2-dimethyl-aminobiphenyl in the induction of intestinal metaplasia, *Cancer Res.*, 27, 708, 1967.

69. **Wittig, G., Wildner, G. P., and Zeibarth, D.,** Der Einfluss der Ingesta auf die Kanzerisierung des Rattendarmes durch Dimethylhydrazin, *Arch. Geschwulstforsch.*, 37, 105, 1971.

70. **Gennaro, A. R., Villaneauva, R., Sukon-Haman, Y., Vathanphas, V., and Rosemond, G. P.,** Chemical carcinogenesis in transposed intestinal segments, *Cancer Res.*, 33, 536, 1973.

71. **Heitmann, D. W., Grubbs, B. G., Heitmann, T. O., and Cameron, I. L.,** Effects of 1,2-dimethylhydrazine treatment and feeding regimen on rat colonic epithelial cell proliferation, *Cancer Res.*, 43, 1153, 1983.

72. **Lotan, R.,** Effects of vitamin A and its analogs on normal and neoplastic cells, *Biochim. Biophys. Acta*, 605, 33, 1980.

73. **Bird, R. P., Schneider, R., Stamp, D., and Bruce, W. R.,** Effects of dietary calcium and cholic acid on the proliferative indices of murine colonic epithelium, *Carcinogenesis*, 7, 1657, 1986.

74. **Jacobs, L. R.,** Inhibition of duodenal carcinogenesis and crypt cell proliferation in rats fed guar gum, *Fed. Proc.*, 46, 585, 1987.

75. **Rampal, P., Nano, J. L., Veyres, B., Rampal, A., and Francois, E.,** Prevention of chemically induced colon cancer by dietary selenium in rats, *Dig. Dis. Sci.*, (New Series) 31 (Suppl. 10), 247S, 1986.

76. **Kingsnorth, A. N., King, W. W., MacCann, P. P., Diekema, K., Ross, J. S., and Malt, R. A.,** Difluoromethylornithine (DMFO) diminishes 1,2-dimethylhydrazine induced colonic carcinogenesis in mice, *Gastroenterology*, 82, 1100, 1982.

77. **Luk, G. D. and Yang, P.,** Polyamines in intestinal and pancreatic adaptation, *Gut*, 28, 95, 1987.

78. **Hosomi, M., Lirussi, F., Stace, N. H., Vaja, S., Murphy, G. M., and Dowling, R. H.,** Mucosal polyamine profile in normal and adapting (hypo- and hyperplastic) intestine: effects of DMSO treatment, *Gut*, 28, 103, 1987.

79. **Deschner, E. E., Cohen, B. I., and Raicht, R. F.,** The kinetics of the protective effect of betasitosterol against MNU-induced colonic neoplasia, *J. Cancer Res. Clin. Oncol.*, 103, 49, 1982.

80. **Deschner, E. E., Cohen, B. I., and Raicht, R. F.,** The acute effect of beta-sitosterol on colonic epithelial cell proliferation: implications for MNU-induced neoplasia, *Cell Tissue Kinet.*, 15, 102, 1982.

81. **Deschner, E. E. and Wattenberg, L. W.,** The proliferative effect of dietary butylated hydroxyanisole on methylazoxymethanol treated colonic mucosa, *Cancer Lett.*, 16, 197, 1982.

82. **Weidema, W. F., Deschner, E. E., Cohen, B. I., and DeCosse, J. J.,** Acute effects of dietary cholic acid and methylazoxymethanol acetate on colonic epithelial cell regeneration: metabolism of bile salts and neutral sterols in conventional and germfree SD rats, *J. Natl. Cancer Instit.*, 74, 665, 1985.

83. **Simanowski, U. A., Seitz, H. K., Czygan, P., Hörner, M., Waldherr, R., Weber, E., and Kommerell, B.,** Chronic ursodesoxycholic acid- and chenodesoxycholic acid feeding induced changes of colon mucosal cell proliferation in rats, *J. Natl. Cancer Instit.*, 79, 163, 1987.

84. **Suzuki, K. and Bruce, W. B.,** Increase by deoxycholic acid of the colonic nuclear damage induced by known carcinogens in C57BL/6J mice, *J. Natl. Cancer Instit.*, 76, 1129, 1986.

85. **Galloway, D. J., Jarrett, F., Boyle, P., Indran, M., Carr, K., Owen, R. W., and George, W. D.,** Morphological and cell kinetic effects of dietary manipulations during colorectal carcinogenesis, *Gut*, 28, 754, 1987.

86. **Mezey, E.,** Effect of ethanol on intestinal morphology, metabolism, and function, in *Alcohol Related Diseases in Gastroenterology*, Seitz, H. K. and Kommerell, B., Eds., Springer-Verlag, Berlin, Heidelberg, New York, 1985, 342.

87. **Seitz, H. K. and Simanowski, U. A.,** Alcohol and carcinogenesis, *Ann. Rev. Nutr.*, 8, 99, 1988.

88. **Seitz, H. K. and Simanowski, U. A.,** Alcohol and cancer: a critical review, in *Alcoholism: A Molecular Perspective*, Palmer, T. N, Ed., NATO ASI Series, Plenum Press, New York, 1991, 275.

89. **Maier, H. and Sennewald, E.,** Risikofaktoren für Plattenepithelkarzinome im Kopf-Halsbereich. Ergebnisse der Heidelberger Fallkontrollstudien. Hauptverband der gewerblichen Berufsgenossenschaften, DCM Druck, 1994.

90. **Seitz, H. K., Simanowski, U. A., and Osswald, B. R.,** Epidemiology and pathophysiology of ethanol-associated gastrointestinal cancer, *Pharmacogenetics*, 2, 278, 1992.

91. **Seitz, H. K., Simanowski, U. A., and Osswald, B. R.,** Gastrointestinal carcinogenesis: ethanol as a risk factor, *Eur. J. Cancer Prev.*, 1, 5, 1992.

92. **Lieber, C. S., Garro, A. J., Leo, M. A., Mak, K. M., and Worner, T. M.,** Alcohol and cancer, *Hepatology*, 6, 1005, 1986.

93. **Maier, H., Born, I. A., Veith, S., Adler, D., and Seitz, H. K.,** The effect of chronic ethanol consumption on salivary gland morphology and function in the rat, *Alcohol. Clin. Exp. Res.*, 10, 425, 1986.

94. **Seitz, H. K. and Suter, P. M.,** Ethanol toxicity and nutritional status, in *Nutritional Toxicity*, Kotsonis, F., Mackey, M., and Hjelle, J., Eds., Raven Press, New York, 1994, 95.

95. **Mueller, P., Hepke, B., Meldau, U., and Raabe, G.,** Tissue damage in the rabbit oral mucosa by acute and chronic direct toxic action of different ethanol concentrations, *Exp. Pathol.*, 24, 171, 1983.

96. **Pikkarainen, P. H., Baraona, E., Jauhonen, P., Seitz, H. K., and Lieber, C. S.,** Contribution of oropharynx microflora and of lung microsomes to acetaldehyde in expired air after alcohol ingestion, *J. Lab. Clin. Med.*, 97, 631, 1979.

97. **Seitz, H. K., Egerer, G., Simanowski, U. A., Waldherr, R., Eckey, R., Agarwal, D. P., Goedde, H. W., and van Wartburg, J. P.,** Human gastric alcohol dehydrogenase activity, effect of age, sex and alcoholism, *Gut*, 34, 1433, 1993.

98. **Yin, S. J., Chou, F. J., Chao, S. F., Tsai, S. F., Liao, C. S., Wang, S. L., Wu, C. W., and Lee, S. C.,** Alcohol and aldehyde dehydrogenases in human esophagus: comparison with the stomach enzyme activities, *Alcoholism: Clin. Exp. Res.*, 17, 376, 1993.

99. **Maier, H., Weidauer, H., Zöller, J., Seitz, H. K., Flentje, M., Mall, G., and Born, I. A.,** Effect of chronic ethanol consumption on the morphology of oral mucosa, *Alcoholism: Clin. Exp. Res.*, 18, 387, 1994.

100. **Wynder, E. L., Hultberg, S., Jacobsson, F., and Bross, I. J.,** Environmental factors in cancer of the upper elimentary tract. Swedish study with special reference to Plummer Vinson (Patterson-Kelly) syndrome, *Cancer*, 10, 470, 1957.

101. **Valentine, J. A., Scott, J., West, C. R., and Hill, C. A. S.,** A histological analysis of the early effects of alcohol and tobacco usage on human epithelium, *Oral. Pathol.*, 14, 654, 1985.

102. **Massa, J.,** Hochdosierte Vitamin A Gabe zur Prävention alkohol- und tabak-induzierter Schäden der Mundschleimhaut der Ratte. Eine morphometrische Analyse, M.D. thesis, University of Heidelberg, Germany, 1994.

103. **Mobarhan, S., Seitz, H. K., Russell, R. M., Mehta, R., Hupert, J., Friedman, H., Layden, T. J., Meydani, M., and Langenberg, P.,** Age related effects of chronic ethanol intake on vitamin A status in Fisher 344 rats, *J. Nutr.*, 121, 510, 1991.

104. **Leo, M. A., Kim, C., and Lieber, C. S.,** Increased vitamin A in esophagus and other extrahepatic tissues after chronic ethanol consumption in the rat, *Alcoholism: Clin. Exp. Res.*, 10, 487, 1986.

105. **Leo, M. A., Seitz, H. K., Maier, H., and Lieber, C. S.,** Carotenoid, retinoid and vitamin E status of the oropharyngeal mucosa in the alcoholic, *Alcohol Alcohol.*, 30, 163, 1994.

106. **Craddock, V. M.,** *Cancer of the Esophagus*, Cambridge University Press, New York, 1993.

107. **Hogan, W. J., deAndrade, S. R. V., and Winship, D. H.,** Ethanol-induced acute esophageal motor dysfunction, *J. Appl. Physiol.*, 32, 755, 1972.

108. **Kaufman, S. E. and Kaye, M. D.,** Induction of gastroesophageal reflux by alcohol, *Gut*, 19, 336, 1978.

109. **Salo, J. A.,** Ethanol induced mucosal injury in rabbit esophagus, *Scand. J. Gastroenterol.*, 18, 713, 1983.

110. **Haentjens, P., DeBacker, A., and Willems, G.,** Effect of an apple brandy from Normandy and of ethanol on epithelial cell proliferation in the esophagus of rats, *Digestion*, 37, 184, 1987.

111. **Mak, K. M., Leo, M. A., and Lieber, C. S.,** Effect of ethanol and vitamin A deficiency on epithelial cell proliferation and structure in the rat esophagus, *Gastroenterology*, 93, 362, 1987.

112. **Simanowski, U. A., Suter, P. M., Stickel, F., Maier, H., Waldherr, R., Smith, D., Russell, R. M., and Seitz, H. K.,** Esophageal epithelial hyperproliferation following long-term alcohol consumption in rats: effect of age and salivary gland function, *J. Natl. Cancer Instit.*, 85, 2030, 1993.

113. **Garfinkel, L., Poindexer, C. E., and Silverberg, E.,** Cancer in black Americans, *CA Cancer J. Clin.*, 30, 39, 1980.

114. **Jankowski, J., Murphy, S., Coghill, G., Grant, A., Wormsley, K. G., Sanders, D. S. A., Kerr, M., and Hopwood, D.,** Epidermal growth factor receptor in the esophagus, *Gut*, 33, 439, 1992.

115. **Mukaisa, H., Toi, M., Hirai, T., Yamashita, Y., and Toge, T.,** Clinical significance of the expression of epidermal growth factor and its receptor in esophageal cancer, *Cancer*, 68, 142, 1991.

116. **Dalke, D. D., Casey, A. A., and Sorrell, M. F.,** Chronic ethanol feeding alters binding and internalization of epidermal growth factor (EGF) in isolated rat hepatocytes, *Gastroenterology*, 92 (Abstr.), A1727, 1987.

117. **Seitz, H. K., Kuhn, B., von Hodenberg, E., Fiehn, W., Conradt, C., and Simanowski, U. A.,** Increased messenger RNA levels for low-density lipoprotein receptor and 3-hydroxy-3-methylglutaryl coenzyme A reductase in rat liver after long-term ethanol ingestion, *Hepatology*, 20, 487, 1994.

118. **Tarnawski, A., Lu, S. Y., Stachura, J., and Sarfeh, I. J.,** Adaptation of gastric mucosa to chronic alcohol administration is associated with increased mucosal expression of growth factors and their receptors, *Scand. J. Gastroenterol.*, Suppl. 193, 59-63, 1992.

119. **Craddock, V. M.,** Metabolism of ethanol and of higher alcohols present in alcoholic drinks and their corresponding aldehydes in subcellular components of rat esophageal mucosa, and relevance for esophageal cancer in man, in *Alcoholism: A Molecular Perspective*, Palmer, T. N., Ed., Plenum Press, New York, 1991, 283.

120. **Craddock, V. M.,** Aetiology of esophageal cancer: some operative factors, *Eur. J. Cancer Prev.*, 1, 89, 1992.

121. **Moreno, A. and Pares, X.,** Purification and characterization of a new alcohol dehydrogenase from the human stomach, *J. Biol. Chem.*, 266, 1128, 1991.

122. **Seitz, H. K., Simanowski, U. A., Egerer, G., Waldherr, R., and Örtl, U.,** Human gastric alcohol dehydrogenase: *in vitro* characteristics and effect of cimetidine, *Digestion*, 51, 80, 1992.

123. **Simanowski, U. A., Suter, P. M., Russell, R. M., Heller, M., Waldherr, R., Ward, R., Peters, T. J., Smith, D., and Seitz, H. K.,** Enhancement of ethanol induced rectal mucosal hyperregeneration with age in F344 rats, *Gut*, 35, 1102, 1994.

124. **Furihata, C., Yamakoshi, A., and Matsushima, T.,** Induction of ornithine decarboxylase and DNA synthesis in rat stomach mucosa by formaldehyde, *Jpn. J. Cancer Res.*, 79, 917, 1988.

125. **Schweinsberg, F., Weissenberger, I., Bruckner, B., Schweinsberg, E., Burkle, V., Wittenberg, H., and Reinecke, H. J.,** Effect of disulfiram on N-nitroso-N-methylbenzylamine metabolism. Biochemical aspects, in *N-Nitroso Compounds, Occurrence, Biological Effects and Relevance to Human Cancer*, O'Neill, J. K., von Borstel, R. C., Miller, C. T., Long, J., and Bartsch, H., Eds., Scientific Publishers, No. 57, IARC, Lyon, 1984, 525.

126. **Nomura, A., Grove, J. S., Stemmerman, G., N., and Severson, R. K.,** A prospective study of stomach cancer and its relation to diet, cigarettes and alcohol consumption, *Cancer Res.*, 50, 627, 1990.

127. **McDonald, W. C.,** Clinical and pathological features of adenocarcinoma of the gastric cardia, *Cancer*, 29, 724, 1972.

128. **Kvietys, P. R., Twohig, B., Danzell, J., and Specian, R. D.,** Ethanol induced injury to the gastric mucosa, *Gastroenterology*, 98, 909, 1990.

129. **Gottfried, E. B., Korsten, M. A., and Lieber, C. S.,** Alcohol induced gastric and duodenal lesions in man, *Am. J. Gastroenterol.*, 70, 578, 1978.

130. **Lev, R., Thomas, E., Parl, F. F., and Pitchumoni, C. S.,** Pathological and histomorphometric study of the effect of alcohol on the human duodenum, *Digestion*, 20, 207, 1980.

131. **Seitz, H. K., Velasquez, D., Waldherr, R., Veith, S., Czygan, P., Weber, E., Deutsch-Diescher, O. G., and Kommerell, B.,** Duodenal gamma-glutamyl-transferase activity in human biopsies: effect of chronic ethanol consumption and duodenal morphology, *Eur. J. Clin. Invest.*, 15, 192, 1985.

132. **Chen, T., Kiernan, T., and Leevy, C. M.,** Ethanol and cell replication in the digestive tract, *Clin. Gastroenterol.*, 10, 343, 1981.

133. **Seitz, H. K., Czygan, P., Kienapfel, H., Veith, S., Schmidt-Gayk, H., and Kommerell, B.,** Changes in gastrointestinal DNA synthesis produced by acute and chronic ethanol consumption in the rat: a biochemical study, *Gastroenterology*, 21, 79, 1983.

134. **Baraona, E., Pirola, R. C., and Lieber, C. S.,** Small intestinal damage and changes in cell population produced by ethanol ingestion in the rat, *Gastroenterology*, 66, 226, 1974.

135. **Simanowski, U. A., Seitz, H. K., Baier, B., Kommerell, B., Schmidt-Gayk, H., and Wright, N. A.,** Chronic ethanol consumption selectively stimulates rectal cell proliferation in the rat, *Gut*, 27, 278, 1986.

136. **Ishii, H., Tatsuta, M., Baba, M., and Taniguchi, H.,** Promotion by ethanol of gastric carcinogenesis induced by N-methyl-N'-nitro-N-nitroso-guanidine in Wistar rats, *Br. J. Cancer*, 59, 719, 1989.

137. **Rubin, E., Rybak, B. J., Lindenbaum, J., Gerson, C. D., Walker, G., and Lieber, C. S.,** Ultrastructural changes in the small intestine induced by ethanol, *Gastroenterology*, 63, 801, 1972.

138. **Zucoloto, S. and Rossi, M. A.,** Effect of chronic ethanol consumption on mucosal morphology and mitotic index in the rat small intestine, *Digestion*, 19, 277, 1979.

139. **Seitz, H. K., Czygan, P., and Kommerell, B.,** Stimulation of thymidine incorporation in isolated rat intestinal mucosal cells by feeding an ethanol-containing liquid diet, *Digestion*, 23, 65, 1982.

140. **Mazzanti, R. and Jenkins, W. J.,** Effect of chronic ethanol ingestion on enterocyte turnover in the small intestine, *Gut*, 28, 52, 1987.

141. **Nano, J. L., Cefai, D., and Rampal, P.,** Effects of ethanol on an intestinal epithelial cell line, *Alcoholism: Clin. Exp. Res.*, 14, 32, 1990.

142. **Seitz, H. K. and Simanowski, U. A.,** Ethanol and colorectal carcinogenesis, in *Colorectal Cancer from Pathogenesis to Prevention*, Seitz, H. K., Simanowski, U. A., and Wright, N. A., Eds., Springer-Verlag, Berlin, Heidelberg, New York, 1989, 177.

143. **Seitz, H. K. and Simanowski, U. A.,** Alcohol and colorectal carcinogenesis, in *Alcohol and Cancer*, Watson, R. R., Ed., CRC Press, Boca Raton, FL, 1992, 167.

144. **Seitz, H. K. and Simanowski, U. A.,** Ethanol and colorectal cancer, in *Alcohol, Immunity and Cancer*, Yirmiya, R. and Taylor, A. N., Eds., CRC Press, Boca Raton, FL, 1993, 211.

145. **Kikendall, J. W., Bowen, P. E., Burgess, M. B., Magnetti, C., Woodward, J., and Langenberg, P.,** Cigarettes and alcohol as independent risk factors for colonic adenomas, *Gastroenterology*, 97, 660, 1989.

146. **Seitz, H. K., Czygan, P., Waldherr, R., Veith, S., Raedsch, R., Kaessmodel, H., and Kommerell, B.,** Enhancement of 1,2-dimethylhydrazine induced rectal carcinogenesis following chronic ethanol consumption in the rat, *Gastroenterology*, 86, 886, 1984.

147. **Seitz, H. K., Simanowski, U. A., Garzon, F. T., Rideout, J. M., Peters, T. J., Koch, A., Berger, M. R., Einecke, H., and Maiwald, M.,** Possible role of acetaldehyde in ethanol-related rectal cocarcinogenesis in the rat, *Gastroenterology*, 98, 406, 1990.

148. **Simanowski, U. A., Arce, L., Knühl, M., Waldherr, R., Weissgerber, U., Stickel, F., and Seitz, H. K.,** Chronic alcohol consumption enhances rectal cell regeneration in man, *Gastroenterology*, 106 (Abstr.), A442, 1994.

149. **Seitz, H. K., Simanowski, U. A., and Peters, T. J.,** (Letter to the Editor), *Hepatology*, 7, 616, 1987.

150. **Jokelainen, K., Renkonen, O. V., Roine, P. R., and Salaspuro, M.,** Alcohol dehydrogenase mediated acetaldehyde production by enteric microbes: possible role in carcinogenesis?, *Gastroenterology*, 106 (Abstr.), A399, 1994.

151. **Brozinski, S., Fami, K., and Grosberg, J. J.,** Alcohol ingestion induced changes in the human rectal mucosa: light and electron microscopic studies, *Dis. Colon Rectum*, 21, 329, 1979.

152. **Simanowski, U. A., Hubaleck, K., Ghatei, M. A., Bloom, S. R., Polak, J. M., and Seitz, H. K.,** Effects of acute and chronic ethanol administration on the gastrointestinal hormones gastrin, enteroglucagon, pancreatic glucagon and peptide YY in the rat, *Digestion*, 42, 167, 1989.

153. **Goodlad, R. A., Lenton, W., Ghatei, M. A., Bloom S. R., and Wright, N. A.,** Effects of an elemental diet, inert bulk and different types of dietary fibre on the response of the intestinal epithelium to refeeding in the rat and relationship to plasma gastrin, enteroglucagon and PYY concentrations, *Gut*, 28, 171, 1987.

154. **Savage, A. P., Matthews, J. L., Ghatei, M. A., and Bloom, S. R.,** Enteroglucagon and experimental intestinal carcinogenesis in the rat, *Gut*, 28, 33, 1987.

155. **Mason, J. B., Greaves, S., and Seitz, H. K.,** Localized folate depletion in the rectum does not occur in chronically alcohol fed rats, *Gastroenterology*, 102 (Abstr.), A376, 1992.

156. **Shaw, S., Jayatilleke, E., Herbert, V., and Colman, N.,** Cleavage of folates during ethanol metabolism: role of acetaldehyde/xanthine oxidase generated superoxide, *Biochem. J.*, 257, 277, 1989.

# 16

## Lipid Metabolism in the Intestinal Tract and Its Modification by Ethanol

Hiroshi Hayashi

## CONTENTS

## 16.1  INTRODUCTION

Numerous studies have been performed on the effect of ethanol on lipid metabolism. At first, the dramatic changes in the liver produced by ethanol, i.e., fatty liver and liver cirrhosis, attracted the attention of investigators because the liver is the largest organ supplying endogenous lipoproteins to the whole body. On the other hand, the hyperlipidemia following ethanol ingestion, so-called alcoholic hyperlipidemia, had been known as another modification of lipid metabolism by ethanol. Thus, the intestine, which produces exogenous lipoproteins exclusively, became one of the major subjects of research on the interaction between ethanol and lipid metabolism. Since the late 1960s, numerous papers have been published in this field and have profoundly advanced our knowledge. Experiments using laboratory animals, especially rats, have revealed the various modes by which ethanol interferes with lipid metabolism in the intestine, and this has also expanded our understanding of the normal metabolic processing of lipids in the intestine.

## 16.2  GENERAL ASPECTS OF INTESTINAL LIPID METABOLISM

### 16.2.1  Dietary Lipids

As much as 40% of the caloric intake in the Western diet is supplied in the form of lipids. Chemically, almost all lipids (approximately 90%), whether of plant or animal origin, are triglycerides (TG), with the remainder consisting of cholesteryl esters, plant sterols, and phospholipids. TGs are triesters of glycerol (triacylglycerols), and the esterified fatty acids are usually long-chain (length $>C_{14}$). Two saturated fatty acids, palmitate (16:0) and stearate (18:0), and two unsaturated fatty acids, oleate (18:1) and linoleate (18:2), are commonly found in TGs. Trace amounts of medium-chain fatty acids ($C_6$ to $C_{14}$) are also present in the diet in plant oils such as palm oil, nutmeg and seed oils, and in animal fats, e.g., milk.

The predominant sterol supplied in the diet is cholesterol, and plant sterols account for 20 to 25% of all total dietary sterols.[1] Phosphatidylcholines (PC) contribute the major class of dietary phospholipids and two-thirds are of animal origin.[2] About 1 to 2 g of PCs enter the intestinal lumen in the diet daily, but endogenous PCs, i.e., biliary PCs, are quantitatively more important, with 11 to 12 g/day being secreted.[3]

### 16.2.2  Lipid Digestion

TG digestion occurs mainly in the duodenum, where TGs are hydrolyzed by pancreatic lipase to form 2-monoglycerides (MG) and fatty acids (FA). TGs must be emulsified to facilitate their hydrolysis by pancreatic lipase, and the initial emulsification occurs in the stomach. Peristaltic waves in the stomach, including propulsion, grinding, and retropulsion, provide the mechanical action needed to emulsify dietary TGs. Another role of the stomach is secretion of gastric lipase.[4] The main products of gastric lipase activity are diglycerides and fatty acids. Crudely emulsified lipids are propelled through the pyloric canal into the duodenum. The diameter of emulsion particles in the upper duodenum is generally less than 0.5 μm.[5] Fat droplets with a core of triglyceride are emulsified with surface (water-oil interface) components such as acid soap (ionized fatty acids), phosphatidylcholine, bile salts, and cholesterol in the duodenum. Pancreatic lipase acts at the water-oil interface of the lipid droplets. Lipolysis occurs slowly in the presence of bile salts above their critical micellar concentration, but inhibition by bile salts can be overcome by another protein present in pancreatic juice, colipase.[6]

Luminal PCs, most of which are secreted in the bile, are hydrolyzed by pancreatic phospholipase $A_2$ to lysophosphatidylcholine (LPC) and fatty acids.[7] Phospholipase $A_2$ has an absolute requirement for $Ca^{2+}$ ions to function.[8] Cholesteryl esters are hydrolyzed to cholesterol by the cholesterol esterase contained in pancreatic juice. Pancreatic cholesterol esterase appears to be the same enzyme as pancreatic nonspecific lipase (carboxylic lipase).[9] The enzyme has broad substrate specificity from water-soluble carboxyl esters to insoluble esters dispersed in bile salt micelles.[10]

### 16.2.3  Lipid Uptake into Enterocytes

Lipid hydrolysis products (2-MGs, fatty acids, cholesterol, and LPC) must make contact with the enterocyte membrane before being absorbed. A series of diffusion barriers exist, including bulk water, the unstirred water layer, mucin gels, and the glycocalyx.[11] The products of lipolysis exist in aqueous and oil phases. In the aqueous phase, they exist mainly as a part of the mixed bile salt micelle. Two other dispersed phases also occur: a phase of large micelles saturated with both mixed lipids and cholesterol and unilamellar vesicles (liposomes) of mixed lipids saturated with bile salts.[12] This micellar solubilization can increase the concentration of MGs and fatty acids markedly, resulting in the formation of a concentration gradient from the lumen toward the cell membrane. This may be one of the mechanisms which facilitates lipid penetration of these barriers.

Fatty acids and MGs have been thought to be absorbed into enterocytes by passive diffusion.[13,14] During transfer through the barriers, luminal micelles lose their integrity and absorption is mediated by the lipid monomers in the interparticle aqueous phase.[11] However, Stremmel has recently shown that an FA-binding protein (FABP) is present in the brush-border membrane of jejunal mucosal cells, and that this protein mediates the uptake of FAs into enterocytes.[15] The answer to the question of whether FA uptake is passive or carrier mediated must await the results of further investigation. The absorption of tristearin is significantly less than that of triolein, and poor lipolysis in the lumen seems to be partially involved.[16]

In contrast to the absorption of TGs, which has generally been accepted as occurring by passive diffusion, cholesterol absorption may be a facilitated process.[17] Cholesterol is absorbed by the intestinal mucosa in the free form, and although the mechanism is unknown, cholesterol absorption is relatively fixed. Thurnhofer and Hauser claimed that cholesterol absorption is catalyzed by an intrinsic protein in the brush-border membrane.[18] Since the cholesterol uptake may depend on the capacity of the brush-border membrane of the absorptive cell to solubilize cholesterol, the amount of sphingomyelin, which has high affinity for cholesterol, present in the brush-border membrane may also regulate the uptake of cholesterol by altering the solubility of cholesterol in the membrane.[19] Luminal PC must be hydrolyzed to LPC prior to being absorbed by enterocytes,[20,21] and uptake of LPC is believed to be passive. However, Stremmel has demonstrated that the FA-binding protein in the brush-border membrane can bind and transport LPC, raising the possibility that LPC transport may also be carrier mediated.[15]

### 16.2.4  Intracellular Metabolism of Absorbed Lipids

Lipids absorbed by the enterocyte, namely, MG, FA, cholesterol, and LPC, must be translocated from the brush-border of the cell where absorption occurs to the endoplasmic reticulum (ER), where lipids are further metabolized. Esterification of these lipids yields TGs, cholesteryl esters, and PCs. Little is known about the mechanism of lipid trafficking, although Ockner and Manning isolated and characterized FABP from the cytosolic fraction of the enterocyte and suggested that this protein may play an important role in intracellular transport of FA.[22] On the other hand, two sterol carrier proteins, SCP-1 (MW 47,000) and SCP-2 (MW 13,500) have been isolated.[23,24] SCP-1 is considered to play an important role in the esterification of cholesterol as well as in the intracellular transport of cholesterol.

Prior to their utilization in the synthesis of TG, FAs must be activated to their CoA derivatives. The enzyme catalyzing this reaction is acyl-CoA synthetase. TGs are synthesized in the enterocyte by two distinct metabolic pathways; the MG pathway and the glycerophosphate pathway. In the MG pathway, absorbed 2-MGs are acylated by acyl-CoA in a stepwise manner with intermediate formation of diacylglycerol (diglyceride) to form TGs. The major enzymes involved in the MG pathway are monoglyceride acyl transferase and diglyceride acyl transferase. The MG pathway is primarily associated with the smooth ER (SER).[25] In the glycerophosphate pathway, glycerophosphate is acylated by acyl-CoA to form phosphatidic acid. Then the phosphatidic acid is hydrolyzed to 1,2-DGs via the action of phosphatidate phosphohydrolase, and DGs are finally acylated to TGs. The glycerophosphate pathway is associated with the rough ER (RER).[25]

The MG pathway is the major pathway of TG production in the enterocyte, although the relative importance of the two pathways depends on the supply of MGs. During normal fat absorption when both MGs and FAs are supplied to the enterocyte, the MGs and FAs absorbed are efficiently converted to TG via the MG pathway. Furthermore, the MG pathway inhibits the glycerophosphate pathway. When the supply of MG is insufficient or absent, however, TGs are mainly synthesized via the glycerophosphate pathway. Interestingly, DGs, the common intermediates of both pathways, do not equilibrate, and two different pools of DGs seem to exist, one from each pathway.[26] Johnston explained this phenomenon by the difference in localization of the two pathways, i.e., the MG pathway is associated with the SER and the glycerophosphate pathway with the RER.[27]

Some of the LPC absorbed is reacylated to form PC, while the remainder is further hydrolyzed to form glycerophosphocholine,[7,20] which is transported out of the intestine to the liver via the portal vein.[28] The enterocyte has a pathway for *de novo* synthesis of PC and does not need to utilize absorbed LPC. It has been shown that one of the major pathways of PC synthesis in the liver, the cytidine pathway (Kennedy pathway), also operates in the intestinal mucosa.[29,30] In the cytidine pathway, CDP-choline activated from phosphocholine binds to DGs to form TGs. The DGs used for PC formation in the cytidine pathway are derived exclusively from DGs synthesized via the glycerophosphate pathway for TG formation, and not from DGs synthesized via the MG pathway.[31]

Absorbed cholesterol is esterified to cholesteryl esters in enterocytes. Two enzymes are involved in the esterification process. The first is cholesterol esterase (cholesteryl ester hydrolase), which is basically the same enzyme as the one secreted by the pancreas.[32,33] Pancreatic cholesterol esterase is somehow incorporated into the enterocyte. The other enzyme is acyl-CoA:cholesterol acyltransferase (ACAT). The relative importance of these two enzymes in the esterification of cholesterol is unknown, but may depend on the dietary cholesterol load.[34-36]

### 16.2.5   Synthesis of Apolipoproteins in the Intestine

Reesterified lipids, namely TGs, PCs, and cholesteryl esters, are assembled into lipoproteins in the enterocyte, and the lipoproteins are then secreted into mesenteric lymph. Major lipoproteins transporting intracellularly synthesized lipids originally derived from the diet are chylomicrons (CM) and very low density lipoprotein (VLDL). CMs and VLDL are defined on the basis of their Svedberg flotation (Sf) rate in the ultracentrifugate; CMs are lipoproteins with an Sf greater than 400 while the Sf of VLDL ranges from 20 to 400.[37] Both lipoproteins have micelles as their common structure. They contain hydrophobic lipids such as TGs and cholesteryl esters as their core component surrounded by bipolar substances such as phospholipids, represented by PC, cholesterol, and apolipoproteins (apoproteins) as the envelope component.

CMs and VLDL in lymph and plasma possess several species of apolipoproteins, including apo A-I, A-II, A-IV, B, Cs, and E, but most apo Cs and E are known to be transferred to CMs and VLDL after they are secreted by the enterocytes. There is little possibility that the intestinal mucosa synthesizes apo E actively,[38,39] and estimates of synthesis of apo Cs by the intestine are also low (<10%).[40] Major apolipoproteins synthesized by enterocytes are apo B, A-I, and A-IV.

There are two species of apo B. In humans, apo B-100, an extremely large protein composed of 4536 amino acids (MW 549,000), is synthesized by the liver and is crucial for the assembly of VLDL. After being secreted by the liver, VLDL is transformed into low density lipoprotein (LDL) in the plasma. Apo B-48, composed of 2152 amino acids (MW 264,000), is synthesized in the intestine and has an obligatory structural role in the formation of CMs and intestinal VLDL. In rats, small apo B, which corresponds to apo B-48 contained in CMs, has a MW of 240,000 vs. a MW of 353,000 for large apo B, which corresponds to the apo B-100 contained in LDL. Interestingly, apo B-48 possesses the same amino terminal 2152 amino acid as apo B-100 and is produced by the intestine as a result of editing a single nucleotide of the apo B mRNA, which changes the codon specifying apo B-100 amino acid 2153 to a premature stop codon.[41-43] Apo B mRNA editing to create an in-frame stop codon occurs not only in human but also in rat and rabbit intestinal apo B mRNA[42,44] and rat liver, which is known to produce both small and large apo Bs.[44,45] Recently, a complementary DNA clone coding apo B mRNA editing protein was isolated from rat small intestine.[46]

While CMs and VLDLs cannot be integrated structurally without apo B, it is not known whether the synthesis of apo B is a rate-limiting step in lipoprotein formation in enterocytes. Synthesis of apo B after lipid infusion has been reported to: (1) increase,[47] (2) increase but not with statistical significance,[48] or (3) not to increase.[49] Our findings suggest that apo B synthesis and secretion are unaffected by lipid infusion.[50] The author therefore suspects that the synthesis of apo B may not be a rate-limiting step in lipoprotein formation.

Apo A-IV has been shown to be actively synthesized in the intestinal mucosa,[40] while the physiological role of apo A-IV is still unclear. When TG-rich lipoproteins secreted by the intestine enter the circulation, apo A-IV is displaced from CMs to high density lipoprotein (HDL) and the lipoprotein-free fraction.[51,52] This characteristic of apo A-IV led the investigator to propose that apo A-IV is the cofactor of an enzyme, lecithin:cholesterol acyltransferase (LCAT),[53,54] or that apo A-IV is a ligand of HDL in binding to the liver[55,56] and aortic endothelial cells.[57] Recently, Fujimoto et al. presented evidence suggesting that apo A-IV acts in the central nervous system to control food intake.[58] While it is well known that synthesis of apo A-IV is dependent on a lipid meal,[59-61] the precise mechanism of how lipid absorption regulates apo A-IV synthesis has not been determined. Hayashi et al. recently suggested that lipid uptake and increased TG content in the enterocyte cannot stimulate apo A-IV synthesis and secretion.[62] They showed that active packaging and secretion of CMs are necessary for apo A-IV synthesis.

Apo A-I has also been shown to be actively produced in the intestinal mucosa.[38-40] Apo A-I is a major component of HDL.[63] Both the intestine and the liver are capable of making apo A-I.[64,65] While intestinal apo A-I secretion into lymph increases after a lipid meal,[65,66] it is less certain whether mucosal synthesis of apo A-I increases after a lipid meal.[67-69] Enterocytes produce a small quantity of apo A-II.[70]

### 16.2.6 Intracellular Assembly and Secretion of Lipoproteins

After reesterification to TGs, FAs become morphologically visible as TG droplets within the cisternae of the smooth ER.[71-74] Since the enzymes involved in the MG pathway of TG synthesis have been demonstrated to be located on the cytoplasmic surface of the ER,[75] TGs must somehow cross the membrane of the ER. Using [$^{14}$C]oleate, [$^3$H]leucine, and [$^{14}$C]glucosamine Kessler et al. found that the lipid, protein, and sugar of intracellular CM precursors are synthesized in the smooth ER, the rough ER, and the Golgi apparatus, respectively.[76] It is suspected that not only apolipoproteins but also phospholipids are synthesized in the rough ER.[27] Thus, it appears that the lipid droplets in the SER become associated with the phospholipids and apolipoproteins synthesized in the RER by a still unknown mechanism and are then transported to the Golgi apparatus, where carbohydrate molecules are thought to be attached to the lipoproteins.

Apo B has a crucial role in the formation of lipoprotein. According to Christensen et al., apo B is synthesized in the rough ER, transferred to the smooth ER, and then added onto the lipoprotein particle.[77] In a rare inherited disorder of lipoprotein metabolism, hypobetalipoproteinemia, homozygous patients have virtually no circulating apo B-containing lipoproteins (CMs, VLDL, or LDL), resulting in a deficiency of fat-soluble vitamins and eventually in spinocerebellar and retinal degeneration. Hypobetalipoproteinemia has been shown to be caused by defects in the apo B gene resulting in the total absence of apo B.[78,79] While hypobetalipoproteinemia is an autosomal codominant disorder, abetalipoproteinemia, whose clinical features cannot be distinguished from those of hypobetalipoproteinemia, is inherited recessively. Apo B has been demonstrated in the hepatocytes and enterocytes of individuals with abetalipoproteinemia.[80-83] Recently, however, microsomal triglyceride transfer protein (MTP) was shown to be defective in patients with abetalipoproteinemia but intact in hypobetalipoproteinemia patients.[84] The absence of MTP is caused by defects in the gene encoding the 97 kDa[85] or 88 kDa[86] subunit of MTP. MTP is a lipid-binding protein that shuttles TGs, cholesteryl esters, and phospholipids between intracellular membranes. The mechanism by which apo B and TG droplets associate to form a mature lipoprotein is not yet fully understood, but these findings strongly suggest that MTP plays a crucial role in the assembly of lipid and apo B. Patients with Anderson's disease (also referred to as chylomicron retention disease) have defects in the assembly or secretion of CMs resulting in the formation of large droplets in enterocytes.[87,88] Interestingly, the synthesis of apo B-48 is not disturbed in this recessively transmitted disorder, and a normal level of TG transfer activity has been demonstrated.[84] Therefore, the site of metabolic impairment in Anderson's disease is different from that of either abetalipoproteinema or hypobetalipoproteinemia.

Assembled lipoproteins are transferred from the ER to the Golgi apparatus. Two mechanisms of transport have been suggested. One is that vesicles containing the lipoprotein particles bud off the smooth ER and fuse with the membrane of the Golgi apparatus.[28,89] The other, proposed by Morrè et al., is that the SER and the Golgi apparatus are connected by tubules that transport the lipoproteins.[90,91]

The Golgi apparatus serves as the final site for lipoprotein assembly and packaging prior to their release from the absorptive cell. The incorporation of a carbohydrate moiety into the lipoprotein is completed in the Golgi apparatus.[92-95] Redgrave isolated lipoproteins from a pellet of Golgi membranes and found that these lipoproteins in the Golgi apparatus, referred to as "prechylomicrons," have a very different phospholipid composition from the CMs isolated from intestinal lymph.[96] Thus considerable modification other than glycosylation occurs in the Golgi apparatus.

After the Golgi cisternae have filled with lipoprotein particles, vesicles containing lipoproteins are pinched off the Golgi apparatus. The vesicles then migrate toward the plasma membrane and release their contents into the intercellular space by exocytosis.[97] The number of apo B molecules contained in CM particles has been shown to be constant,[98] which also seems to be true for intestinal VLDL, in view of the fact that plasma VLDL has only one apo B molecule per particle.[99] Based on this evidence, Hayashi et al. measured lymphatic apo B output during various phases of lipid metabolism in the intestine to determine the number of lipoprotein particles in lymph.[50] They concluded that the number of CM particles produced by the intestine remains relatively constant during both fasting and active lipid uptake and transport. During active lipid absorption, instead of increasing the number of CMs, the enterocytes expand the size of the CM particles to transport absorbed lipid in the lymph.

In many secretory cells microtubules have been found to be essential to the intracellular transport and release of secretory material. Ultrastructural studies have revealed that microtubules also play an important role in intracellular lipid trafficking and in the secretion of CMs by enterocytes.[97,100] Glickman et al. observed a striking decrease of lipids in the lymph of rats treated with colchicine, an inhibitor of microtubular assembly.[101] Pavelka and Gang showed that colchicine treatment decreases microtubules and displaces such subcellular organelles as the ER and Golgi apparatus which are necessary for the formation and transport of CM.[102]

Although the major lipoproteins secreted by the intestine are CMs and VLDL, the rat intestine also secretes discoidal HDL into the lymph.[103] Its major apoprotein is apo A-I, with a little apo E. Magun et al. examined the intracellular distribution of apo A-I in the rat intestine.[104] Following a lipid meal, the percentage of total intracellular mass accounted for by HDL-associated apo A-I tripled. Bisgaier and Glickman resolved mesenteric lymph HDL into discrete fractions, including a discoidal fraction, a spherical fraction similar in size to plasma HDL, and a small spherical particle fraction not present in plasma and originating in the intestine.[105] HDL has also been reported to be present in human intestinal lymph[106] and may be of intestinal origin. No definite evidence is available, however.

### 16.2.7   Separate Pathways for CM and VLDL Formation

As mentioned, the intestine produces two species of TG-rich lipoproteins: CMs and VLDL. It has been shown that lymph from fat-fed rats contains a continuous spectrum of TG-rich lipoproteins ranging in size from 300 to 4300 Å.[107] VLDLs have therefore been called "small chylomicrons,"[108] although several findings suggest that CMs and VLDLs are two distinct populations of lipoproteins. Mahley et al., for example, showed that Golgi vesicles contain either CMs or VLDLs with little mixing of particle sizes.[109] Recently Tso and co-workers presented evidence that CMs and VLDLs are formed via different metabolic pathways.[110,111] They found that Pluronic L-81 (L-81), a hydrophobic surfactant, prevented the lymphatical transport of TG by blocking the formation of CMs in enterocytes. They also found that when rats are intraduodenally infused with egg PC and L-81, the lipids infused are transported in lymph as VLDL, and no

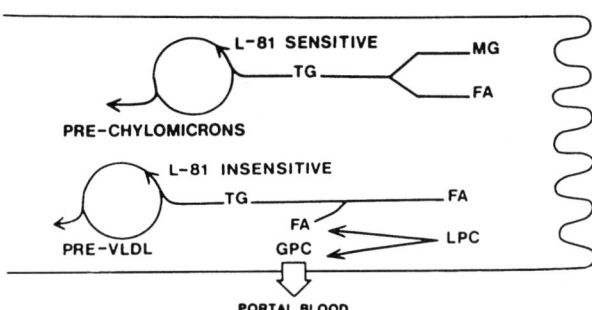

**FIGURE 16.1** Formation of intestinal pre-chylomicrons (pre-CM) and pre-very low density lipoprotein (pre-VLDL) particles. This diagram depicts packaging of pre-CM and pre-VLDL particles by enterocytes of the small intestine. Absorbed monoglycerides (MG) and fatty acids (FA), major digestion products of triglycerides (TG), are reconstituted in the cell to form TGs via the monoglyceride pathway, and then subsequently packaged into predominantly pre-CM particles. This pathway is inhibited by the presence of Pluronic L-81 (L-81). In contrast, absorbed FAs and FAs derived from hydrolysis of absorbed lysolecithin are used to form TGs via the glycerophosphate pathway, and then packaged into pre-VLDL particles. Unlike the formation of pre-CM, this pathway is not sensitive to L-81. (From Tso, P., Drake, D. S., Black, D. D., and Sabesin, S. M., *Am. J. Physiol.*, 247, G599, 1984. With permission.)

inhibition by L-81 is observed.[112] They therefore proposed that different synthetic pathways for CM and VLDL exist in enterocytes, and that the pathway for CM formation is sensitive to inhibition by L-81 while the pathway for VLDL formation is insensitive (Figure 16.1). The mechanism of action of L-81 is now being investigated.

### 16.2.8   Lipid Transport in the Portal Vein

While absorbed long-chain FAs are transported in intestinal lymph as CMs or VLDL, the major route of absorbed medium- and short-chain FAs from the intestine to the liver is the portal vein.[113,114] In some cases, however, absorbed long-chain FAs have been reported to be transported in the portal vein. The increase in portal vein transport of absorbed oleic acids has been observed in the bile-fistula rat, which has deficient reesterification of FAs because of the absence of bile acids.[115] McDonald et al. showed that a substantial amount of absorbed long-chain FAs are transported in the portal vein in bile-intact rats.[116] They infused long-chain FAs at a low infusion rate (0.3 μmol/h). Recently, Mansbach et al. reported that 39% of absorbed oleate is transported in the portal vein when lipids are infused at a high rate (135 μmol/h of triolein).[117] Mansbach et al. also reported that the rate of portal transport of oleate was 16.5% of the input rate when triolein was infused at a low rate (27 μmol/h) and that when 9 μmol/h of PC was infused together with triolein the portal transport of oleate decreased to 1.4% at a high infusion rate (135 μmol/h) and to 0.5% at a low infusion rate (9 μmol/h).[118] They further found that there is no net transport of fatty acids in the portal vein, i.e., the amount of lipid in the portal vein and the amount in the carotid artery is approximately the same under these three experimental conditions. Clearly much work remains to be done to determine whether the portal vein contributes substantially to the transport of absorbed long-chain FAs in the physiological state.

## 16.3   MODIFICATION OF INTESTINAL LIPID METABOLISM BY ETHANOL

### 16.3.1   Alcoholic Hyperlipidemia and the Intestine

It has been well known for several decades that alcohol can affect lipid metabolism throughout the entire body. Zieve, for example, described a syndrome consisting of hyperlipidemia, jaundice, and hemolytic anemia in patients with alcoholic liver dysfunction.[119] The prominent disorders of lipid metabolism which develop in response to the ingestion of alcohol are fatty liver and hyperlipidemia. The latter, so-called alcoholic hyperlipidemia, not only occurs in humans but also can be reproduced in experimental animals, such as the rat.[120] There have been numerous reports on alcoholic hyperlipidemia in humans. Schapiro et al. reported striking elevation of serum TGs in 10 chronic alcoholics when challenged with alcohol in increasing doses over a 24-day period.[121] Brewster et al. demonstrated that fatty meals containing ethanol cause hyperlipidemia in humans.[122] Verdy and Gattereau also concluded that dietary lipid is necessary for the promotion of alcoholic hyperlipidemia,[123] and their findings were supported by those of Barboriak and Meade.[124] Wilson and Arkey showed that pre-beta lipoprotein (corresponding to VLDL) on agarose gel electrophoresis increases after the administration of fat and ethanol to human subjects.[125] Moreover, Wilson and co-workers demonstrated that patients with endogenous hyperlipidemia are particularly subject to ethanol-induced augmentation of alimentary lipemia.[126]

The absorption of dietary lipids into the intestinal mucosa is followed by the formation of intestinal lipoproteins. Intestinal lipoproteins transport absorbed lipid into the bloodstream via the lymph. Hyperlipidemia is caused by either the overproduction of lipoprotein or decreased catabolism of lipoprotein or by both. The liver and intestine serve as two major sites of lipoprotein production. Based on these findings, investigators have hypothesized that alcohol enhances the production of intestinal lipoproteins thereby leading to alcoholic hyperlipidemia. Many experiments have been performed to test this hypothesis, especially in laboratory animals. This chapter will examine the results of earlier experiments on each category of lipid metabolism in the intestine in the following sections and ultimately evaluate the original hypothesis.

### 16.3.2  Triglyceride Synthesis

One of the earliest systematic studies on the effects of ethanol on the synthesis of TGs in the intestine was reported by Carter et al.[127] Rats were acutely or chronically infused with ethanol, 7.5 g/kg of body weight. Slices of excised intestine or microsomes prepared from intestinal mucosa were incubated with [$^{14}$C] palmitate to measure the synthesis of TGs. The results showed a significant increase in [$^{14}$C] incorporation into TGs. In microsomes, acute and chronic exposure to ethanol caused a 17-fold and 25- to 54-fold increase, respectively, of microsomal conversion of [$^{14}$C] palmitate into TG. They also demonstrated that direct addition of 2.6% ethanol to untreated, normal intestinal slices produced a significant increase in TG synthesis of 30%. These enhancing effects of alcohol on TG synthesis were diminished both *in vivo* and *in vitro* by pyrazole, an inhibitor of alcohol dehydrogenase, indicating that the findings observed are specific to ethanol. Carter et al. claimed that the ability of the intestinal mucosa to esterify FA to TG is enhanced by intestinal infusion with ethanol and that this effect of ethanol is partly caused by direct contact between ethanol and the intestinal mucosa.

It was predicted that the TG content in the intestinal mucosa would increase as a result of the enhanced esterification of FAs. This was tested by Mistilis and Ockner by infusing the duodenum of rats with ethanol (0.63 g/kg/h), or isocaloric amounts of glucose as a control, for 8 h (the total ethanol dose was 5 g/kg).[128] Mucosal TG levels in the small intestine increased fourfold after ethanol infusion. This indicates that enhanced ability to esterify FAs to TGs actually resulted in an increased TG content in the intestinal mucosa. Mistilis and Ockner showed that when ethanol is injected intravenously, the increase in the mucosal TG level is twofold, less than in the case of intraluminal administration of ethanol. This means that not only an elevated concentration of ethanol in the blood but direct contact between intraluminal ethanol and the intestinal mucosa can enhance esterification of FA and increase the TG content of the mucosa.

In the study by Mistilis and Ockner, ethanol was infused into the intestine in saline solution without any lipid, and thus the question is the source of the mucosal FAs utilized to esterify the TGs. Bile and shed gastrointestinal epithelium, both of which are present intraluminally, contain FAs and are capable of supplying them to the mucosa. There are also other possible sources of

FA supply; the intestinal mucosa can synthesize FAs[129] and also utilize FAs in the blood because plasma free fatty acids are incorporated into lymph TGs.[130] Gangl and Ockner investigated the intestinal metabolism of plasma-derived FAs.[131] They intravenously injected rats with [$^{14}$C] palmitate when ethanol was infused intraduodenally at a dose of 333 mg/kg/h for 15 h. They found that mucosal oxidation of plasma-derived palmitate was inhibited 53% and that incorporation of palmitate into TG increased by 86% in response to intraluminal ethanol. Thus, it can be said that unless lipid is supplied to the intestinal lumen, some FAs are derived from the blood when TG synthesis in the intestinal mucosa is enhanced by intraluminal administration of ethanol.

The pathway by which TGs are synthesized in the intestinal mucosa involves many enzymes, as already described. Rodgers and O'Brien assessed the effect of ethanol on acyl-CoA synthetase, the enzyme which activates FAs and is common to both the MG pathway and the glycerophosphate pathway, and on monoglyceride acyltransferase in the MG pathway.[132] They infused rats intraduodenally with 5 g/kg of ethanol for 5 h and then with saline overnight. The activity of both the enzymes was measured in samples prepared from an intestinal homogenate. The results showed that the activity of both enzymes increased in the jejunum and that the activity of acyl-CoA synthetase increased in the ileum in comparison with the controls infused with isocaloric glucose. Although the MG pathway may not have predominated under their experimental conditions because of the lack of an intraluminal MG supply, their findings mean that the enhancement of TG synthesis may be caused by stimulation of enzymes involved in the TG esterification pathway.

The hypothesis mentioned above, that intraluminal ethanol increases TG synthesis in the intestinal mucosa, was then challenged by Baraona et al.[133] They followed basically the same experimental design as Carter et al.[127] In an *in vivo* experiment, Baraona et al. investigated the metabolism of [$^{14}$C]palmitate in intestinal slices from untreated rats at various concentrations of ethanol. Incorporation of the palmitate label into $^{14}$CO$_2$ was inhibited by ethanol at concentrations of 2.5 g/dl or greater.[133] The incorporation of [$^{14}$C]palmitate to TG was unaffected by 0.5 g/dl of ethanol, but, surprisingly, it was significantly inhibited by ethanol in concentrations of 1 g/dl or greater (5 g/dl is the maximum concentration tested). In contrast, they found a significant increase in labeled ethylpalmitate in response to ethanol in concentrations of 2.5 g/dl or greater. Sixty percent of the labeled compound was recovered in ethylpalmitate in 5 g/dl of ethanol. Carter et al., on the other hand, reported a 30% increase in TG synthesis after adding 2.6% ethanol, as already described.[127] This large discrepancy between the two experiments was interpreted by Baraona et al. as possibly being explained by contamination of the TG fraction by labeled ethylpalmitate, causing an apparent increase in TG synthesis in the experiment by Carter et al. We need to await the results of further investigations to resolve this controversy.

The results of the *in vivo* experiments by Baraona et al.[133] also differ somewhat from those by Carter et al.[127] To acutely administer ethanol, Baraona et al. infused rats with 3 g/kg of ethanol in a liquid diet via an intragastric tube. One hour after administration, [$^{14}$C]palmitate was incubated with the intestinal slices to measure $^{14}$CO$_2$ production and [$^{14}$C]-labeled TG synthesis. Acute intragastric administration of ethanol decreased the ability of the jejunal slices to oxidize palmitate and to synthesize TGs, while no such changes were found in slices taken from the ileum. Baraona et al. attributed the inhibition of TG synthesis by ethanol to the high concentration of intraluminal ethanol causing tissue damage. Carter et al., on the other hand, reported enhancement of TG synthesis after acute administration of 7.5 g/kg of ethanol, more than twice the dosage used by Baraona et al. How can this discrepancy be explained? There seem to be very important differences between the experimental conditions in the two studies. Carter et al. excised the intestine 18 h after administering ethanol, whereas Baraona et al. excised it 1 h after ethanol treatment. In the former study, ethanol was intended to affect intestinal metabolism not only from the intestinal lumen but from the bloodstream. Mistilis and Ockner showed that high concentrations of ethanol in the blood increased TG synthesis in the intestine.[128] The next difference between them was whether ethanol was administered with or without a meal which included lipids. Carter et al. infused ethanol in saline solution alone. In contrast, Baraona et al. infused ethanol with lipids, and a large amount of FAs must have been supplied to the lumen. Thus, the metabolic situations in terms of the supply of material required for TG synthesis were considerably different. The other point to be noted is the route of intraluminal administration of ethanol. Baraona et al. infused ethanol via a gastric tube, and ethanol is known to be rapidly absorbed in the stomach,[134] whereas the exact route of administration of ethanol was not mentioned in the report by Carter et al.

The results of the experiment involving chronic *in vivo* administration of ethanol by Baraona et al.[133] basically agreed with those of Carter et al.[127] Baraona et al. found increased $CO_2$ production and TG synthesis in slices of jejunum and ileum from rats chronically fed ethanol. This was associated with a 44% increase in acyl-CoA (palmitoyl-CoA in this case) synthetase in the jejunum, and to a lesser extent, in the ileum. These investigators' findings indicate that chronic dietary supplementation with ethanol gives rise to enhanced ability to synthesize TG in the intestinal mucosa.

Shakir et al. performed an *in vitro* experiment to assess lipid metabolism in the intestine using isolated rat intestinal cells instead of intestinal slices or microsomes prepared from intestinal homogenates.[135] They incubated intestinal cells with [$^{14}$C]acetate and $^3H_2O$. Incorporation of [$^{14}$C]acetate into cellular lipids was six- to eightfold greater in crypt cells than in villus cells. Ethanol (10 m*M*) tripled $^3H_2O$ incorporation into cellular lipids which were not fractionated into classes and, interestingly, had no effect on [$^{14}$C]acetate incorporation. Although Shakir et al. did not have any reasonable explanation for the discrepancies in the effect of ethanol on labeled acetate and $^3H_2O$ incorporation into cellular lipids, they concluded that ethanol stimulated intestinal lipid synthesis in isolated cells.

While there is considerable controversy in regard to the *in vitro* effect of ethanol on mucosal ability to synthesize TGs and the *in vivo* effect of acute administration of ethanol on TG synthesis, all these findings are based on observations in rats. Unfortunately, thus far very few investigations have been performed to assess the effect of ethanol on ability to synthesize lipid in the human intestine. Zimmerman et al. incubated human duodenojejunal biopsy specimens from healthy subjects.[136] The medium contained a micellar lipid solution with [$^{14}$C]oleate supplemented with ethanol in concentrations of 0.1, 1.0, and 5.0%. The results showed that tissue TG synthesis was decreased by 52.0, 57.0, and 81.3%, respectively. Since the 1.0 and 5.0% solutions of ethanol increased the osmolality of the medium, Zimmerman et al. suspected that the inhibitory effect of 1.0 and 5.0% ethanol on TG synthesis might in large part be a reflection of increased osmolality; however, as the osmolality of the medium containing 0.1% ethanol was similar to that of the control medium, they concluded that the inhibition of TG synthesis observed in the 0.1% solution was specific to ethanol. This conclusion is consistent with the conclusion made by Baraona et al. from the results of the experiments in rats.

Barros et al. obtained human jejunal tissue from nonalcoholic subjects by peroral biopsy.[137] The biopsy specimens were transferred to culture medium to perform organ culture. [$^3$H]arachidonate and [$^{14}$C]linoleate were added to the medium with or without 100 mmol/l of ethanol. After 1-h culture, labeled material in the tissue was measured, and a significantly higher amount of [$^3$H]arachidonate was found to have been incorporated into phospholipids, and more [$^{14}$C]linoleate incorporated into TGs in the control experiment. When ethanol was present in the medium, there was a significant decrease in the incorporation of both fatty acids into tissue lipids, especially into phospholipids. Although the results obtained by Zimmerman et al. and Barros et al. both showed that ethanol does not exhibit an enhancing effect on TG synthesis in human intestinal biopsy specimens, few studies are available to provide a basis for discussing whether there is a species difference in ethanol modification of TG synthesis in the intestinal mucosa.

### 16.3.3   Cholesterol Synthesis

Enterocytes obtain cholesterol not only from the dietary intraluminal cholesterol supply but from the endogenous supply. Endogenous cholesterol is derived both from nondietary intraluminal cholesterol and from *de novo* synthesized cholesterol.[138] The effect of ethanol on *de novo* cholesterol synthesis was investigated by Middleton et al.[139] Rats were fed 7.5 g/kg of ethanol by intragastric tube. Intestinal slices were prepared after fasting with free access to water for 18 h. Incorporation of [[14]C]acetate into cholesterol was significantly higher in the intestinal slices from the rats given ethanol, but no enhancement of cholesterogenesis was observed when rats were chronically fed ethanol for 3 to 4 weeks. Since ethanol intake ceased 24 h before preparing the intestinal slices in the chronic ethanol administration experiment, Middleton et al. attributed the difference between the effect of acutely and chronically administered ethanol on cholesterogenesis to the dependence of enhancing effect on recent ethanol ingestion and to a direct effect of ethanol on the intestinal mucosa. We need to await the results of further investigations to confirm their hypothesis.

### 16.3.4   Lipid Absorption

One of the simplest ways to measure the absorption of dietary lipids in the intestine is to collect feces and material remaining in the intestinal lumen. Subtraction of lipid excreted and remaining in the lumen from the amount of lipid administered represents the amount of lipid absorbed by the mucosa. Using this method, Lieber et al. assessed the effect of ethanol on lipid absorption in the intestine.[140] They infused rats with ethanol as 36% of the calories in a coconut liquid diet containing [[3]H]palmitate via a gastric tube. Sixteen hours later, they excised the gastrointestinal tract (from cardia to rectum) and found no significant difference between the amount of total labeled lipid remaining in the gut wall and lumen in the ethanol group and the control group to which sucrose was adminstered instead of ethanol. The effect of ethanol on lipid absorption much earlier after ingestion was tested by Baraona and Lieber.[141] They administered the same dose of ethanol (36% of calories) to rats with a diet containing [[3]H]palmitate and measured the radioactivity remaining in the gastrointestinal tract 0, 30, 60, 90, 120 min and 6 h after administration. There were no differences in radioactivity between the ethanol-fed and the control group at any of the points in time measured. The conclusion of these investigators that ethanol does not affect lipid absorption in the intestine was supported by Rodrigo et al.[142] They infused ethanol (16% of calories) to rats for 24 days and collected feces for 4 days preceding sacrifice. Ethanol feeding did not significantly change the amount of fecal fat excretion compared with the control.

Boquillon claimed that ethanol causes retention of fat in the stomach, but that the final absorption of lipid in the intestine under the influence of ethanol was comparable to the results in controls without ethanol.[143] A test meal of 100 mg corn oil plus 3.2 g/kg of ethanol was administered to mesenteric lymph-fistula rats by intubation. The corn oil was labeled with [[3]H]oleate, and labeled lipids in the gastrointestinal lumen and lymph were measured. Ingestion of ethanol led to marked retention of radioactivity in the stomach: more than 25% of the radioactivity fed to the rats remained 8 h later after feeding whereas less than 10% remained 6 h after feeding in the control. In contrast, about 68% and 12% of the radioactivity were recovered in the control and alcohol-treated rats, respectively, during the first 6 h of lymph collection, although the quantity of endogenous and exogenous lipids in lymph collected during the 24 h after feeding were similar in both groups. While the issue of the overall effect of ethanol on the stomach was discussed in detail in the previous chapter, the results of the experiment by Boquillon are consistent with the hypothesis that ethanol does not affect the absorption of dietary lipid in the intestine.

This hypothesis was then challenged by Thomson and co-workers.[144] They performed an *in vitro* experiment to assess the uptake of lipid into the rabbit jejunum. They also assessed the resistance of the unstirred water layer. When the bulk phase was unstirred, the unstirred layer resistance was about fivefold higher. Although acute exposure of the jejunum to 4% ethanol had no effect on the uptake of the medium-chain fatty acids, C6:0, 8:0, and 10:0, ethanol altered the permeability of the jejunum to longer-chain FAs. The addition of increasing concentrations of ethanol to the medium was associated with a progressive decline in the uptake of C12:0, 14:0, and 16:0 FAs. They also found that ethanol increased cholesterol uptake in their experimental system. Thomson performed experiments to assess the effect of chronic ethanol feeding on *in vitro* lipid uptake in the rabbit jejunum.[145] The uptake of various chain-length FAs and cholesterol was assessed in rabbits fed ethanol by providing them with drinking water which contained 15% ethanol for 6 to 7 weeks and was compared to a first control group fed *ad libitum*, a second control group in which food intake was restricted to match their body weight gain to that of the ethanol-fed group, and a third control group whose food intake was restricted to match the food intake of the ethanol-fed group. The results indicated that the uptake of C4:0 to 12:0 FAs was similar in all four groups. While food restriction and chronic ethanol feeding were associated with a decline in unstirred layer resistance, they caused a rise in the true passive permeability properties of the jejunum toward short- and medium-chain length FAs. In contrast, uptake of the long-chain C14:0, 16:0, and 18:0 FAs was lower in the ethanol-fed group than in the control groups. This was interpreted as meaning that the true permeability properties of the intestine for long-chain FA decreased more in the chronic ethanol-fed animals than the lowering of effective resistance of the unstirred layer. While the observation that the addition of ethanol causes a decline in the uptake of long-chain FAs in the jejunum in the *in vitro* experiment was reproduced in intact animals fed ethanol chronically, the results for cholesterol uptake were the opposite. In the same chronic ethanol feeding experimental system, Thomson et al. found that cholesterol uptake in the rabbit jejunum decreased in the ethanol-administered group and concluded that the effect of ethanol on passive uptake is probably secondary to changes in membrane structure and/or composition, perhaps as an adaptive response to chronic ethanol exposure.

Thomson et al. then assessed whether ethanol affects lipid uptake in the rat intestine in the same manner as in the rabbit jejunum and examined whether the species of lipid, namely, saturated FAs and polyunsaturated FAs, fed with ethanol can modify the effect of ethanol.[146] Rats were given 15% ethanol in their drinking water for 4 weeks and were then fed a diet rich in either saturated or polyunsaturated FAs with ethanol for the next 2 weeks. The uptake of C8:0, 10:0, 12:0, 14:0, 16:0, 18:1, and 18:2 FAs and cholesterol in the jejunum was measured. The results showed that when the diet was rich in polyunsaturated FAs, ethanol feeding reduced lipid uptake as compared with the control animals, whereas when the diet was rich in saturated FAs, ethanol feeding increased lipid uptake compared with the control rats. After 2 weeks of feeding with a diet rich in either saturated or polyunsaturated FAs without ethanol, C18:2 uptake in rat jejunum was assessed with or without adding 5% ethanol to the medium to investigate the acute effect of ethanol. Again, feeding polyunsaturated FAs was associated with a reduction in C18:2 uptake when compared with animals fed saturated FAs. Thomson et al. concluded that feeding rats a diet rich in saturated FAs prevents the inhibitory effect of acute and chronic ethanol exposure on the *in vitro* jejunal uptake of lipids observed in animals fed a polyunsaturated diet.

### 16.3.5   Lipid Transport in Lymph

As already described in Section 16.3.2, Mistillis and Ockner showed that mucosal TG synthesis in fasting rats is increased by intraduodenal infusion of ethanol.[128] They also collected lymph from the intestinal lymph-fistula rats to observe the metabolism of the TGs synthesized.[128,147] Rats were infused with ethanol (0.63 g/kg/h) for 8 h. While mucosal TG levels in the small intestine increased fourfold after ethanol infusion, lymph TG output in ethanol-treated rats was 25% greater at 8 to 16 h and 50% greater at 16 to 24 h than in the control rats infused with isocaloric glucose. Lymphatic TGs were carried primarily in VLDL. On the basis of this experiment, they concluded that the increased production and secretion of endogenous TG-rich lipoprotein (VLDL) caused by intraduodenal ethanol infusion contributes to ethanol-induced hyperlipidemia.

Baraona and Lieber, however, did not find any difference in lymphatic lipid output between lymph-fistula rats infused with one 0.75 g/kg dose of ethanol and the control rats infused with isocaloric glucose.[148] The amount of ethanol infused in their experiment may not have been sufficient to enhance endogenous TG synthesis and lipoprotein transport. Baraona and co-workers, on the other hand, obtained interesting findings when they added ethanol to the diet or a lipid meal and fed it to rats.[148,149] In rats not previously given alcohol, acute administration of a single dose 3 g/kg of ethanol in the diet or in emulsions containing palmitate (46 mg), glycerol monoleate, and taurocholate, significantly increased lymphatic lipid output and incorporation of dietary fat into lymph lipids 1 h after ethanol administration. In contrast, previous feeding of ethanol abolished the stimulatory effect of acute administration of ethanol on lymph lipid output. Lymph lipid output after a test meal, whether it contained 3 g/kg of ethanol or not, was no higher in rats fed a diet with ethanol as 36% of total calories for 3 to 4 weeks than in pair-fed controls. It was also noticed that while lymphatic lipid output did not increase in rats fed ethanol chronically, postprandial hyperlipidemia developed in the same rats after a single dose meal. Baraona et al. concluded that under their experimental conditions, alcoholic hyperlipidemia does not result from changes in intestinal lymph lipids, but possibly from changes in hepatic lipid metabolism. Baraona and co-workers demonstrated that acute ethanol administration has an enhancing effect on the transport of dietary fat, and that chronic ethanol feeding inhibits it.

The observation of Baraona and co-workers that acute ethanol feeding with dietary lipid results in increased output of lymphatic lipid was supported by the findings of Mendenhall et al., who infused one dose of emulsions containing 10 mg of radiolabeled tripalmitin and 2.5 g/kg of ethanol into rats whose thoracic duct had been cannulated.[150] Chyle was collected from the thoracic duct for 24 h after administration of a test meal. The radiolabeled lipid recovered in chyle after ethanol administration was twice as great in the controls fed glucose instead of ethanol.

Long-chain FAs may be transported in the portal vein instead of lymph in certain situations, as described above (see the "Lipid Transport in the Portal Vein" section). One such situation is when FAs are infused into the intestine at a very low rate, as demonstrated by McDonald et al.[116] As a result, Saunders et al. hypothesized that ethanol may enhance lymphatic lipid transport more than portal vein transport when oleate is infused at a very low rate.[151] The results of their experiments, however, did not support this hypothesis. They collected lymph during a 4-h infusion of a total dose of 8 μmol (2 μmol/h) of radiolabeled oleate with or without ethanol. There was no difference in radioactivity between the ethanol-administered rats and the control rats in the lymphatic lipid transport. They also administered a high dose oleate. When 360 μmol/4 h of oleate was infused, 162 and 144 μmol of labeled lipid were collected in the ethanol-treated and control rats, respectively. On the basis of these findings, they concluded that ethanol enhances lymphatic lipid transport when a high dose of lipid is administered. However, there does not seem to be any statistically significant difference between the two groups of rats in the presented figure in their report.

Lymphatic lipid transport was measured in lymph-fistula rats whose mesenteric lymph or thoracic duct had been cannulated by investigators mentioned thus far. It is known to take 3 or 4 h to achieve stable lymphatic transport when lipid is infused into lymph-fistula rats. Hayashi et al. observed the effect of intraduodenally administered ethanol on the stable lymphatic transport of lipid in mesenteric lymph-fistula rats.[152] They divided lymph-fistula rats to three groups. In group A (control rats), 120 μmol/h of oleate was infused over 8 h, while in group B 120 μmol/h of oleate with 0.75 g/kg/h of ethanol was infused over 8 h. In group C rats, 120 μmol/h of oleate was infused for the first 4 h then replaced with 120 μmol/h of oleate plus 0.75 g/kg/h of ethanol for the next 4 h. Lymphatic TG output is shown in Figure 16.2. In the control (group A), TG output reached a plateau of more than 30 μmol/h after 3-h infusion. The concomitant infusion of ethanol with oleate (group B) inhibited lymphatic lipid transport to two-thirds of the control in the stable transport phase. Interestingly, the addition of ethanol to rats transporting lymphatic lipid stably (group C) also decreased lymphatic TG output to two-thirds of the control by 2 h of infusion. This experiment clearly shows that ethanol exhibits an inhibitory effect on lymphatic lipid transport. In the experiment by Hayashi et al., lymphatic TG output in

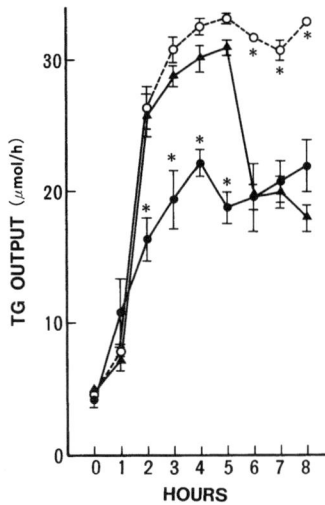

**FIGURE 16.2**  Lymphatic triglyceride output. Each group is depicted as: group A (··○··), B (–●–) and C (–▲–). Lipid was extracted from lymph and triglyceride was measured chemically. Values are expressed as means ± SEM. If SEM is not given, it's because it was too small to be displayed in this figure. Significant differences among groups (*) were seen in B vs. A and C from 2 h to 5 h and in A vs. B and C from 6 h to 8 h. (Reprinted from Hayashi, H., Nakata, K., Motohashi, Y., and Takano, T., *Alcohol Alcohol.*, 27, 627, 1992. With permission.)

group B at 1 h was higher than in group A (control), although the difference was not significant. Thus, lipid transport may be enhanced only very early during ethanol administration, as demonstrated by Baraona and co-workers.[148,149]

## 16.3.6  Alcohol Consumption and Hyperlipidemia

Although a huge number of investigations have already reported on the effect of ethanol on intestinal lipid metabolism under various experimental conditions, it seems that much controversy and confusion will remain until definite conclusions are drawn from the studies described above. However, we can summarize these experimental studies in several directions if appropriate key factors are introduced to interpret them. First of all, we need to apply this laboratory research to events in human subjects occurring both under physiological and pathological conditions influenced by alcohol. Since the major role of the intestine in the body is to absorb food, the effect of alcohol must be considered under each of the conditions when the gut is performing its absorptive function, namely, when eating, and when it is at relative rest, namely, during fasting. These may correspond to the actual situations of human subjects drinking alcohol with or without food.

Drinking alcohol without food seems to enhance lipoprotein production in the intestine in certain situations. VLDL is the lipoprotein produced under these circumstances, as demonstrated by Mistillis and Ockner.[128] The sources of lipids used to form lipoproteins are not food. Not only intraluminally supplied lipid, such as bile and shed gastrointestinal epithelium, but plasma-derived FAs may serve as the essential material for lipoprotein production. In any event, however, drinking without food cannot be said to directly lead to the overproduction of intestinal lipoprotein. There are many controversies regarding the effect of a single dose of alcohol. The results of measurements of the activity of enzymes involved in lipid synthesis in the intestinal mucosa also conflict. Differences in the doses of ethanol in the individual study may be responsible for the discrepancies between them. There is relatively convincing data that continuous alcohol feeding increases lipid synthesis in the mucosa and transport in the lymph. Moreover, in rats fed alcohol chronically, lipid synthetic activity in the intestinal mucosa is enhanced. The question is whether the overproduction of intestinal lipoprotein caused by continuous drinking without food leads to hyperlipidemia. While the amount of lipid transported from the intestine to the bloodstream increases in response to continuous drinking, it is assumed that the amount of lipid transported from the intestine after food intake is much larger than that. Therefore the overproduction of intestinal lipoprotein alone is not sufficient to cause hyperlipidemia during drinking.

Drinking while eating, probably a more common situation in society, seems to affect intestinal lipid metabolism differently than drinking alone. The absorption of intraluminal lipids derived from food can be inhibited to some extent by alcohol. Thomson and co-workers demonstrated this in rabbits[144,145] and rats.[146] As a result, feces contain more lipid when drinking than when not drinking. Clinical steatorrhea complicating alcoholism may be partly attributable to this phenomenon. A single dose of alcohol and food may temporarily increase lymphatic lipid transport very early after administration, but Hayashi et al. showed that continuous drinking and eating inhibit lymphatic lipid transport instead.[152] Moreover, in chronically alcohol-fed animals, the addition of alcohol to meals has no effect on lymphatic lipid output, as demonstrated by Baraona et al.[148,149] It is reasonable to assume that the inhibition of lipid absorption by alcohol is related to the unchanged or decreased lipid transport in lymph. In summary, it is rather difficult to postulate that the supply of lipid from the intestine to the entire body is enhanced by alcohol when a substantial amount of food is supplied.

All of these data discourage the idea that alcoholic hyperlipidemia is caused by the overproduction of intestinal lipoproteins. It is beyond the scope of this chapter to discuss the pathogenesis of alcoholic hyperlipidemia in detail, but a few comments can be added to facilitate our understanding of this issue. Hyperlipidemia is caused by enhanced production or delayed clearance of plasma lipoprotein. If the intestine is not involved in the etiology of hyperlipidemia, the other possibilities are alteration of lipid metabolism in the liver and/or delayed catabolism of lipoprotein in the plasma. Actually, Lieber pointed out about 30 years ago that the secretion of endogenous lipoproteins by the liver is unaffected by ethanol, and that ethanol instead causes a delay in the clearance of lipoprotein from the plasma.[153] One of the characteristics of alcohol-induced hyperlipidemia is an elevation of plasma HDL-cholesterol,[154] and as already mentioned, the intestine synthesizes HDL. The possibility that ethanol may enhance HDL production in the intestine remains, but no experimental data are available thus far to provide a basis for discussion. On the other hand, the activity of cholesteryl ester transport protein (CETP) has been shown to be reduced in alcoholics.[155] CETP facilitates the transfer of cholesteryl esters from HDL to LDL and VLDL in the plasma. Therefore, defective activity of CETP leads to the high HDL-cholesterol levels.

## 16.4 CONCLUDING REMARKS

In the 1980s, the molecular biology techniques were introduced into the field of lipid metabolism research and to other fields related to medicine, or to put it another way, lipidology was one of the earliest applied sciences in which bimolecular methods demonstrated their revolutionary power in the discovery and development of scientific information. This has also been the case in research on lipid metabolism in the intestine. Many aspects of regulation in intestinal lipid metabolism can now be described in molecular biological terms. However, progress based on the molecular biology has not necessarily been associated with a basic understanding of intestinal lipid metabolism either under physiological or pathological conditions. Modification by alcohol may be one of those areas where many fields of researchers are provided with future possibilities. We do not have enough information in humans to test the hypotheses based on the results of studies in laboratory animals. There has not been sufficient examination of the effects of alcohol on intestinal lipid metabolism from the standpoint of molecular sciences, nor has there been any reasonable hypothesis on colon cancer, which is one of the greatest problems regarding the interaction between alcohol and gastrointestinal system from the standpoint of lipid metabolism. Nevertheless, progress in this field over the past three decades has been enormous and outstanding. Our present understanding of how lipids are metabolized in the intestine was described first in this chapter. It may not been known at present how certain topics are related to alcohol, and they will provide readers with suggestions for future research.

## 16.5 ACKNOWLEDGMENTS

The author dedicates this chapter to Professor Chikayuki Naito and Professor Patrick Tso in gratitude for their instruction in lipidology research. The author would like to acknowledge and thank his colleagues in the Department of Internal Medicine, Yokohama Red Cross Hospital, which is headed by Dr. Takanori Amakawa, for their sincere support in the production of the manuscript. The author also wants to express his gratitude to Dr. Haruhiko Yoshinaga for his editorial assistance.

## REFERENCES

1. **Tso, P.,** Gastrointestinal digestion and absorption of lipid, *Adv. Lipid Res.,* 21, 143, 1985.
2. **Rizek, R. L., Friend, B., and Page, L.,** Fat in today's food supply-level of use and source, *J. Am. Oil. Chem. Soc.,* 51, 244, 1974.
3. **Northfield, T. C. and Hofman, A. F.,** Biliary lipid output during three meals and an overnight fast. I. Relationship to bile acid pool size and cholesterol saturation of bile in gallstone and control subjects, *Gut,* 16, 1, 1975.
4. **Helander, H. F. and Olivecrona, T.,** Lipolysis and lipid absorption in the stomach of the suckling rat, *Gastroenterology,* 59, 22, 1970.
5. **Senior, J. R.,** Intestinal absorption of fats, *J. Lipid Res.,* 5, 495, 1964.
6. **Borgström, B. and Erlanson, C.,** Pancreatic lipase and colipase. Interactions and effects of bile salts and other detergents, *Eur. J. Biochem.,* 37, 60, 1973.
7. **Nilsson, Å.,** Intestinal absorption of lecithin and lysolecithin by lymph fistula rats, *Biochim. Biophys. Acta,* 152, 379, 1968.
8. **van Deenen, L. L. M., deHaas, G. H., and Heemskerk, C. H. T.,** Hydrolysis of synthetic mixed phosphatides by phospholipase A from human pancreas, *Biochim. Biophys. Acta,* 67, 295, 1963.
9. **Patton, J. S.,** Gastrointestinal lipid digestion, in *Physiology of the Gastrointestinal Tract,* Johnston, L. R., Ed., Raven Press, New York, 1981, 1123.
10. **Lombardo, D. and Guy, O.,** Binding of human pancreatic carboxylic ester hydrolase to lipid interfaces, *Biochim. Biophys. Acta,* 659, 401, 1981.
11. **Thomson, A. B. R. and Dietschy, J. M.,** Intestinal lipid absorption: major extracellular and intracellular events, in *Physiology of the Gastrointestinal Tract,* Johnston, L. R., Ed., Raven Press, New York, 1981, 1147.
12. **Carey, M. C., Small, D. M., and Bliss, C. M.,** Lipid digestion and absorption, *Ann. Rev. Physiol.,* 45, 651, 1983.
13. **Mishkin, S. and Kessler, J. I.,** The uptake and release of bile salt and fatty acid by hamster jejunum, *Biochim. Biophys. Acta,* 202, 222, 1970.
14. **Schulthess, G., Lipka, G., Compassi, S., Boffelli, D., Weber, F. E., Paltauf, F., and Hauser, H.,** Absorption of monoacylglycerols by small intestinal brush border membrane, *Biochemistry,* 33, 4500, 1994.
15. **Stremmel, W.,** Uptake of fatty acids by jejunal mucosal cells is mediated by a fatty acid binding membrane protein, *J. Clin. Invest.,* 82, 2001, 1988.
16. **Bergstedt, S. E., Hayashi, H., Kritchevsky, D., and Tso, P.,** A comparison of glycerol tristearate and glycerol trioleate by rat small intestine, *Am. J. Physiol.,* 259, G386, 1990.
17. **Bosner, M. S., Gulick, T., Riley, D. J., Spilburg, C. A., and Lange, L. G., III,** Receptor-like function of heparin in the binding and uptake of neutral lipids, *Proc. Natl. Acad. Sci. U.S.A.,* 85, 7438, 1988.
18. **Thurnhofer, H. and Hauser, H.,** Uptake of cholesterol by small intestinal brush border membrane is protein-mediated, *Biochemistry,* 29, 2142, 1990.
19. **Chen, H., Born, E., Mathur, S. N., Johlin, F. C., Jr., and Field, F. J.,** Sphingomyelin content of intestinal cell membranes regulates cholesterol absorption. Evidence for pancreatic and intestinal cell sphingomyelinase activity, *Biochem. J.,* 286, 771, 1992.
20. **Scow, R. O., Stein, Y., and Stein, O.,** Incorporation of dietary lecithin and lysolecithin into lymph chylomicrons in the rat, *J. Biol. Chem.,* 242, 4919, 1967.
21. **Parthasarathy, S., Subbaiah, P. V., and Ganguly, J.,** The mechanism of intestinal absorption of phosphatidyl-choline in rats, *Biochem. J.,* 140, 503, 1974.
22. **Ockner, R. K. and Manning, J. A.,** Fatty acid binding protein in small intestine. Identification, isolation and evidence for its role in cellular fatty acid transport, *J. Clin. Invest.,* 54, 326, 1974.
23. **Srikantaiah, M. V., Hansbury, E., Loughram, E. D., and Scallen, T. J.,** Purification and properties of sterol carrier protein, *J. Biol. Chem.,* 251, 5496, 1976.

24. **Scallen, T. J., Noland, B. J., Gavey, K. L., Bass, N. M., Ockner, R. K., Chanderbhan, R., and Vahouny, G. V.,** Sterol carrier protein 2 and fatty acid-binding protein. Separate and distinct physiological functions, *J. Biol. Chem.,* 260, 4733, 1985.

25. **Higgins, J. A. and Barrnett, R. J.,** Fine structural localization of acyltransferases: the monoglyceride and α-glycerophosphate pathways in intestinal absorptive cells, *J. Cell Biol.,* 50, 102, 1971.

26. **Johnston, J. M., Paltauf, F., Schiller, C. M., and Schultz, L. D.,** The utilization of the α-glycerophosphate and monoglyceride pathways for phosphatidylcholine biosynthesis in the intestine, *Biochim. Biophys. Acta,* 218, 124, 1970.

27. **Johnston, J. M.,** Esterification reactions in the intestinal mucosa and lipid absorption, in *Disturbances in Lipid and Lipoprotein Metabolism,* Dietschy, J. M., Gotto, A. M., Jr., and Ontko, J. A., Eds., American Physiological Society, Bethesda, MD, 1978, 57.

28. **Weiss, J. M.,** The role of the Golgi complex in fat absorption as studied with the electron microscope with observations on the cytology of duodenal absorptive cells, *J. Exp. Med.,* 102, 116, 1955.

29. **Gurr, M. I., Brindley, D. N., and Hübscher, G.,** Metabolism of phospholipids. VIII. Biosynthesis of phosphatidylcholine in the intestinal mucosa, *Biochim. Biophys. Acta,* 98, 486, 1965.

30. **O'Doherty, P. J. A.,** Phospholipid synthesis in differentiating cells of rat intestine, *Arch. Biochem. Biophys.,* 190, 508, 1978.

31. **Johnston, J. M., Rao, G. A., and Lowe, P. A.,** The separation of the α-glycerophosphate and monoglyceride pathways in the intestinal biosynthesis of triglycerides, *Biochim. Biophys. Acta,* 137, 578, 1967.

32. **Gallo, L. L., Chiang, Y., Vahouny, G. V., and Treadwell, C. R.,** Localization and origin of rat intestinal cholesterol esterase determined by immunocytochemistry, *J. Lipid Res.,* 21, 537, 1980.

33. **Field, F. J.,** Intestinal cholesterol esterase: intracellular enzyme or contamination of cytosol by pancreatic enzymes, *J. Lipid Res.,* 25, 389, 1984.

34. **Heider, J. G., Pickens, C. E., and Kelly, L. A.,** Role of acyl CoA:cholesterol acyltransferase in cholesterol absorption and its inhibition by 57-118 in the rabbit, *J. Lipid Res.,* 24, 1127, 1983.

35. **Gallo, L. L., Bennett Clark, S., Meyers, S., and Vahouny, G. V.,** Cholesterol absorption in rat intestine: role of cholesterol esterase and acyl coenzyme A:cholesterol acyltransferase, *J. Lipid Res.,* 25, 604, 1984.

36. **Bennett Clark, S. and Tercyak, A. M.,** Reduced cholesterol transmucosal transport in rats with inhibited mucosal acyl CoA:cholesterol acyltransferase and normal pancreatic function, *J. Lipid Res.,* 25, 148, 1984.

37. **Lindgren, F. T., Jensen, L. C., and Hatch, F. T.,** The isolation and quantitative analysis of serum lipoproteins, in *Blood Lipids and Lipoproteins: Quantitation, Composition and Metabolism,* Nelson, G. J., Ed., Wiley, New York, 1972, 181.

38. **Imaizumi, K., Havel, R. J., Fainaru, M., and Vigne, J. L.,** Origin and transport of the A-I and arginine-rich apolipoproteins in mesenteric lymph of rats, *J. Lipid Res.,* 19, 1038, 1978.

39. **Riley, J. W., Glickman, R. M., Green, P. H., and Tall, A. R.,** The effect of chronic cholesterol feeding on intestinal lipoproteins in the rat, *J. Lipid Res.,* 21, 942, 1980.

40. **Wu, A. L. and Windmueller, H. G.,** Relative contributions by liver and intestine to individual plasma apolipoproteins in the rat, *J. Biol. Chem.,* 254, 7316, 1979.

41. **Chen, S. H., Habib, G., Yang, C. Y., Gu, Z. W., Lee, B. R., Weng, S., Silberman, S. R., Cai, S. J., Deslypere, J. P., Rosseneu, M., Gotto, A. M., Jr., Li, W. H., and Chan, L.,** Apolipoprotein B-48 is the product of a messenger RNA with an organ-specific in-frame stop codon, *Science,* 238, 363, 1987.

42. **Powell, L. M., Wallis, S. C., Pease, R. J., Edwards, Y. H., Knott, T. J., and Scott, J.,** A novel form of tissue-specific RNA processing produces apolipoprotein-B48 in intestine, *Cell,* 50, 831, 1987.

43. **Hospattankar, A. V., Higuchi, K., Law, S. W., Meglin, N., and Brewer, H. B., Jr.,** Identification of a novel in-frame translational stop codon in human intestine apoB mRNA, *Biochem. Biophys. Res. Commun.,* 148, 279, 1987.

44. **Davidson, N. O., Powell, L. M., Wallis, S. C., and Scott, J.,** Thyroid hormone modulates the introduction of a stop codon in rat liver apolipoprotein B messenger RNA, *J. Biol. Chem.,* 263, 13482, 1988.

45. **Tennyson, G. E., Sabatos, C. A., Higuchi, K., Meglin, N., and Brewer, H. B., Jr.,** Expression of apolipoprotein B mRNAs encoding higher- and lower-molecular weight isoproteins in rat liver and intestine, *Proc. Natl. Acad. Sci. U.S.A.,* 86, 500, 1989.

46. **Teng, B., Burant, C. F., and Davidson, N. O.,** Molecular cloning of an apolipoprotein B messenger RNA editing protein, *Science,* 260, 1816, 1993.

47. **Renner, F., Samuelson, A., Rogers, M., and Glickman, R. M.,** Effect of saturated and unsaturated lipid on the composition of mesenteric triglyceride-rich lipoproteins in the rat, *J. Lipid Res.,* 27, 72, 1986.

48. **Krause, B. R., Sloop, C. H., Castle, C. K., and Roheim, P. S.,** Mesenteric lymph apolipoproteins in control and ethinyl estradiol-treated rats: a model for studying apolipoproteins of intestinal origin, *J. Lipid Res.,* 22, 610, 1981.

49. **Davidson, N. O., Magun, A. M., Brasitus, T. A., and Glickman, R. M.,** Intestinal apolipoprotein A-I and B-48 metabolism: effects of sustained alterations in dietary triglyceride and mucosal cholesterol flux, *J. Lipid Res.,* 28, 388, 1987.

50. **Hayashi, H., Fujimoto, K., Cardelli, J. A., Nutting, D. F., Bergstedt, S., and Tso, P.,** Fat feeding increases size, but not number, of chylomicrons produced by small intestine, *Am. J. Physiol.,* 259, G709, 1990.

51. **Fidge, N. H.,** The redistribution and metabolism of iodinated A-IV in rats, *Biochim. Biophys. Acta*, 619, 129, 1980.

52. **Ohta, T., Fidge, N. H., and Nestel, P. J.,** Studies on the *in vivo* and *in vitro* distribution of apolipoprotein A-IV in human plasma and lymph, *J. Clin. Invest.*, 76, 1252, 1985.

53. **DeLamatre, J. G., Hoffmeier, C. A., Lacko, A. G., and Roheim, P. S.,** Distribution of apolipoprotein A-IV between the lipoprotein and the lipoprotein-free fractions of rat plasma: possible role of lecithin:cholesterol acyltransferase, *J. Lipid Res.*, 24, 1578, 1983.

54. **Bisgaier, C. L., Sachdev, O. P., Lee, E. S., Williams, K. J., Blum, C. B., and Glickman, R. M.,** Effect of lecithin:cholesterol acyltransferase on distribution of apolipoprotein A-IV among lipoproteins of human plasma, *J. Lipid Res.*, 28, 693, 1987.

55. **Ghiselli, G., Crump, W. L., III, and Gotto, A. M., Jr.,** Binding of apo A-IV-phospholipid complexes to plasma membranes of rat liver, *Biochem. Biophys. Res. Commun.*, 139, 122, 1986.

56. **Dvorin, E., Gorder, N. L., Benson, D. M., and Gotto, A. M., Jr.,** Apolipoprotein A-IV. A determinant for binding and uptake of high density lipoproteins by rat hepatocytes, *J. Biol. Chem.*, 261, 15714, 1986.

57. **Savion, N. and Gamliel, A.,** Binding of apolipoprotein A-I and apolipoprotein A-IV to cultured bovine aortic endothelial cells, *Arteriosclerosis*, 8, 178, 1988.

58. **Fujimoto, K., Fukagawa, K., Sakata, T., and Tso, P.,** Suppression of food intake by apolipoprotein A-IV is mediated through the central nervous system in rats, *J. Clin. Invest.*, 91, 1830, 1993.

59. **Green, P. H. R., Glickman, R. M., Riley, J. W., and Quinet, E.,** Human apolipoprotein A-IV. Intestinal origin and distribution in plasma, *J. Clin. Invest.*, 65, 911, 1980.

60. **Weinberg, R. B., Dantzker, C., and Patton, C. S.,** Sensitivity of serum apolipoprotein A-IV levels to changes in dietary fat content, *Gastroenterology*, 98, 17, 1990.

61. **Harim, I. E., Befort, J. J., Balafrej, A., Lahrichi, M., and Girard-Globa, A.,** Lipids and lipoproteins of malnourished children during early renutrition: apolipoprotein A-IV as a potential index of recovery, *Am. J. Clin. Nutr.*, 58, 407, 1993.

62. **Hayashi, H., Nutting, D. F., Fujimoto, K., Cardelli, J. A., Black D., and Tso, P.,** Transport of lipid and apolipoprotein A-I and A-IV in intestinal lymph of the rat, *J. Lipid Res.*, 31, 1613, 1990.

63. **Schaefer, E. J., Eisenberg, S., and Levy, R. I.,** Lipoprotein apoprotein metabolism, *J. Lipid Res.*, 19, 667, 1978.

64. **Rooke, J. A. and Skinner, E. R.,** The biosynthesis of rat serum apolipoproteins by liver and intestinal mucosa, *Biochem. Soc. Trans.*, 4, 1144, 1976.

65. **Glickman, R. M. and Green, P. H. R.,** The intestine as a source of apolipoprotein A1, *Proc. Natl. Acad. Sci. U.S.A.*, 74, 2569, 1977.

66. **Imaizumi, K., Fainaru, M., and Havel, R. J.,** Composition of proteins of mesenteric lymph chylomicrons in the rat and alterations produced upon exposure of chylomicrons to blood serum and serum proteins, *J. Lipid Res.*, 19, 712, 1978.

67. **Schonfeld, G., Bell, E., and Alpers, D. H.,** Intestinal apoproteins during fat absorption, *J. Clin. Invest.*, 61, 1539, 1978.

68. **Alpers, D. H., Lancaster, N., and Schonfeld, G.,** The effects of fat feeding on apolipoprotein A-I secretion from rat small intestinal epithelium, *Metabolism*, 31, 784, 1982.

69. **Gordon, J. I., Smith, D. P., Andy, R., Alpers, D. H., Schonfeld, G., and Strauss, A. W.,** The primary translation product of rat intestinal apolipoprotein A-I mRNA is an unusual preproprotein, *J. Biol. Chem.*, 257, 971, 1982.

70. **Gordon, J. I., Budelier, K. A., Sims, H. F., Edelstein, C., Scanu, A. M., and Strauss, A. W.,** Biosynthesis of human preproapolipoprotein A-II, *J. Biol. Chem.*, 258, 14054, 1983.

71. **Strauss, E. W.,** Electron microscopic study of intestinal fat absorption *in vitro* from mixed micelles containing linolenic acid, monoolein, and bile salt, *J. Lipid Res.*, 7, 307, 1966.

72. **Jersild, R. A., Jr.,** A time sequence study of fat absorption in the rat jejunum, *Am. J. Anat.*, 118, 135, 1966.

73. **Cardell, R. R., Jr., Badenhausen, S., and Porter, K. R.,** Intestinal triglyceride absorption in the rat. An electron microscope study, *J. Cell Biol.*, 34, 123, 1967.

74. **Friedman, H. I. and Cardell, R. R., Jr.,** Effects of puromycin on the structure of rat intestinal epithelial cells during fat absorption, *J. Cell Biol.*, 52, 15, 1972.

75. **Bell, R. M., Ballas, L. M., and Coleman, R. A.,** Lipid topogenesis, *J. Lipid Res.*, 22, 391, 1981.

76. **Kessler, J., Narcessian, P., and Mauldin, D. P.,** Biosynthesis of lipoproteins by intestinal epithelium. Site of synthesis and sequence of association of lipid, sugar and protein moieties, *Gastroenterology*, 68, 1058, 1975.

77. **Christensen, N. J., Rubin, C. E., Cheung, M. C., and Albers, J. J.,** Ultrastructural immunolocalization of apolipoprotein B within human jejunal absorptive cells, *J. Lipid Res.*, 24, 1229, 1983.

78. **Collins, D. R., Knott, T. J., Pease, R. J., Powell, L. M., Wallis, S. C., Robertson, S., Pullinger, C. R., Milne, R. W., Marcel, Y. L., Humphries, S. E., Talmud, P. J., Lloyd, J. K., Miller, N. E., Muller, D., and Scott, J.,** Truncated variants of apolipoprotein B cause hypobetalipoproteinaemia, *Nucleic Acids Res.*, 16, 8361, 1988.

79. **Young, S. G., Northey, S. T., and McCarthy, B. J.,** Low plasma cholesterol levels caused by a short deletion in the apolipoprotein B gene, *Science*, 241, 591, 1988.

80. **Lackner, K. J., Monge, J. C., Gregg, R. E., Hoeg, J. M., Triche, T. J., Law, S. W., and Brewer, H. B., Jr.,** Analysis of the apolipoprotein B gene and messenger ribonucleic acid in abetablipoproteinemia, *J. Clin. Invest.*, 78, 1707, 1986.

81. **Dullaart, R. P., Speelberg, B., Schuurman, H. J., Milne, R. W., Havekes, L. M., Marcel, Y. L., Geuze, H. J., Hulshof, M. M., and Erkelens, D. W.,** Epitopes of apolipoprotein B-100 and B-48 in both liver and intestine. Expression and evidence for local synthesis in recessive abetalipoproteinemia, *J. Clin. Invest.*, 78, 1397, 1986.

82. **Talmud, P. J., Lloyd, J. K., Muller, D. P., Collins, D. R., Scott, J., and Humphries, S.,** Genetic evidence from two families that the apolipoprotein B gene is not involved in abetalipoproteinemia, *J. Clin. Invest.*, 82, 1803, 1988.

83. **Huang, L. S., Janne, P. A., de Graaf, J., Cooper, M., Deckelbaum, R. J., Kayden, H., and Breslow, J. L.,** Exclusion of linkage between the human apolipoprotein B gene and abetalipoproteinemia, *Am. J. Hum. Genet.*, 46, 1141, 1990.

84. **Wetterau, J. R., Aggerbeck, L. P., Bouma, M. E., Eisenberg, C., Munck, A., Hermier, M., Schmitz, J., Gay, G., Rader, D. J., and Gregg, R. E.,** Absence of microsomal trigyceride transfer protein in individuals with abetalipoproteinemia, *Science*, 258, 999, 1992.

85. **Shoulders, C. C., Brett, D. J., Bayliss, J. D., Narcisi, T. M. E., Jarmuz, A., Grantham, T. T., Leoni, P. R. D., Bhattacharya, S., Pease, R. J., Cullen, P. M., Levi, S., Byfield, P. G. H., Purkiss, P., and Scott, J.,** Abetalipoproteinemia is caused by defects of the gene encoding the 97 kDa subunit of a microsomal triglyceride transfer protein, *Hum. Mol. Genet.*, 2, 2109, 1993.

86. **Sharp, D., Blinderman, L., Combs, K. A., Kienzle, B., Ricci, B., Wager-Smith, K., Gil, C. M., Turck, C. W., Bouma, M. E., Rader, D. J., Aggerbeck, L. P., Gregg, R. E., Gordon, D. A., and Wetterau, J. R.,** Cloning and gene defects in microsomal triglyceride transfer protein associated with abetalipoproteinaemia, *Nature*, 365, 65, 1993.

87. **Levy, E., Marcel, Y., Deckelbaum, R. J., Milne, R., Lepage, G., Seidman, E., Bendayan, M., and Roy, C. C.,** Intestinal apoB synthesis, lipids, and lipoproteins in chylomicron retention disease, *J. Lipid Res.*, 28, 1263, 1987.

88. **Roy, C. C., Levy, E., Green, P. H. R., Sniderman, A., Letarte, J., Buts, J. P., Orquin, J., Brochu, P., Weber, A. M., Morin, C. L., Marcel, Y., and Deckelbaum, R. J.,** Malabsorption, hypocholesterolemia, and fat-filled enterocytes with increased intestinal apoprotein B. Chylomicron retention disease, *Gastroenterology*, 92, 390, 1987.

89. **Friedman, H. I. and Cardell, R. R., Jr.,** Alterations in the endoplasmic reticulum and Golgi complex of intestinal epithelial cells during fat absorption and after termination of this process: a morphological and morphometric study, *Anat. Rec.*, 188, 77, 1977.

90. **Morrè, D. J., Keenan, T. W., and Huang, C. M.,** Membrane flow and differentiation: origin of Golgi apparatus membranes from endoplasmic reticulum, in *Advances in Cytopharmacology*, Vol. 2, Ceccarelli, B., Clementi, F., and Weldolesi, J., Eds., Raven Press, New York, 1974, 107.

91. **Morrè, D. J.,** Golgi apparatus and membrane biogenesis, *Cell Surf. Rev.*, 4, 1, 1977.

92. **Neutra, M. and Leblond, C. P.,** Synthesis of carbohydrates of mucus in the Golgi complex as shown by electron microscope radioautography of goblet cells from rats injected with glucose, *J. Cell Biol.*, 30, 119, 1966.

93. **Neutra, M. and Leblond, C. P.,** Radioautographic comparison of the uptake of galactose-$H^3$ and glucose-$H^3$ in the Golgi region of various cells secreting glycoproteins or mucopolysaccharides, *J. Cell Biol.*, 30, 137, 1966.

94. **Schachter, H.,** The subcellular site of glycosylation, *Biochem. Soc. Symp.*, 40, 57, 1974.

95. **Kessler, J. I., Narcessian, P., and Mauldin, D. P.,** Biosynthesis of lipoproteins by intestinal epithelium. Site of synthesis and sequence of association of lipid, sugar and protein moieties, *Gastroenterology*, 68, 1058, 1975.

96. **Redgrave, T. G.,** Association of Golgi membrane with lipid droplets (pre-chylomicrons) from within intestinal epithelial cells during absorption of fat, *Aust. J. Exp. Biol. Med. Sci.*, 49, 209, 1971.

97. **Sabesin, S. M. and Frase, S.,** Electron microscopic studies of the assembly, intracellular transport, and secretion of chylomicrons by rat intestine, *J. Lipid Res.*, 18, 496, 1977.

98. **Bhattacharya, S. and Redgrave, T. G.,** The content of apolipoprotein B in chylomicron particles, *J. Lipid Res.*, 22, 820, 1981.

99. **Elovson, J., Chatterton, J. E., Bell, G. T., Schumaker, V. N., Reuben, M. A., Puppione, D. L., Reeve, J. R., Jr., and Young, N. L.,** Plasma very low density lipoproteins contain a single molecule of apolipoprotein B, *J. Lipid Res.*, 29, 1461, 1988.

100. **Reaven, E. P. and Reaven, G. M.,** Distribution and content of microtubules in relation to the transport of lipid. An ultrastructural quantitative study of the absorptive cell of the small intestine, *J. Cell Biol.*, 75, 559, 1977.

101. **Glickman, R. M., Perrotto, J. L., and Kirsh, K.,** Intestinal lipoprotein formation: effect of colchicine, *Gastroenterology*, 70, 347, 1976.

102. **Pavelka, M. and Gangl, A.,** Effects of colchicine on the intestinal transport of endogenous lipid, *Gastroenterology*, 84, 544, 1983.

103. **Green, P. H. R., Tall, A. R., and Glickman, R. M.,** Rat intestine secretes discoid high density lipoprotein, *J. Clin. Invest.*, 61, 528, 1978.

104. **Magun, A. M., Mish, B., and Glickman, R. M.,** Intracellular apoA-I and apoB distribution in rat intestine is altered by lipid feeding, *J. Lipid Res.*, 29, 1107, 1988.

105. **Bisgaier, C. L. and Glickman, R. M.,** Intestinal synthesis, secretion, and transport of lipoproteins, *Annu. Rev. Physiol.*, 45, 625, 1983.

106. **Anderson, D. W., Bronzert, T. J., Schaefer, E. J., Niblack, G. D., Zech, L., Forte, T., and Brewer, H. B., Jr.,** Evidence for recirculation of apolipoproteins A-I and A-II between plasma and human thoracic duct lymph, *Clin. Res.*, 27, 362, 1979.

107. **Zilversmit, D. B., Sisco, P. H., Jr., and Yokoyama, A.,** Size distribution of thoracic duct lymph chylomicrons from rats fed cream and corn oil, *Biochim. Biophys. Acta*, 125, 129, 1966.

108. **Havel, R. J.,** Lipoprotein biosynthesis and metabolism, in *Lipoprotein Structure*, Scanu, A. M. and Landsberger, F. R., Eds., New York Academy of Science, New York, 1980, 16.

109. **Mahley, R. W., Bennett, B. D., Morrè, D. J., Gray, M. E., Thistlethwaite, W., and LeQuire, V. S.,** Lipoproteins associated with the Golgi apparatus isolated from epithelial cells of rat small intestine, *Lab. Invest.*, 25, 435, 1971.

110. **Tso, P., Balint, J. A., Bishop, M. B., and Rodgers, J. B.,** Acute inhibition of intestinal lipid transport by Pluronic L-81 in the rat, *Am. J. Physiol.*, 241, G487, 1981.

111. **Tso, P. and Balint, J. A.,** Formation and transport of chylomicrons by enterocytes to the lymphatics, *Am. J. Physiol.*, 250, G715, 1986.

112. **Tso, P., Drake, D. S., Black, D. D., and Sabesin, S. M.,** Evidence for separate pathways of chylomicron and very low density lipoprotein assembly and transport by rat small intestine, *Am. J. Physiol.*, 247, G599, 1984.

113. **Kiyasu, J. Y., Bloom, B., and Chaikoff, I. L.,** The portal transport of absorbed fatty acids, *J. Biol. Chem.*, 199, 415, 1952.

114. **Carlier, M. and Bazard, J.,** Electron microscope autoradiographic study of intestinal absorption of decanoic and octanoic acids in the rat, *J. Cell Biol.*, 65, 383, 1975.

115. **Saunders, D. R. and Dawson, A. M.,** The absorption of oleic acid in the bile fistula rat, *Gut*, 4, 254, 1963.

116. **McDonald, G. B., Saunders, D. R., Weidman, M., and Fisher, L.,** Portal venous transport of long-chain fatty acids absorbed from rat intestine, *Am. J. Physiol.*, 239, G141, 1980.

117. **Mansbach, C. M., II, Dowell, R. F., and Pritchett, D.,** Portal transport of absorbed lipids in rats, *Am. J. Physiol.*, 261, G530, 1991.

118. **Mansbach, C. M., II and Dowell, R. F.,** Portal transport of long acyl chain lipids: effect of phosphatidylcholine and low infusion rates, *Am. J. Physiol.*, 264, G1082, 1993.

119. **Zieve, L.,** Jaundice, hyperlipemia and hemolytic anemia: a heretofore unrecognized syndrome associated with alcoholic fatty liver and cirrhosis, *Ann. Intern. Med.*, 48, 471, 1958.

120. **DiLuzio, N. R. and Poggi, M.,** Abnormal lipid tolerance and hyperlipemia in acute ethanol-treated rats, *Life Sci.*, 10, 751, 1963.

121. **Schapiro, R. H., Scheig, R. L., Drummey, G. D., Mendelson, J. H., and Isselbacher, K. J.,** Effect of prolonged ethanol ingestion on the transport and metabolism of lipids in man, *N. Engl. J. Med.*, 272, 610, 1965.

122. **Brewster, A. C., Lankford, H. G., Schwartz, M. G., and Sullivan, J. F.,** Ethanol and alimentary lipemia, *Am. J. Clin. Nutr.*, 19, 255, 1966.

123. **Verdy, M. and Gattereau, A.,** Ethanol, lipase activity, and serum-lipid level, *Am. J. Clin. Nutr.*, 20, 997, 1967.

124. **Barboriak, J. J. and Meade, R. C.,** Enhancement of alimentary lipemia by preprandial alcohol, *Am. J. Med. Sci.*, 255, 245, 1968.

125. **Wilson, D. E. and Arky, R. A.,** Changes in the disposition of alimentary fat induced by ethanol, *Diabetes*, 17, 306, 1968.

126. **Wilson, D. E., Schreibman, P. H., Brewster, A. C., and Arky, R. A.,** The enhancement of alimentary lipemia by ethanol in man, *J. Lab. Clin. Med.*, 75, 264, 1970.

127. **Carter, E. A., Drummey, G. D., and Isselbacher, K. J.,** Ethanol stimulates triglyceride synthesis by the intestine, *Science*, 174, 1245, 1971.

128. **Mistilis, S. P. and Ockner, R. K.,** Effects of ethanol on endogenous lipid and lipoprotein metabolism in small intestine, *J. Lab. Clin. Med.*, 80, 34, 1972.

129. **Franks, J. J., Riley, E. M., and Isselbacher, K. J.,** Synthesis of fatty acids by rat intestine *in vitro*, *Proc. Soc. Exp. Biol. Med.*, 121, 322, 1966.

130. **Havel, R. J. and Goldfien, A.,** The role of the liver and of extrahepatic tissues in the transport and metabolism of fatty acids and triglycerides in the dog, *J. Lipid Res.*, 2, 389, 1961.

131. **Gangl, A. and Ockner, R.,** Intestinal metabolism of plasma free fatty acids (FFA), *Gastroenterology*, 66, 841, 1974.

132. **Rodgers, J. B. and O'Brien, R. J.,** The effect of acute ethanol treatment on lipid-reestrifying enzymes of the rat small bowel, *Dig. Dis.*, 20, 354, 1975.

133. **Baraona, E., Pirola, R. C., and Lieber, C. S.,** Acute and chronic effects of ethanol on intestinal lipid metabolism, *Biochim. Biophys. Acta*, 388, 19, 1975.

134. **Mansbach, C. M., II,** Effect of ethanol on intestinal lipid absorption in the rat, *J. Lipid Res.*, 24, 1310, 1983.

135. **Shakir, K. M. M., Sundaram, S. G., and Margolis, S.,** Lipid synthesis in isolated intestinal cells, *J. Lipid Res.*, 19, 433, 1978.

136. **Zimmerman, J., Gati, I., Eisenberg, S., and Rachmilewitz, D.,** Ethanol inhibits triglyceride synthesis and secretion by human small intestinal mucosa, *J. Lab. Clin. Med.*, 107, 498, 1986.

137. **Barros, H., Chen, Q., Florèn, C. H., and Nilsson, Å.,** Arachidonic acid absorption in human jejunum in organ culture: effects of ethanol, *Eur. J. Clin. Invest.,* 20, 506, 1990.

138. **Wilson, J. D. and Lindsey, C. A., Jr.,** Studies on the influence of dietary cholesterol on cholesterol metabolism in the isotopic steady state in man, *J. Clin. Invest.,* 44, 1805, 1965.

139. **Middleton, W. R. J., Carter, E. A., Drummey, G. D., and Isselbacher, K. J.,** Effect of oral ethanol administration on intestinal cholesterogenesis in the rat, *Gastroenterology,* 60, 880, 1971.

140. **Lieber, C. S., Spritz, N., and DeCarli, L. M.,** Role of dietary, adipose, and endogenously synthesized fatty acids in the pathogenesis of the alcoholic fatty liver, *J. Clin. Invest.,* 45, 51, 1966.

141. **Baraona, E. and Lieber, C. S.,** Effects of chronic ethanol feeding on serum lipoprotein metabolism in the rat, *J. Clin. Invest.,* 49, 769, 1970.

142. **Rodrigo, C., Antezana, C., and Baraona, E.,** Fat and nitrogen balances in rats with alcohol-induced fatty liver, *J. Nutr.,* 101, 1307, 1971.

143. **Boquillon, M.,** Effect of acute ethanol ingestion on fat absorption, *Lipids,* 11, 848, 1976.

144. **Thomson, A. B. R., Man, S. F. P., and Shnitka, T.,** Effect of ethanol on intestinal uptake of fatty acids, fatty alcohols, and cholesterol, *Dig. Dis. Sci.,* 29, 631, 1984.

145. **Thomson, A. B. R.,** Effect of chronic ingestion of ethanol on *in vitro* uptake of lipids and glucose in the rabbit jejunum, *Am. J. Physiol.,* 246, G120, 1984.

146. **Thomson, A. B. R., Keelan, M., and Clandinin, M. T.,** Feeding rats a diet enriched with saturated fatty acids prevents the inhibitory effects of acute and chronic ethanol exposure on the *in vitro* uptake of hexoses and lipids, *Biochim. Biophys. Acta,* 1084, 122, 1991.

147. **Mistilis, S. P. and Ockner, R. K.,** Alcohol-induced fatty liver: importance of endogenous intestinal lipoproteins, *J. Clin. Invest.,* 49, 66a, 1970.

148. **Baraona, E. and Lieber, C. S.,** Intestinal lymph formation and fat absorption: stimulation by acute ethanol administration and inhibition by chronic ethanol feeding, *Gastroenterology,* 68, 495, 1975.

149. **Baraona, E., Pirola, R. C., and Lieber, C. S.,** Pathogenesis of postprandial hyperlipemia in rats fed ethanol-containing diets, *J. Clin. Invest.,* 52, 296, 1973.

150. **Mendenhall, C. L., Greenberger, P. A., Greenberger, J. C., and Julian, D. J.,** Dietary lipid assimilation after acute ethanol ingestion in the rat, *Am. J. Physiol.,* 227, 377, 1974.

151. **Saunders, D. R., Sillery, J., and McDonald, G. B.,** Effect of ethanol on transport from rat intestine during high and low rates of oleate absorption, *Lipids,* 17, 356, 1982.

152. **Hayashi, H., Nakata, K., Motohashi, Y., and Takano, T.,** Acute inhibition of lipid transport in rat intestinal lymph by ethanol administration, *Alcohol Alcohol.,* 27, 627, 1992.

153. **Lieber, C. S.,** Metabolic derangement induced by alcohol, *Annu. Rev. Med.,* 18, 35, 1967.

154. **Castelli, W. P., Doyle, J. T., Gordon, T., Hames, C. G., Hjortland , W. C., Halley, S. B., Kagan, A., and Zukel, W. J.,** Alcohol and blood lipids, the cooperative lipoprotein phenotyping study, *Lancet,* 2, 153, 1977.

155. **Savolainen, M. J., Hannuksela, M., Seppänen, S., Kervinen, K., and Kesäniemi, Y. A.,** Increased high-density lipoprotein cholesterol concentration in alcoholics is related to low cholestryl ester transfer protein activity, *Eur. J. Clin. Invest.,* 20, 593, 1990.

# 17

# Alcohol's Promotion of Gastrointestinal Carcinogenesis

Siraj I. Mufti

## CONTENTS

## 17.1   INTRODUCTION

Alcohol is a major cancer risk factor. The association is particularly strong with cancers of the upper aerodigestive tract — 75% of esophageal cancers and 50% of oral cavity cancers in the U.S. are attributed to alcohol consumption.[1] The existing evidence further indicates that the degree of cancer risk increases synergistically when alcohol consumption is combined with tobacco use. For example, McCoy and Wynder[2] observed that the relative risk of developing oral and laryngeal cancers in the U.S. among individuals who consumed seven or more ounces of alcohol and more than one pack of cigarettes a day increased 20- to 27-fold compared to nondrinkers and nonsmokers. Recently, Maier and co-workers[3] carried out a case-control study at the University of Heidelberg and Giessen (FRG) and found that the risk of head and neck cancers increased with tobacco and alcohol use in a dose-dependent fashion. In heavy smokers (20 cigarettes per day) adjusted for alcohol use (about 20 g/day), there was a relative risk of 23.4. The subject of upper aerodigestive cancers and alcohol has been reviewed in recent articles by us.[4,5] Epidemiological studies also show an association of chronic alcohol consumption, particularly beer, with cancer of the large bowel. However, the association appears significant for the rectum but far less for the colon (for a review see reference 6).

Despite an abundance of epidemiological evidence associating alcohol ingestion with cancers, however, none of the experimental studies has shown that alcohol (ethanol) by itself is a carcinogen. Thus, in cancer causation, ethanol must act in concert with other environmental carcinogens such as those that are derived from tobacco or nutritional factors that are often deficient in alcoholics (for a review of nutritional factors involved see Reference 7). Such an effect could be exerted at the preinitiation, initiation, or postinitiation promotion and progression stages of carcinogenesis. Preinitiation and initiation effects by their very nature would be limited in duration while promotion/progression effects would occupy a longer duration of the carcinogenic process and are of significance because of their amenability to intervention and other remedial measures. This chapter discusses the effects of ethanol and their underlying mechanisms with a special focus on ethanol promotion/progression effects in the light of our recent findings.

## 17.2    ETHANOL'S EFFECT ON PREINITIATION AND INITIATION STAGES

Ethanol may influence the preinitiation stage because it is an effective inducer of the cytochrome P-450 microsomal enzymes[8] that are involved in converting procarcinogens into their DNA reactive electrophilic intermediates[9] that are mutagenic.[10] The treatment of animals with microsomal enzyme inducers such as phenobarbital, chrysene,[11] or ethanol[12] causes increased metabolism of azoxymethane (AOM), the colorectal carcinogen. That pretreatment with ethanol would increase tumor incidence was shown by Seitz et al.,[13] who pair fed Sprague-Dawley rats a Lieber-DeCarli ethanolic diet for 4 weeks before treating them with the rectal carcinogen 1,2-dimethylhydrazine dihydrochloride (DMH). At the time of DMH treatment the Lieber-DeCarli diet was replaced by a standard laboratory chow diet. The results of necropsy after 32 weeks showed a significant increase of rectal tumors in ethanol-fed rats. However, since the feeding regimen was repeated postinitiation, the positive results may at least partially be due to ethanol-induced promotion also.

On the other hand, if ethanol is administered at the same time as the procarcinogen, it inhibits carcinogenesis. Such an inhibition was apparent when we treated Sprague-Dawley rats with N-nitrosomethylbenzylamine (NMBzA) and pair fed them the Lieber-DeCarli ethanolic diet before and during treatment with NMBzA.[14] The results showed that the frequency of total esophageal lesions as well as tumors was significantly decreased with this ethanol administration. Hamilton et al.[15] pair fed Fischer-344 rats beer and ethanol for 3 weeks before treating them with AOM. Necropsy results showed that with ethanol and beer providing 18% and 23% of total caloric intake, the incidence of tumors was significantly reduced in the right colon. The suppression of colonic carcinogenesis with 22% and 33% of ethanol given before and during different doses of AOM administered was confirmed in other studies by Hamilton and co-workers.[16,17] Inhibition occurs because given together ethanol competes in the same detoxification pathway with the procarcinogen for its metabolism thus decreasing the availability of reactive carcinogenic metabolites. Thus ethanol is found to be a competitive inhibitor of the demethylase enzyme that is involved in the breakdown of nitrosamines.[18,19] The more lipophilic compounds such as NMBzA are inhibited weakly compared to compounds that have low lipophilicity such as N-nitrosodimethylamine. There may be a similar inhibition of the microsomal cytochrome P-450-dependent N-hydroxylase that catalyses conversion of AOM to methylazoxymethanol in the liver[11] and the colon.[20-22] Hamilton et al.[15-17] found that exhalation of $^{14}CO_2$ was decreased in ethanol-fed rats, supporting the notion that a suppression of AOM metabolism occurred and a change from ethanol to nonethanol diet 12 h prior to AOM injection increased the rate of metabolism, indicating loss of this suppression. Furthermore, with coadministration of ethanol and AOM there was also a reduction of $O^6$-methylguanine and $N^7$-methylguanine 24 h after AOM injection. Similarly, agents which inhibit DMH metabolism are found to inhibit the related colorectal carcinogenesis.[23]

Yet ethanol also interferes with first-pass clearance of carcinogens and is known to alter their tissue specificity[24] such that with coadministration while tumors may be inhibited at one place they may appear spontaneously at other susceptible sites. Furthermore, with chronic consumption, when ethanol is withdrawn, an increased activation of procarcinogens may still occur as shown for AOM by Sohn et al.[12]

## 17.3    ETHANOL'S EFFECTS ON POSTINITIATION PROMOTION/
## PROGRESSION STAGES

For studies of the ethanol effect on carcinogenesis in the esophagus, the tissue at most risk in alcoholics,[1] we selected NMBzA, a potent esophagus-specific carcinogen that occurs naturally in areas of high incidence for esophageal neoplasia in China.[25] To delineate the promotion from initiation effects a low dose of this complete carcinogen was used such that a high proportion (about 70%) of experimental animals would be exposed to only a subcarcinogenic dose of the carcinogen thus providing a background on which the promoting potential of ethanol could be studied. This experimental strategy is essentially a modification of the technique used by Slaga et al.,[26] who could use a 100% subcarcinogenic dose of a complete carcinogen because they used a stronger promoter, tetradecanoylphorbolacetate (TPA) compared to ethanol (we could thus also save on an otherwise larger population of test animals). Our preliminary studies determined that 2.5 mg/kg of NMBzA given 3 times a week for 3 weeks would induce esophageal tumors in about 30% of male Sprague-Dawley rats. The results from animals necropsied at 18 months showed that when ethanol was administered as a tumor promoter there was a remarkable sixfold increase in the incidence of esophageal tumors.[14] Subsequently, these promotional effects of ethanol on NMBzA-induced esophageal carcinogenesis were verified in C57Bl/6 female mice showing a significant increase in both the frequency and size of esophageal tumors.[27]

In the rat study described above, it was observed that although the total number of NMBzA-induced esophageal lesions (focal areas + nodules + tumors) was not substantially different in ethanol vs. control-fed rats, yet an extensive dysplastic proliferation of these lesions increased development of tumors with ethanol consumption, suggesting that ethanol played a significant role in promotion to progression stages.[14] A careful following examination of the lesions showed that with ethanol more of the cells infiltrated into the inner epithelial wall of the esophagus and exhibited focal areas of polymorphonuclear cell hemorrhage in the subcutaneous tissue.[28] These observations suggest that ethanol causes promotion by allowing extensive proliferation and malignant development of the chemically induced esophageal lesions.

In other studies, 1% 7,12-dimethylbenzanthracene (DMBA) was used to paint right buccal pouch mucosa of Syrian golden hamsters, three times for one week. At necropsy, the incidence of oral epidermoid carcinomas, their multiplicity and size was found to significantly increase with ethanol consumption.[29] Ethanol promotion was observed to cause an increase in incidence and size of tumors induced in the oral cavity and esophagus (also lungs and liver) of male Fischer-344 rats treated with N-nitrosonornicotine (NNN) and N-nitrosaminomethylpyridylbutanone (NNK), the two potent carcinogens derived from tobacco.[30] Thus using different oral and esophageal carcinogens our studies confirm the results of a number of other investigations recently reviewed by us[31] indicating that ethanol acts as a tumor promoter.

The results of ethanol effect on promotion of colorectal carcinogenesis are less clear, however. Hamilton et al.[16] found that chronic ethanol consumption after AOM administration had no effect on tumor outcome regardless of the quantity of ethanol consumed. However, positive results were obtained by Seitz et al.[13] with DMH-induced rectal carcinogenesis, which, as discussed above, may at least partially be ascribed to ethanol-induced promotion. Further studies are needed to clarify these contradictory observations.

## 17.4  ETHANOL-INDUCED LIPID PEROXIDATION AND TUMOR PROMOTION

Ethanol generates free radicals when it or its metabolites are oxidatively metabolized. The author recently reviewed different mechanisms of ethanol oxidation which could generate oxygen-free radicals.[32] Of these mechanisms the ethanol induction of the endoplasmic reticulum (ER)-associated microsomal ethanol oxidizing system (MEOS) is of particular significance. The MEOS is a NADPH-dependent system which is linked to the cytochrome P-450 mono-oxygenases[33,34] and an ethanol-inducible form of the cytochrome P-450 called the cytochrome P-450 2E1 or CYP2E1 plays a significant role in generating reactive oxygen species (ROS). Microsomes isolated from ethanol-fed rats reduce dioxygen to oxygen-derived radicals and $H_2O_2$.[35,36] Since most ROS have half-lives of $10^{-9}$ to $10^{-5}$ s and are difficult to measure, the stable products formed by their reactions with lipids are often measured. In initial studies the author confirmed that ethanol metabolism induces lipid peroxidation measured by such indices as ethane exhaled by ethanol-fed animals and by the hepatic production of malondialdehyde, diene conjugates, and lipid fluorescence.[37,38] This observation of increased lipid peroxidation was confirmed by administration of vitamin E, a potent antioxidant, which caused an inhibition of ethanol-induced lipid peroxidation.[38,39] On the other hand, administration of polyunsaturated fatty acids (PUFA) (e.g., fish oil) caused a further increase in lipid peroxidation and this enhancement was also inhibited by vitamin E administration.[40]

The following observations support that lipid peroxidation or generation of oxygen-free radicals plays a role in tumor promotion: (1) peroxidant-promoters are structurally unrelated compounds that cause lipid peroxidation; (2) many antioxidants that suppress lipid peroxidation are also antipromoters; (3) stable endoperoxide analogs of prostaglandins promote transformation of mouse skin cells; (4) promotion of mouse epidermal cells *in vitro* is accompanied by oxidation; and (5) lipid hydroperoxides and their degradation products act as clastogenic factors (probably modulating expression of genes involved in tumor promotion and progression by gene rearrangement).[41,42]

When rodents treated with NMBzA, NNN, or NNK were examined for indices of lipid peroxidation, i.e., ethane exhalation and hepatic malondialdehyde, diene conjugates and lipid fluorescence, an increase was found to occur with ethanol consumption in intact animals as well as in the liver, which is the main site for carcinogen metabolism and generation of lipid peroxides.[27,30,43] In addition, lipid peroxidation indices were determined in the target tissues, i.e., the esophagus of the NMBzA-treated rats, the buccal mucosa of the DMBA-treated hamsters, and the oral cavity and esophagus (as well as the lungs and liver) of the NNN or NNK-treated rats. The results indicated that, overall, there was significant increase in lipid peroxidation products in the target tissues also, and the largest increases were seen when carcinogen and ethanol consumption were combined.[30,44] Thus, ethanol-induced promotion of carcinogen-induced lesions was associated with increased lipid peroxidation. Furthermore, supplemental feeding of the antioxidant vitamin E to NMBzA-treated and ethanol-fed mice inhibited tumor incidence along with an inhibition of lipid peroxidation.[27] Positive as well as negative evidence for the association of ethanol-related lipid peroxidation with ethanol-induced tumor promotion was obtained by using the two hepatocarcinogens: N-nitrosodiethylamine (NDEA) and aflatoxin $B_1$ ($AFB_1$). Whereas both hepatic tumors[45] and lipid peroxidation[46,47] are increased with ethanol consumption in $AFB_1$-induced hepatocarcinogenesis, there was an absence of such increase in hepatic enzyme-altered foci or tumors[48-51] as well as in lipid peroxidation with ethanol metabolism in NDEA-induced hepatocarcinogenesis.[50,51] The absence of increase with the NDEA protocol could be explained by the observations of Garcea et al.[52] which indicate that the NDEA treatment causes functional alterations in the ER and on the basis of our results suggesting that ethanol could not induce the ER-associated MEOS under these conditions.[50]

An increase in lipid peroxidation with tumor promotion occurring with ethanol metabolism may be followed by a subsequent decline when tumors appear as shown by us in DMBA-induced oral carcinogenesis in hamsters.[29] At 22 weeks of the start of study an increase was observed in all the indices of lipid peroxidation measured in buccal mucosa but at 35 weeks these indices had either returned to intermediate levels or were no different than the untreated controls of 22 weeks. The cellular phospholipids provide the major substrate for lipid peroxidation and with an increase in lipid peroxidation, the proportion of cholesterol to phospholipids in buccal mucosa was found to be significantly increased at 22 weeks. An increase in cholesterol is associated with loss of membrane fluidity as suggested by Dianzani[53] and this may account at least partially for the subsequent decline in lipid peroxidation. Along with altered proportion of phospholipids vs. cholesterol, increased levels of vitamin E in buccal mucosa were also observed at 22 weeks, possibly due to increased mobilization from hepatic stores by ethanol, and an increase in this vitamin may also cause a decline in lipid peroxidation. Patel and Edwards[54] observed that an increase in vitamin E was associated with decreased membrane fluidity, and Dianzani[53] and

Cheeseman and co-workers[55] suggested that increase in vitamin E may also be responsible for decreased lipid peroxidation observed in hepatic tumor cells. A low rate of lipid peroxidation in hepatic tumors was first demonstrated by Thiele and Huff[56] and may present an adaptive response of such cells to reduce damage due to oxidative stress.

Mizui and Doteuchi[57] observed that when absolute ethanol was administered orally to rats it resulted in increased lipid peroxide levels and decreased nonprotein sulfhydryl levels in the gastric mucosa. Mizui et al.[58] and Zselenyi and Brune[59] also found that antiperoxidative drugs reduced the severity of alcohol-induced gastric mucosal injury. That ROS were involved was confirmed in cultured mucosal cells since exposure to ethanol led to increased generation of superoxide anions and to the extent of cell damage, in a dose-dependent manner, while pretreatment with desferrioxamine decreased the injury.[60] The association of ROS or lipid peroxidation with gastric or lower alimentary tract carcinogenesis has yet to be studied, however.

## 17.5 CHANGES IN FATTY ACID PROFILE WITH ALCOHOL-INDUCED PROMOTION

The fatty acid profile of phospholipids (PL) and cholesterol esters (CE) isolated from the buccal mucosa of hamsters treated with DMBA and fed ethanol or isocaloric control diet was determined in our experiments. DMBA treatment combined with ethanol consumption caused the most significant alterations, and the fatty acids that were altered most were: oleate, palmitate, linoleate, and arachidonate. The mechanism for the changes appears to be related to the increased formation of ROS during ethanol metabolism. Since ROS are primarily generated in the ER where enzymes that alter fatty acid structures (i.e., elongases, desaturases, esterifying enzymes for glycerophosphate and CE) reside, the data suggest that ROS are reacting with these enzymes, significantly decreasing their activities and causing changes in the fatty acid profiles of both the PL and CE of oral mucosa.[61]

The hepatic and esophageal PL fatty acid analysis carried out on NMBzA-treated rats that were fed ethanol for 10 months provided further elucidation of the changes brought about with ethanol-induced promotion. While the overall saturated vs. unsaturated PL fatty acid profile was not substantially altered in the liver with regard to their peroxidizability, it was significantly altered toward increased polyunsaturated fatty acids (PUFA) in the esophageal PLs with ethanol metabolism.[44] ROS react readily with PUFA of cell membranes producing conjugated dienes and trienes and cleaving PUFA-hydrocarbon chains to produce aldehydes (nonal, nonenal, malondialdehyde, etc.). Since increased ROS generation is associated with ethanol metabolism, decreased PUFA are expected in tissues undergoing ethanol metabolism but this was not observed in this study. The increase in esophageal PUFA with ethanol metabolism may be due to increased cellularity with chronic ethanol consumption[62] or clonal expansion of the carcinogen-induced lesions. Other factors involved may be decreased activity of ROS due to increased vitamin E observed in the esophagus or increased uptake from plasma lipoproteins to meet esophageal tumorigenic requirements.

Since tumor promotion by ethanol occurs only with prior treatment with a carcinogen, of interest were the alterations that took place when ethanol use was observed in combination with NMBzA treatment. Thus, increased PUFA in esophageal PL suggest that such cell membranes are more fluid than normal esophageal cells. Furthermore, while hepatic PL showed a substantial increase in linolenate (C18:3) but no change in arachidonate (C20:4), there was a pronounced increase in the levels of C18:3, C20:2, C20:3, C20:3′, and C22:6 along with a significant increase in arachidonate in esophageal PL when ethanol consumption was combined with NMBzA treatment.[44] Docosahexanoic acid (C22:6) is derived from linolenate while C20:3 is derived from linoleate (C18:2). Linoleic and linolenic acids constitute two classes of PUFA which are essential fatty acids required by humans and other mammals. These parent essential fatty acids undergo chain elongation and desaturation to produce long chain derivatives with 3 to 6 double bonds. The conversion of linoleate to arachidonate is a necessary step in lipid metabolism involved in a variety of physiological processes and this enables synthesis of eicosanoids that are required for cell proliferation. The process of eicosanoid production in normal cells is well regulated but gets exaggerated in neoplasia,[63] and an eicosanoid metabolic disorder has been reported in several malignancies, including mammary and colon cancers[63,64] and alcoholic liver disease.[65]

Based on the above observations, the following hypothesis was proposed for tumor promotion effects of ethanol: that ethanol metabolism during tumor promotion causes excessive cell proliferation by a disorder in eicosanoid metabolism and this could induce selective outgrowth and clonal expansion of the carcinogen-initiated cells. This model is supported by the observation that chronic ethanol consumption leads to hyperregeneration[62] and that excessive cell proliferation is conducive to exacerbate genetic errors in carcinogenesis.[66]

## 17.6 SUPPORTING EVIDENCE FOR ETHANOL-INDUCED HYPERREGENERATION

It appears that although the biliary bile acid output is increased,[67] the fecal bile acid excretion and pattern do not change with ethanol consumption.[13,68] Thus ethanol may not be involved in affecting bile acids that are generally considered as promoters of colorectal carcinogenesis.[69]

However, the existing evidence supports the hypothesis that hyperregeneration of colorectal mucosa may be involved in alcohol-induced promotion. An important feature of the chemical carcinogens that induce colorectal tumors is their capacity to increase cellular regeneration in colorectal mucosa.[70] Simanowski et al.[71] used the metaphase arrest technique utilizing vincristine and measured cell proliferation by the rate of crypt cell production after 4 weeks of feeding rats either the isocaloric ethanol or carbohydrate control diet. Cell proliferation selectively increased in the rectal mucosa of ethanol-fed rats with a concomitant increase in the size of the proliferative compartment. A concomitant increase in the proliferative compartment of the crypt toward the intestinal lumen could be used as a biomarker in the identification of high-risk groups for colorectal cancer.[72]

Polyamines appear to play an important role in cell proliferation and ornithine decarboxylase (ODC) is the first and rate-limiting enzyme involved in their biosynthesis. An increase in colonic mucosal ODC activity occurs in colonic carcinogenesis and in AOM-treated rats. Hamilton and Luk[73] observed a significant increase in ODC activity in colonic mucosa of rats after 3 weeks of chronic ethanol consumption. Other gastrointestinal hormones may be involved in the process of hyperregeneration. In a study done by Simanowski et al.,[74] it was found that while there was no significant change in the levels of gastric and peptide YY, pancreatic glucagon and enteroglucagon were significantly elevated both after acute and chronic ethanol feeding in rats.

Growth factors play a critical role in cell growth and invasion and a number of growth factors are reported to be synthesized or overexpressed in cancerous cells. Two of the most studied are the epidermal growth factor (EGF) and the transforming growth factor-$\alpha$ (TGF-$\alpha$) that exhibits structural homology to EGF. Both polypeptides share a common membrane receptor.[75] Of interest is the recent report of Tarnawski et al.[76] that adaptation of gastric mucosa to chronic ethanol consumption was associated with increased cell proliferation along with increased expression of mucosal EGF, TGF-$\alpha$, and their common receptors. Similarly, the role of protein kinases and the secondary messengers such as cAMP that are involved in regulating a diverse variety of cell functions needs to be elucidated in ethanol-induced tumor promotion. Protein kinase C (PKC) is actively involved in cell proliferation and differentiation through phosphorylation. Phorbol ester tumor promoters and related compounds bind to and activate PKC while inhibitors of PKC act as antipromoters (for a review see reference 77). Of interest is the association of altered intracellular cAMP turnover with alcoholism in humans. Abstinent alcoholics have reduced cAMP accumulation compared with normal subjects.[78] Furthermore, ethanol depresses human platelet cAMP levels, which is overcome by an inhibitor of PKC, suggesting that ethanol may be acting through activation of PKC.[79]

In this regard, the role of oncogenes in ethanol-induced tumor promotion also needs to be studied. Normal products of these genes are such essential cell constituents as kinases, growth factor receptors, guanyl-nucleotide-binding proteins, and nuclear proteins; all these products conferring selective growth advantage on cells committed to transformation. Of interest are the recent findings by Wilson and co-workers[80] showing that even a single acute dose of ethanol caused transient rapid induction of several oncogenes including myc and fos. A similar early rapid and transient expression of c-*fos* and c-*myc* genes occurs after TPA application.[81] Immediate early or competence genes such as c-*fos* and c-*myc* play a role in cell growth and differentiation and an overexpression of these genes is presumably related to hyperplasia and an inflammatory response.[82] JB6 mouse epidermal cells that were treated with either xanthine/xanthine oxidase or TPA caused an induction of c-*fos*.[83] Recently, Amstad et al.[84] showed that active oxygen was required for a transcriptional induction of c-*fos*. While the c-*fos* is found to increase during differentiation, the c-*myc* is switched off.[85] High levels of c-*myc* are associated with progression of malignancy and, therefore, as such are an aberrant expression. An overexpression could possibly occur during chronic inflammation and ROS generated under such conditions would provide a stimulus to chromosomal translocation that is associated with c-*myc* function, resulting in its constitutive expression. Thus, ROS may be involved in early stages of tumor promotion as well as in progression and metastasis. Therefore, the role that the differential induction of such genes plays in carcinogen-initiated promotion by ethanol needs to be understood.

## 17.7  CONCLUSIONS

Although alcohol could influence the preinitiation and initiation stages of the carcinogenic process, its effect on the longer duration promotion and progression stages are of greater significance since they could be subjected to intervention and other possible remedies. Our studies using animals as models of oral and esophageal carcinogenesis support the hypothesis that alcohol (ethanol) acts as a tumor promoter. The author and his co-workers have also obtained positive as well as negative *in vivo* evidence relating ethanol's ability to cause lipid peroxidation with its tumor promoting potential. This offers the possibility that the tumor promoting effects of ethanol could be combatted by using antioxidants such as vitamin E. The author's studies also suggest that ethanol promotion is caused by disordered lipid and eicosanoid metabolism which could induce selective outgrowth and clonal expansion of the carcinogen-initiated lesions. Initial data obtained by others on the colorectal carcinogenesis supports this model. Future studies would strengthen this assumption as well as elucidate the role played by antipromoters in inhibiting or reversing the damage induced by promoters.

## 17.8  ACKNOWLEDGMENTS

The research described in this article that was carried out in the author's laboratory was supported by a grant (No. CA51088) by the U.S. National Institutes of Health. The author wishes to thank Char Prytula for her diligent assistance in the preparation of the manuscript for this paper.

## REFERENCES

1.  **Rothman, K., Garfinkel, L., Keller, A. Z., et al.,** The proportion of cancer attributable to alcohol consumption, *Rev. Med.,* 9, 174, 1980.

2.  **McCoy, G. D. and Wynder, E. L.,** Etiological and preventive implications in alcohol carcinogenesis, *Cancer Res.,* 39, 2844, 1979.

3.  **Maier, H., Dietz, A., Gewelke, U., et al.,** Tobacco and alcohol and the risk of head and neck cancer, *Clin. Invest.,* 70, 320, 1992.

4.  **Mufti, S. I., Garewal, H. S., and Watson, R. R.,** Role of environment, drugs of abuse and nutritional factors in the etiology and prevention of cancers of oral cavity and esophagus, in *Biochemistry and Physiology of Substance Abuse,* Vol. II, Watson, R. R., Ed., CRC Press, Boca Raton, FL, 1990, 1.

5. **Mufti, S. I.,** Alcohol and cancers of the esophagus and liver, in *Alcohol, Immunity and Cancer*, Yirmiya, R. and Taylor, A. N., Eds., CRC Press, Boca Raton, FL, 1993, 159.

6. **Seitz, H. K. and Simanowski, U. A.,** Ethanol and colorectal cancer, in *Alcohol, Immunity and Cancer*, Yirmiya, R. and Taylor, A. N., Eds., CRC Press, Boca Raton, FL, 1993, 211.

7. **Mufti, S. I.,** Prevention of alcohol-induced disease and cancer by nutrition, in *Nutrition and Cancer Prevention*, Watson, R. R. and Mufti, S. I., Eds., CRC Press, Boca Raton, FL, in press, 1995.

8. **Rubin, E. and Lieber, C. S.,** Hepatic microsomal enzymes in men and rat: induction and inhibition by ethanol, *Science*, 162, 690, 1968.

9. **Miller, J. A. and Miller, E. C.,** Ultimate chemical carcinogens as reactive mutagenic electrophiles, in *Origins of Human Cancer*, Hiat, H. H., Watson, J. P., and Winsten, J. A., Eds., Cold Spring Harbor Laboratory, NY, 1977, 607.

10. **Garro, A. J., Seitz, H. K., and Lieber, C. S.,** Enhancement of dimethylnitrosamine metabolism and activation to a mutagen following chronic ethanol consumption, *Cancer Res.*, 41, 120, 1981.

11. **Fiala, E. S.,** Investigations into the metabolism and mode of action of the colon carcinogen 1,2DMH and azoxymethane, *Cancer*, 40, 4236, 1977.

12. **Sohn, O. A., Fiala, E. S., Puz, C., et al.,** Enhancement of rat liver microsomal metabolism of azoxymethane to methylazoxymethanol by chronic ethanol administration: similarity to the microsomal metabolism of N-nitrosomethylamine, *Cancer Res.*, 47, 3123, 1987.

13. **Seitz, H. K., Czygan, P., Waldherr, R., et al.,** Enhancement of 1,2-dimethylhydrazine induced rectal carcinogenesis following chronic ethanol consumption in the rat, *Gastroenterology*, 86, 886, 1984.

14. **Mufti, S. I., Becker, G., and Sipes, I. G.,** Effect of chronic dietary ethanol consumption in the initiation and promotion chemically-induced esophageal carcinogenesis in experimental rats, *Carcinogenesis*, 10, 303, 1989.

15. **Hamilton, S. R., Hyland, J., McAvinchey, D., et al.,** Effects of chronic dietary beer and ethanol consumption on experimental colonic carcinogenesis by azoxymethane in rats, *Cancer Res.*, 47, 1551, 1987.

16. **Hamilton, S. R., Sohn, O. S., and Fiala, E. S.,** Effects of timing and quantity of chronic dietary ethanol consumption on azoxymethane-induced colonic carcinogenesis and azoxymethane metabolism in Fischer-344 rats, *Cancer Res.*, 47, 4305, 1987.

17. **Hamilton, S. R., Sohn, O. S., and Fiala, E. S.,** Inhibition by dietary ethanol of experimental colonic carcinogenesis induced by high-dose azoxymethane in F-344 rats, *Cancer Res.*, 48, 3313, 1988.

18. **Phillips, J. C., Lake, B. G., Gangolli, S. D., et al.,** Effect of pyrazole and 3-amino-1,2,4-triazole on the metabolism and toxicity of dimethylnitrosamine in the rat, *J. Natl. Cancer Instit.*, 58, 629, 1977.

19. **Miller, K. W. and Yang, C. S.,** Studies of induction of N-nitrosodimethylamine demethylase by fasting, acetone and ethanol, *Arch. Biochem. Biophys.*, 229, 483, 1984.

20. **Wargovich, M. J. and Felkner, I. C.,** Metabolic activation of DMH by colonic microsomes: a process influenced by dietary fat, *Nutr. Cancer*, 4, 146, 1982.

21. **Glauert, H. P. and Bennink, M. R.,** Metabolism of 1,2-dimethylhydrazine by cultured rat colon epithelial cells, *Nutr. Cancer*, 5, 78, 1983.

22. **Oravec, C. T., Jones, C. A., and Huberman, E.,** Activation of the colon carcinogen DMH in a rat colon cell-mediated mutagenesis assay, *Cancer Res.*, 46, 5068, 1986.

23. **Wattenberg, L. W.,** Inhibition of dimethylhydrazine-induced neoplasia of the large intestine by disulfiram, *J. Natl. Cancer Instit.*, 54, 1005, 1975.

24. **Swann, P. F.,** Effect of ethanol on nitrosamine metabolism and distribution. Implications for the role of nitrosamines in human cancer and for the influence of alcohol consumption on cancer incidence, in *N-nitroso-compounds: Occurrence, Biological Effects and Relevance to Human Cancer*, O'Neill, K., Von Borstel, R. C., Miller, C. T., et al., Eds., IARC Scientific Pub. No. 57, Lyon, 1984, 501.

25. **Yang, C. S.,** Research on esophageal cancer in China: a review, *Cancer Res.*, 40, 2633, 1980.

26. **Slaga, T. J., O'Connell, J., Rotstein, J., et al.,** Critical genetic determinants and molecular events in multistage skin carcinogenesis, in *Critical Molecular Determinants of Carcinogenesis*, Becker, F. F., Slaga, T. J., Eds., University of Texas Press, Austin, 1987, 31.

27. **Odeleye, O. E., Eskelson, C. D., Mufti, S. I., and Watson, R. R.,** Vitamin E inhibition of lipid peroxidation and ethanol mediated promotion of esophageal tumorigenesis, *Nutr. Cancer*, 17, 223, 1992.

28. **Mufti, S. I.,** Effect of long-term ethanol consumption on malignant development of methylbenzylnitrosamine-induced esophageal lesions, *Alcoholism: Clin. Exp. Res.*, 15, 349, 1991.

29. **Nachiappan, V., Mufti, S. I., and Eskelson, C. D.,** Ethanol-medicated promotion of oral carcinogenesis in hamsters: association with lipid peroxidation, *Nutr. Cancer*, 20, 293, 1993.

30. **Nachiappan, V., Mufti, S. I., Chakravarti, A., Eskelson, C. D., and Rajasekharan, R.,** Lipid peroxidation and ethanol related tumor promotion in Fischer-344 rats treated with tobacco-specific nitrosamines, *Alcohol Alcohol.*, 29, 565, 1994.

31. **Mufti, S. I., Darban, H., and Watson, R. R.,** Ethanol, cancer and immunomodulation, *Crit. Rev. Oncol. Hematol.*, 9, 234, 1989.

32. **Mufti, S. I., Eskelson, C. D., Odeleye, O. E., and Nachiappan, V.,** Alcohol-associated generation of oxygen-free radicals and tumor promotion, *Alcohol Alcohol.*, 28, 621, 1993.

33. **Koop, D. R., Morgan, E. T., Tarr, G. E., and Coon, M. J.,** Purification and characterization of a unique isozyme of cytochrome P-450 from liver microsomes of ethanol-treated rabbits, *J. Biol. Chem.*, 257, 8472, 1982.

34. **Koop, D. R. and Coon, M. J.,** Role of P-450 oxygenase (APO) in microsomal ethanol oxidation, *Alcohol*, 2, 23, 1985.

35. **Ingelman-Sundberg, M. and Johansson, I.,** Mechanisms of hydroxyl radical formation and ethanol oxidation by ethanol-inducible and other forms of rabbit liver microsomal cytochrome P-450, *J. Biol. Chem.*, 259, 6447, 1984.

36. **Gorsky, L. D., Koop, D. R., and Coon, M. J.,** On the stoichemistry of the oxidase and monooxygenase reaction catalyzed by liver microsomal cytochrome P450, *J. Biol. Chem.*, 259, 6812, 1984.

37. **Szebeni, J., Eskelson, C. D., Mufti, S., Watson, R. R., and Sipes, I. G.,** Inhibition of ethanol induced ethane exhalation by carcinogenic pretreatment of rats 12 months earlier, *Life Sci.*, 39, 2587, 1986.

38. **Odeleye, O. E., Eskelson, C. D., Watson, R. R., Mufti, S. I., et al.,** Effect of ethanol consumption and vitamin E supplementation on *in vivo* lipid peroxidation in rats, *Nutr. Res.*, 11, 1177, 1991.

39. **Mufti, S. I. and Eskelson, C. D.,** Alcohol-related cancers may be inhibited by dietary vitamin E, *Ann. N.Y. Acad. Sci.*, 625, 824, 1991.

40. **Odeleye, O. E., Eskelson, C. D., Watson, R. R., Mufti, S. I., et al.,** Vitamin E reduction of lipid peroxidation products in rats fed cod liver oil and ethanol, *Alcohol*, 8, 273, 1991.

41. **Cerutti, P. A.,** Prooxidant states and tumor promotion, *Science*, 227, 375, 1985.

42. **Fisher, S. M., Floyd, R. A., and Copeland, E. S.,** Oxygen radicals in carcinogenesis, *Cancer Res.*, 48, 3882, 1988.

43. **Mufti, S. I.,** Free radicals generated in ethanol metabolism may be responsible for tumor promoting effects of ethanol, *Adv. Exp. Med. Biol.*, 283, 777, 1991.

44. **Mufti, S. I., Nachiappan, V., and Eskelson, C. D.,** Ethanol-mediated promotion of esophageal carcinogenesis: association with lipid peroxidation and changes in phospholipid fatty acid profile of the target tissue, submitted, 1995.

45. **Tanaka, T., Nishikawa, A., Iwata, H., et al.,** Enhancing effect of ethanol on aflatoxin $B_1$-induced hepatocarcinogenesis in male AC1/N rats, *Jpn. J. Cancer Res.*, 80, 526, 1989.

46. **Toskulkao, C. and Glinsukon, T.,** Hepatic lipid peroxidation and intracellular calcium accumulation in ethanol potentiated aflatoxin $B_1$ toxicity, *J. Pharmacobiodyn.*, 11, 191, 1988.

47. **Nachiappan, V. and Mufti, S. I.,** Ethanol related tumor promotion is positively correlated with lipid peroxidation in aflatoxin-induced hepatocarcinogenesis, *Proc. Am. Assoc. Cancer Res.*, 34, 181, 1993.

48. **Schmahl, D., Thomas, C., Sattler, W., and Scheld, G. F.,** Experimental studies of syncarcinogenesis: III. Attempts to induce cancer in rats by administering di-ethylnitrosamine and $CCl_4$ (or ethyl alcohol) simultaneously. In addition, an experimental contribution regarding "alcoholic cirrhosis", *Z. Krebsforsch.*, 66, 526, 1965.

49. **Habs, M. and Schmahl, D.,** Inhibition of the hepatocarcinogenic activity of diethylnitrosamine (DENA) by ethanol in rats, *Hepatogastroenterology*, 28, 242, 1981.

50. **Mufti, S. I. and Sipes, I. G.,** A reduction in mixed function oxidases and in tumor promoting effects of ethanol in a NDEA-initiated hepatocarcinogenesis model, *Adv. Exp. Med. Biol.*, 283, 347, 1991.

51. **Mufti, S. I.,** Tumor promoting effects of long term ethanol consumption, *Adv. Biosci.*, 86, 361, 1993.

52. **Garcea, R., Canuto, R. A., Biocca, M. E., et al.,** Functional alterations of the endoplasmic reticulum and the detoxification systems during diethylnitrosamine carcinogenesis in rat liver, *Cell Biochem. Funct.*, 2, 171, 1984.

53. **Dianzani, M. N.,** Lipid peroxidation and cancer: a critical reconsideration, *Tumorigenesis*, 75, 351, 1989.

54. **Patel, J. M. and Edwards, D. A.,** Vitamin E membrane order and antioxidant behavior in lung microsomes and reconstituted lipid vesicles, *Toxic Appl. Pharmacol.*, 96, 101, 1988.

55. **Cheeseman, K. H., Burton, G. W., Ingold, K. V., and Slater, T. F.,** Lipid peroxidation and lipid antioxidants in normal and tumor cells, *Toxicol. Pathol.*, 12, 235, 1984.

56. **Thiele, E. H. and Huff, J. W.,** Lipid peroxide production and inhibition by tumor mitochondria, *Arch. Biochem. Biophys.*, 88, 208, 1960.

57. **Mizui, T. and Doteuchi, M.,** Lipid peroxidation: a possible role in gastric damage induced by ethanol in rats, *Life Sci.*, 38, 2163, 1986.

58. **Mizui, T., Sato, H., Hirose, F., and Doteuchi, M.,** Effect of antiperoxidative drugs on gastric damage induced by ethanol in rats, *Life Sci.*, 41, 755, 1987.

59. **Zselenyi, I. and Brune, K.,** Possible role of oxygen free radicals in ethanol-induced gastric mucosal damage in rats, *Dig. Dis. Sci.*, 33, 865, 1988.

60. **Mutoh, H., Hiraishi, H., Ota, S., et al.,** Role of oxygen radicals in ethanol-induced damage to cultured gastric mucosal cells, *Am. J. Physiol.*, 258, G603, 1990.

61. **Eskelson, C. D., Nachiappan, V., and Mufti, S. I.,** Ethanol-mediated promotion of oral carcinogenesis in hamsters. 2. Changes in fatty acid profile of phospholipids and cholesterol esters, submitted, 1995.

62. **Mak, K. M., Leo, M. A., and Lieber, C. S.,** Effect of ethanol and vitamin A deficiency on epithelial cell proliferation and structure in the rat esophagus, *Gastroenterology*, 93, 362, 1987.

63. **Karmali, R. A.,** Eicosanoids in neoplasia, *Prev. Med.*, 16, 493, 1987.

64. **Fischer, S. M., Conti, C. J., Locniskar, M., et al.,** The effect of dietary fat on the rapid development of mammary tumors induced by 7,12-dimethylbenz(a) anthracene in SENCAR mice, *Cancer Res.,* 52, 662, 1992.

65. **French, S. W.,** Nutrition in the pathogenesis of alcoholic liver disease, *Alcohol Alcohol.,* 28, 97, 1993.

66. **Cohen, S. M. and Ellwein, L. B.,** Genetics errors, cell proliferation, and carcinogenesis, *Cancer Res.,* 51, 6493, 1991.

67. **Sieg, A. and Seitz, H. K.,** Increased production hepatic conjugation, and biliary secretion of bilirubin in the rat following chronic ethanol consumption, *Gastroenterology,* 93, 261, 1987.

68. **Cohen, B. I. and Raicht, R. F.,** Sterol metabolism in the rat: effect of alcohol on sterol metabolism in two strains of rats, *Alcoholism,* 5, 225, 1981.

69. **Cohen, B. I. and Deschner, E. E.,** The role of bile acid in colorectal carcinogenesis, in *Colorectal Cancer,* Seitz, H. K., Simanowski, U. A., and Wright, N. A., Eds., Springer-Verlag, Berlin, 1989, 125.

70. **Simanowski, U. A., Wright, N. A., and Seitz, H. K.,** Increased cellular regeneration in colorectal carcinogenesis, in *Colorectal Cancer,* Seitz, H. K., Simanowski, U. A., and Wright, N. A., Eds., Springer-Verlag, Berlin, 1989, 225.

71. **Simanowski, U. A., Seitz, H. K., Baier, B., et al.,** Chronic ethanol consumption selectivity stimulates rectal cell proliferation in the rat, *Gut,* 27, 278, 1986.

72. **Lipkin, M.,** Biomarkers in the identification of high risk groups, in *Colorectal Cancer,* Seitz, H. K., Simanowski, U. A., and Wright, N. A., Eds., Springer-Verlag, Berlin, 1989, 73.

73. **Hamilton, S. R. and Luk, G. D.,** Induction of colonic mucosal ornithine decarboxylase activity by chronic dietary ethanol consumption in the rat, *Gastroenterology,* 92 (Abstr.), 1423, 1987.

74. **Simanowski, U. A., Hubalek, K., Ghatei, M. A., et al.,** Effects of acute and chronic ethanol administration on the gastrointestinal hormones gastrin, enteroglucagon, pancreatic glucagon and PYY in the rat, *Digestion,* 42, 167, 1989.

75. **Derynck, R.,** Transforming growth factor-$\alpha$: structure and biological activities, *J. Cell Biochem.,* 32, 293, 1986.

76. **Tarnawski, A., Lu, S. Y., Stachura, J., and Sarfeh, I. J.,** Adaptation of gastric mucosa to chronic alcohol administration is associated with increased mucosal expression of growth factors and their receptor, *Scand. J. Gastroenterol.,* Suppl. 193, 59, 1992.

77. **Kikkawa, U., Kishimoto, A., and Niskizuka, Y.,** The protein kinase C family: heterogeneity and its implications, *Annu. Rev. Biochem.,* 58, 31, 1989.

78. **Diamond, I., Wrubel, B., Estrin, W., and Gordon, A.,** Basal and adenosine receptor stimulated levels of cAMP are reduced in lymphocytes from alcoholic patients, *Proc. Natl. Acad. Sci. U.S.A.,* 84, 1413, 1987.

79. **DePetrillo, P. B. and Swift, R. M.,** Ethanol exposure results in a transient decrease in human platelet cAMP levels: evidence for a protein kinase C mediated process, *Alcoholism: Clin. Exp. Res.,* 16, 290, 1992.

80. **Wilson, D. M., Halloran, M., Tentler, J., et al.,** The *in vitro* effect of acute ethanol (ETOH) exposure on proto-oncogene gene expression, Alcohol. Clin. Exp. Res., 15 (Abstr.), 345, 1992.

81. **Rahmsdorf, H. J and Herrlich, P.,** Regulation of gene expression by tumor promoters, *Pharmacol. Ther.,* 48, 157, 1990.

82. **Rose, J. S., Furstenberger, G., Krieg, P., et al.,** Differential effects of phorbol esters on c-*fos* and c-*myc* and ornithine decarboxylase gene expression in mouse skin *in vivo, Carcinogenesis,* 9, 665, 1988.

83. **Crawford, D., Zbinden, I., Amstad, P., and Cerutti, P.,** Oxidant stress induces the proto-oncogenes c-*fos* and c-*myc* in mouse epidermal cells, *Oncogene,* 3, 27, 1988.

84. **Amstad, P. A., Krupitza, G., and Cerutti, P. A.,** Mechanisms of c-*fos* induction by active oxygen, *Cancer Res.,* 52, 3952, 1992.

85. **Dmitrovsky, E., Kuehl, W. M., Hollis, G. R., et al.,** Expression of a transfected human c-*myc* oncogene inhibits differentiation of a mouse erythroleukemia cell line, *Nature,* 322, 748, 1986.

# 18

# Nutritional Implications of Hepatointestinal Disorders

Jeremy Powell-Tuck

## CONTENTS

In this book we have seen that alcohol can cause or be implicated in the pathophysiology of many gastrointestinal diseases. Some of these are listed in Table 18.1 and each is covered in previous chapters. How might we expect such diseases to affect nutrition and metabolism? There is little in the literature to help us answer the question for alcohol-induced gastrointestinal disease specifically so we must first look at the effect of similar conditions not necessarily caused by alcohol. We shall next consider the prevalence of nutrient deficiencies in alcohol abusers, and consider briefly what pathophysiological effects these may have before discussing nutritional treatment.

## 18.1  NUTRITIONAL AND METABOLIC EFFECTS OF SOME GASTROINTESTINAL DISORDERS

Keeping in mind that the gastrointestinal tract plays a major part in determining appetite and satiety, and that gut disorders often give rise to abdominal pain and discomfort, vomiting,

**TABLE 18.1    Principal Gastrointestinal Disease Related to Alcohol Intake**

**Mouth**
Salivary gland secretory abnormalities
**Esophagus**
Esophagitis, esophageal carcinoma
**Stomach**
Gastritis, gastric carcinoma
**Pancreas**
Acute, chronic pancreatitis
**Liver**
Steatosis, hepatitis, cirrhosis, carcinoma
**Small Intestine**
Villous abnormalities, increased permeability, bacterial overgrowth; salt and water handling
**Large Intestine**
Colorectal cancer

diarrhea, social embarrassment, isolation, and depression, it is no revelation to state that such disorders often give rise to reduced food intake. Some of the ways in which alcohol-related intestinal disease can interrelate with nutrition are depicted in Figure 18.1. Not only can alcohol result in micronutrient deficiency by reduced intake or malabsorption, but the deficiency induced may, in turn, cause or increase the risks of intestinal disease. Mood, which is so important for food intake, will be affected not only by alcohol but also by the diseases it causes or enables.

### 18.1.1    Gastritis and Dyspepsia

Alcoholics commonly suffer from gastritis and dyspepsia. Harju[1] studied, with a structured questionnaire and a 7-day diary, the food intake of 54 patients after various gastrointestinal operations and 33 with gastritis, peptic ulcer, or undefined abdominal pain. The patients who had had previous surgery disclosed more food intolerance than the others, but in both groups the problem was frequent (78 vs. 64%). Fatty foods, coffee, and meat, in general, were well tolerated but milk, beans, cabbage, other vegetables, bread, and fried foods were often avoided, though

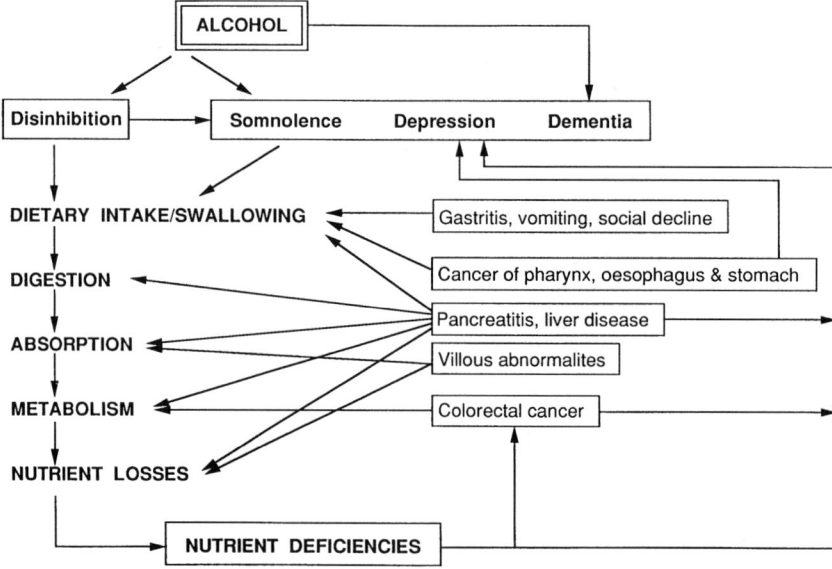

**FIGURE 18.1**    Some ways by which alcohol and its associated gastrointestinal diseases can affect nutrition.

their avoidance did not result in a symptom-free life and may have represented merely common foods in the Finnish diet; the results may well therefore not be as specific to food types as they seem. A study[2] of diet comparing patients with organic (endoscopically demonstrated peptic ulcer disease) and functional dyspepsia with controls has shown how patients with both types of dyspepsia tend to avoid citrus fruits, onions, fatty and spicy foods. Patients with organic dyspepsia tend to drink more milk. This pattern of eating tends to reduce the dietary intake of fiber, iron, vitamin C, and folic acid. In functional dypepsia, females in particular reduce their intake of energy, carbohydrate, fat, percentage protein energy, and vitamin C. Gastric dysmotility may result in diminished food intake. In a recent comparison[3] of the diets of 24 patients with idiopathic gastroparesis (defined as a gastric half-emptying time of more than 111 min using a technetium-labeled egg meal) with age- and sex-matched controls, the intake of energy, vitamins $B_{12}$ and C, folate, thiamine, niacin, magnesium, phosphorus, and zinc were all diminished in patients, although proportions of energy as carbohydrate, fat, and protein were not altered. The rate of gastric emptying was inversely proportional to the intake of protein, potassium, iron, and niacin which argues against this being a problem of underreporting of food intake, but the patients were of normal weight. Total energy intake did not show such inverse relationship and so interpretation of this interesting study remains difficult.

### 18.1.2   Oropharyngeal, Esophageal, and Gastric Malignancy

While reduced intake in malignant diseases of the esophagus and upper stomach may be due primarily to mechanical obstruction to swallowing, the effects of the tumor itself on appetite and the psychological aspects of having cancer may also decrease appetite and food intake. The relative contributions of these factors can best be assessed by a comparison of the effects on intake of benign and malignant stricture, and of esophagogastric malignancy with malignancy elsewhere, for example, the pancreas. Seventeen patients with unresectable carcinoma of the esophagus and cardia were studied[4] before and following endoscopic intubation of the tumor to enable ingestion of a soft diet. At the time of the intubation, they had lost a median (range) of 8 (0 to 28) kg. Mean daily energy intake increased from 802 kcal (0 to 2065) to 1843 (500 to 2617 kcal) 1 month after the procedure with two patients gaining 8.4 and 9.4 kg, respectively, over this period. However five patients failed to gain weight, and after a few months weight loss often recurred more as a result of anorexia than of dysphagia. In a study,[5] however, of 42 patients with gastrointestinal malignancies and 24 with benign disease in comparable sites little difference was found either in weight loss or in food intake between those with benign or malignant disease. Reduction in food intake associated with gastrointestinal disease seemed more significant in women than in men. There was a trend for increased tumor bulk to be associated with reduced food intake.

### 18.1.3   Other Gastrointestinal Malignancies

In addition to oropharyngeal, esophageal and gastric neoplasms, alcohol intake, particularly in the form of beer, is associated with colorectal carcinomas. As well as effects on food intake, patients with solid tumors have modestly elevated resting energy expenditure before weight loss is apparent.[6] Heart rate is a powerful predictor of this and adrenergic mechanisms are thought likely to be involved.

### 18.1.4   Therapeutic Diets

Another potent cause for reduction in nutrient intake is the therapeutic use of diets. Clinicians all too often forget that alterations of one part of the diet often result in changes, sometimes unwanted, in another part. Thus a low-fat diet almost invariably results in a reduction in total energy too because of the different energy densities of fat and starchy foods; this unwanted reduction in total calories can outweigh the potential advantage of reducing the fat as has been well demonstrated in the context of cystic fibrosis.[7,8] High-fiber diets tend to have the same effect.

### 18.1.5   Pancreatic Disease and Digestion

Balance studies in patients secreting less than 10% of normal pancreatic enzymes in response to CCK eating 32 kcal/kg of which 100 g was fat and an unspecified amount was nitrogen were reported.[9] In the absence of treatment, stool weights averaged 463 g/24 h, stool nitrogen excretion was 9 g/d and mean fat excretion was about 60 g/d. These results compare with earlier work[10] in three patients in whom the pancreatic duct had been ligated and in whom fecal losses of fat and protein were about 65 g/d and 50 g/d on daily intakes of 102 and 118 g, respectively. The nutritional significance of such losses is great: if 0.6 g protein/kg/d is taken as a reasonable minimum intake in the normal for balance, losses of this degree would demand intakes of about 95 g protein/d minimum for balance. A fecal loss of 60% of ingested fat calories on a 100 g intake implies a malabsorptive loss of 540 kcal/d as fat alone — roughly one-quarter of total ingested energy in a 65 kg individual eating 32 kcal/kg. However pancreatin supplementation was effective in both studies cited in reducing fecal losses, in Regan et al.'s study[9] to 2.1 N g/d and about 28 g fat/d or less, an effect which could be increased by adding cimetidine.

There is a striking functional reserve as far as pancreatic exocrine excretion is concerned. DiMagno et al.[11] demonstrated that fecal fat excretion increased only when lipase secretion was less than about 10% of normal and that fecal nitrogen increased in patients with less than 10% of normal trypsin output into the duodenum. The functional reserve has also been demonstrated in patients submitted to 90 or 75% pancreatectomy for chronic pancreatitis with 80% of dietary fat absorbed after 95% resection and normal fat absorption in a patient treated with 75% resection.[12] In pancretic insufficiency lingual and gastric lipase is preserved, and perhaps because it is not itself digested by pancreatic trypsin, is demonstrable in the upper small intestine at higher concentrations than normal. Under these conditions it may represent roughly 85 to 90% of all the lipolytic activity present in the upper jejunum in contrast with less than 10% in control subjects.[13]

Maintenance of good nutrition despite little or no pancreatic exocrine function is well demonstrated in the follow-up studies among patients undergoing pancreatoduodenectomy and Neoprene injection into the duct of Wirsung — a group in whom pancreatic endocrine function is maintained.[14] It is much more difficult, however, to eradicate steatorrhea completely, an objective which is likely to have more significance for specific micronutrients and for aesthetic reasons than for the maintenance of protein-calories nutrition.

### 18.1.6   Villous Abnormalities and Absorption

As with pancreatic exocrine function, there is a large reserve of small bowel absorptive function. Apart from fluid and electrolytes, and bile salts and vitamin $B_{12}$ which are specifically absorbed in the terminal ileum, most nutrient absorption is completed in the first 100 cm of the small intestine. Acute ingestion of alcohol as whisky can produce hemorrhagic erosions of the tips of the villi, an effect thought to be toxic rather than osmotic.[15] In addition, more chronically, there may be increased mucosal cell turnover. The villous height and cell number are decreased with associated increases in crypt cell numbers. Alcohol ingestion acutely impairs thiamine absorption by inhibition of basolateral membrane ATPase[16] and increases mucosal permeability.

Steatorrhea due to gastrointestinal diseases other than pancreaticobiliary disease or short bowel syndrome may vary widely in severity. Thus fecal fat excretion on prescribed intakes of 90 to 100 g fat/d ranged from 13 to 180 g/d.[17] Patients had relatively modest steatorrhea following partial gastrectomy (mean $25 \pm 8$ sd g/d; $n = 10$) and more severe steatorrhea with coeliac disease (mean $65 \pm 52$ sd g/d; $n = 8$). For a given degree of steatorrhea fecal weight tended to be higher in gastrointestinal disease than in pancreatic insufficiency indicating a concomitant abnormal handling of water by the intestine when it is diseased and perhaps also the increased effect of partially hydrolyzed lipid within the gut lumen in gastrointestinal compared with pancreatic disease.

## 18.1.7   Intestinal Bacterial Overgrowth

Alcohol has profound effects on intestinal muscle protein and its turnover.[18-20] Abnormalities of gut muscle function and intestinal motility can give rise to bacterial overgrowth within the small intestine. Bacterial overgrowth most notably results in $B_{12}$ deficiency, which may classically be associated (though often it isn't) with high circulating folate levels as a result of bacterial folate release into the intestine. Steatorrhea too, caused by poor formation of micelles resulting from deconjugation of bile salts and reduced concentrations of them in the lumen, can be a problem with its tendency to cause deficiencies of the fat soluble vitamins and calcium. Unabsorbed fat too can be metabolized by intestinal bacteria to hydroxy fatty acids which cause diarrhea rather like ricinoleic acid in castor oil and may result in electrolyte and water losses. Carbohydrate malabsorption, as evidenced by an abnormal xylose absorption test, is sometimes present. Protein loss from the intestine is at least one factor in the hypoalbuminemia which is seen. Degradation of protein to nitrogen containing substances available for urea but not for protein synthesis is another.

## 18.1.8   Chronic Hepatitis and Cirrhosis

The energy consumption of patients with primary biliary cirrhosis has been studied;[21] about 40% of such patients are undernourished though they are said to have a normal food intake. Fasting fat oxidation among PBC patients was nearly twice control and was also relatively elevated after a standard meal. Diet-induced thermogenesis was prolonged in PBC patients. BMR expressed per kg body weight was about 20 to 30% raised in patients with primary biliary cirrhosis compared with normals and controls who had undergone hepatic transplantation a mean of 16 (7 to 23) months previously. In the PBC patients the BMR correlated significantly with the child Pugh score of disease severity. Though the posttransplantation patient–controls and the normal controls were matched with patients for age, sex, and height, patients were a mean 14 kg less than their posttransplant counterparts.

Muller et al.[22] studied the body composition and resting energy expenditure (REE) in 123 patients with cirrhosis under consideration for transplantation. In general, body composition was within normal limits but is difficult to assess because data for men and women are not presented separately, and, for example, in the case of primary biliary cirrhosis, females predominate. Twenty-one patients were classified "hypermetabolic" on the basis of an energy expenditure of >40 kcal/kg fat free mass per d and 37 were regarded as hypometabolic, i.e., REE <30 kcal/kg fat free mass per d. There was no clear link between type of cirrhosis and metabolic expenditure, though patients with child class C disease tended to have higher REE than others. This paper and others have shown that resting respiratory quotient (RQ) is lower in cirrhotics than normal. This reflects the increased combustion of fat compared with carbohydrate seen in cirrhotic patients after an overnight fast occurring probably as a result of reduced hepatic glycogen storage in these patients, whose energy metabolism in early starvation mimics that of normals subjected to more prolonged fasting.[23] A review[24] summarizes this; studies of gluconeogenesis suggest that whereas in the normal patient after an overnight fast only 20% of splanchnic glucose production derives from gluconeogenesis, in the cirrhotic patient it provides 67%. Glycogen storage is reduced in the cirrhotic with the result that total splanchnic glucose production after an overnight fast (gluconeogenesis + glycogenolysis) is about 62% of normal. It is compensated for energetically by increased lipolysis. Hyperinsulinemia and insulin resistance (as far as glucose is concerned) is well recognized in cirrhosis. Though there is some evidence on the basis of insulin:C peptide ratios that there is some hypersecretion of insulin in cirrhosis, the hyperinsulinemia appears mainly to be due to reduced hepatic degradation of insulin, as a result of both intrahepatic portasystemic shunting and hepatocellular dysfunction; extrahepatic shunting has little effect *per se* on circulating insulin concentrations. In these patients intolerance to an oral glucose load is initially related to diminished first-pass uptake of glucose by the liver, with the effect of decreased glucose disappearance becoming dominant after about 20 min.[25] Metabolic clearance of the ingested glucose is delayed in cirrhosis. The hyperinsulinemia is associated with a characteristic but nonspecific pattern of plasma amino acid concentrations in which the levels of the branched chain amino acids valine, leucine, and isoleucine are reduced, and those of the aromatic amino acids phenylalanine, tyrosine, and methionine are increased.[26]

In hepatic disease, as in other conditions, surgical trauma modestly increases REE in the first few days, by amounts up to about 10%; but since the postoperative period is characterized by relative immobility, total energy expenditure is seldom higher than in the preoperative phase; the transient increase in REE is of little clinical significance.

Whole body protein turnover has been measured using [13C]-leucine infusions in stable cirrhosis; though turnover, synthesis, and breakdown did not differ from age- and sex-matched controls, rates of leucine oxidation were reduced by about one-quarter in the cirrhotics. This reduction correlated with the reduced plasma leucine concentration seen in the cirrhotics.[27] The reduced protein oxidation was reflected by reductions in total urinary urea and nitrogen excretion.

## 18.2   UNDERNUTRITION AND ALCOHOL ABUSE

When alcoholics develop gastrointestinal disease they are at risk, as outlined above, of becoming undernourished as a result of that disease.[28] Of course many alcoholics suffer only relatively mild GI disease. Alcoholics fall into two groups: the underweight derelict and those who remain well fed. Though weight loss in alcoholism is often attributed to impaired nutrient intake, nutritional status of alcohol abusers depends on food intake, digestion and absorption, metabolic abnormalities arising from the alcohol itself and its derivatives, and from resultant diseases which include not only damage to gut, liver, pancreas, but also to organs such as brain and muscle. A normal body weight for height can obscure a multitude of mineral and micronutrient deficiencies which need to be considered in the management of such patients, and may arise to a greater or lesser extent independently of alcohol-induced gastrointestinal disease.

### 18.2.1   Prevalence of Undernutrition Among Abusers of Alcohol

#### 18.2.1.1   Protein-Energy Status

Abusers of alcohol are far from a homogeneous group in this respect and it is easy to conjure caricature figures such as the obese beer-swilling barman, the alcoholic journalist (or doctor) of normal weight for height, and the wasted derelict. Perhaps then it is more worthwhile to consider the prevalence of lean tissue wasting or loss in alcohol abusers and in particular consider muscle mass and structure. Martin et al.[29] found that 60% of 151 consecutive patients admitted for alcoholism to have myopathic changes on muscle biopsy mainly of type IIb fiber atrophy; 5% exhibited acute alcoholic myopathy. This myopathy was not related to the social class of the patients and could not be linked with the dereliction caricature. Though muscle or lean body mass was not measured Quetelet index was; taking the lower limit of normal as 20 kg/m$^2$ for females and 19 kg/m$^2$ for males, 24% of patients were underweight. Though W/H$^2$ correlated with type II fiber atrophy factors, these factors were not statistically significantly smaller in the patients regarded as undernourished: low Quetelet index accounted for 17% of the variance of the atrophy factors. Thus it seems that alcoholic myopathy is only slightly related to weight loss and presumably loss of lean body mass. A consecutive study was made of 50 asymptomatic men attending an outpatient alcohol dependency unit, all consuming more than 100 g alcohol per d and free of overt alcohol-related or other diseases.[30] This group (mean age 38.5 years, mean daily ethanol intake 268 g over 16 years) was compared with a control healthy group of similar mean age and male sex, who drank less than a mean of 20 g alcohol per d. Though the data on body weight, fat free mass, skinfolds, and arm circumferences unfortunately were not given in the paper, mean triceps skinfold measurements were less in the alcohol abusers than in the controls.

None of the alcoholic patients had clinical or laboratory evidence of undernutrition; anthropometric measurements of the arm circumference were done, and triceps skinfold allowed calculation of fat free body mass, defined as abnormal if it was more than 10% below normal values given by Blackburn and co-workers.[31] Food intake was assessed and considered normal. Despite this lack of weight loss and arm muscle wasting 23 of 50 patients subjected to muscle biopsy exhibited evidence of myopathy. The mean cardiac radionuclide ejection fractions of the 46 alcoholics studied in this way were significantly lower than the controls; left ventricular mass of the alcohol abusers was positively correlated with lifetime alcohol consumption. Total lifetime dose of alcohol correlated negatively with muscular strength. Thus alcohol abuse is associated with cardiomyopathy, myopathy, and muscle weakness in the relative absence of wasting of lean body mass. This is a paradoxical finding because, as muscle forms a very major part of lean body mass, it implies that there can be little muscle wasting in these patients; yet every clinician recognizes muscle wasting as part of alcoholism. More work is needed in this field.

### 18.2.1.2   Micronutrient Deficiencies

If it is difficult to categorize the protein energy status of alcohol abusers, can we generalize better with respect to micronutrients? The vitamins in alcoholism have been reviewed extensively in a series of papers by Bonjour.[32-38] In a study of 121 anemic predominantly African American patients[39] admitted with alcoholism and its complications, nearly all were consuming more than 100 g ethanol/d (mean 5.6 g ethanol/kg body weight/d). At the time of admission 70% had been consuming one meal per d or less during the previous week. Aggregated macrophage iron, suggesting the anemia of chronic disease was present in 81%, megaloblastic bone marrow changes occurred in 34%, and absent iron stores in 13%. Plasma folate was less than 2.1 ng/ml in 36 of 119 patients tested and red cell folate was less than 150 ng/ml in 23 of 55 tested.

Blood levels of B vitamins have been assessed[40] in 172 alcoholic patients: 57 with a normal liver, 47 with fatty change, and 68 with cirrhosis on liver biopsy. It is not clear from the paper whether they were inpatients or not, nor what the criteria for inclusion in the study were. All but 18 were considered to have grossly deficient diets. Folic acid deficiency occurred in nearly one-half of those with cirrhosis, 40% of those with fatty liver and 30% of those without liver abnormality. Vitamin $B_6$ deficiency occurred in about 40% of cirrhotics and 25% of those with normal liver histology, with those with fatty livers intermediate. This pattern of increased likelihood of deficiency for cirrhotics was repeated for $B_1$ (about 35%), riboflavin (about 25%) and nicotinic acid (about 30%) though significant proportions even of those with normal livers had deficiencies too. Vitamin $B_{12}$ deficiency occurred in about 10% as did biotin deficiency. In this series clinical stigmata of hypovitaminosis were regularly elicited: 40 of 44 patients with peripheral neuropathy had a low thiamine level, 2 had a low pantothenic acid level, and low pyridoxine and nicotinic acid accounted for 1 each. Glossitis, cheilitis (sic), and/or atrophy of lingual papillae were accompanied by low nicotinic acid and/or low riboflavin levels in 80% of 60 patients; 7 patients with Wernicke's encephalopathy had low thiamine levels; 5 patients had characteristic symptoms and signs of pellagra confirmed by a low serum nicotinic acid level.

A study[41] of 31 patients all with histologically proven liver disease revealed that there was biochemical evidence for thiamine deficiency in 18 (58%). There was a significantly higher incidence in alcoholic patients (71%) than in nonalcoholic patients (43%). In another study[42] both erythrocyte transketolase and thiamine pyrophosphate (TPP) effect were measured in 64 patients with a daily alcohol intake of more than 1 g/kg body weight for 5 or more years, referred to the Royal Free Hospital's liver unit for investigation of suspected liver disease. Transketolase activity was below 2 SD of control in 19 patients, of whom 6 had the expected abnormally high TPP effect to confirm thiamine deficiency, but 10 had a normal and 3 a low TPP effect. Eight patients had normal transketolase but a low TPP effect. Thus unequivocal thiamine deficiency could be said to have been present in about 10% of the patients. However there is evidence that thiamine deficiency in alcoholism and liver disease can produce a low erythrocyte transketolase

(ETK) with a low TPP effect because low levels of apoenzyme (ETK) exist in a near saturation state with coenzyme (TPP).[35] When the energy intake from alcohol was ignored the dietary composition as judged by dietary history was similar between these patients and a control group. The patients seemed therefore to be adding the alcohol to their normal food intake rather than replacing calories with alcohol. Under these circumstances it is perhaps surprising that the patients were all within 10% of their ideal body weights, but this lack of expected weight gain in chronic alcoholism is well documented and discussed elsewhere.[43] None of the patients exhibited symptoms or signs of thiamine deficiency. Though scurvy is not reported in alcoholics, vitamin C status is often impaired compared with control subjects.[32] Circulating and hepatic concentrations of vitamin A are depressed in alcoholic patients with liver disease, but occur also in patients with other causes of liver injury.[37] Vitamin A is poorly absorbed in pancreatic steatorrhea of whatever etiology. There is conflicting evidence on the effect of alcohol *per se* on vitamin A absorption but in practice malabsorption is probably not the dominant cause of the rapid redistribution and depletion of the hepatic stores of this vitamin during alcohol abuse. Intake is commonly depressed but the principal effect is likely to be metabolic.[38] Abnormal visual dark adaptation is common in alcoholics and this may respond partially or completely to cautious vitamin A repletion though zinc may be an important cofactor particularly in the production of retinol binding protein.

## 18.3    WHAT PATHOPHYSIOLOGICAL EFFECTS DOES THE MALNUTRITION ASSOCIATED WITH ALCOHOL INTAKE AND ABUSE HAVE?

It is clear that while alcohol is sometimes associated with social dereliction and therefore protein calorie undernutrition, muscle weakness, and such wasting as there is, is much more common; the wasting of undernutrition is not the dominant cause of weakness and myopathy in alcoholism. Fat stores may be great or slight. Glycogen storage will be impaired with major implications for physical endurance. Gluconeogenesis may be inhibited, which together with deficient glycogen stores may result in hypoglycemia.[44]

The micronutrient defects may be associated with specific deficiency syndromes, the best known of which are the Wernicke/Korsakoff syndromes. Anemias, neuropathies, and cardiac muscle abnormalities all arise as a result of water soluble vitamin and trace element deficiencies. Vitamin A deficiency has been implicated in the abnormal spermatogenesis, and may also produce abnormalities of taste and smell. The effect of the vitamin C deficiencies is poorly investigated but may reduce drug metabolism and reduce alcohol dehydrogenase activity in the liver. Reduced antioxidant status with carcinogen activation by alcohol may predispose to cancers and atheroma *inter alia*.

### 18.3.1    Liver Disease

The production of hepatic pathology seems hastened in the presence of vitamin A deficiency though such deficiency is not necessary for it. Alcohol produces other substrate deficiencies within the liver such as S-adenosyl methionine and phosphatidylcholine. Its metabolism results in the excess generation of reducing equivalents especially NADH. Lactic acidosis, hyperuricemia, and hyperlipidemia result from this, as well as the tendency for the liver to accumulate fat. The complex interrelations of nutrition with alcoholic liver disease have been widely reviewed; good recent examples being the papers by Lieber[45] and by Thompson.[46]

## 18.4    NUTRITIONAL TREATMENT

The nutritional management of the alcoholic patient can for the most part be summarized as the cessation of the alcohol and the encouragement of a well-balanced diet. Obesity may respond well to alcohol withdrawal; undernutrition may need supplemental oral or enteral artificial feeding until a good spontaneous intake is achieved. The success of such an apparently simple strategy will be bound up in psychosocial factors beyond the scope of this chapter; its simplicity in concept belies the huge difficulties of implementing such changes in practice.

Specific deficiencies of folate and the water soluble vitamins need urgent replacement, particularly in the presence of macrocytic anemia or Wernicke's encephalopathy but the use of more chronic artificial supplementation of vitamins is more questionable. A case can certainly be made for the provision of extra water soluble vitamins to alcoholics on the grounds that they are commonly deficient; however, whether this is a more cost efficient approach than responding to specific or suspected deficiencies in individuals chosen on clinical grounds in unclear. Nicotinic acid might reduce the hypertriglyceridemia seen in alcohol abuse but its effect on the hepatic steatosis is less clear; there may be unwanted potentiation. Fat soluble vitamins may need replacement, though with these there is a greater risk of toxicity if used in excess; in particular doses of vitamin A above standard daily requirements may result in enhanced hepatic damage. There has been recent interest in dietary supplementation of patients with alcoholic liver disease by methionine, S-adenosyl methionine, and phosphatidylcholine.

# REFERENCES

1. **Harju, E.,** Dietary and supplementary intake of nutrients by patients with gastrointestinal diseases, *J. Clin. Gastroenterol.,* 8, 661, 1986.
2. **Mullan, A., Kavanagh, P., O'Mahony, P., Gleeson, F., and Gibney, M. J.,** Food and nutrient intakes and eating patterns in functional and organic dypepsia, *Eur. J. Clin. Nutr.,* 48, 97, 1994.
3. **Ogorek, C. P., Davidson, L., Fisher, R. S., and Krevsky, B.,** Idiopathic gastroparesis is associated with a multiplicity of severe dietary deficiencies, *Am. J. Gastroenterol.,* 86, 423, 1991.
4. **Fellows, I. W., Greensmith, J., and Atkinson, M.,** The nutritional effects of endoscopic intubation for carcinoma of the oesophagus and cardia, *Clin. Nutr.,* 2, 167, 1984.
5. **Burke, M., Bryson, E. I., and Kirk, A. E.,** Dietary intakes, resting metabolic rates and body composition in benign and malignant gastrointestinal disease, *Br. Med. J.,* 1, 211, 1980.
6. **Gelin, J. and Lundholm, K.,** The metabolic response to cancer, *Proc. Nutr. Soc.,* 51, 279, 1992.
7. **Chase, H. P., Long, M. A., and Lavin, M. J.,** Cystic fibrosis and malnutrition, *J. Pediatr.,* 95, 337, 1979.
8. **Pencharz, P. B.,** Energy intakes and low fat diets in children with cystic fibrosis and malnutrition, *J. Pediatr. Gastroenterol. Nutr.,* 2, 400, 1983.
9. **Regan, P. T., Malagelada, J.-R., DiMagno, E. P., Glanzman, S. L., and Go, V. L. W.,** Comparative effects of antacids, cimetidine, and enteric coating on the therapeutic response to oral enzymes in severe pancreatic insufficiency, *N. Engl. J. Med.,* 297, 854, 1977.
10. **Wollaeger, E. E., Comfort, M. W., Clagett, O. T., and Osterberg, A. E.,** Efficiency of gastrointestinal tract after resection of head of pancreas, *JAMA,* 137, 838, 1948.
11. **DiMagno, E. P., Go, V. L. W., and Summerskill, W. H. J.,** Relations between pancreatic enzyme outputs and malabsorption in severe pancreatic insufficiency, *N. Engl. J. Med.,* 288, 813, 1973.
12. **Kalser, M. H., Leite, C. A., and Warren, W. D.,** Fat assimilation after massive distal pancreatectomy, *N. Engl. J. Med.,* 279, 570, 1968.
13. **Abrams, C. K., Hamosh, M., Dutta, S. K., Hubbard, V. S., and Hamosh, P.,** Role of non-pancreatic lipolytic activity in exocrine pancreatic insufficiency, *Gastroenterology,* 92, 125, 1987.
14. **Braga, M., Cristallow, M., De Franchis, R., Mangiagalli, A., Agape, D., Primignani, M., and Di Carlo, V.,** Correction of malnutrition and maldigestion with enzyme supplementation in patients with surgical suppression of exocrine pancreatic function, *Surg. Gynecol. Obstet.,* 167, 485, 1988.
15. **World, M. J., Ryle, P. R., and Thomson, A. D.,** Alcoholic malnutrition and the small intestine, *Alcohol Alcohol.,* 2, 89, 1985.
16. **Hoyumpa, A. M., Strickland, R., Sheeham, J. J., Yarborough, G., and Nichols, S.,** Dual system of intestinal thiamine transport in humans, *J. Lab. Clin. Med.,* 99, 701, 1982.
17. **Bo-Linn, G. W. and Fordtran, J. S.,** Fecal fat concentration in patients with steatorrhoea, *Gastroenterology,* 87, 319, 1984.
18. **Neale, G., Gompertz, D., Schonsby, H., Tabaqchali, S., and Booth, C. C.,** The metabolic and nutritional consequences of bacterial overgrowth in the small intestine, *Am. J. Clin. Nutr.,* 25, 1409, 1972.
19. **Isaacs, P. E. T. and Kim, Y. S.,** Blind loop syndrome and small bowel bacterial contamination, *Clin. Gastroenterol.,* 12, 395, 1983.
20. **Preedy, V. R., Marway, J. S., Siddiq, T., Ansari, F. A., Hashim, I. A., and Peters, T. J.,** Gastrointestinal protein turnover and alcohol misuse, *Drug Alcohol Depend.,* 34, 1, 1993.

21. **Green, J. H., Bramley, P. N., and Losowsky, M. S.,** Are patients with primary biliary cirrhosis hypermetabolic? A comparison between patients before and after liver transplantation and controls, *Hepatology*, 14, 464, 1991.

22. **Muller, J., Lautz, H. U., Plogmann, B., Burger, M., Korber, J., and Schmidt, F. W.,** Energy expenditure and substrate oxidation in patients with cirrhosis: the impact of cause, clinical staging, and nutritional state, *Hepatology*, 15, 782, 1992.

23. **Owen, O. E., Reichle, F. A., Mozzoli, M. A., Kreulen, T., Patel, M. S., Elfenbein, I. B., Golsorkhi, M., Chang, K. H. Y., Rao, N. S., Sue, H. S., and Boden, G.,** Hepatic, gut and renal substrate flux rates in patients with hepatic cirrhosis, *J. Clin. Invest.*, 68, 240, 1981.

24. **Morgan, M. Y.,** Nutritional aspects of liver and biliary disease, in *Oxford Textbook of Clinical Hepatology*, McIntyre, N., Benhamou, J.-P., Bircher, J., Rizzetto, M., and Rodes, J., Eds., Oxford University Press, Oxford, 1991.

25. **Kruszynska, Y. T., Meyer-Alber, A., Darakhshan, F., Home, P. D., and McIntyre, N.,** Metabolic handling of orally administered glucose in cirrhosis, *J. Clin. Invest.*, 91, 1057, 1993.

26. **Munro, H. N., Fernstrom, J. D., and Wurtman, R. J.,** Insulin, plasma amino acid imbalance, and hepatic coma, *Lancet*, i, 722, 1975.

27. **Mullen, K. D., Denne, S. C., McCullough, A. J., Savin, S. M., Bruno, D., Tavill, A. S., and Kalhan, S. C.,** Leucine metabolism in stable cirrhosis, *Hepatology*, 6, 622, 1986.

28. **Powell-Tuck, J., Ed.,** Review in depth: alcohol and nutrition, *Eur. J. Gastroenterol. Hepatol.*, 2, 393, 1990.

29. **Martin, F., Ward, K., Slavin, G., Levi, J., and Peters, T. J.,** Alcoholic skeletal myopathy, a clinical and pathological study, *Q. J. Med.*, 55, 233, 1985.

30. **Urbano-Marquez, A., Estruch, R., Navarro-Lopez, F., Grau, J. M., Mont, L., and Rubin, E.,** The effects of alcoholism on skeletal and cardiac muscle, *N. Engl. J. Med.*, 320, 409, 1989.

31. **Blackburn, G. L., Bistrian, B. R., Maini, B. S., Schlamm, H. T., and Smith, M. F.,** Nutritional and Metbolic assessment of the hospitalized patient, *J. Parenter. Enter. Nutr.*, 1, 11, 1977.

32. **Bonjour, J. P.,** Vitamins and alcoholism: I Ascorbic acid, *Int. J. Vitam. Nutr. Res.*, 49, 434, 1979.

33. **Bonjour, J. P.,** Vitamins and alcoholism: II Folate and vitamin B12, *Int. J. Vitam. Nutr. Res.*, 50, 96, 1980.

34. **Bonjour, J. P.,** Vitamins and alcoholism: III Vitamin B6, *Int. J. Vitam. Nutr. Res.*, 50, 215, 1980.

35. **Bonjour, J. P.,** Vitamins and alcoholism: IV Thiamin, *Int. J. Vitam. Nutr. Res.*, 50, 321, 1980.

36. **Bonjour, J. P.,** Vitamins and alcoholism: V Riboflavin; VI Niacin; VII Pantothenic acid; VIII Biotin, *Int. J. Vitam. Nutr. Res.*, 50, 425, 1980.

37. **Bonjour, J. P.,** Vitamins and alcoholism: IX Vitamin A, *Int. J. Vitam. Nutr. Res.*, 51, 166, 1981.

38. **Bonjour, J. P.,** Vitamins and alcoholism: X Vitamin A; XI Vitamin E; XII Vitamin K, *Int. J. Vitam. Nutr. Res.*, 51, 307, 1981.

39. **Savage, D. and Lindebaum, J.,** Anemia in alcoholics, *Medicine*, 65, 322, 1986.

40. **Leevy, C. M., Baker, H., tenHove, W., Frank, O., and Cherrick, G. R.,** B-complex vitamins in liver disease of the alcoholic, *Am. J. Clin. Nutr.*, 16, 339, 1965.

41. **Rossouw, J. E., Labadarios, D., Krasner, N., Davis, M., and Williams, R.,** Red blood cell transketolase activity and the effect of thiamine supplementation in patients with chronic liver disease, *Scand. J. Gastroenterol.*, 13, 133, 1978.

42. **Camilo, M. E., Morgan, M. Y., and Sherlock, S.,** Erythrocyte transketolase activity in alcoholic liver disease, *Scand. J. Gastroenterol.*, 16, 273, 1981.

43. **Lieber, C. S.,** Perspectives: do alcohol calories count?, *Am. J. Clin. Nutr.*, 54, 976, 1991.

44. **Palmer, T. N.,** Fuel homeostasis and alcohol abuse, *Eur. J. Gastroenterol. Hepatol.*, 2, 406, 1990.

45. **Lieber, C. S.,** A personal perspective on alcohol, nutrition, and the liver, *Am. J. Clin. Nutr.*, 58, 430, 1993.

46. **Thompson, R. P. H.,** Alcohol, nutrition and the liver, *Eur. J. Gastroenterol. Hepatol.*, 2, 417, 1990.

# 19

## Objectives for Future Research in Understanding the Effects of Ethanol on the Gastrointestinal Tract

Victor R. Preedy and Ronald R. Watson

### CONTENTS

### 19.1 INTRODUCTION

This chapter will briefly summarize some of the effects of ethanol on the gastrointestinal tract and to identify some areas that merit further investigation. Some deficiencies in present knowledge have also been highlighted in individual chapters. Nevertheless, to mention every potential process thought to be of importance would be an enormous undertaking, particularly as there are some rapidly expanding fields and their significance in the etiology of disease is currently speculative. To circumvent such a problem, a few key disciplines that require investigation have been identified and attention is focused on protein metabolism. The terms protein synthesis, protein turnover or protein metabolism may conjure up gross physiological processes. To a certain extent this is both an over simplification and a misconception, as they also encompass molecular events. Villus atrophy, loss of contractile or membrane proteins, the reductions in the relative amounts of a single protein (i.e., a key enzyme) or groups of proteins (i.e., such as those pertaining to the subcellular organelles) all involve changes in protein pool size and thus by implication protein turnover. The latter may involve changes in mRNA encoding specific proteins or amino acid supply, the availability of initiation factors, or subcellular assembly and processing.

The metabolic and functional lesions that arise in the liver are well characterized and, compared to the intestinal tract, have been thoroughly investigated.[1-3] Epidemiological studies have clearly shown that a number of intestinal pathologies also arise as a consequence of excessive ethanol intake. These include cancers of the orocavity, esophagus, and large bowel, as well as gastric lesions.[4-7] Pancreatitis and salivary gland abnormalities (the latter involving sialadenosis and impaired saliva excretion) also occur.[8,9] There are also cellular and biochemical changes, including alterations in protein synthesis,[10] cell turnover,[11] and lipid metabolism.[12] Some of these effects may be mediated by endocrine abnormalities[13] and to this extent Marway et al.[10] have clearly shown that protein synthesis in the small bowel of ethanol treated rats is modulated by prevailing endocrine status. Reactive oxygen species are also important in that they may also cause damage to intestinal tissues.[14] Functional abnormalities include defects in motility, malabsorption, and permeability.[15-17] These functional abnormalities, together with defects in intermediary metabolism, may contribute to the impaired nutritional status of alcohol abusers which will have profound consequences for morbidity.[18]

The above intestinal pathologies should not detract from the fact that the function of the liver in ethanol metabolism is central to some of ethanol's deleterious effects. For example, hepatic metabolism is responsible for the generation of acetaldehyde which has been shown to be an important intestinal perturbant. Thus, raising circulating acetaldehyde levels with the metabolic inhibitor cyanamide reduces protein synthesis in the jejunum.[10] Both contractile and noncontractile proteins are affected. However, although alcohol and acetaldehyde dehydrogenases are present in gastrointestinal tissues,[19] an important question relates to the extent to which local and hepatic derived acetaldehyde exert their deleterious effects. It would not be unreasonable for intestinally derived acetaldehyde to form localized protein-adducts or to alter key metabolic processes such as protein synthesis. It should be remembered, however, that the effects on protein metabolism are only one facet of acetaldehyde's deleterious effects. Other effects include organelle dysfunction, membrane changes, lipid peroxidation. Indeed, it is probably a truism that many of the effects of ethanol or its derived metabolites on the liver may also occur in the ethanol-exposed intestinal tract. However, while there is evidence of ethanol- and acetaldehyde-induced damage in the seromuscular layer of ethanol treated rats, there is a paucity of data derived from clinical studies and this is an area that merits some investigation. The problem is: how does one investigate this on a routine basis? A study of smooth muscle actin elements in the villus may be of benefit in this regard or even by use of biochemical markers (for example, 3-methylhistidine content).

## 19.2   METABOLIC SUPERIMPOSITION

There is sufficient epidemiological evidence to suggest that increased numbers of esophago-gastrointestinal cancers occur when then there is concomitant alcohol abuse and cigarette smoking, compared to the incidence due to alcohol ingestion or cigarette smoking alone. Other associations are still being made; for example, Hansson et al.[20] for gastric cancer. Certainly, moderate to heavy alcohol intake is correlated with incremental cigarette smoking.[4] If we consider that cigarette smoking is a component of the addiction phenomenon then there are clearly areas of polydrug abuse that merit serious concern. Thus, cocaine abuse is evident in 5% of the U.S. adult population and a combination of cocaine and ethanol induces the formation (in the liver) of cocaethylene. This product is toxic to myocardial cells.[21] Further, it is becoming increasingly evident that cocaine is immunosuppressive as well as being directly toxic to intestinal tissues.[22] However, the synergistic effect of ethanol and cocaine on the intestine is little understood, and merits further investigation, as do other forms of polydrug misuse on intestinal structure and function.

It is also well known that a substantial proportion (some studies suggest half) of alcoholics are malnourished with regard to one or more macro- or micronutrients. This, of course will arise as a direct consequence of the toxic effects of ethanol on the intestine, but also due to caloric displacement and socioeconomic consequences in some subjects. It should be remembered that some ethanol-related abnormalities are not directly a result of impaired nutritional intake, particularly skeletal and cardiac muscle disease.[23-27] However, information regarding the metabolic interactions of ethanol and malnutrition on pathological processes in the intestine is lacking.

Thus, while ethanol undoubtedly impairs nutrient absorption, many studies have been carried out in normal animals without regard to interacting phenomena such as nutritional status. The relationship between ethanol and nutrition is not a simple one, however, as both effect the immune response.[28] Thus, a clear need exists to pursue studies into the complex associations, such as sepsis, with alcohol and malnutrition. Each of these injurious insults affect the intestine by specific processes such as increased cell turnover in sepsis.[29]

## 19.3   SUITABLE MODELS AND METHODS

A repeated theme in this book is the need to adopt and apply suitable methodologies. The applicability of this is evident from the original work by Lieber and DeCarli in devising their liquid diet feeding regime (reviewed in Reference 30). Although simple in concept, profound implications arise from the notion that data from laboratory models are dependent on whether due consideration has been made to the model of feeding. Thus, specific attention has also been focused on the methods for measuring protein synthesis[10] and intestinal permeability.[16] Although, *in vitro* models have provided the backbone of biomedical research, there is a substantial amount of data that can be ascertained from measurements made in intact laboratory animals or in humans *in vivo*. (Nevertheless, advances are still being made in the application of *in vitro* methodology.[31]) The transition from invasive to noninvasive technologies can be exemplified by blood flow measurements. What used to be measured with radiolabeled microspheres or other invasive procedures[32] can now be measured noninvasively by laser-Doppler techniques[33] and these type of transitions need to be applied to understanding the pathophysiology of intestinal disorders. A cautionary note is required: while many studies have entailed the use of young growing animals, they do not mimic the nongrowing states of the adult or aged person. This implies that there is a need to investigate the ethanol-induced pathologies in aged laboratory animals.[34] However, there is still a great deal to learn about the normal physiology of the gut and especially its role in nutrient processing.[35]

Several chapters have considered the phenomena of malabsorption, albeit in passing or in greater detail.[17] However, when considering whether alcohol is perturbing digestive or absorptive function in isolated or *in vivo* systems, it is essential to determine if this will give rise to *functional* malabsorption. As has been described,[35] diarrhea is a colonic phenomena which may comprise primary defects in water and/or electrolyte salvage. Alternatively, diarrhea may arise secondary to nutrient malabsorption, as is the case with osmotic diarrhea. If stool output of carbohydrate, fat, or protein is not measured it is difficult to determine the primary cause of the diarrhea or its metabolic significance. Thus, in patients with cystic fibrosis, the pancreatic lesion gives rise to fat malabsorption with a consequent increase in fat in stool output. Alcohol, in contrast, may lead to a partial downregulation of specific nutrient transporters or digestive functions. This may not be sufficient, however, to reduce the global "safety margin" of the small intestine to the extent where significant amounts of macronutrients are malabsorbed and enter the colon. This emphasizes the need to perform simple assessment of stool volume and composition before arriving at a diagnosis of alcohol-related malabsorption. In this regard, it may be profitable to use the approach described by Grimble et al.[36] in investigating malabsorption, which defines the degree of functional impairment of digestive and absorptive steps with a variety of techniques, such as breath hydrogen to quantify carbohydrate malabsorption.

## 19.4   STUDIES IN THE PRESENCE AND ABSENCE
##         OF CIRCULATING ETHANOL

Of merit is the recent study by Hirsch et al.[37] which has also been reviewed by Preedy et al.[38] They studied the impact of alcoholic cirrhosis on whole body leucine kinetics and ascertained that markedly different conclusions were obtained when abstinent alcoholics were compared to subjects who did not refrain from ethanol consumption. This raises questions as to the relevance of some studies which, for ethical and practical reasons, have carried out investigations in the absence of circulating ethanol.[39] The study by Pacy et al.[39] showed that reduced rates of muscle protein synthesis were obtained in alcoholics without circulating ethanol, compared to normal controls, implicating a defect in tissue biochemistry *per se*. This illustrates that meaningful data can still be obtained from a comparison on abstinent alcoholics and normal abstinent controls. In contrast, in innumerable animal studies, measurements have been carried out in the presence of circulating ethanol. Although these issues may seem trivial, the implications for strategies and treatments are clearly not an insignificant matter and some degree of sophistication is needed in controlling prevailing ethanol levels while measurements are being carried out and comparing data derived from periods of abstinence. The possibility that the nonabstinent to abstinent transition has a modulating influence on metabolism has received some attention, for example, in the study of brain blood flow,[40] liver metabolism,[41] plasma lipids,[42] and esophageal motor function[43] but the proportion of these studies to those investigating the effect of alcohol toxicity *per se* are comparatively rare.

## 19.5 MOLECULAR EVENTS

These can be approached at various levels. With reference to genetic polymorphism, there is a growing body of literature relating to the addiction process and hepatic damage.[44] This emphasizes the need to correlate polymorphism with the indices of intestinal damage, including both gross cellular lesions as well as cancers, although some studies have been carried out relating to alcoholic pancreatic disease.[45] Transcriptional control mechanisms are clearly important but their role in mediating intestinal damage are again little understood. Furthermore, where mRNA levels have been assessed in response to ethanol, there is a lack of concordant data on the relative amounts of those proteins that mRNA encodes, and the levels of mRNA. Finally, there is a paucity of translational and transcriptional correlates. Certainly, increases in mRNA encoding contractile proteins are of importance in the smooth muscle hypertrophy in infection such as that induced by *Trichinella spiralis* and in intestinal bypass.[46,47] It is possible that a downregulation of genes encoding smooth muscle proteins is a contributing mechanism in the reduced contractile protein apparatus seen in response to chronic ethanol feeding.[10] However, this still begs the question of whether the ethanol impaired alterations will be mediated directly by ethanol, or if they are secondary to other process such as free radical-mediated injury.[14]

## 19.6 CONCLUSION

A few areas that necessitate investigation have been highlighted in a number of reviews. There is a clear need to understand the mechanisms at the molecular level and to carry out these studies with appropriate models that encompass the superimposition of additional pathologies.

## 19.7 ACKNOWLEDGMENTS

Part of the work was carried out in The Rayne Institute, Coldharbour Lane, London SE5 9NU, UK. The support of Professor T. J. Peters and the advice of Dr. H. J. F. Why and Dr. G. K. Grimble are gratefully acknowledged.

## REFERENCES

1. **Lieber, C. S. and DeCarli, L. M.,** Hepatotoxicity of alcohol, *J. Hepatol.*, 12, 394, 1991.
2. **Lieber, C. S. and Leo, M. A.,** Alcohol and the liver, in *Medical and Nutritional Complications of Alcoholism. Mechanisms and Management*, Lieber, C. S., Ed., Plenum Publishing Corporation, New York, 1992, 185.

3. **Lieber, C. S.,** The metabolism of alcohol and its implication for the pathogenesis of disease, in *Alcohol and the Gastrointestinal Tract*, Preedy, V. R. and Watson, R. R., Eds., CRC Press, Boca Raton, FL, 1995, 19.

4. **Kato, I.,** The extent of the problems and the epidemiology of alcohol drinking, in *Alcohol and the Gastrointestinal Tract*, Preedy, V. R. and Watson, R. R., Eds., CRC Press, Boca Raton, FL, 1995, 1.

5. **Beck, I. T.,** Small bowel injury by ethanol, in *Alcohol and the Gastrointestinal Tract*, Preedy, V. R. and Watson, R. R., Eds., CRC Press, Boca Raton, FL, 1995, 163.

6. **Konturek, S. J., Stachura, J., and Konturek, J. W.,** Gastric cytoprotection and adaptation to ethanol, in *Alcohol and the Gastrointestinal Tract*, Preedy, V. R. and Watson, R. R., Eds., CRC Press, Boca Raton, FL, 1995, 123.

7. **Mufti, S. I.,** Alcohol's promotion of gastrointestinal carcinogenesis, in *Alcohol and the Gastrointestinal Tract*, Preedy, V. R. and Watson, R. R., Eds., CRC Press, Boca Raton, FL, 1995, 311.

8. **Norton, I. D. and Wilson, J. S.,** Alcoholic pancreatitis, in *Alcohol and the Gastrointestinal Tract*, Preedy, V. R. and Watson, R. R., Eds., CRC Press, Boca Raton, FL, 1995, 143.

9. **Proctor, G. B. and Shori, D. K.,** The effects of ethanol on salivary glands, in *Alcohol and the Gastrointestinal Tract*, Preedy, V. R. and Watson, R. R., Eds., CRC Press, Boca Raton, FL, 1995, 111.

10. **Marway, J. S., Bonner, A. B., Peters, T. J., and Preedy, V. R.,** Protein synthesis in the gastrointestinal tract and its modification by ethanol, in *Alcohol and the Gastrointestinal Tract*, Preedy, V. R. and Watson, R. R., Eds., CRC Press, Boca Raton, FL, 1995, 255.

11. **Seitz, H. K. and Simanowski, U. A.,** Cell turnover in the gastrointestinal tract and the effect of ethanol, in *Alcohol and the Gastrointestinal Tract*, Preedy, V. R. and Watson, R. R., Eds., CRC Press, Boca Raton, FL, 1995, 273.

12. **Hayashi, H.,** Lipid metabolism in the intestinal tract and its modification by ethanol, in *Alcohol and the Gastrointestinal Tract*, Preedy, V. R. and Watson, R. R., Eds., CRC Press, Boca Raton, FL, 1995, 289.

13. **Ojeas, H. S., Harty, R. F., and Van Thiel, D.,** Endocrine changes in alcoholism with special reference to gastrointestinal hormones, in *Alcohol and the Gastrointestinal Tract*, Preedy, V. R. and Watson, R. R., Eds., CRC Press, Boca Raton, 1995, 69.

14. **Albano, E. and Clot, P.,** Free radicals and ethanol toxicity, in *Alcohol and the Gastrointestinal Tract*, Preedy, V. R. and Watson, R. R., Eds., CRC Press, Boca Raton, FL, 1995, 57.

15. **Keshavarzian, A. and Fields, J. Z.,** Gastrointestinal motility disorders induced by ethanol, in *Alcohol and the Gastrointestinal Tract*, Preedy, V. R. and Watson, R. R., Eds., CRC Press, Boca Raton, FL, 1995, 235.

16. **Bjarnason, I. and Macpherson, A.,** Alcohol and small intestinal permeability, in *Alcohol and the Gastrointestinal Tract*, Preedy, V. R. and Watson, R. R., Eds., CRC Press, Boca Raton, FL, 1995, 219.

17. **Thomson, A. D., Heap, L. C., and Ward, R. J.,** Alcohol-induced malabsorption in the gastrointestinal tract, in *Alcohol and the Gastrointestinal Tract*, Preedy, V. R. and Watson, R. R., Eds., CRC Press, Boca Raton, FL, 1995, 203.

18. **Powell-Tuck, J.,** Nutritional implications of hepato-intestinal disorders, in *Alcohol and the Gastrointestinal Tract*, Preedy, V. R. and Watson, R. R., Eds., CRC Press, Boca Raton, FL, 1995, 34.

19. **Parés, X. and Farrés, J.,** Alcohol and aldehyde dehydrogenases in the gastrointestinal tract, in *Alcohol and the Gastrointestinal Tract*, Preedy, V. R. and Watson, R. R., Eds., CRC Press, Boca Raton, FL, 1995, 41.

20. **Hansson, L. E., Baron, J., Nyren, O., Bergstrom, R., Wolk, A., and Adami, H. O.,** Tobacco, alcohol and the risk of gastric cancer. A population-based case-control study in Sweden, *Int. J. Cancer*, 57, 26, 1994.

21. **Welder, A. A., Dickson, L. J., and Melchert, R. B.,** Cocaethylene toxicity in rat primary myocardial cell cultures, *Alcohol*, 10, 285, 1993.

22. **Gourgoutis, G. and Das, G.,** Gastrointestinal manifestations of cocaine addiction, *Int. J. Clin. Pharmacol. Ther.*, 32, 136, 1994.

23. **Urbano-Marquez, A., Estruch, R., Navarro-Lopez, F., Grau, J. M., Mont, L., and Rubin, E.,** The effect of alcoholism on skeletal and cardiac muscle, *N. Engl. J. Med.*, 320, 409, 1989.

24. **Preedy, V. R., Peters, T. J., Patel, V. B., and Miell, J. P.,** Chronic alcoholic myopathy: transcriptional and translational alterations, *FASEB J.*, in press, 1994.

25. **Preedy, V. R., Patel, V. B., Why, H. J. F., Corbett, J. M., Dunn, M. J., and Richardson, P. J.,** Alcohol and the heart: biochemical alterations, *Cardioscience*, in press, 1995.

26. **Reilly, M. E., Preedy, V. R., and Peters, T. J.,** Investigations into the toxic effects of alcohol on skeletal muscle, *Adverse Drug React. Toxicol. Rev.*, 14, 117, 1995.

27. **Preedy, V. R. and Richardson, P. J.,** Ethanol-induced cardiovascular disease, *Br. Med Bull.*, 50, 152, 1994.

28. **Watzl, B. and Watson, R. R.,** Nutrition and alcohol-induced immunomodulation, in *Nutrition and Alcohol*, Watson, R. R. and Watzl, B., Eds., CRC Press, Boca Raton, FL, 1992, 429.

29. **Rafferty, J. F., Noguchi, Y., Fischer, J. E., and Hasselgren, P.-O.,** Sepsis in rats stimulates cellular proliferation in the mucosa of the small intestine, *Gastroenterology*, 107, 121, 1994.

30. **Lieber, C. S.,** 1986 update. The feeding of ethanol in liquid diets, *Alcoholism: Clin. Exp. Res.*, 10, 550, 1986.

31. **Nagy, L., Szabo, S., Morales, R. E., Plebani, M., and Jenkins, J. M.,** Identification of subcellular targets and sensitive tests of ethanol-induced damage in isolated rat gastric mucosal cells, *Gastroenterology*, 107, 907, 1994.

32. **Preedy, V. R., Venkatesan, S., Peters, T. J., Nott, D. M., Yates, S., and Jenkins, S. A.,** The effect of chronic ethanol ingestion on tissue RNA and blood flow in skeletal muscle with comparative reference to blood flow in bone and tissues of the gastrointestinal tract of the rat, *Clin. Sci.*, 72, 243, 1989.

33. **Preedy, V. R., Cook, E. B., and Siddiq, T.,** Non-invasive laser-Doppler assessment of cutaneous blood-flow in alcohol studies: effects of chronic ethanol consumption on peripheral blood-flow in unanaesthetised rats, *Alcohol Alcohol.,* 27, 165, 1992.

34. **Simanowski, U. A., Suter, P., Russell, R. M., Heller, M., Waldherr, R., Ward, R., Peters, T. J., Smith, D., and Seitz, H. K.,** Enhancement of ethanol induced rectal mucosal hyper regeneration with age in F344 rats, *Gut,* 35, 1102, 1994.

35. **Grimble, G. K.,** The physiology of digestion, absorption and metabolism in the gastrointestinal tract, in *Alcohol and the Gastrointestinal Tract,* Preedy, V. R. and Watson, R. R., Eds., CRC Press, Boca Raton, FL, 1995, 79.

36. **Grimble, G. K., Bowling, T. E., and Silk, D. B. A.,** Intestinal digestion and absorption of nutrients, in *Surgical Nutrition,* Fischer, J. E., Ed., W. B. Saunders, London, in press, 1995.

37. **Hirsch, S., de la Maza, P., Petermann, M., Iturriaga, H., Ugarte, G., and Bunout, D.,** Protein turnover in abstinent and non-abstinent patients with alcoholic cirrhosis, *J. Am. Coll. Nutr.,* 14, 99, 1995.

38. **Preedy, V. R., Reilly, M. E., Why, H. J. F., Bonner, A. B., and Richardson, P. J.,** Protein turnover in alcoholism: should it be considered as a whole body event or tissue specific phenomena?, *J. Am. Coll Nutr.,* 14, 7, 1995.

39. **Pacy, P., Preedy, V. R., Peters, T. J., Read, M., and Halliday D.,** The effects of chronic alcohol ingestion on whole-body and muscle protein synthesis — a stable isotope study, *Alcohol Alcohol.,* 26, 503, 1991.

40. **Newman, L. M., Hoffman, W. E., Miletich, D. J., and Albrecht, R. F.,** Regional blood flow and cerebral metabolic changes during alcohol withdrawal and following midazolam therapy, *Anesthesiology,* 63, 395, 1985.

41. **Hadengue, A., Moreau, R., Lee, S. S., Gaudin, C., Rueff, B., and Lebrec, D.,** Liver hypermetabolism during alcohol withdrawal in humans. Role of sympathetic overactivity, *Gastroenterology,* 94, 1047, 1988.

42. **Lamisse, F., Schellenberg, F., Bouyou, E., Delarue, J., Benard, J. Y., and Couet, C.,** Plasma lipids and alcohol consumption in alcoholic men: effect of withdrawal, *Alcohol Alcohol.,* 29, 25, 1994.

43. **Keshavarzian, A., Polepalle, C., Iber, F. L., and Durkin, M.,** Esophageal motor disorder in alcoholics: results of alcoholism or withdrawal?, *Alcoholism: Clin. Exp. Res.,* 14, 561, 1990.

44. **Sherman, D. I. N. and Williams, R.,** Liver damage: mechanisms and management, *Br. Med. Bull.,* 50, 124, 1994.

45. **Takada, A., Tsutsumi, M., and Kobayashi, Y.,** Genotypes of ALDH2 related to liver and pulmonary disease and other genetic factors related to alcoholic liver disease, *Alcohol Alcohol.,* 29, 719, 1994.

46. **Lai, M., Thomason, D. B., and Weisbrodt, N. W.,** Effects of intestinal bypass on the expression of actin mRNA in ileal smooth muscle, *Am. J. Physiol.,* 258, R39, 1990.

47. **Weisbrodt, N. W., Lai, M., Bowers, R. L., Harari, Y., and Castro, G. A.,** Structural and molecular changes in intestinal smooth muscle induced by *Trichinella spiralis* infection, *Am. J. Physiol.,* 266, G856, 1994.

# Index